Whiplash

Whiplash

Edited by

Gerard A. Malanga, MD
Director
Sports, Spine, and Orthopedic Rehabilitation
Kessler Institute for Rehabilitation, West Orange
Associate Professor
Department of Physical Medicine and Rehabilitation
University of Medicine and Dentistry of New Jersey–
    New Jersey Medical School
Newark, New Jersey

Scott F. Nadler, DO
Director of Sports Medicine
Associate Professor
Department of Physical Medicine and Rehabilitation
University of Medicine and Dentistry of New Jersey–
    New Jersey Medical School
Newark, New Jersey

Hanley & Belfus, Inc. / Philadelphia
An Imprint of Elsevier

Publisher: HANLEY & BELFUS, INC.
              An Imprint of Elsevier
              Medical Publishers
              210 South 13th Street
              Philadelphia, PA 19107
              (215) 546-7293; 800-962-1892
              FAX (215) 790-9330
              Web site: http://www.hanleyandbelfus.com

Library of Congress Cataloging-in-Publication Data

Whiplash / edited by Gerard A. Malanga, Scott Nadler.
     p. ; cm.
   Includes bibliographical references and index.
   ISBN-13: 978-1-56053-438-9   ISBN-10: 1-56053-438-9(alk. paper)
     1. Whiplash injuries. 2. Spine—Wounds and injuries. I. Malanga, Gerard A.
   II. Nadler, Scott, 1964-
   [DNLM: 1. Whiplash Injuries. WE 725 W5723 2001]
   RD 533.5.W48 2002
   617.5'3044—dc21

                                                              2001039767

ISBN-13: 978-1-56053-438-9
ISBN-10: 1-56053-438-9(alk. paper)

Whiplash

Permissions may be sought directly from Elsevier's Health Sciences
Rights Department in Philadelphia, PA, USA: phone: (+1) 215 239 3804,
fax: (+1) 215 239 3805, e-mail: healthpermissions@elsevier.com. You
may also complete your request on-line via the Elsevier homepage
(http://www.elsevier.com), by selecting 'Customer Support' and then
'Obtaining Permissions'.

Transferred to Digital Printing in 2012

Table of Contents

Contributors

Leslie Barnsley, Bmed, Grad Dip Epid, PhD, FRACP, FAFRM (RACP)
Associate Professor, Department of Medicine, University of Sydney; Senior Staff Specialist, Concord Hospital, Concord, New South Wales, Australia

Andrea J. Boon, MD
Assistant Professor, Department of Physical Medicine and Rehabilitation/Department of Neurology, Mayo Clinic, Rochester, Minnesota

Nikolai Bogduk, MD, PhD, DSc
Professor, Department of Anatomy and Musculoskeletal Medicine, University of Newcastle, Newcastle; Director, Newcastle Bone and Joint Institute, Royal Newcastle Hospital, Newcastle, New South Wales, Australia

Christopher M. Bono, MD
Spine Fellow, Department of Orthopedic Surgery, University of California, San Diego, California

Donald S. Ciccone, PhD
Assistant Professor, Department of Psychiatry, University of Medicine and Dentistry of New Jersey–New Jersey Medical School, Newark, New Jersey

David W. Chow, MD
Director, Interventional Spine, and Assistant Professor, Department of Physical Medicine and Rehabilitation, University of Cincinnati, Cincinnati, Ohio

Ann C. Cotter, MD
Clinical Assistant Professor, Department of Physical Medicine and Rehabilitation, University of Medicine and Dentistry of New Jersey–New Jersey Medical School, Newark; Medical Director, Atlantic Mind Body Center, Morristown Memorial Hospital, Atlantic Health System, Morristown, New Jersey

Ronald Patrick Dellanno, DC
Chiropractor, Director of Spinal Biophysics Research Center, Bloomfield; President, Cervigard, Inc., Bloomfield, New Jersey

Todd A. Edelson, MA, PT, Dip MDT
Associate Faculty, New York Medical College, Valhalla, New York; Faculty, McKenzie Institute International, Waikanae, New Zealand; Owner/Director, Montclair Physical Therapy Associates, Montclair, New Jersey

Deborah K. Elliott, BS
Research Specialist, Department of Psychiatry, University of Medicine and Dentistry of New Jersey–New Jersey Medical School, Newark, New Jersey

Joseph D. Fortin, DO
Clinical Professor, Department of Physical Medicine and Rehabilitation, Indiana University School of Medicine, Fort Wayne; Medical Director, Spine Technology and Rehabilitation, Fort Wayne, Indiana

Michael B. Furman, MD, MS
Clinical Assistant Professor, Department of Physical Medicine and Rehabilitation, Temple University, Philadelphia; The Center for Pain Management and Rehabilitation, York, Pennsylvania

Ralph E. Gay, MD, DC
Instructor, Department of Physical Medicine and Rehabilitation, Mayo Clinic, Mayo School of Medicine, Rochester, Minnesota

Roy C. Grzesiak, PhD
Clinical Associate Professor, Department of Psychiatry, University of Medicine and Dentistry of New Jersey–New Jersey Medical School, Newark; Consulting Psychologist, New Jersey Pain Institute, UMDNJ, New Brunswick, New Jersey

Robert F. Heary, MD
Director, The Spine Center of New Jersey, Neurological Institute of New Jersey, University Hospital, Newark; Associate Professor, Department of Neurological Surgery, University of Medicine and Dentistry of New Jersey–New Jersey Medical School, Newark, New Jersey

Gary M. Heir, DMD
Associate Clinical Professor, Department of Oral Pathology, Biology, and Diagnostic Services, University of Medicine and Dentistry of New Jersey, Newark; Attending Physician, St. Barnabas Medical Center, Livingston, New Jersey

Nancy Kim, MD
Chief Resident, Department of Physical Medicine and Rehabilitation, University of Medicine and Dentistry of New Jersey–New Jersey Medical School, Newark, New Jersey

Steven C. Kirshblum, MD
Associate Professor, Department of Physical Medicine and Rehabilitation, University of Medicine and Dentistry of New Jersey–New Jersey Medical School, Newark; Kessler Institute for Rehabilitation, West Orange, New Jersey

Robert S. Levine, MD
Clinical Associate Professor, Department of Orthopedic Surgery, Wayne State University School of Medicine; Adjunct Associate Professor and Medical Director, Bioengineering Center, College of Engineering, Wayne State University, Detroit, Michigan

Craig Liebenson, DC
Private Practice, Los Angeles, California

Susan M. Lord, BmedSc, Bmed, PhD
Division of Anaesthesia, Intensive Care, and Pain Management, John Hunter Hospital, Newcastle, New South Wales, Australia

Gerard A. Malanga, MD
Director, Sports, Spine, and Orthopedic Rehabilitation, Kessler Institute for Rehabilitation, West Orange; Associate Professor, Department of Physical Medicine and Rehabilitation, University of Medicine and Dentistry of New Jersey–New Jersey Medical School, Newark, New Jersey

Paul Robert McCrory, MBBS, PhD, FRACP, FACSP, FACSM, FASMF, Grad Dip Epid Stats
Director, Head Injury and Headache Clinics, Box Hill Hospital, Melbourne; Brain Research Institute and Centre for Sports Medicine Research and Education, University of Melbourne, Parkville

Pietro A. Memmo, MD
Chief Resident, Department of Physical Medicine and Rehabilitation, University of Medicine and Dentistry of New Jersey–New Jersey Medical School, Newark, New Jersey

Gregory J. Mulford, MD
Chairman, Department of Rehabilitation Medicine, Morristown Memorial Hospital, Morristown, New Jersey; Assistant Clinical Professor, Department of Rehabilitation Medicine, Columbia University College of Physicians and Surgeons, New York, New York

Scott F. Nadler, DO
Director of Sports Medicine, and Associate Professor, Department of Physical Medicine and Rehabilitation, University of Medicine and Dentistry of New Jersey–New Jersey Medical School, Newark, New Jersey

Benjamin N. Nguyen, MD
Assistant Professor, Department of Physical Medicine and Rehabilitation, University of Cincinnati Medical Center, Cincinnati, Ohio

Yong I. Park, MD
Staff Physiatrist, Department of Physical Medicine and Rehabilitation, Kessler Institute for Rehabilitation, West Orange, New Jersey

Kirk M. Puttlitz, MD
The Center for Pain Management and Rehabilitation, York, Pennsylvania

Steven Roman, MD
Resident, Department of Physical Medicine and Rehabilitation, University of Medicine and Dentistry of New Jersey–New Jersey Medical School, Newark, New Jersey

Scott R. Ross, DO, DC
Senior Associate Consultant, Department of Physical Medicine and Rehabilitation, Anesthesiology/Pain Medicine, Mayo Clinic, Rochester, Minnesota

Richard B. Rubenstein, JD
Faculty, Institute for Continuing Legal Education, National Business Institute, Livingston, New Jersey

Allan Peter Shapiro, MS, PhD
Adjunct Professor, Department of Physical Medicine and Rehabilitation, University of Western Ontario, London; Psychologist, St. Joseph's Health Centre and London Health Sciences Centre, London, Ontario, Canada

Clayton D. Skaggs, DC
Adjunct Faculty, Washington University School of Medicine, St. Louis, Missouri

Curtis W. Slipman, MD
Director, Penn Spine Center, Chief, Division of Musculoskeletal Rehabilitation, Associate Professor, Departments of Rehabilitation Medicine and Orthopedics, University of Pennsylvania, Philadelphia, Pennsylvania

Jay Smith, MD
Assistant Professor, Department of Physical Medicine and Rehabilitation, Mayo Clinic, Rochester, Minnesota

Robert W. Teasell, BSc, MD, FRCPC
Chief and Chair, Professor of Medicine, Department of Physical Medicine and Rehabilitation, St. Joseph's Health Centre and London Health Sciences Centre, University of Western Ontario, London, Ontario, Canada

Edward C. Weber, DO
Adjunct Associate Professor, Department of Anatomy, Fort Wayne Center for Medical Education, Indiana University School of Medicine, and the Imaging Center, Fort Wayne, Indiana

J. Bradley Williams, PhD
Co-Director, Pain Management Program, Kessler Institute for Rehabilitation, East Orange; Assistant Professor, Department of Physical Medicine and Rehabilitation, University of Medicine and Dentistry of New Jersey–New Jersey Medical School, Newark, New Jersey

Stuart A. Yablon, MD
Assistant Professor, Departments of Neurology and Neurosurgery, and Director, The Brain Injury Program, University of Mississippi School of Medicine, Jackson, Mississippi

Acknowledgements

With great thanks to my coauthor, Scott Nadler, an admired colleague
and friend
With love to Carrie, Tara, Grace, and Luke
With deep respect to my father and with great admiration of my
mother's inner strength

G.A.M

To my wife Jodi and daughter Sydni, who bring meaning to my life
To my parents, who instilled in me the confidence and work ethic to
complete this book
To my teacher, mentor, and friend Liz Narcessian, MD, who believed
in me—you will never be forgotten

S.F.N.

Preface

The topic of whiplash continues to be surrounded by controversy and heated debate. As in many facets of life, each of us brings some bias—based on our prior experiences, our training as professionals, and our beliefs arising from what we have heard, read, and seen. In the case of whiplash injuries, treating practitioners may be biased due to their training and exposure as therapists, chiropractors, primary care physicians, physiatrists, pain specialists, or surgeons. Our behavior may also be reinforced by factors including praise from patients, recognition by fellow practitioners, and monetary gain.

Because of the many issues influencing treatment decisions, we must not forget the importance of basing our medical decisions on good science. Over time, however, many treatments based on nonscientific medicine have become accepted as the standard of care. This process continues even when there is evidence suggesting that the treatment may be no more effective than the passage of time, and in some instances may even be harmful to patients. Generally, normalization of activity after a whiplash injury is in the best interest of the patient. Overemphasis on passive treatment may in reality disable the patient. Physician education is the key to solving this difficult problem.

The purpose of this book is to provide a current review of the important issues facing practitioners who encounter patients who have suffered whiplash injuries. A multidisciplinary consortium of authors was employed to accomplish this task. They were instructed to provide current, scientific information and not their opinions or anecdotal experiences. We would like to thank the contributing authors of this book for their excellent chapters. We believe that this textbook will be a valuable asset to those involved in the care of patients with whiplash injuries. We hope that the information provided will ultimately lead to improved outcome in those who have suffered these injuries.

Gerard A. Malanga, MD
Scott F. Nadler, DO
EDITORS

1

Whiplash Injury: A Continuing Dilemma In the 21st Century

Scott F. Nadler, D.O., and Gerard A. Malanga, M.D.

Whiplash is a common occurrence associated with any hyperflexion-extension injury. The mechanism of injury is an acceleration-deceleration event such as may occur in a motor vehicle accident or within contact sporting activities. Injury occurs to multiple structures, including muscle, tendon, ligament, bone, joint, and nerve tissue, and can therefore result in significant impairment and disability. Diagnosing these injuries can be a source of some controversy because there are often limited objective findings. Subjective complaints need to be carefully reviewed for many reasons but most importantly to avoid missing a potentially serious injury and to avoid overdiagnosing and treating a more simple condition. Unfortunately, the monetary potential associated with motor vehicle accidents creates an environment of mistrust, false expectations, and inappropriate care. Whiplash in rare circumstances causes severe life-threatening or life-altering conditions, such as spinal cord and traumatic brain injury. These injuries are the source of significant economic and social burden, most commonly because of the limited resources allocated for the most traumatically injured individuals. Many states have adopted a monetary cap on how much the victim of a motor vehicle accident is entitled to for treatment of injuries. This system is a result of the multitude of frivolous lawsuits brought about in the quest for dollars. This is a disturbing phenomenon for such a highly advanced society and, unfortunately, the truly injured individual suffers as a result.

Making the appropriate diagnosis and providing the correct treatment is the goal of any clinician who manages patients suffering from whiplash injury. Taking a proper history and performing a comprehensive physical assessment is the hallmark of any such evaluation. The history is invaluable because the treating provider can ascertain factors such as the mechanism of injury, preexisting problems that may have been aggravated, and steps the individual has taken in regard to self-treatment. The physical examination needs to include a comprehensive neurologic assessment, which should incorporate elements of strength, sensation, reflexes, and other provocative maneuvers.

Unfortunately, there is wide variation with regard to the performance of the physical examination and interpretation of findings. Education is the key to solving this problem. Ultimately, without a proper physical examination, diagnostic testing is ordered based on subjective complaints alone. This strategy is fraught with problems, and this is most especially apparent in individuals with significant psychosocial overlay. Overinterpretation of complaints in these individuals may set in place a vicious cycle of inappropriate testing, treatment, and risk of iatrogenic injury. An example of this phenomenon is an individual who presents 1 month after a motor vehicle accident and complains of isolated neck pain. The treating clinician takes an x-ray, which is negative, and does not perform a comprehensive physical examination. Based on the patient's complaints of neck pain, the treating provider orders magnetic resonance imaging (MRI) of the cervical spine. The MRI is reviewed by a radiologist who, without a clinical assessment, interprets any possible findings. In light of a significant false-positive rate in asymptomatic subjects,[1,3] a diagnosis of a herniated disc is made based only on the MRI finding of subtle disc bulging. The treating provider initiates a treatment program of passive modalities, including traction, electrical stimulation, massage, and ultrasound for the patient; it feels good during therapy, but the patient is in reality getting no better. The patient is next referred for various injections, which do not provide much in the way of subjective improvement. Finally, the patient ends up as a surgical candidate.

This case follows a paradigm in which a nonspecific history and physical leads to nonspecific diagnostic testing, nonspecific treatment strategies, and ultimately to a nonspecific (poor) outcome. An evidence-based approach to this case would not support MRI testing based on subjective complaints of axial pain. A program that may consist of flexibility exercises, strengthening, mobilization/manipulation, and the use of an appropriate analgesic or anti-inflammatory drug would first be indicated.[2] The use of modalities such as electrical stimulation and ultrasound would not be supported as providing any significant impact on functional recovery and therefore would not be the focus of treatment.[2,4] Appropriate therapeutic spinal injections may be of some potential benefit in an individual who has failed treatment, but they would have no place in an individual who has had no progressive, goal-directed program. Finally, surgical intervention should be reserved for carefully selected patients with objective findings without superimposed psychological issues. As clinicians, we must cautiously evaluate the diagnostic and treatment we recommend because inappropriate utilization can lead to disastrous outcomes.

This book is a compendium of knowledge regarding whiplash injury. We believe that prevention should ultimately be the focus in this century. The automobile industry must be at the forefront in this regard. Newer, more biomechanically sound head and neck restraints and, also, seating systems with specialized crush zones to absorb the forces generated at impact need to be developed and implemented. Newer technology should additionally focus on the structure and materials used to construct the underlying frame of the automobile to make it better able to absorb impact. Finally, these changes need to be made to all automobiles manufactured and should not be reserved for the privileged few who can afford the more expensive, technologically advanced automobiles. Prevention is the goal; however, in the face of injury we need proper assessment through detailed history and physical examination, judicious use of diagnostic testing, and treatments that have some scientific evidence of efficacy.

References

1. Boden SD, McCowin PR, Davis DO, et al: Abnormal magnetic-resonance scans of the cervical spine in asymptomatic subjects. A prospective investigation. J Bone Joint Surg Am 72: 1178–1184, 1990.
2. Bogduk N: Whiplash: "Why pay for what does not work?" J Musculoskel Pain 8:29–53, 2000.
3. Jensen MC, Brant-Zawadski MN, Obuchowski N, et al: Magnetic resonance imaging of the lumbar spine in people without back pain. N Engl J Med 331:69–73, 1994.
4. Spitzer WO, Skovron ML, Salmi LR, et al: Scientific monograph of the Quebec Task Force on Whiplash-Associated Disorders: redefining "whiplash" and its management. Spine 20(8 suppl):1S–73S, 1995.

2
Anatomy of the Cervical Spine

Scott R. Ross, D.O, D.C.

CERVICAL VERTEBRAE

The cervical spine is composed of seven vertebrae, including three atypical and four typical vertebrae. The typical cervical vertebrae, C3-C6, are composed of a vertebral body and a vertebral arch and possess several processes for articulations and muscular attachments (Fig. 1). The vertebral body comprises the anterior aspect of the vertebrae and supplies the strength and support for two-thirds of the vertebral load. The body of a typical cervical vertebra is elongated transversely so that its width is approximately 50% greater than its anteroposterior dimension. The upper surface is concave from side to side and convex in an anterior-to-posterior direction. The concavity is deepened by an uncinate process. The uncinate processes (*uncus* is Latin for "a small hook") are bony excrescences that project upward from the posterior lateral aspect of the rim of the body on C3-C7. The uncinate process predated the evolution of the extremities and evolved from the reptilian and avian costovertebral joints, which joined the ribs to the vertebrae. The lower surface is convex from side to side and concave in the anterior-to-posterior direction, with the anterior lip of the concavity often overlapping the vertebrae below. The inferior and slightly posterolateral aspects of the cephalic vertebral body are beveled and lie in apposition to the uncinate process of the vertebrae below. These articulations are known as the uncovertebral joints or joints of Luschka.

Projecting from the posterolateral aspect of the vertebral body are the pedicles. The pedicles of the lower cervical vertebrae are short and combine with the laminae to form the vertebral arch. The pedicles have a height of approximately 7 mm and a width of 6 mm.[22] Laminae project posteromedially from the pedicles and join in the midline to form the spinous process. Arising from the junction of the pedicle and laminae are the lateral masses. The lateral masses give rise to the superior and inferior articulating processes, or zygapophyseal joints. The superior articulating process, or facet, faces upward and posteriorly at 45 degrees while the inferior articulating process faces downward and anteriorly at 45 degrees. The inclination becomes more vertical at the lower cervical zygapophyseal joints.[14] The cervical zygapophyseal joints are planar, true synovial joints. Each articular process bears a circular or ovoid facet that is covered by articular cartilage; each joint is enclosed by a fibrous joint capsule lined by a synovial membrane. The cervical zygapophyseal joints are relatively flat with only minimal concavity or convexity. The orientation of the articular process allows for complex movements of the cervical spine, including flexion-extension, rotation, and lateral flexion. However, by facing upward and posteriorly, the superior articulating processes resist both forward and downward displacement of

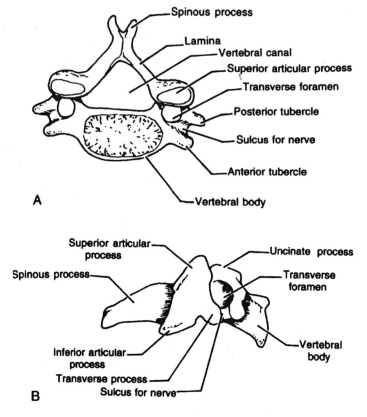

Figure 1.   Fifth cervical vertebra: **A,** cranial view; **B,** lateral view. (From Borenstein DG, Wiesel SW, Boden SD: Anatomy and biomechanics of the cervical spine. In Neck Pain: Medical Diagnosis and Comprehensive Management. Philadelphia, WB Saunders, 1996, pp 3–25; with permission.)

the vertebrae they support. Each cervical zygapophyseal joint from C3/C4 to C7/T1 is innervated from the medial branches of the dorsal rami from the branch above and below that joint.[5] The C2/C3 joint is largely innervated from the third occipital nerve, which is the superficial medial branch of the C3 dorsal ramus. The third occipital nerve continues around the lower lateral and dorsal surface of the C2/C3 joint, embedded in the connective tissue that invests the joint capsule.[5,7] The cervical zygapophyseal joint volume is usually 1 mL or less.[1,6,7] Each joint is lined with hyaline cartilage and may contain a meniscus.[8,27] The fibrous capsule is richly innervated with both mechanoreceptors and nociceptors[20,25,26] and forms superior and inferior capsular recesses. The ligamentum flavum covers the internal margin of the joint capsule.[3]

A transverse process projects laterally from the junction of each pedicle and laminae and is composed of two elements. The anterior element of the transverse process, developmentally a rib or costal process, arises from the lateral aspect of the vertebral body. The posterior element is a true transverse process and arises from the junction of the laminae and pedicle. These elements fuse.

However, between them persists the foramen transversarium that allows passage of the vertebral artery. The transverse process contains a gutter for the spinal nerves that runs obliquely from back to front. The anterior tubercle of C6 is large and is known as the carotid tubercle or Chassaignac's tubercle.

At each of the typical cervical segments, nerve roots exit from the spinal canal through short tunnels called the intervertebral foramen. The intervertebral foramen is bordered superiorly and inferiorly by the pedicles, posteriorly by the zygapophyseal joints, and anteriorly by the vertebral body, intervertebral discs, and uncovertebral joints. The foramina open obliquely forward, laterally, and inferiorly at an angle of 10 to 15 degrees downward. The average vertical diameter of the intervertebral foramen is approximately 10 mm, the horizontal diameter is 4 mm, and the average length is 5 mm.[11] The foramina are the largest at the C2-C3 level. They decrease in size progressively to the C6-C7 level.

The intervertebral foramina enclose and transmit the lateral termination of the anterior and posterior nerve root, spinal radicular arteries, intervertebral veins and plexuses, and an extension of the epidural space with areolar and fatty tissue. Small arteries, veins, and lymphatics provide a protective cushion for the nerves. The roots occupy one-fourth to one-third of the foraminal space.[4] All of the cervical spinal nerves except the first and second are contained within the intervertebral foramina. The nerves of the cervical spine take the name of the pedicle above which they exit. For example, the C6 nerve root exits between the fifth and the sixth cervical vertebrae. The exception is the eighth cervical nerve root, which exits between the seventh cervical and first thoracic vertebrae. In contrast to the thoracic and lumbar spine, the cervical nerve roots pass almost directly lateral at each level to exit from the spinal canal at the same foraminal level as their origin from the spinal cord.

The first, second, and seventh cervical vertebrae are considered atypical. The first cervical vertebra, also known as the atlas, lacks a body and a spinous process. It is a ringlike structure consisting of a short anterior arch and longer posterior arch joining to form the lateral masses that bear the superior and inferior articulating processes (Fig. 2). It is the widest cervical vertebra. A tubercle is located on the anterior aspect of the anterior arch for attachment of the anterior longitudinal ligament (ALL) and the longus colli muscle. The posterior arch corresponds to the lamina of other vertebrae. On the superior surface of the posterior arch is an oblique groove for the vertebral artery after it has wound around the outside of the articular mass. The attachment of the posterior atlantooccipital membrane arches over the artery at this point. This arch is sometimes outlined completely or incompletely by bone to form the arcuate foramen. The clinical significance of this bony arch is that it renders the atheromatous, tortuous vertebral artery more vulnerable to compression on rotation of the cervical spine.

The superior and inferior articulating processes arise from the lateral masses. The superior articulating processes are kidney shaped and face medially and cephalad to articulate with the occipital condyles. The inferior articulating processes are more ovoid and face caudally as well as medially to articulate with the second cervical vertebra. The transverse processes of the atlas are wider than those of other cervical vertebrae because of muscular attachments

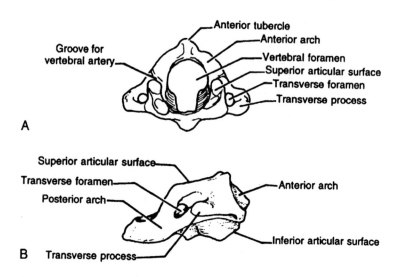

Figure 2. First cervical vertebra (atlas): **A**, cranial view; **B**, lateral view. (From Borenstein DG, Wiesel SW, Boden SD: Anatomy and biomechanics of the cervical spine. In Neck Pain: Medical Diagnosis and Comprehensive Management. Philadelphia, WB Saunders, 1996, pp 3–25; with permission.)

and the leverage needed to rotate the head. The transverse processes also possess a foramina transversarium for passage of the vertebral artery, veins, and sympathetic nerve fibers. These transverse processes are the only ones in the cervical spine that are not grooved to allow exit of a nerve root.

The second cervical vertebra, or axis, is identified by an odontoid process or dens that projects upward from the body of C2 to articulate with posterior aspect of the anterior arch of the first cervical vertebra (Fig. 3). The transverse ligament extends between the tubercles located on the medial aspect of each C1 lateral mass and holds the odontoid process of the second cervical vertebra against the posterior aspect of the anterior arch of the first cervical vertebra. The dimensions of the dens are variable; its mean height is 37.8 mm, its external transverse diameter is 9.3 mm, internal transverse diameter 4.5 mm, mean anteroposterior external diameter 10.5 mm, and internal diameter 6.2 mm.16 Lateral to the dens, on the body of the second cervical vertebra, are the superior articulating surfaces. The superior articulating surfaces are large, slightly convex, and face cephalad and laterally.

The superior articulating surfaces are not true processes because they arise directly from the body and pedicle lateral to the dens. On the under surface of the body are the inferior articulating processes, which are forward-facing and articulate with the superior articulating processes of the third cervical vertebra. The lamina of C2 are thick, and the spinous process is large and bifed. Another distinctive feature is that the C2 spinal nerve exits posterior to the superior articulating surface of C2 rather than anterior to the articulating processes, as spinal nerves do at other levels.

The seventh cervical vertebra is the transitional vertebra of the cervicothoracic region. The C7 vertebra has anatomic characteristics similar to those of

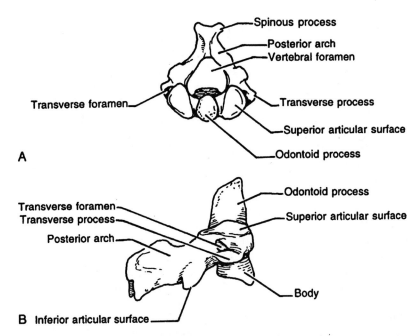

Figure 3. Second cervical vertebra (axis): **A,** cranial view; **B,** lateral view. (From Borenstein DG, Wiesel SW, Boden SD: Anatomy and biomechanics of the cervical spine. In Neck Pain: Medical Diagnosis and Comprehensive Management. Philadelphia, WB Saunders, 1996, pp 3–25; with permission.)

the first thoracic vertebra. The spinous process is single and usually larger than the process associated with the first thoracic vertebra and thus has been given the name *vertebral prominens*. The transverse process is large and rarely is there a foramen transversarium, and although the costal component is small it may give rise to a cervical rib.

INTERVERTEBRAL DISCS
The intervertebral discs make up approximately one-fourth of the length of the spinal column. They are the major structural link between adjacent vertebrae. The discs are biconvex and conforming to the concavity of the vertebral bodies. The discs in the cervical spine are thicker anteriorly. The sum of their anterior heights is 8 mm greater than the sum of their posterior height, which accounts for the cervical lordosis and anterior convexity.[4] Discs are relatively thick in the cervical spine. This thickness contributes to the flexibility of the cervical spine. The thickest disc is at the C6-C7 level. The ratio of disc to vertebral body height ranges from 1:3 to 1:2.[4] The discs absorb stress along the vertebral column. The viscoelastic nucleus changes its shape and distributes forces equally and uniformly in all directions; it converts longitudinal forces to horizontal forces and transmits them radially to the circumferential annuli.

The disc is made up of the annulus fibrosus and nucleus pulposus. The annulus fibrosus makes up the outer aspect of the disc. It is composed of fibrocartilage and fibrous protein and made up of crisscrossing concentric lamellae that provide strength and stability. The annulus is reinforced in front and behind by the anterior and posterior longitudinal ligament (PLL). Laterally, about the circumference of the vertebral body the annulus blends with the periosteum and is bound to bone. With age these anular fibers deteriorate and can become fissured and lose their capacity to restrain the nucleus. The nucleus of the disc is a water-rich mixture of proteoglycan gel and a lattice of collagen fibers. The nucleus is not in the center of the disc but lies a little anterior to the center and has a volume of 0.2 mL and is approximately 0.7 cm in diameter.[4] The nucleus over time loses its hydrophilic properties, becoming more fibrocartilaginous with increasing age until it eventually resembles the remainder of the disc.[4]

LIGAMENTS OF THE CERVICAL SPINE

A complex system of ligaments is found in the cervical spine (Fig. 4). The ALL is a broad, strong ligament that tightly adheres to the anterior and anterolateral aspect of the vertebral bodies and loosely blends with each annulus as it crosses the disc space from the atlas to the sacrum. Superiorly the ALL extends upward and is known as the anterior atlantooccipital membrane connecting the anterior margin of the foramen magnum to the anterior arch of the atlas. The PLL lies on the posterior aspect of the vertebral bodies from the axis to the sacrum. The posterior ligament, to the contrary, is firmly bound to each disc but is only loosely bound to the posterior concavity of the vertebral body. By only having loose attachment to the vertebral bodies, the PLL allows the spinal canal to be a smooth walled tube. However, any pathological thickening or ossification of the ligament may compromise the diameter of the canal. The tectorial membrane is continuation of the PLL to the basiocciput, and its fibers blend with the dura mater. The PLL is wider in the upper cervical spine than in the lower cervical spine.[15,24]

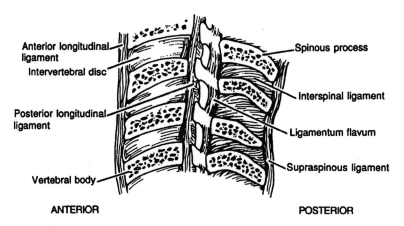

Anterior longitudinal ligament
Intervertebral disc
Posterior longitudinal ligament
Vertebral body
ANTERIOR

Spinous process
Interspinal ligament
Ligamentum flavum
Supraspinous ligament
POSTERIOR

Figure 4. Lateral view of the cervical spine demonstrating the ligaments that support the anterior (anterior longitudinal, posterior longitudinal) and the posterior (supraspinous, interspinal) elements of the vertebral column. Note the position of the ligamentum flavum forming a smooth posterior wall of the neural foramen. (From Borenstein DG, Wiesel SW, Boden SD: Anatomy and biomechanics of the cervical spine. In Neck Pain: Medical Diagnosis and Comprehensive Management. Philadelphia, WB Saunders, 1996, pp 3–25; with permission.)

The osseous and ligamentous structures of the cervical spine are surrounded by a network of interlacing nerve fibers. The ventral plexus of the ALL and the dorsal plexus of the PLL are connected at the level of the intervertebral foramina by branches of rami communicantes.[15] These nerves receive contributions from the sympathetic trunk rami communicantes and the perivascular nerve plexus of the segmental arteries. Anteriorly, branches may reach the ALL by coursing both superiorly and deep to the longus colli muscle. The PLL receives innervation via the sinuvertebral nerve,[9,15] which after its origin from the ventral ramus courses back through the intervertebral foramina anterior to the spinal nerve and posterior to the vertebral artery. It arrives at the posterior aspect of the disc, and the vertebral body then branches cephalad and caudally along the borders of the PLL, branching to the periosteum, intraspinal veins, and outer third of the annulus. The sinuvertebral nerve of cervical nerve C3 ascends cephalad, crossing the dorsal surface of the tectorial membrane, and enters the cranial fossa and supplies dura of the clivus. It joins the sinuvertebral nerve of C1 and C2 to innervate the ligaments of the atlantoaxial joint.

The articulations between the posterior arches in the cervical spine are maintained by the ligamentum nuchae, which is the continuation of the supraspinous ligament in the cervical spine, the interspinous ligaments, the ligamentum flavum, the synovial facet joints, and capsules. The ligamentum nuchae extends from the vertebral prominens to the external occipital protuberance. It is considered rudimentary in humans compared with its configuration in quadrupeds but is a stabilizer of the head and neck. Its deeper fibers attach to the interspinous ligament. The interspinous ligaments attach adjacent spinous processes. These ligaments attach in an oblique orientation from the posterior inferior aspect of the superior spinous process to the anterior superior aspect of the spinous process below.

The ligamenta flava are strong elastic ligaments spanning the space between laminae in pairs. The ligamenta flava attach the anteroinferior surface of the laminae above to the posterosuperior margin of the laminae below. They stretch laterally to the zygapophyseal joint and enter the fibrous composition of the capsule. They lie at approximately the same level as the intervertebral discs. Their function is supporting the neck in erect posture, aiding the muscles to extend the flexed neck, limiting the motion of the zygapophyseal joints, as well as restraining abrupt vertebral movements.

The articulation of the occiput, atlas, and axis differs considerably enough from that of the lower cervical spine that it needs to be considered separately. In addition to the anterior and posterior atlantooccipital membrane discussed earlier, the stability of the upper cervical spine is maintained by a group of ligaments between the occiput, atlas, and axis (Fig. 5).

The cruciate (cruciform ligament) is composed of the transverse ligament of the atlas and the superior and inferior ligamentous extensions that connect it to the anterior aspect of the foramen magnum and posterior aspect of the C2 vertebral body, respectively. The transverse ligament attaches laterally to tubercles located on the posterior aspect of the anterior arch of C1, where it blends with the lateral mass.[12] The length of the transverse ligament averages 21.9 mm and holds the odontoid process to the anterior arch of the atlas.[23]

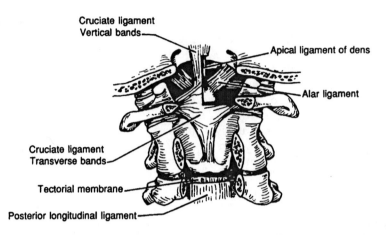

Figure 5. Coronal view of the skull and upper cervical spine shows the transverse cruciate ligaments, the primary stabilizers of the odontoid process. Secondary stabilizers of the odontoid are the alar ligament, which arises from the sides of the dens to the condyles of the occipital bone, and the apical ligament, which arises from the apex of the dens to the foramen magnum as a remnant of the notochord. (From Borenstein DG, Wiesel SW, Boden SD: Anatomy and biomechanics of the cervical spine. In Neck Pain: Medical Diagnosis and Comprehensive Management. Philadelphia, WB Saunders, 1996, pp 3–25; with permission.)

The alar ligaments are short, strong bundles of fibrous tissue directed obliquely upward and laterally from either side of the upper part of the odontoid process of the axis to the medial aspect of the occipital condyles with a small insertion also on the lateral mass of the atlas. The length of the alar ligaments averages 10.3 mm. The apical ligament extends from the tip of the odontoid process to the anterior edge of the foramen magnum. The apical ligament has an average length of 23.5 mm and a 20-degree anterior tilt.[23]

SPINAL CANAL

The cervical spinal canal is triangular in transverse section with rounded edges. The lateral diameter of the canal is significantly greater than the anteroposterior diameter at all levels. The spinal canal is widest at the atlantoaxial level, with sagittal diameters averaging between 20 to 23 mm at the C1-C2 level. In comparison, the average diameter at the C3-C6 ranges between 17 to 18 mm and is decreased to 15 mm at the C7 level.[22] The posterior aspect of the vertebral body is the base of the triangle. The pedicles, lamina, zygapophyseal joints, ligamentum flavum, and intervertebral foramina make up the sides of the triangle.

The cervical canal is fairly roomy from the atlas to the C3 level where the cervical enlargement of the cord begins. The cervical enlargement extends from C3 to T2 and corresponds to the large number of nerve roots innervating the upper limbs. The cervical cord nearly fills the canal more here than at any other level in the spine. The sagittal diameter of the spinal canal and the size of the spinal cord differ significantly among individuals, and a factor in the pathogenesis of cervical myelopathy is the size of the spinal canal relative to the cord. The vertebral canal is narrower in women than in men.[4]

SPINAL CORD

The spinal cord is surrounded by three meninges, the outermost being the spinal dura mater, which slightly adheres to the foramen magnum, and the C2 and C3 vertebral bodies. The dura merges with periosteum of the skull inside the foramen magnum where it continues as the dura mater of the brain. Between the dura mater and the posterior vertebral wall lies the epidural space. The epidural space contains fat, loose connective tissue and a venous plexus.

Spinal roots enter a tubular prolongation of the dura mater called the dural sheath as they approach the intervertebral foramina. At approximately the level of the spinal ganglia, the sheaths of the two roots blend to form a sheath that continues into the epineurium of the spinal nerve. The arachnoid is a delicate membrane that lies inside the dura mater and is continuous with the cerebral arachnoid through the foramen magnum. Laterally it continues with the dural sheath for a short distance. The subdural space is a potential space between the arachnoid and dura.

The subarachnoid space is filled with cerebrospinal fluid as well as blood vessels and nerve rootlets and is the interval between the arachnoid and the pia. The pia mater covers the spinal cord and forms a linear fold that runs the length of the cord. This fold is the source of the dentate ligaments that line both sides of the cord. The dentate ligaments extend between the dorsal and ventral nerve roots to attach to the dura and suspend the spinal cord in the spinal fluid. This organization of ligaments limits the motion of the spinal cord while allowing movement of the dura.

NERVE ROOTS

Each spinal nerve is composed of an anterior (ventral, predominately motor) root and a posterior (dorsal, predominately sensory) root. The posterior root, which is composed of the central processes of afferent neurons, breaks up into 12 or more rootlets that attach in a linear series to the dorsolateral sulcus of the cord (Fig. 6A). These sensory fibers enter the Lissauer tract and then plunge into the dorsal and ventral horns. The sensory rootlets peripherally converge into two bundles, the fasciculi radiculi, which in turn unite just proximal to the dorsal root ganglion. The anterior root arises from the ventrolateral sulcus of the cord by a smaller number and a less regular series of rootlets. Normally the posterior root is three times thicker than the anterior root (except at C1 and C2) because of the much greater amount of neural sensory traffic and the consequently greater number of neural fibers (Fig. 6B).

Each rootlet is covered by pia mater and, as they coalesce and form the two roots, the rootlets become enclosed within a funnel-shaped sac of the pia dura, the "root pouch," which tapers toward the intervertebral foramina (Fig. 6C). Within the spinal canal each root is separately enclosed in an arachnoid-dural sleeve, with each sleeve being separated by the interradicular septum. The dural root sleeves are attached to the bony margin of the intervertebral foramina, adhering more firmly with age and with pathological processes such as osteoarthritis.[4]

As they pass through the short intervertebral foramina, the anterior roots are in intimate contact with the Luschka joint and the annulus of the disc, which

A

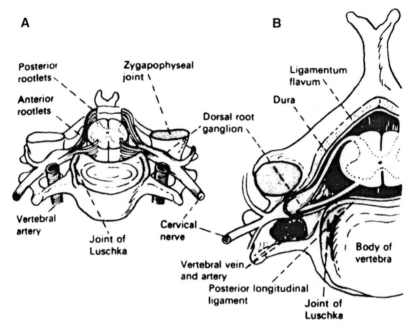

Posterior
rootlets

Zygapophyseal
joint

Anterior
rootlets

Dorsal root
ganglion

Vertebral
artery

Cervical
nerve

Joint of
Luschka

Vertebral vein
and artery

Posterior longitudinal
ligament

B

Ligamentum
flavum

Dura

Body of
vertebra

Joint of
Luschka

C

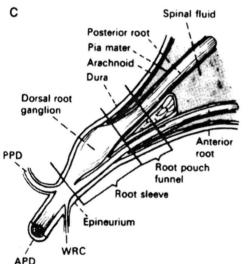

Spinal fluid

Posterior root
Pia mater
Arachnoid
Dura

Dorsal root
ganglion

PPD

Anterior
root

Root pouch
funnel

Root sleeve

Epineurium

WRC

APD

Figure 6. Transverse sections of the cervical spine. **A,** The spinal cord and anterior and posterior rootlets join to form the spinal nerve. Note the relationship of the nerves to the Luschka and zygapophyseal joints and the two vertebral arteries, which pass through the transverse foramina and are located just anterior to the nerve. (Adapted from Bland JH [ed]: Disorders of the Cervical Spine: Diagnosis and Medical Management. Philadelphia, WB Saunders, 1987.) **B,** Cross-section of a cervical vertebra showing some details of the relationship of the posterior root to the lateral aspect of the ligamentum flavum, which covers the zygapophyseal joint just posterior to it. The anterior root and its dural covering are close to the lateral part of the PLLs and to the capsules of the joint of Luschka. The proximal portion of the dorsal root ganglion is in the outer portion of the intervertebral foramen, whereas the remainder is in the gutter of the transverse process. **C,** Detailed anatomy of a nerve root and its meningeal covering. Note the extent of the root pouch and root sleeve. Just distal to the joining of the anterior and posterior roots is the short spinal nerve covered by epineurium (the continuation of the dura), which promptly divides into the anterior primary division (APD) and posterior primary division (PPD) and gives off white rami communicantes (WRC). (B and C modified from Cailliet R: Neck and Arm Pain, 2nd ed. Philadelphia, FA Davis, 1981.)

is covered by the lateral portion of the PLL. The posterior root lies close to the articular process and the zygapophyseal joint capsule of the adjacent vertebrae. The roots occupy only one-fourth to one-third of the foramina. As each root passes distally beyond the foramina, it enters the "gutter" of the sulcus of the transverse process, where the arachnoid and dura blend with the nerve sheath. The arachnoid, and subsequently the cerebrospinal fluid that envelops the nerve roots, ends at the outer part of the intervertebral foramina. The dura continues more distally, and at the point beyond the joining of the two roots into the formed spinal nerve it blends with the epineurium of the formed nerve.

Just beyond the dorsal root ganglion and usually just outside the intervertebral foramina, the cervical spinal nerves divide into dorsal and ventral primary rami. The first cervical nerve exits the vertebral canal through an orifice in the posterior atlantooccipital membrane just above the posterior arch of the C1 vertebra and posteromedially to the lateral mass of the C1 vertebra. The dorsal primary ramus of C1 enters the suboccipital triangle, and its terminal branches supply the muscles of that region. There is usually no cutaneous branch of dorsal primary ramus of C1, also known as the *suboccipital nerve*. The second cervical nerve emerges between the posterior arch of C1 and the lamina of C2 just posterior to its lateral mass. The medial branch of the dorsal rami, or greater occipital nerve, runs transversely in the soft tissue dorsal to C2 laminae, turning cephalad and eventually entering the scalp with the occipital artery through an opening above the aponeurotic sling between the trapezius and the sternocleidomastoid.

The principle branch of the third cervical dorsal rami is the *third occipital nerve*, which curves dorsally and medially around the superior articular process of C3 and crosses behind the C2-C3 zygapophyseal joint, supplying it. It runs medially toward the midline, where it turns dorsally and superiorly, supplying the posterior cervical musculature and terminating in cutaneous branches for the occiput and mastoid regions. The dorsal rami for the cervical nerves C4-C8 arise from the spinal nerve just outside the intervertebral foramina and divide into medial and lateral branches. The medial branches of these nerves have an overlapping cutaneous innervation supplying the multifidus and interspinal muscles and send branches to the zygapophyseal joints rostral and caudal to it. The lateral branches of C4-C7 supply the longissimus cervices and splenius cervicis, with the lateral branches supplying the iliocostalis cervicis.[5] Immediately after emerging from the spinal canal, each nerve receives one, two, or more gray rami communicantes from the cervical sympathetic ganglia. The superior cervical sympathetic ganglion contributes fibers to the upper four cervical spinal nerves. The middle and intermediate ganglia contribute fibers to the fifth and sixth nerves, and the inferior (stellate) ganglion to the seventh and eighth nerves, while the first thoracic sends gray rami communicantes over to the eighth cervical and first thoracic nerves. The anterior rami of C1-C4 form the cervical plexus and from C5-T1 form the brachial plexus.

The cervical plexus is arranged in a series of loops from which peripheral branches arise. This arrangement results in overlap of the cutaneous sensory distribution. A loop formed between branches of the first through third cervical nerves gives branches that form the ansa cervicalis. The superior root of the ansa cervicalis is formed between the first and second cervical nerves and gives off a branch to the hypoglossal nerve. The inferior root consists of fibers of cervical nerves C2 and C3. The ansa cervicalis lies superficial to the carotid sheath and supplies all the strap or infrahyoid muscles except for the thyrohyoid. The cervical plexus also gives rise to superficial cutaneous branches, including the lesser occipital, greater auricular, and transverse cervical nerves. The lesser occipital nerve is derived from the anterior primary division of the second cervical nerve or from a loop derived from the second or third cervical nerve. It ascends along the sternocleidomastoid muscle, curving around its posterior border and, near the insertion of the muscle on the cranium, it perforates the deep fascia to continue cephalad along the side of the head, behind the ear to supply the skin of this part of the scalp.

The greater auricular nerve, larger than the lesser occipital nerve, arises from the second or third cervical nerves, winds around the posterior border of the sternocleidomastoid and, after perforating the deep fascia, ascends on the surface of that muscle deep to the platysma and divides into an anterior and posterior branch. The anterior (facial) is distributed to the skin of the face over the parotid gland and communicates with the facial nerve within the substance of the gland. The posterior (mastoid) branch supplies the skin over the mastoid process in back of the auricula, except its upper part. A filament of the nerve pierces the auricula to reach its lateral surface. The nerve communicates with the lesser occipital nerve, the auricular branch of the vagus, and the posterior auricular branch of the facial nerve. The cervical plexus also communicates with cranial nerves X, XI, and XII and to the sympathetic chain via rami communicantes.

As stated, the ventral rami of C5-T1 form the brachial plexus. After exiting the intervertebral foramina, they proceed anterolaterally and inferiorly to occupy the interval between the anterior and middle scalene muscles within the posterior triangle under the cover of the platysma and deep fascia.

VERTEBRAL ARTERIES

The vertebral arteries are a major source of blood supply to the cervical spine and the cervical portion of the spinal cord. These arteries are usually the first branches of the subclavian artery, arising medially to the scalenus anterior, and ascend behind the common carotid artery between the longus colli and the scalenus anterior. The vertebral arteries pass cephalad by coursing through the foramen transversarium of C6-C1, where they are directly in front of the cervical nerves and medial to the intertransverse muscle. Accompanying each artery are the vertebral plexus of veins and the postganglionic sympathetic fibers originating in the inferior (stellate) ganglion. After passing through the C1 foramen transversarium, the vertebral arteries turn posteromedially, coursing transversely behind the superior articular process, and lie within a groove on the upper surface of the posterior arch of the atlas. The arteries then pass through the posterior atlantooccipital membrane, turning anterior and cephalad through the foramen magnum into the cranium and join to form the basilar artery. The vertebral arteries give off spinal branches that pass into the foramina to supply ligament, dura, and bone as well as communicate with the posterior spinal arteries that supply the spinal cord. Most vertebral arteries are unequal in size. The diameter of the left vertebral artery is often larger than that of the right vertebral artery.[4] One vessel may be congenitally absent.

ARTERIAL SUPPLY TO THE VERTEBRAL BODY, SPINAL CORD, AND ROOTS

The arterial supply to the vertebral bodies arises from segmental vessels off the vertebral arteries. At each level these segmental branches pass beneath the longus colli muscle and course to the anterior vertebral body and the ALL. Other segmental branches enter the intervertebral foramina and supply the posterior vertebral body, PLL, and lamina as well as radicular branches to the spinal cord. The dens receive its arterial supply via paired ascending anterior and posterior arteries that arise from the vertebral arteries that eventually form an anastomosis with the carotid system.

The arterial blood supply to the spinal cord arises from three longitudinal channels on the surface of the spinal cord[13] (Fig. 7). One channel is positioned anteromedially, and the other two are posterior laterally positioned. Just before joining, one or both of the vertebral arteries give off a branch that joins with the branch from the other side and descends as the anterior spinal artery in a caudal direction in the ventral median fissure on the anterior surface of the spinal cord. The anterior spinal artery is reinforced along its course by medullary arteries from the vertebral arteries. The two posterior spinal arteries arise from either the vertebral arteries or from the posterior inferior cerebellar arteries. They are positioned on the posterolateral aspect of the spinal cord and are reinforced by medullary arteries derived primarily from the spinal branches of the ascending cervical arteries, deep cervical arteries, and vertebral

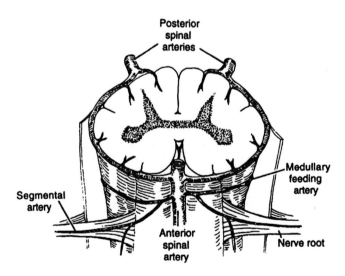

Figure 7. The anterior and posterior spinal artery blood supply to the spinal cord. A medullary feeding artery, originating from the segmental artery, also contributes to the vascularity of the spinal cord. (From Borenstein DG, Wiesel SW, Boden SD: Anatomy and biomechanics of the cervical spine. In Neck Pain: Medical Diagnosis and Comprehensive Management. Philadelphia, WB Saunders, 1996, pp 3–25; with permission.)

arteries. The dorsal and ventral nerve roots receive their arterial supply via radicular branches of the spinal arteries.

The spinal veins have a distribution somewhat similar to that of the spinal arteries. There are usually three anterior and three posterior spinal veins. These veins are arranged longitudinally, communicating freely with each other, and are drained by numerous radicular veins.[18,19] Veins of the cervical vertebral column have a continuous series of plexuses in the extradural space. The importance of these plexuses in the spread of malignant disease has long been known through Batson's study of veins now known for him.[2] The anterior and posterior spinal veins and vertebral venous plexuses drain into the intervertebral veins, and then into the vertebral veins and deep cervical veins. These venous systems drain into the brachiocephalic veins.

MUSCLES OF THE CERVICAL SPINE

A high degree of finely coordinated muscle balance is required to support and move the head and neck. Because the cervical spine is the most mobile section of the spine, it contains the most elaborate and specialized muscle system of the spine. The musculature of the neck and cervical spine can be divided into the anterolateral and posterior muscle groups.

The anterolateral cervical muscles function to flex and rotate the head and neck. The anterolateral muscular group can be further subdivided into the superficial cervical, lateral cervical, suprahyoid, infrahyoid, anterior vertebral, and lateral vertebral groups.[10,17]

The superficial cervical muscles include the platysma and trapezius. The platysma is a broad, thin muscle originating from the superior fascia of the pectoral and deltoid region. It inserts on the inferior border of the mandible and the subcutaneous tissue and skin of the lower face. Its action tenses the skin of the neck, draws the corner of the mouth inferiorly, and assists in depressing the mandible inferiorly. When the entire muscle contracts, it wrinkles the skin of the neck in an oblique direction and widens the aperture of the mouth. The innervation of the platysma comes from a cervical branch of the facial nerve (CN VII).

The sternocleidomastoid muscle is the key muscular landmark in the neck (Fig. 8). The sternocleidomastoid muscle originates from the anterior surface of the manubrium and superior surface of the medial third of the clavicle to rise superior and laterally across the anterior lateral neck and insert into the lateral surface of the mastoid process. The sternocleidomastoid covers the great vessels of the neck and the cervical plexus of nerves. Its action is to bend the head laterally to the same side and rotate the head to the opposite side. When contracting together its anterior fibers flex the neck and its posterior fibers extend the head. It is innervated by the spinal accessory nerve (CN XI) and the second and third cervical nerve.

The sternocleidomastoid muscle is the dividing boundary for the anterior and posterior triangles of the neck. The anterior triangle is bounded by the midline of the neck, the lower border of the mandible superiorly, and the sternocleidomastoid posteriorly. It can be further divided into the submental, submandibular, muscular, and carotid triangles. The submandibular or digastric triangle, bound by the two bellies of the digastric muscle and the inferior

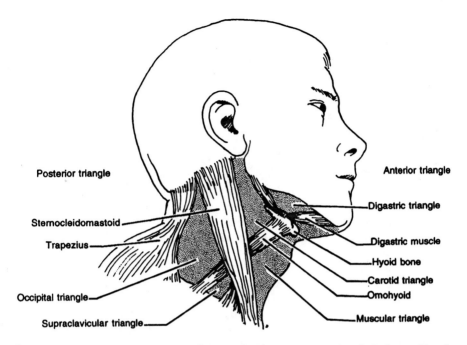

Figure 8. Triangle organization of the neck. The posterior triangle is formed by the trapezius, clavicle, and sternocleidomastoid, with the omohyoid muscle dividing this triangle into the occipital and supraclavicular areas. The midline of the neck, the lower border of the mandible, and the sternocleidomastoid bound the anterior triangle. The anterior triangle is subdivided by the digastric and omohyoid muscles. (From Borenstein DG, Wiesel SW, Boden SD: Anatomy and biomechanics of the cervical spine. In Neck Pain: Medical Diagnosis and Comprehensive Management. Philadelphia, WB Saunders, 1996, pp 3–25; with permission.)

border of the mandible, contains the submandibular gland, facial artery and vein, and mylohyoid artery and nerve as well as a portion of the parotid gland and external carotid artery. The internal carotid artery, jugular vein, glossopharyngeal, and vagus nerves reside deeper in the triangle. The carotid triangle is a vascular area bound by the superior belly of the omohyoid, the posterior belly of the digastric, and the anterior border of the sternocleidomastoid muscle. It contains the common carotid artery; its bifurcation; the internal jugular vein; the superior thyroid, lingual, and facial branches of the external carotid artery; portions of cranial nerves X, XI, and XII; the larynx; pharynx; and the superior laryngeal nerve as well as the ansa cervicalis.

The posterior triangle of the neck is bounded posteriorly by the anterior border of the trapezius muscle, anteriorly by the posterior border of the sternocleidomastoid muscle, and inferiorly by the clavicle. The floor of the posterior cervical triangle is formed by the splenius capitis muscle, levator scapulae muscle, and the scalenus medius and scalenus posterior muscles. The contents of the posterior cervical triangle include the accessory nerve, a portion of the brachial plexus, the third part of the subclavian artery, the dorsal scapular nerve, the long thoracic nerve, the nerve to the subclavius, the suprascapular nerve, a portion of the lesser occipital nerve, the greater auricular nerve, the suprascapular artery, and a portion of the occipital artery.

The suprahyoid muscles include the stylohyoid, mylohyoid, geniohyoid, and digastric muscle. As a group they raise the hyoid bone during swallowing and help in opening the mouth when the hyoid bone is stabilized by the infrahyoid muscles. The stylohyoid muscle originates from the styloid process of the temporal bone and inserts on the body of the hyoid bone. It is supplied by the facial nerve (CN VII). The mylohyoid are thin, flat muscles that form a sling inferior to the tongue that supports the floor of the mouth. It originates from the mylohyoid line on the medial aspect of the mandible and inserts on the raphe and body of the hyoid bone. It is innervated by the trigeminal nerve (CN V). The geniohyoid muscle lies medial to the mylohyoid, originating from the inferior mental spine of the mandible, and inserts onto the body of the hyoid. It is supplied by the ventral ramus of C1 hypoglossal nerve (CN XII). The digastric consists of an anterior and posterior belly, which originate from the lower border of the mandible and mastoid notch of the temporal bone, respectively. The digastric inserts on the body in the greater horn of the hyoid bone via a common intermediate tendon. The anterior belly is innervated by a branch of the inferior alveolar nerve, and the posterior belly is innervated by the facial nerve (CN VII).

The infrahyoid muscles act as group to depress the larynx and hyoid after these structures have been raised with the pharynx during swallowing. They consist of four muscles and because of their ribbonlike appearance are often referred to as the strap muscles (Fig. 9). The sternohyoid is a thin, narrow muscle that arises from the posterior manubrium and medial clavicle to insert on the

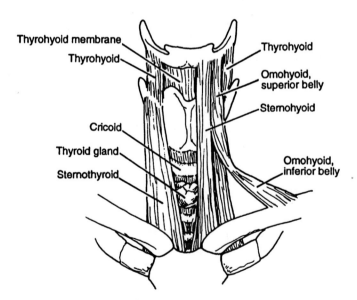

Figure 9.   Anterior view of the deeper anterior muscles of the cervical spine. (From Borenstein DG, Wiesel SW, Boden SD: Anatomy and biomechanics of the cervical spine. In Neck Pain: Medical Diagnosis and Comprehensive Management. Philadelphia, WB Saunders, 1996, pp 3–25; with permission.)

body of the hyoid. The sternothyroid muscle is located posterior to the sternohyoid and arises from the posterior surface of the manubrium and first costal cartilage. It inserts on the oblique line of the thyroid cartilage. Both the sternohyoid and sternothyroid muscles receive their innervation from branches of the ansa cervicalis (C1-C3). The thyrohyoid appears as the superior continuation of the sternothyroid muscle. It inserts on the great horn of the hyoid bone. It acts to depress the hyoid and elevate the thyroid cartilage.

The innervation to the thyrohyoid muscle is the ventral rami of the first cervical nerve via the hypoglossal nerve (CN X11). The omohyoid muscle has two bellies that are united by an intermediate tendon. The inferior belly arises from the superior border of the scapula near the suprascapular notch. It ends in the intermediate tendon, from which the superior belly arises: This belly inserts into the inferior border of the hyoid bone. It depresses, retracts, and steadies the hyoid bone in swallowing and speaking. It receives innervation from branches of the superior root of the ansa cervicalis (C1) and by the ansa cervicalis itself (C2 and C3).

The anterior (prevertebral) muscles of the neck are covered anteriorly by prevertebral fascia (Fig. 10). They flex the neck and head on the neck and are supplied by ventral rami of the cervical nerves. The anterior muscles include

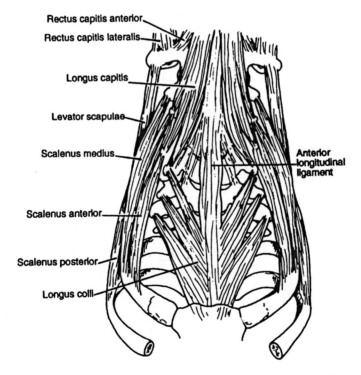

Rectus capitis anterior
Rectus capitis lateralis
Longus capitis
Levator scapulae
Scalenus medius
Scalenus anterior
Scalenus posterior
Longus colli
Anterior longitudinal ligament

Figure 10. Anterior view of the superficial muscles of the cervical spine. (From Borenstein DG, Wiesel SW, Boden SD: Anatomy and biomechanics of the cervical spine. In Neck Pain: Medical Diagnosis and Comprehensive Management. Philadelphia, WB Saunders, 1996, pp 3–25; with permission.)

the longus colli and the longus capitis. The longus colli muscle is the longest and most medial of the prevertebral muscles. It extends from the anterior tubercle of the atlas to the body of the third thoracic vertebra. It also attaches to the bodies of the vertebrae between C1 and C3 and to the transverse processes of the third to sixth cervical vertebrae. The longus capitis muscle arises from the anterior tubercles of the third through sixth cervical transverse processes and inserts on the base of the occiput, where it is supplemented by the rectus capitis anterior and rectus capitis lateralis. They are flexors of the upper cervical spine and head.

The scalenus anterior lies deep to the sternocleidomastoid and arises from the anterior tubercle of the transverse of C3-C6 and inserts on the scalene tubercle on the inner and upper ridge of the first rib. It is innervated by the ventral rami of C5 and C6. The phrenic nerve overlies the anterior scalene muscle and provides motor to the diaphragm via ventral rami of C3-C5. The scalenus medius arises from the posterior tubercle of the transverse process of C2-C7 and inserts on the upper first rib behind the subclavian groove. It is supplied by the ventral rami of C3-C8. The brachial plexus arises from the neck in the interval between the anterior and middle scalenes. The scalenus posterior arises from the posterior tubercle of the transverse processes of C4-C6 and inserts on the outer surface of the second rib just deep to the attachment of the scalenus anterior. It is innervated by C7 and C8. These muscles act as group to flex and rotate the neck while raising the rib on which they insert.

The musculature of the posterior aspect of the neck can be divided into superficial and deep groups. The most superficial muscle on the posterior aspect of the neck is the trapezius (Fig. 11). It originates from the medial third of the

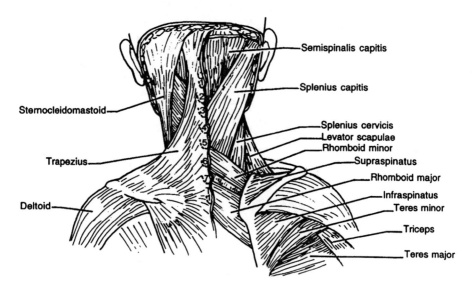

Figure 11.   Posterior view of the superficial muscles of the cervical spine. (From Borenstein DG, Wiesel SW, Boden SD: Anatomy and biomechanics of the cervical spine. In Neck Pain: Medical Diagnosis and Comprehensive Management. Philadelphia, WB Saunders, 1996, pp 3–25; with permission.)

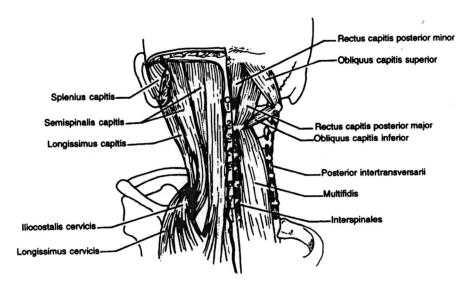

Splenius capitis

Semispinalis capitis

Longissimus capitis

Rectus capitis posterior minor

Obliquus capitis superior

Rectus capitis posterior major

Obliquus capitis inferior

Posterior intertransversarii

Multifidis

Interspinales

Iliocostalis cervicis

Longissimus cervicis

Figure 12. Posterior view of the deeper muscles of the cervical spine. (From Borenstein DG, Wiesel SW, Boden SD: Anatomy and biomechanics of the cervical spine. In Neck Pain: Medical Diagnosis and Comprehensive Management. Philadelphia, WB Saunders, 1996, pp 3–25; with permission.)

superior nuchal line, the external occipital protuberance, ligamentum nuchae, and spinous process of C7-T12. It inserts on the lateral aspect of the clavicle (superior fibers), acromion and spine of the scapula (middle fibers), and base of the scapular spine (inferior fibers). The superior fibers act to elevate the scapula, the middle fibers retract the scapula, and the inferior fibers lower the shoulder. The trapezius receives innervation from the spinal accessory nerve (CN XI) and the third and fourth cervical nerves.

The deep muscles of the posterior cervical musculature can be divided into two groups: a superficial layer and deep layer (Fig. 12). The superficial layer of the deep cervical musculature consists of four muscles and is known as the transversocostal group. All are innervated by dorsal rami of the cervical nerves. The splenius capitis and splenius cervicis originate from the ligamentum nuchae and the spinous processes of C7-T6. The splenius capitis inserts into the mastoid process, and the splenius cervicis inserts into transverse processes of the superior four cervical vertebrae. They act to laterally bend and rotate the head to the same side. Contracting together they extend the head. The iliocostalis and longissimus are part of the erector spinae muscles. They act to extend, laterally flex, and rotate the spine in the cervicothoracic region All receive innervation via dorsal rami of the spinal nerves.

The deep layer of the deep cervical musculature is termed the transversospinal group and is composed of the semispinalis capitis, semispinalis cervicis, multifidi, and rotatores. The semispinalis capitis forms the largest muscle mass in the posterior aspect of the neck. It arises from the transverse processes of C7-T6 and from the articular processes of C4-C6 and inserts on the superior and inferior nuchal line of the occiput. The semispinalis cervicis lies deep to the semispinalis capitis. It arises from the transverse processes of T1-T5 and inserts on the spinous processes of C2-C5. The semispinalis cervicis extends and rotates the vertebral column to the opposite side, whereas the semispinalis capitis extends and rotates the head to the opposite direction. The innervation to both the semispinalis capitis and semispinalis cervicis is via dorsal primary rami of spinal nerves. The multifidi lie deep to the semispinalis cervicis in the cervical spine and arise from the articular processes of the lower four cervical vertebrae. The muscles ascend obliquely, two to five vertebral levels, and insert on the spinous processes at the higher levels. The multifidi are innervated by dorsal primary rami of the cervical spinal nerves and act to extend, laterally bend, and rotate the neck to the opposite side. The rotatores are just deep to the multifidi and are short muscles that arise from the transverse processes and ascend to insert on the spinous processes of the next superior vertebra. They also assist in rotation of the neck to the opposite side and receive innervation from dorsal rami of the spinal nerves.

The muscles of the suboccipital region consist of four small muscles lying deep to the semispinalis capitis. They extend and rotate the head. All the muscles of the suboccipital region receive innervation via a branch of the dorsal rami of the suboccipital nerve. The rectus capitis posterior major originates from the spinous process of the axis, whereas the rectus capitis posterior minor arises from the posterior tubercle of the atlas. These muscles insert, side by side, onto the occiput inferior to the inferior nuchal line. The oblique capitis inferior is a thick muscle that arises from the spinous process of the axis and runs obliquely superiorly and anteriorly to insert onto the tip of the transverse process of the atlas. The oblique capitis superior is a flat triangular muscle that arises from the tip of the transverse process of the atlas and runs obliquely superiorly and posteriorly to insert onto the occiput between the superior and inferior nuchal lines. It acts to extend and rotate the head to the same side.

CONCLUSIONS

The anatomy of the cervical spine is complex and allows for a high degree of motion while serving as a protective conduit for the spinal cord and nerve roots. A thorough understanding of this intricate anatomy is essential before attempting to diagnosis and treat the myriad conditions that can affect this region.

References

1. Aprill C, Bogduk N: The prevalence of cervical zygapophyseal joint pain. A first approximation. Spine 17:744–747, 1992.
2. Batson OV: The vertebral vein system. Am J Roentgenol 78:195,1957.
3. Bland JH: Anatomy and biomechanics. In Bland JH (ed): Disorders of the Cervical Spine: Diagnosis and Medical Management. Philadelphia, WB Saunders, 1987, pp 9–63.
4. Bland JH (ed): Disorders of the Cervical Spine: Diagnosis and Medical Management, 2nd ed. Philadelphia, WB Saunders, 1994.
5. Bogduk N: The clinical anatomy of the cervical dorsal rami. Spine 7:319–330, 1982.
6. Bogduk N: Back pain: zygapophysial blocks and epidural steroids. In Cousins MJ, Bridenbaugh PO (eds): Neural Blockade in Clinical Anesthesia and Management of Pain. Philadelphia, Lippincott, 1989, pp 935–954.
7. Bogduk N, Marsland A: On the concept of third occipital headache. J Neurol Neurosurg Psychiatry 49:75–78, 1986.
8. Bogduk N, Marsland A: The cervical zygapophysial joints as a source of neck pain. Spine 13:610–617, 1988.

9. Bogduk N, Windsor M, Inglis A: The innervation of the cervical intervertebral discs. Spine: 13:2–8, 1988.
10. Clemente C (ed): Gray's Anatomy, 30th American ed. Philadelphia, Lea and Febiger, 1985.
11. Czervionke LF, Daniels DL, Ho PSP, et al: Cervical neural foramina: correlative anatomic and MR imaging study. Neuroradiology 169:753–759, 1988.
12. Daniels DL, Williams AL, Haughton VM: Computed tomography of the articulations and ligaments at the occipito-atlantoaxial region. Radiology 146:709–716, 1983.
13. Dommisse GF: The blood supply of the spinal cord. J Bone Joint Surg Br 56:225–235, 1974.
14. Dvorak J, Dvorak V: Biomechanics and functional examination of the spine. In Manual Medicine-Diagnostics, 2nd ed. New York, Thieme Medical Publishers, 1990, pp 1–34.
15. Hayashi K, Yabuki T, Kurokawa T, et al: The anterior and the posterior longitudinal ligaments of the lower cervical spine. J Anat 124:633–636, 1977.
16. Heller JG, Alson MD, Schaffler MB, et al: Quantitative internal dens morphology. Spine 17:861–966, 1992.
17. Hollingshead WH: Anatomy for Surgeons, Vol 3. 3rd ed. Philadelphia, Harper and Row, 1982.
18. Kubo Y, Waga S, Kojima T: Microsurgical anatomy of the lower cervical spine and cord. Neurosurgery 34:895–902, 1994.
19. Lang J: Clinical Anatomy of the Cervical Spine. New York, Thieme Medical Publishers, 1993.
20. McLain R: Mechanoreceptor endings in human cervical facet joints. Spine 9:495–502, 1994.
21. [Reference deleted].
22. Panjabi M, Duranceau J, Goel V, et al: Cervical human vertebrae. Quantitative three-dimensional anatomy of the middle and lower regions. Spine 16:861–869, 1993.
23. Panjabi M, Oxland T, Parks E. Quantitative anatomy of the cervical spine ligaments. Part I: upper cervical spine. J Spinal Disord 4:270–276,1991.
24. Parke WW, Sherk HH: Normal adult anatomy. In Sherk HH, Dunn EJ, Eismont FJ, et al (eds): The Cervical Spine, 2nd ed. Philadelphia, JB Lippincott, 1988, pp 11–32.
25. Woodring JH, Goldstein SJ: Fractures of the articular processes of the cervical spine. Am J Roentgenol 139:341–344, 1982.
26. Wyke B: Articular neurology-A review. Physiotherapy 58:563–580, 1981.
27. Yu S, Sether L, Haughton VM: Facet joint menisci of the cervical spine: correlative MR imaging and cryomicrotomy study. Radiology 164:79–82, 1987.

3

The Biomechanics of Whiplash

Ralph E. Gay, M.D., D.C., and Robert Levine, M.D.

The concept of *whiplash* as a mechanism of injury has been surrounded by controversy almost since Crowe coined the word.[1] The term is most often used to refer to a complex and variable set of circumstances arising out of a rear-end motor vehicle crash. It has long been accepted that, due to the large forces generated, injury to the spine may occur with high-speed impacts of this type. The ability of low-speed impact to cause injury remains controversial.[2] This type of collision is felt to be responsible for a variety of signs and symptoms know as whiplash-associated disorders.[3] Whiplash-associated symptoms have been reported with various impact mechanisms but occur most often after rear-end collisions.[4,5] For this reason, most research has concentrated on impacts that occur when a vehicle at rest (the target vehicle) is hit from the rear by a moving vehicle (the bullet vehicle) traveling at low speed (8 to 12 km/h). This chapter reviews normal biomechanics of the cervical spine and then considers the biomechanics of low-speed, rear-end automobile collisions.

NORMAL BIOMECHANICS OF THE CERVICAL SPINE
To understand the mechanism of whiplash, one must be familiar with normal cervical spine function. The following definitions will help in this understanding.

Definitions

Kinematics is the study of motion of rigid bodies *without* consideration of the forces involved.[6] In the spine, the rigid bodies are the vertebral bodies. To communicate movement of the vertebra, a coordinate system of axes and planes is used (Fig. 1). This coordinate system is used extensively by investigators in the impact engineering field who study whiplash but differs from that proposed by White and Panjabi.

Kinetics is the study of motion of rigid bodies *with* consideration of the forces involved. Forces acting on the cervical spine may be intrinsic (eg, muscles, ligaments) or extrinsic (eg, gravity, acceleration). The neck is exposed to various forces that influence its movement, including the head, which it supports.

Translation occurs when all parts of a body move along a curvilinear path without rotation. An example might be a cup sliding across a table without tipping or spinning. Convention dictates that vertebral translation occurs in a positive (anterior or forward) or negative (posterior or backward) direction. Therefore, anterior translation of a vertebra is movement in the +x direction.

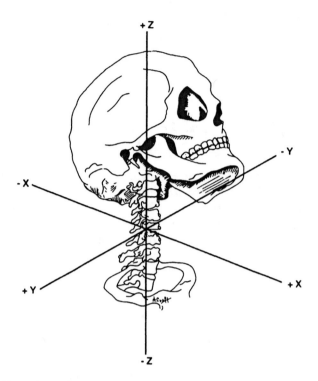

Figure 1. Central coordinate system used in impact engineering studies of whiplash. (Adapted from Foreman SM, Croft AC: Whiplash Injuries: The Cervical Acceleration/Deceleration Syndrome. Baltimore, Williams & Wilkins, 1988.)

Rotation occurs when all parts of an object move about an instantaneously stationary axis. Rotation may be represented by a cup spinning on a table but not sliding along the table. Vertebral rotation occurs about the y-axis during head flexion or about the z-axis during right and left rotation. Rotation is denoted by the theta symbol (θ), with clockwise rotations being $+\theta$ and counterclockwise rotations being $-\theta$. Right rotation is therefore represented by $+\theta z$ and pure forward flexion by $+\theta y$. Thus, there are 6 degrees of freedom in the cervical spine: rotation around three axes (x, y, z) and translation in three planes (sagittal, coronal, axial).

A *functional spinal unit* (also known as a *motion segment*) consists of two adjacent vertebrae and the nonbony tissues that hold them together. Motion of any one vertebra is described relative to the subjacent vertebra. The pattern of movement that occurs between cervical vertebrae is a result of the shape of the vertebrae, the orientation of the zygapophyseal (facet) joints, the state of the intervertebral disc, and the influence of soft tissues acting on the motion segment (eg, muscles, ligaments).

The *instantaneous axis of rotation* (IAR) is an axis passing through the center of motion of a vertebra at any instant of time during motion. At that single instance, the IAR does not move (it is the point around which the vertebra is moving), but if the IAR is calculated at multiple points in an arc of vertebral motion, its position will change.

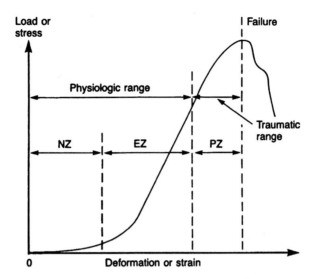

Figure 2. A typical load-deformation curve of a ligament, obtained in a materials testing machine. One end of the ligament is displaced with respect to the other, while the load and deformation of the ligament are continuously recorded. The deformation, being the independent parameter, is plotted on the horizontal axis. This load-deformation curve may be divided into physiologic and traumatic ranges. The physiologic range may be further divided into two parts. A ligament deformation around the neutral position where very little effort is required to deform the ligament is called the neutral zone (NZ). In the second part, a more substantial effort is needed to deform the ligament; this is called the elastic zone (EZ). In the trauma range there is microtrauma with increasing load, eventually leading to failure. This has been designated as the plastic zone (PZ). (From White AA, Panjabi MM: Kinematics of the spine. In Clinical Biomechanics of the Spine, 2nd ed. Philadelphia, JB Lippincott, 1978; with permission.)

Coupling occurs when motion around one axis is consistently accompanied by simultaneous motion around another axis. For instance, if a cervical vertebra is laterally flexed, there is always simultaneous rotation of the same vertebra so that the spinous process moves toward the convexity of the developing curve.

The *neutral zone* is that degree of movement that can occur between two vertebrae in any one plane (during either translation or rotation) without physiologic resistance to motion (Fig. 2).

The *elastic zone* is that degree of movement that occurs between the end of the neutral zone (ie, when resistance begins) and the end of the range of physiologic motion (Fig. 2).

Paradoxical motion occurs when the motion pattern of a vertebra is opposite that demonstrated by its adjacent vertebra. For instance, a cervical vertebra may move in a pattern of extension when the adjacent vertebra is moving into flexion. Although this is often discussed relative to motion in the sagittal plane, it can theoretically occur in other planes.

Spinal stability has been defined in numerous ways. A definition that incorporates the concept of *spinal clinical stability* is that state in which the spine is able to function under physiologic loads to maintain its pattern of displacement so that there is no initial or additional neurologic deficit, no major deformity, and no incapacitating pain.[6]

Motion of the Upper Cervical Spine (C0-C2)

Most authors divide the cervical spine into two functional regions: the upper (C0-C2) and lower (C3-C7). As a result of the unique and complicated anatomic characteristics of the upper cervical spine, the normal biomechanics are much different than observed in the lower cervical spine. The C0-C1 joints contribute approximately 25 degrees of combined flexion/extension and 5 degrees of lateral bending to each side. They apparently allow a small amount of rotation (3-8 degrees).[6] Paradoxical motion in the upper cervical spine was first described by Gutmann, who noted extension of C0-C1 during the end phase of cervical flexion.[7] This motion pattern has since been observed during flexion of the cervical spine in most young, normal persons, suggesting that it is a normal phenomenon.[8]

The C1-C2 articulations allow about 20 degrees of combined flexion/extension and 5 degrees of lateral flexion. They also allow 40 degrees of rotation to each side, which is about half of the axial rotation in the cervical spine. Although it is generally accepted that a strong coupling pattern exists between C1-C2 rotation and vertical translation of C1, some controversy exists as to the exact mechanism.[6]

Motion of the Middle and Lower Cervical Spine (C3-C7)

Lysell published the most exhaustive study of the kinematics of the lower cervical spine. Movement in the sagittal plane (ie, flexion/extension) is a combination of translation and rotation with a similar pattern of motion observed throughout the middle and lower functional spinal units.[9] Computer-assisted evaluation of cervical flexion/extension radiographs has been used to calculate the representative centers of rotation for each cervical motion segment, as shown in Figure 3.[10] The representative values for angular displacement in middle and lower cervical functional spinal units are listed in Table 1. Cadaveric studies have demonstrated sagittal plane translation under loads simulating physiologic flexion and extension to be about 2 mm, with a maximum of 2.7 mm (measured at the anteroinferior corner of the moving vertebra).[11] Based on these findings, it has been recommended that the upper limits of normal as measured on lateral cervical radiographs should be 3.5 mm (which allows for an estimated 25% magnification due to radiographic technique).

A strong coupling pattern exists in the lower cervical spine between lateral flexion and rotation. When the neck is laterally bent, there is rotation of the vertebrae so that the spinous processes move toward the convexity of the curve (as viewed in the frontal plane). The ratio of rotation to lateral flexion (in degrees) varies depending on the spinal level observed, with a gradual decrease in the amount of axial rotation associated with each degree of lateral flexion from C2 to C7. These ratios range from 0.67 at C2 (2 degrees of rotation for every 3 degrees of lateral flexion) to 0.13 at C7 (1 degree of rotation for every 7.5 degrees

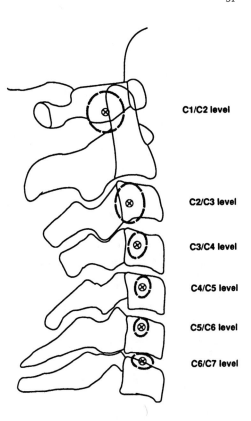

Figure 3. The positions of the centers of rotations for each motion segment. The marker shows a mean position, and the dashed line encloses the area of two standard deviations of this mean. Positions are marked as center of rotation of level/with respect to level (ie, C3/C4, COR of C3 with respect to C4). (From Dvorak J, Panjabi MM, Novotny JE, Antinnes JA: In vivo flexion/extension of the normal cervical spine. J Orthop Res 9:828–834, 1991; with permission.)

of lateral flexion).[9] Likewise, there is coupled lateral flexion when rotation is induced in the cervical spine.[12]

Table 1. Limits of Representative Values of Ranges of Rotation of the Middle and Lower Cervical Spine

Interspace	Combined Flexion/ Extension (± x-axis rotation)		One Side Lateral Bending (z-axis rotation)		One Side Axial Rotation (y-axis rotation)	
	Limits of Ranges (degrees)	Representative Angle (degrees)	Limits of Ranges (degrees)	Representative Angle (degrees)	Limits of Ranges (degrees)	Representative Angle (degrees)
Middle						
C2–3	5–16	10	11–20	10	0–10	3
C3–4	7–26	15	9–15	11	3–10	7
C4–5	13–29	20	0–16	11	1–12	7
Lower						
C5–6	13–29	20	0–16	8	2–12	7
C6–7	6–26	17	0–17	7	2–10	6
C7–T1	4–7	9	0–17	4	0–7	2

From White AA, Panjabi MM: Kinematics of the spine. In Clinical Biomechanics of the Spine, 2nd ed. Philadelphia, JB Lippincott, 1978; with permission.

THE BIOMECHANICS OF WHIPLASH

Definition of Whiplash

In their comprehensive monograph on whiplash-associated disorders, the Quebec Task Force defined whiplash as "... an acceleration-deceleration mechanism of energy transfer to the neck."[3] Although the task force went on to state that it may result from rear-end or side-impact motor vehicle collisions, as well as diving accidents and similar mishaps, it is unlikely that the kinematics are the same for all of these mechanisms. In a rear-impact collision, there is a rapid forward acceleration of the torso relative to the head with an initial flexion response, whereas in diving accidents (and similar injuries) force is usually applied to the head first and then transferred to the neck and upper torso. For the purposes of this chapter. we restrict the use of the term *whiplash* to the events that occur when a vehicle is hit by another vehicle from the rear. Barnsley and colleagues have summarized the sequence of events after such a rear-end impact: "The head, with no force acting upon it, remains static in space, resulting in forced extension of the neck as the shoulders travel anteriorly under the head. Following extension, the inertia of the head is overcome and [it] is also accelerated forward. The neck then acts as a lever to increase the forward acceleration of the head and force the neck into flexion."[13] In fact, the events are more complicated than this description infers.

The Biomechanics of Low-speed, Rear-end Collision

Numerous models have been used to study the kinematics of whiplash. Severy and colleagues performed controlled rear-end automobile collisions with a human volunteer in the 1950s.[14] Macnab later strapped anesthetized monkeys to a steel platform and dropped them from varying heights (causing sudden extension of the neck).[15] Many advances in methodology and technology have occurred since those early reports. Various experimental models are now used, including sled models (with animals, live humans, or cadavers), vehicle collision (live humans, anthropomorphic dummies, or cadavers), and mathematical models. Although useful information can be obtained from these studies, we concentrate on those using live or cadaveric human subjects in real or simulated low-speed collisions because they are most likely to provide an accurate understanding of the whiplash mechanism.

It is not our intent to address concepts of accident reconstruction, but a basic understanding of collision factors is necessary. These factors can be generally divided into vehicle factors and human factors. Human factors include variables such as body size and posture of the occupant. Vehicle factors include variables such as the weight, size, and velocity of each vehicle; the characteristics of seating and restraint systems; and the ability of the vehicles to absorb and transfer impact energy.

To explore the mechanism of whiplash logically, we first consider the sequence of biomechanical events known to occur in a typical rear-end collision. These events are listed in Table 2 and depicted in Figure 4. We then examine the variables that may alter those events.

Table 2.   Typical Sequence of Events in Rear-End Collisions
1. Impact of bullet vehicle into rear of target vehicle
2. Sudden acceleration of target vehicle
3. Seat back contact with torso of occupant
4. Simultaneous forward and upward acceleration of torso
5. Extension/compression of lower cervical spine and flexion/compression of upper cervical spine causing an S curve
6. Head contact with head restraint
7. Cervical spine extension and rearward head rotation
8. Forward acceleration of head past shoulders
9. Flexion of complete cervical spine.

Impact of the Bullet Vehicle into the Rear of the Target Vehicle

In vivo simulation studies usually assume that the target vehicle is not moving. If the target vehicle is moving in the same direction as the bullet vehicle prior to a rear-end collision, the difference in their speeds will determine the effective impact velocity. Rear impact results in a sudden acceleration of the target vehicle. The degree of acceleration is a function of the mass and velocity of the bullet vehicle, the mass and velocity of the target vehicle, and the energy-absorbing properties of the vehicle contact regions. The change in velocity of the target vehicle is known as *delta V*. The forces acting on an occupant are more a function of delta V than simply the speed or mass of the vehicles. Low-speed collision testing typically involves impact velocities of 8 to 15 km/h, or 4.8 to 9 mph, resulting in delta Vs of 8 to 10 km/h (4.8 to 6 mph).[16,17]

The risk of injury to an occupant in a target vehicle that sustains a forward delta V less than 5 mph is felt to be small.[17,18] The delta V may be influenced by the energy-absorbing bumper systems used on most modern cars. These systems are designed to absorb the forces of an 8 km/h (or 5 mph) fixed barrier impact so that minimal vehicle damage occurs.[19] They were not designed to decrease the delta V caused by an impact. Theoretically, if rebound occurs as a result of a malfunctioning energy-absorption system, the target vehicle could experience greater acceleration than if such a system was not present.

Forward and Upward Acceleration of the Torso

As the target vehicle is accelerated forward, the seat back first contacts the lumbopelvic region, causing the seat to deflect backward, away from the upper torso. This causes the seat back and head restraint to be lowered relative to the stationary torso of the occupant. The rearward tilting of the seat back causes a "ramping" effect, resulting in vertical displacement of the torso almost immediately after impact. Because the head remains stationary, there is compression of the cervical spine. This compression occurs before there is significant forward acceleration of the torso.[20]

Flattening of the thoracic kyphosis due to contact of the seat back with the thoracic spine has been proposed as an additional mechanism that may cause cervical compression.[21]

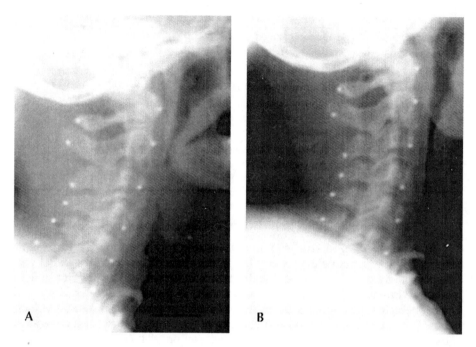

Figure 4. Sequential high-speed x-rays of a rear-end collision using a whole cadaver and impact sled. Time from impact: (A) 0 ms, (B) 152 ms, (C) 176 ms, (D) 192 ms, (E) 208 ms, (F) 224 ms. (Courtesy of Bing Deng, Paul Begeman, King Yang, Scott Tashman, and Albert King.)   (C, D, E, and F on next page.)

Extension/Compression Loading of the Lower Cervical Spine and Flexion/Compression Loading of the Upper Cervical Spine

The cervical spine is initially in a flexed posture due to forward movement of the torso. Forward acceleration and compression forces affect the lower neck first and then build quickly in the upper neck. Although the neck appears to be erect in high-speed photographic studies,[18] cineradiographic studies of human volunteers using a sled device have demonstrated that extension and forward motion of C5 and C6 occur while there is still flexion of the mid and upper cervical spine. Similar findings have been noted in studies using whole cadavers.[20,21] This produces an S-shaped cervical curve (Fig. 5). Kaneoka noted that the IAR of C6 shifted upward into the lower C5 body (compared with the normal IAR), causing downward movement of the inferior C5 facet into the superior C6 facet. This compression has been hypothesized as a possible mechanism of facet injury (Fig. 6).[22]

Grauer et al found the same S configuration to be present during testing of fresh cadaveric spines. They noted peak vertebral rotations at C6-C7 and C7-T1 that exceed maximum physiologic extension. These rotations occurred at the same time as the S-shaped curvature.[23] Deng et al and Ono et al have documented the relative rotation of each cervical vertebra and noted that the head flexes relative to the neck; C2-C3 is in relative flexion, and C3-C4, C4-C5 and

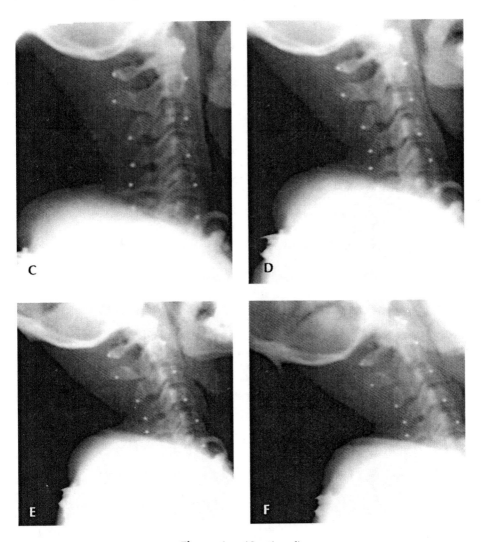

Figure 4. *(Continued).*

C5-C6 assume relative extension.[20,24] Available data indicate that muscle activation does not occur until about the time the S-shaped curvature is seen. Full muscle tension does not develop for 60 to 70 ms after onset of contraction.[17]

Head Contact with Head Restraint

In live crash studies by Siegmund et al head restraint contact occurred with the head still in its initial flexed and retracted position (relative to C7). Backward head rotation/extension did not begin until after head restraint contact. The peak horizontal acceleration of the head (relative to the ground) occurred during head restraint contact, with the average being 1.9 times the delta V of the target vehicle.[16] Peak relative displacements between vertebrae likely

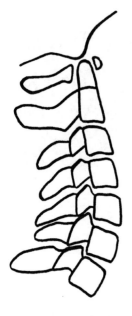

Figure 5.   An S-shaped cervical curve results from extension/compression of the lower cervical spine and flexion/compression of the upper cervical spine.

occur prior to the head contacting the head restraint.[20] These observations indicate that the forces most likely to cause injury (lower cervical compression and extension) occur early, before extension of the neck is apparent.

Whether the head contacts the headrest is likely a function of the distance from the base of the skull to the headrest (known as setback) and the acceleration

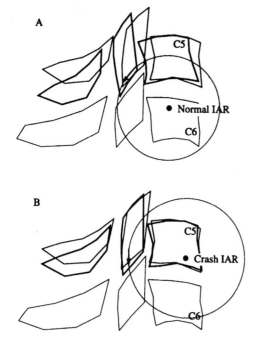

Figure 6.   **A,** In the normal extension motion, the C5 inferior articular facet surface rotated and slid smoothly around the normal instantaneous axis of rotation. **B,** In the impact motion, the posterior edge of the C5 inferior articular facet showed downward movement toward the C6 facet surface and tended to collide with it (facet impingement). (From Kaneoka K, Ono K, Inami S, Hayashi K: Motion analysis of cervical vertebrae during whiplash loading. Spine 24:763–770, 1999; with permission.)

to which the head is exposed. McConnell et al noted that when delta V exceeded 8 km/h, the head restraints were driven downward on their adjustable mountings. They also noted that seated height influenced head restraint contact, with taller people contacting the head restraint more on the upper surface and shorter people contacting more on the forward surface.[18]

Backward Head Rotation and Neck Extension

The momentum of the torso induces forward acceleration of the cervical spine but the mass of the head causes it to lag. This results in cervical extension and rearward head rotation. Maximum total neck extension (45-50 degrees) has been noted to be less than the maximum voluntary extension measured prior to impact testing.[18] Similar amounts of total cervical extension have been noted in sled models using cadaver cervical spines and whole cadavers.[20,25] This brings into doubt the theory that neck injury is related to maximal neck extension. Deng et al calculated peak facet capsular strains in their study (using cadavers) and noted that the average maximal strain observed during low-speed, rear-end impacts was 60%. They suggested that capsular ligaments might undergo stretch exceeding tolerance limits and be a cause of pain.[20]

Forward Head Acceleration and Cervical Spine Flexion

As the torso and base of the neck are accelerated forward with the cervical spine in maximal extension, the head follows in forward acceleration. In the study by McConnell et al, rearward head rotation continued for 60 to 90 ms before it slowed as the entire head was pulled forward (the "ball and chain effect"). The head then approaches the "over the top" position and accelerates past the lower cervical spine, causing cervical flexion. The forward acceleration of the head is actively slowed by the neck muscles with measured decelerations of 1.5-2.5 g.[18] Despite this, the head continues forward relatively faster than the shoulders.

Human Factors

Differences in seating posture and head-neck configuration may affect forces in the neck. Ono et al pre-positioned subjects necks in flexion, neutral, or extension prior to impact using a sled without a head restraint. They computed bending, shear, and axial compression forces and concluded that a kyphotic configuration of the cervical spine (caused by flexion prior to impact) may result in greater injury.[24] Deng et al found that a 20-degree seat-back angle resulted in less initial cervical lordosis and more upward ramping of the thoracic spine. This resulted in more cervical compression and increased the relative rotation of each cervical motion segment as compared with tests with a 0-degree (vertical) seat-back angle.[20]

Taller people are more likely to contact the top of the head restraint and may be exposed to increased cervical extension, but it is unclear if there is a greater risk of injury as a result of this. Croft has suggested that rotation of the neck reduces the available extension range of the cervical spine by 50% and increases the likelihood of extension injury.[26] Cadaveric studies using static loading have shown that pretorque of capsular ligaments (caused by rotation) increases capsular strain, which may in turn increase the risk of subcatastrophic facet injury.[27]

Epidemiologic studies have reported that women have a higher risk of symptomatic injury from whiplash than men.[4,28,29] Although several explanations have been proposed for this phenomenon, its cause is unclear. The higher risk of injury from whiplash does not appear to be due to a higher risk of injury in general but, rather, a specific cervical spine factor.[30]

Vehicle Factors

The mass and speed of the involved vehicles are the primary determinants of delta V. The overall risk of injury in rear-end collisions tends to increase with delta V.[16] Differences in seat-back inclination and stiffness will affect the forces transmitted to the cervical spine. Both a stiff seat and increased rearward tilt of the seat back (prior to impact) will increase the upward compressive load on the cervical spine.[20] Conversely, a softer seat cushion, though reducing the compression, will result in more torso rebound and increase the shear force in the lower cervical spine.[24] The position of the head restraint has been thought to be a risk factor in whiplash-associated disorders. A head restraint is considered properly positioned if the top is aligned with the top of the head.[31] A setback (the distance from the front of the head restraint to the back of the head) greater than 10 cm has been correlated with increased neck injuries.[32] Despite this, the role of the headrest is controversial. Because most of the peak forces thought to be responsible for neck injury occur early, McConnell et al feel it is unlikely that passive head restraints will have a significant effect on injury rate even when properly positioned.[18] A new headrest design that accelerates the head forward simultaneously with the thorax would potentially reduce cervical injury.

Low back injury has been considered unlikely due to the relative lack of differential motion observed in the lumbar spine.[18] Because compression of the lumbar spine occurs as a result of the ramping effect (more pronounced with greater seat-back tilt), there may be insult to lumbar structures. These forces have not yet been reported.

Seat restraint systems in current use (seat belt and shoulder harness) do not appear to play a significant role in occupant response to low-speed, rear-end impacts. Newer restraint systems discussed in this text may play a role in reducing injury occurrence related to vehicle factors.

SUMMARY
The mechanism of whiplash is much more complicated than the simple hyperextension injury proposed by early investigators. Many factors, both human and vehicle, influence the kinematic response of occupants to the sudden acceleration caused by rear impact. Only by studying "whole-body" dynamics will we understand how injury may be produced. This chapter outlines a complex sequence of events that produces an S-shaped cervical curvature (hyperextension in the lower region and flexion in the upper region) resulting in significant stress on the lower cervical motion segments. These events occur before the head contacts the head restraint and prior to full cervical extension. Understanding the influence of human and vehicle biomechanical factors is key to solving the puzzle of whiplash injury.

References

1. Crowe H: A new diagnostic sign in neck injuries. Calif Med 100:12–13, 1964.
2. Howard RP, Harding RM, Krenric SW: The biomechanics of "whiplash" in low velocity collisions. International Body Engineering Conference & Exposition. Detroit, MI, September 1999.
3. Spitzer WO, Skovron ML, Salmi LR, et al: Scientific monograph of the Quebec Task Force on Whiplash-Associated Disorders: redefining "whiplash" and its management [see comments] [published erratum appears in Spine 20:2372, 1995. Spine 20(8 suppl):1S–73S, 1995.
4. Otremski I, Marsh JL, Wilde BR, et al: Soft tissue cervical spinal injuries in motor vehicle accidents. Injury 20:349–351, 1989.
5. Sturzenegger M, DiStefano G, Radanov BP, Schnidrig A: Presenting symptoms and signs after whiplash injury: the influence of accident mechanisms. Neurology 44:488–693, 1994.
6. White AA, Panjabi MM: Clinical Biomechanics of the Spine, 2nd ed. Philadelphia, JB Lippincott, 1990.
7. Gutmann G: Die Wirbelblockierung and ihr radiologischer Nachweis. Die Wirbelsaule in Forschung und Prazis 15:83–102, 1960.
8. Penning L: Normal kinematics of the cervical spine. In Giles LGF, Singer KP (eds): Clinical Anatomy and Management of Cervical Spine Pain, Vol 3. Oxford, Butterworth-Heinemann, 1998, pp 51–55.
9. Lysell E: Motion in the cervical spine. An experimental study in autopsy specimens. Acta Orthop Scand 123(suppl):1+, 1969.
10. Dvorak J, Panjabi MM, Novotny JE, Antinnes JA: In vivo flexion/extension of the normal cervical spine. J Orthop Res 9:828–834, 1991.
11. White AA III, Johnson RM, Panjabi MM, Southwick WO: Biomechanical analysis of clinical stability in the cervical spine. Clin Orthop 109:85–96, 1975.
12. Panjabi MM, Summers DJ, Pelker RR, et al: Three-dimensional load displacement curves of the cervical spine. J Orthop Res 4:152–161, 1986.
13. Barnsley L, Lord S, Bogduk N: The pathophysiology of whiplash. Spine State Art Rev 7:329–353, 1993.
14. Severy DM, Mathewson JH, Bechtol CO: Controlled automobile rear-end collisions, an investigation of related engineering and medical phenomena. Can Serv Med J 11:727–759, 1955.
15. Macnab I: Acceleration injuries of the cervical spine. J Bone Joint Surg Am 46:1797–1799, 1964.
16. Siegmund GP, King DJ, Lawrence JM: Head/neck kinematic response of human subjects in low-speed rear-end collisions. Lake Buena Vista, FL, 41st Stapp Car Crash Conference, Society of Automotive Engineers, paper no. 973341, November 1997.
17. Szabo TJ, Welcher JB: Human subject kinematics and electromyographic activity during low speed rear impacts. Albuquerque, NM, 40th Stapp Car Crash Conference, Society of Automotive Engineers, paper no. 962432, November 1996.
18. McConnell WE, Howard RP, Van Poppel J, et al: Human head and neck kinematics after low velocity rear-end impacts: Understanding "whiplash." San Diego, CA, 39th Stapp Car Crash Conference, Society of Automotive Engineers, paper no. 952724, November 1995.
19. West DH, Gough JP, Harper GTK: Low speed rear-end collision testing using human subjects. Accid Reconstr J 5:22–26, 1993.
20. Deng B, Begeman PC, Yang KH, et al: Kinematics of human cadaver cervical spine during low speed rear-end impacts. Stapp Car Crash J 44:171–188, 2000.
21. Luan F, Yang KH, Deng B, et al: Qualitative analysis of neck kinematics during low-speed rear-end impact. Clin Biomecbh 15:649–657, 2000.
22. Kaneoka K, Ono K, Inami S, Hayashi K: Motion analysis of cervical vertebrae during whiplash loading. Spine 24:763–770, 1999.
23. Grauer JN, Panjabi MM, Cholewicki J, et al: Whiplash produces an S-shaped curvature of the neck with hyperextension at lower levels. Spine 22:2489–2494, 1997.
24. Ono K, Kaneoka K, Wittek A, Kajzer J: Cervical injury mechanism based on the analysis of human cervical vertebral motion and head-neck-torso kinematics during low speed rear impacts. Lake Buena Vista, FL, 41st Annual Stapp Car Crash Conference, Society of Automotive Engineers, paper no. 973340, November 1997.
25. Panjabi MM, Cholewicki J, Nibu K, et al: Simulation of whiplash trauma using whole cervical spine specimens. Spine 23:17–24, 1998.
26. Croft AC: Biomechanics. In Pine JW Jr (ed): Whiplash Injuries. Baltimore, Williams & Wilkins, 1988.
27. Winkelstein BA, Nightingale RW, Richardson WJ, Myers BS: The cervical facet capsule and its role in whiplash injury. Spine 25:1238–1246, 2000.

28. O'Neill B, Haddon W, Kelley AB, Sorenson WW: Automobile head restraints—frequency of neck injury in relation to the presence of head restraints. Am J Public Health 62:399–406, 1972.
29. Versteegen GJ, Kingma J, Meijler WJ, ten Duis HJ: Neck sprain after motor vehicle accidents in drivers and passengers. Eur Spine J 9:547–552, 2000.
30. Temming J: Human factors data in relation to whiplash injuries in rear end collisions of passenger cars. Detroit, MI, SAE International Congress and Exposition, paper no. 981191, February 1998.
31. Walz FH, Muser MH: Biomechanical assessment of soft tissue cervical spine disorders and expert opinion in low speed collisions. Accid Anal Prev 32:161–165, 2000.
32. Nygren A, Gustafsson H, Tingvall C: Effects of different types of headrests in rear-end collisions. 10th Experimental Safety Vehicle Conference, Washington, DC, 1985.

4

The Pathophysiology of Whiplash

Leslie Barnsley, Ph.D., Susan M. Lord, Ph.D., and Nikolai Bogduk, M.D., Ph.D., DSc

This chapter is reprinted from **Spine: State of the Art Reviews** *12(2):209–242, 1998, published by Hanley & Belfus, Inc.*

One thing is certain about whiplash—it is something that happens in a motor vehicle accident. Every other aspect of whiplash has been controversial, or remains so in some quarters. However, that controversy stems largely from preconceived attitudes and beliefs that stand in contrast to the ever increasing body of scientific knowledge about this phenomenon.

The very term *whiplash* has been criticized, on the grounds that it is poorly defined, misrepresented, and invokes connotations of medicolegal claims that cloud the clinical and scientific issues. Alternative terms such as "acceleration-deceleration injury" and "cantilever injury" have been suggested to more accurately describe the inferred mechanism of injury, but these terms have not found favor. "Whiplash" remains the most attractive term colloquially and in the medical literature.

Whiplash entails three components. The *whiplash event* is a biomechanical process suffered by occupants of a vehicle that is struck by another vehicle. The *whiplash injury* is the impairment that ostensibly results from the whiplash event. The *whiplash syndrome* is the constellation of symptoms that are attributed to the supposed whiplash injury.

Controversies concerning whiplash have focused on what specifically constitutes the whiplash event, but more so on the nature of the supposed whiplash injury and even if it occurs at all, and the legitimacy of ascribing symptoms to this injury. However, research into whiplash, particularly during the last decade, has dispelled many of the myths and concerns about it. There is now an impressive body of knowledge about its biomechanics, pathology, and the mechanism of symptoms.

DEFINITION

By usage, whiplash is a term focused on the behavior of the head and neck of occupants of a motor vehicle struck by another vehicle. However, emerging research indicates that parts of the body other than the neck are involved, and the classical definition may change in the future. Nevertheless, the conventional view is that whiplash is an inertial response of the body to the forces delivered to it, in which the head and neck undergo an excursion, but in which neither

Table 1. The Incidence of Various Types of Impact Reported by Whiplash Patients

Source	Number	Proportion of Patients (%) by Direction of Impact				
		Rear	*Front*	*Rear + Front*	*Side*	*Other*
178	117	37	27	23		13
131	68	59	29		12	
182	100	76	24			
65	4640	38	14	37	11	
141	102	46	23	14		17
203	3014	30	15		19	36
104	97	45	22		11	16

the head nor the neck suffer any direct blow. It is this latter feature that distinguishes whiplash from other events that may occur in a motor vehicle accident.

Classical descriptions restricted the definition to movements of the neck in the sagittal plane following rear-end impact collisions. However, contemporary usage also embraces other patterns of movement such as those resulting from head-on and side collisions. Restricting the definition to rear-end collisions does not distinguish patients in terms of reported symptoms or prognosis. Reciprocally, extending the definition to allow any direction of impact does not confound the clinical picture. Although rear-end collisions remain the single most common pattern of impact reported by patients, other patterns constitute substantial proportions (Table 1).

ETIOLOGY AND PATHOGENESIS

Early clinical reports suggested that rear-end impacts resulted in forced flexion of the neck.[86] This belief was questioned in subsequent experimental studies[45,196] and computer models[147,226] that suggested that the cardinal movement after rear-end impact was extension of the neck. This emphasis on extension held sway for over 40 years. However, recent experiments require that this be reconsidered, for they have revealed that the movements are more complex than was previously suspected. In particular, it has been found that axial compression and unnatural, double curvatures of the cervical spine are important and potentially damaging components of the response of the cervical spine to inertial loading.

Cadaver experiments have demonstrated that upon impact, the lower cervical spine is thrust upwards and forwards.[94] The cervical spine is, therefore, compressed from below, and the lower cervical segments are extended while the upper segments are relatively flexed. As a result, the cervical spine assumes an S shape during the first 50–75 ms after impact. Thereafter, all segments are progressively extended until the head is thrown backwards into extension.

In experiments on normal volunteers, one study using high-speed photography[145] determined in detail the excursions of the neck after rear-end impacts at 3–8 km/h. For the first 50 ms the body remained motionless while the vehicle and driver's seat moved forwards about 5–8 cm. After another 10 ms, the seat back began to push the subject's hips and low back forwards and upwards, while the upper part of the seat back declined backwards. By 100 ms the seat back reached its maximum declination of about 10° and the subject's upper trunk began moving forwards and upwards. At 120 ms, as the subject's hips and trunk rose upwards and backwards along the declined seat back, while the neck was axially compressed and straightened as the top of the cervical spine began moving upwards and backwards. At this point the head moved for the first time, rotating upwards and backwards. By 160 ms the forward and upward movement of the trunk began to pull the base of the neck forwards, while the head continued to extend. At 200 ms the upward movement of the trunk and shoulders ceased after an excursion of about 9 cm, and the extension of the head stopped after about 45°, the top of the cervical spine had risen about 1.25 cm. At this time the head started to reverse its motion. By 250 ms the head had not yet assumed a vertical position, but the trunk, neck, and head were descending along the seat back. After 300 ms the descent of the trunk was completed, the head had reached a vertical position and continued its forward movement but was being decelerated, ostensibly by tension in the posterior neck muscles. By 400 ms the head had reached its most forward position, and began a return movement to its normal upright position over the shoulders. By 450 ms all parts of the body were moving at the same velocity as the vehicle, and all body parts had returned to their preimpact positions.

During these movements, the top of the neck underwent accelerations ranging from 0.3 to 3.5 g whose vectors changed direction progressively with time from upwards, to upwards and forwards, downwards and forwards, backwards, and finally backwards and upwards. The emphasis of the results of this experiment was that substantial compressive forces were exerted on the cervical spine. At the low impacts involved, no subject experienced motion beyond the range of normal motion, but several experienced mild discomfort following the impacts. The threshold for mild injury was inferred to be 8 km/h.

Similar observations were reported in experiments in which normal volunteers were studied using high-speed cineradiography during simulated collisions of approximately 5 km/h.[144] The authors again emphasized the compression imparted to the cervical spine. Key additional observations from this study were that the pattern of motion varied with initial body position. If the subject was leaning forwards or stooped, rear-end impact caused extension of the thoracic spine and an upward axial acceleration of the cervical spine. This produced compression loading of the neck so that its length was shortened. At the same time, the cervical lordosis was straightened, and slight cervical flexion occurred before extension. In contrast, if the subject was reclined on the seat back, the chest and shoulders descended as the seat back deflected rearwards, and the cervical spine was not subjected to upward acceleration and compression. In these experiments, the subjects reported mild discomfort and neck pain that lasted 2–4 days, but none had any long-term sequelae.

A series of detailed cineradiographic studies of normal volunteers described the motion of individual cervical segments during the extension phase of whiplash.[120] The volunteers were subjected to an 8 km/h impact that resulted in a 4 g acceleration. The initial movement of the trunk was upwards, driving the C6 vertebra upwards. As it moved, the C6 vertebra extended underneath the rest of the cervical spine which had not yet moved. The extension of C6 forced each of the segments above to undergo a small initial flexion, of

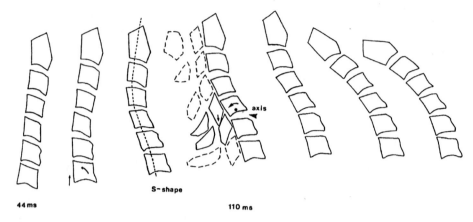

Figure 1. The appearance of sequential radiographs of the cervical spine during the extension phase of whiplash. At 110 ms the C5 vertebra rotates about an abnormally high axis of rotation, causing the vertebral body to separate anteriorly from C6 (*arrowhead*), and the inferior articular process of C5 to chisel into the superior articular process of C6 (*arrows*). (Based on Kaneoka K, Ono L, Inami S, Hayashi K: Abnormal segmental motion of the cervical spine during whiplash loading. J Jap Orthop Assoc 71:S1680, 1997.)

some 2–5° in amplitude, before undergoing extension. Each of the three segments immediately above C6 then extended in sequential order from below. The segments achieved peak initial flexion between 50 and 110 ms after impact, and peak extension between 100 and 200 ms after impact. The net result of these movements was that the cervical spine assumed an S shape at about 100 ms, as lower segments commenced extension while higher segments were still undergoing initial flexion (Fig. 1). Segments at the junction of the extending curve and the flexing curve underwent deformation as they rotated around abnormal axes of rotation. Instead of lying in the vertebral body below,[4] the axis of movement was on the inferior endplate of the extending vertebra. This indicates that the motion was a pure rotation, there being no element of translation. As a result, the anterior end of the vertebra separated from the vertebral body below, and posteriorly the tip inferior articular process chiseled into the supporting superior articular process. Subsequently, the cervical spine underwent extension, as described in the classic model.

These studies on normal volunteers provide data on the qualitative aspects of whiplash injury; they show how the cervical spine can be injured, but understate the severity of possible injury. Perforce, they were limited to studying low-impact collisions, with velocity changes of the order of 4–8 km/h resulting in accelerations of only 2–4 g. Other experiments indicate that in collisions with velocity changes of 32 km/h the human head reaches a peak acceleration of some 12 g.[196] With such greater forces, the propensity for injury would be greater.

All mathematical models and experimental data on rear-impact collisions have assumed that the impact force is transmitted directly along the long axis of the vehicles and that the victim's head is in the anatomical position, looking straight ahead. By implication, this would produce acceleration forces exclusively in the sagittal plane. However, in real life situations, this is unlikely to be the case. If the head is in slight rotation, a rear-end impact will force the head further into rotation before extension occurs.[62] This has important consequences in that cervical rotation prestresses various cervical structures, including the capsules of the zygapophyseal joints, intervertebral discs, and the alar ligament complex,[61,62,134] rendering them more susceptible to injury when subjected to an additional extension force.

There are fewer data on the response of the neck and head to side or frontal impact, since these impacts are more likely to lead to injuries to other body parts[76] and, therefore, fail to attract attention as "classic" whiplash injuries. However, the reported data from computer models and cadaver experiments are consistent with the predictions derived from simple physics and extrapolation from the data on rear-end accidents. Frontal impacts rapidly decelerate the motor vehicle. The body of the passenger, having momentum, continues forwards until decelerated by the seat belt. The head, which has not yet had a force act upon it, will continue moving forwards until decelerated by the neck itself, with the force being applied at the occipitoatlantal joint and then at C6.[45] Since this force is eccentric to the direction of movement of the head, the head rotates forwards, forcibly flexing the neck. There is then a degree of recoil as the elastic properties of the posterior neck structures pull the head out of flexion, extending the neck. Experimental and mathematical models of frontal impact have demonstrated that the head is subject to marked rotational acceleration at the occipital condyles in the first 25 ms after impact, followed by a reversal of the direction of acceleration as extension occurs.[53] The forces involved are again considerable, with models indicating that at an impact speed of 63.5 km/h resulting in a vehicle deceleration of 90 g, the head is subject to a negative acceleration of 46 g. Consequently, the neck dissipates force initially through shear and then torque which can easily exceed the known tolerance levels of bone and ligament, leading to neck injury even in the absence of head injury.[53]

Regardless of the direction of impact, one key feature of whiplash is that the neck moves passively. The muscles that normally control the direction and amplitude of neck motion do not have time to respond to the forces applied to the motion segments.[77,190] The lack of muscle control and the abnormal direction of forces applied to the neck result in movements around abnormal axes of rotation,[79,118,119,120,134,169] which subjects the restraining elements to abnormal stresses.

MODE OF INJURY

Although modern studies have emphasized compression as the cardinal force exerted on the cervical spine, this does not imply that crush fractures should be the expected injury. Rather, the emphasis is that axial compression causes abnormal modes of extension. In particular, when extension occurs about an abnormally high axis of rotation, the vertebra rotates without translation. This results in abnormal separation of the anterior elements of the neck and abnormal patterns of compression posteriorly.

The anterior structures principally at risk are the esophagus, anterior longitudinal ligament, anterior cervical muscles, odontoid process, and the intervertebral discs. Under tension, these structures can fail, resulting in tears of the muscles, ligaments, or discs, or avulsion of the disc from the vertebral body. The odontoid process bears the weight of the head in extension and may fail by fracture. The posterior structures at risk are the spinous processes and the zygapophyseal joints. When extension occurs around an elevated axis of rotation,[120] the zygapophyseal joints do not glide across their supporting articular surfaces. Instead, the inferior articular processes are driven into the superior articular facets (see Fig. 1). This can result in compression fractures of the articular cartilage or the subchondral bone, or in tears of the intra-articular meniscoids.

When the cervical spine recoils into flexion, compression forces are applied to the anterior elements of the neck and tensile forces to the posterior elements. Because they are designed to sustain compression loads, the vertebral bodies are unlikely to fail under the compression loads incurred during whiplash, but under impaction in extreme flexion, the upper corners of the articular pillars may be susceptible to fracture. Under tension, the capsules of the zygapophyseal joints, the ligamentum nuchae, and the posterior neck muscles may be susceptible to sprain. Flexion at the atlantoaxial joint will stress the alar ligament complex as the atlas and head attempt to rotate anteriorly over the axis.

Lateral flexion of the cervical spine between C2 and C7 is strictly coupled to rotation at the cervical disc and is determined by the orientation of the cervical zygapophyseal joints.[169] If an external force laterally flexes the neck, the structures at risk of injury will be determined by the extent to which coupling occurs. If the force simply reproduces physiological movements, the zygapophyseal joint capsules on both sides and the intervertebral discs will be most at risk from axial torque, whereas, if there is little coupling, lateral flexion will compress the ipsilateral zygapophyseal joint and distract the contralateral joint.

Notwithstanding these theoretical considerations as to which structures are mechanically at risk, the actual likelihood of a lesion occurring cannot be extrapolated from such analysis alone. The exact distribution of force and the specific tolerances of different tissues, as well as any interactions, would need to be considered. Consequently, in the absence of such precise and comprehensive data, predictions of pathological lesions from biomechanical observations need to be ratified by experimental or observational studies.

PATHOLOGY

Since whiplash injuries leading to chronic symptoms are nonfatal, no formal pathological studies are available from which to determine the site or nature of any lesions. Therefore, evidence for pathological entities has been obtained through indirect means, including animal experiments, cadaver experiments, post mortem studies, clinical observations, and radiographic studies. Each of these approaches has limitations, which must be borne in mind when evaluating any findings.

Animal studies are limited by the extent to which lesions produced in the animals reflect those sustained by human beings in actual accidents. Unfortunately, there is no reliable means of ascertaining the representativeness of a given animal model because of the large number of interacting variables that must be considered, including size, weight, and morphology.

Cadaver experiments are accurate in terms of gross anatomic relationships but do not simulate the mechanical properties of living tissues, cadaveric matter being usually stiffer.

Postmortem studies are available either from individuals who have whiplash injuries but die from other, unrelated causes or from victims of fatal trauma who have injured their necks. The former patients are unusual, amounting to only 15 cases in the literature.[2,181,191,212] It may be argued that the latter group constitute severely injured individuals whose injuries are not representative of those surviving trauma. However, motor vehicle accidents typically produce increasingly severe injuries with increasing forces. The likelihood of death depends in part on qualitative factors, such as the exact part of the body injured, but is typically proportional to the forces involved.[45] Victims of fatal accidents have typically sustained a head injury or an injury to the C1 segment. This, indeed, is the pattern of injuries seen at post mortem.[117] In these cases, if the obvious cause of death is disregarded, the other, nonlethal injuries of the neck are a reasonable indication of what might have occurred had the victim been subjected to forces just short of those that were lethal.

Clinical observations are limited to those lesions that can be detected on clinical examination or at operation. Other than bruising, bleeding, or swelling, there is little that can be detected on clinical examination, and even then the findings are limited to superficial tissues. Few patients with whiplash injuries are treated by surgery, and if operations are performed it is late in the course of the disease, so that any findings may not necessarily be related to the initial trauma. Findings on plain x-rays are limited to osseous injuries and changes in soft tissue shadows, particularly the prevertebral space.[168,198] Even so, several studies attest to the insensitivity of plain films for detecting significant bony injury, particularly of the articular pillars and zygapophyseal joints.[1,2,19,44,117,201,225,229,232]

Notwithstanding these limitations, marshaling the evidence from clinical, animal, cadaver, and post mortem studies can indicate trends and concordance to support one or more putative pathological lesions (Fig. 2).

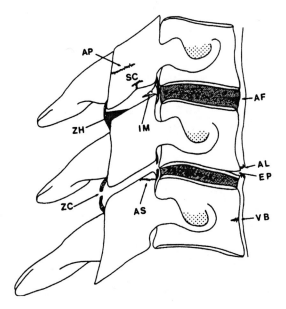

Figure 2. A sketch of the more common lesions affecting the cervical spine following whiplash. AP, articular pillar fracture; SC, fracture of the subchondral plate; AF, tear of the anulus fibrosus of the intervertebral disc; ZH, hemarthrosis of the zygapophyseal joint; IM, contusion of the intraarticular meniscus of the zygapophyseal joint; AL, tear of the anterior longitudinal ligament; EP, endplate avulsion/fracture; ZC, rupture or tear of the zygapophyseal joint capsule; AS, fracture involving the articular surface; VB, vertebral body fracture.

Zygapophyseal Joints

Evidence that the cervical zygapophyseal joints are damaged in whiplash injury is compelling. There is striking consistency between experimental data from cadavers, radiographic findings, operative findings, and post mortem studies. Fractures of the joints themselves or the supporting articular pillar have been noted in several clinical studies,[2,3,19,44,116,127,201,229] and identical fractures have been produced in cadavers.[1,45] Moreover, post mortem examination of a patient with a recent history of extension injury and neck pain, but who died of unrelated causes 4 months later, has revealed a typical healing fracture of the articular pillar on the side of the pain.[2] Other post mortem studies have found similar lesions.[117,213]

Even using optimal imaging parameters in cadavers, the soft tissue elements of the cervical zygapophyseal joints are poorly seen with plain x-ray, CT, or MRI.[74] Consequently, there are no imaging studies of the pathology of these structures. However, tears of the joint capsules have been identified at operation on several occasions[37,114,116] and similar injuries have been found at post mortem[36,117,148,213] and in cadaver studies.[45] Animal experiments have produced damage and hemarthroses in the zygapophyseal joints in a significant proportion of the animals examined.[126,138,228]

Of interest in the setting of chronic pain after whiplash injury, is the report of a single case of severe and isolated arthritic change in a cervical zygapophyseal joint found at post mortem. The patient had severe, disabling, and refractory neck pain for many years after a whiplash injury, culminating in suicide.[181] It is an appealing hypothesis, consistent with known biological models, that injuries to the osseous or soft tissues of a joint predispose it to premature, painful, osteoarthritic change.[142] Such a hypothesis could explain the tragic sequence of events in this and other cases.

Intervertebral Discs

Injuries to the intervertebral discs have been reported from a number of sources. The typical lesions are avulsion of the disc from the vertebral end-plate and tears of the anterior anulus fibrosus of the disc. Separation of the disc from the vertebra or fractures of the vertebral end-plate have been seen on plain x-rays and MRI,[49,121,170] found at surgery,[37,136] reproduced in animal experiments,[126,228] and found at post mortem.[117] Lesions in the anterior anulus of the disc have been identified on MRI scan.[49] Tears at corresponding sites have been identified at surgery,[37] and have been a consistent finding in post mortem studies which have included some patients who survived the initial injury before coming to autopsy.[117,212,213] Other studies have reported disc injury or narrowing without specifying the precise site or nature of the lesion.[17,36,126] A carefully conducted study of whiplash injuries to cadavers has produced anterior disc lesions and noted that they were more common after hyperextension than hyperflexion.[45] Such lesions are consistent with the recent biomechanical evidence that eccentric rotation is an important component of the cervical spine's response to rear-end impact (see Fig. 1).[94,118,119,120,144]

A further piece of evidence indicating damage to the discs or zygapophyseal joints in whiplash injury is the observation that in a group of patients with significant symptoms after ten years, all patients had developed degenerative changes on their x-rays.[223] Furthermore, the age-adjusted prevalence of degenerative changes was significantly higher in those patients who had suffered whiplash than in control groups. These findings are consistent with initial, occult injury to the cervical spine leading to later osteoarthritic change.

Muscles

Muscle tears and sprains have been implicated by clinical examination,[79,116] and have also been visualized on ultrasound examination[143] and MRI.[170] Muscle damage has been seen in animal experiments[126,136,228] and post mortem examinations.[117] The typical pathology observed is as predicted from the forces involved, with muscles demonstrating partial and complete tears and hemorrhage. No studies have addressed the question of the existence and presence of any chronic, painful muscle pathology following trauma in whiplash patients, and indeed there is little basis for such an entity in conventional pathology teaching. The usual expectation would be that sprains or tears of muscles would heal in a matter of weeks, forming a scar within the muscle but leaving the patient with no residual pain.

Trigger Points and Myofascial Pain

The notion of trigger points and myofascial pain enjoys a considerable degree of popularity, particularly in North America. It provides a generic, theoretical basis for chronic pain ostensibly stemming from muscles in many regions of the body.[220] The neck is one such region and many practitioners seem convinced that trigger points and myofascial pain can develop after whiplash.[71,80,214] It is not the purpose nor the intention of this chapter to review the theory of myofascial pain in general, but there is a duty to explore its pertinence in the context of whiplash.

In the first instance, there are no epidemiologic data on the prevalence of myofascial pain in patients with whiplash. Even a recent review provides no such data.[80] It reiterates the theory of trigger points and explains how they can be diagnosed and treated. It opens with a statement that "myofascial pain...is one of the most common causes of persistent pain following flexion-extension injuries," but cites no data in support of this statement. No studies using an appropriate inception cohort, and using specific, diagnostic criteria have been conducted to verify the impression that myofascial pain is common after whiplash. Yet there are reasons to doubt that it is so common.

Formal studies have shown that myofascial experts have difficulty in agreeing as to the very presence of a trigger point—the cardinal feature of regional myofascial pain syndromes.[228] Although they might agree on the presence of tenderness, they could not agree on the presence of the other diagnostic features of trigger points. The theory of trigger points, therefore, lacks demonstrated internal validity. Less expert practitioners may well be finding tenderness in the neck muscles of patients with whiplash injuries, but there is no evidence that this tenderness indicates a trigger point or a primary myofascial diathesis.

More specifically, it is conspicuous that several of the classical trigger points of the neck muscles lack the statutory diagnostic features of a trigger point.[30] Tenderness is present but not the palpable band nor the twitch response. Since they do not satisfy the formal definition of a trigger point these sites cannot be held to be trigger points. It is furthermore conspicuous that, topographically, the so-called trigger points of the neck overlie the cervical zygapophyseal joints and that the reported pain patterns of cervical trigger points are identical to those of referred pain from the zygapophyseal joints.[30] There are grounds, therefore, to believe that what may have been misrepresented as cervical trigger points after whiplash actually represent painful, tender zygapophyseal joints.

Whatever might be written or believed about myofascial pain in general, there is no explicit, reliable data on its occurrence after whiplash, yet there is data that casts doubt on the reliability of diagnosis of trigger points in general, and of trigger points in the neck in particular.

Ligaments

Ligamentous injuries of the neck cannot be diagnosed clinically. However, tears of the anterior longitudinal ligament have been consistently reported in major series of animal experiments,[136,228] found at surgery,[37,110] identified at post mortem,[36,148] and found in cadaver experiments.[45] Magnetic resonance imaging has also confirmed the presence of such lesions in patients not subjected to surgery.[49] Anatomical studies have indicated that the anterior longitudinal ligament merges imperceptibly with the anterior anulus of the intervertebral disc,[180] indicating that ligamentous injuries may be frequently associated with disc injuries. Injuries to the interspinous ligament have also been identified on MRI,[49] at surgery,[114,116] at post mortem, and in animal experiments.[228] However, the significance of any injury to this ligament is questionable since in normal humans it constitutes a delicate, thin fascial sheet, separating the muscular compartments of the left and right of the posterior neck.[180] Damage to the posterior longitudinal ligament and the ligamentum flavum from whiplash injury has never been reported at operation or from any imaging studies, but has been seen in animal experiments,[228] cadaver experiments,[45] and at post mortem.[36,117] These are both highly elastic structures and injury to them would reflect severe trauma with large, destructive, and probably lethal excursions of the cervical vertebrae.

Atlantoaxial Complex

Fractures of the atlas or axis may be dramatic events resulting in death or serious neurologic injury,[128] and it is therefore not surprising to find such injuries in post mortem studies.[36,117] However, more subtle, occult injuries may occur in the setting of whiplash. Fractures of the odontoid peg have been detected clinically,[195,199] and produced in animal experiments.[227] Evidence of bony injury to other parts of C2, including the laminae and superior articular process, have been obtained from radiographic[48,194,199] and surgical[48,199] assessments. Atlas injuries are reported less frequently, but have been found on plain x-rays and reproduced in cadaver experiments.[1,2] The most comprehensive post mortem data come from a controlled study of injuries to the atlantoaxial complex from Australia.[191] Three groups of patients were studied, 30 patients with immediately fatal injuries, 11 patients with a period of survival after the index injury, and 10 control patients with no history of neck injury. The most common finding in the acute death group was bruising around and including the second spinal nerve, found in over half the cases. The next most common injury was bruising of the intra-articular synovial folds of the lateral atlantoaxial joint, which was found in exactly half the cases. Three of eleven cases in the survivor group showed evidence of previous bruising and trauma to the synovial folds of the atlantoaxial joint, and three others had evidence of posterior extracapsular hematoma around the C2 nerve. One patient had evidence of an anterior capsular rupture. Fractures of the lateral masses were observed only in the acute death group.

The atlantoaxial joints permit a wide range of axial rotation,[62] and their integrity is maintained by ligaments, particularly the alar and transverse ligaments.[61,63,188] These structures would appear to be susceptible to injury on the basis of post mortem studies,[117] but demonstration of injuries in vivo is difficult. However, a controlled series involving the elegant application of functional CT scanning has permitted the detection of pathological hypermobility due to disruption of the alar ligaments in patients with pain after whiplash injury.[60]

Cervical Vertebrae

Overt and major fractures of the vertebrae below C2 are uncommon in whiplash, but the incidence of lesser, more subtle fractures may be underestimated, for they are difficult to detect on conventional radiographs. Experimental studies in animals and cadavers[2,45,228] as well as post mortem observations[36,117] have confirmed that vertebral fractures can occur as a result of whiplash. When carefully sought with specialized views, fractures of the pedicles and laminae have been seen in patients.[2] There are also isolated reports of transverse process fractures[117,158] and compression fractures of the vertebral bodies themselves.[40,158] Fracture of the spinous processes appears to be a rare event, but has been noted on plain radiographs and produced in a cadaver experiment.[87]

Brain

Careful animal experiments have demonstrated hemorrhage in and around the brain from acceleration injuries without direct trauma to the head.[126,161,189,228] Subdural hematoma has also been noted following whiplash injury in a human.[162] It is likely that cerebral injuries from whiplash are underreported as the presence of a significant head injury, irrespective of how it was acquired, will distract attention from any neck symptoms and therefore any association between brain injury and whiplash injury may not be apparent. In addition, subtle injuries to the brain may be beyond resolution using conventional imaging.

Temporomandibular Joint

Injuries to the temporomandibular joint from whiplash have been suspected on clinical grounds for many years,[78,184] and two reviews attest to the considerable support for the view that the temporomandibular joint can be injured in whiplash accidents.[35,69] However, much of the supporting evidence stems from clinics specializing in temporomandibular joint pain, and the data is retrospective, not prospective. Many patients with temporomandibular pain report a history of cervical trauma, but these studies do not indicate the prevalence of temporomandibular problems after whiplash.

One study[224] reported an uncontrolled, referral-based series of 28 patients in which internal derangements were detected in 22 of 25 patients investigated with arthrography, and amongst whom pathology was confirmed in 10 patients who proceeded to surgery. This sample, however, lacked a control group and is not likely to be representative, an important consideration when evaluating such a common condition.[125]

On the other hand, other investigators have brought contrary evidence to bear. Heise et al.[99] followed an inception cohort of patients with whiplash, seen at a surgical trauma emergency department, and found the incidence of temporomandibular joint symptoms to be very low. Of 155 patients, 22 reported masticatory and temporomandibular pain when first seen, and none had persistent symptoms at follow-up after one year. In a retrospective, but nonetheless comprehensive, review of 2,198 subjects with whiplash claims, Probert et al.[172] found only 11 who claimed temporomandibular injury in the absence of associated face or skull injuries.

In the absence of direct injury to the face or jaws, temporomandibular joint injury is an exceedingly rare association with whiplash injury. Doubtless, specialists in temporomandibular pain do see patients with a history of cervical trauma, but for a controversial condition that otherwise has variously be ascribed to causes as diverse as depression, myofascial pain, and trauma,[66] a causative link to whiplash has still to be demonstrated.[123]

Other Structures

Injuries to various other structures have been reported following whiplash injury, usually in the form of case reports. Accordingly, they do not constitute common injuries but are examples of serious or unexpected injuries that can occur. They include avulsion of the occipital bone,[40] fracture of an occipital condyle,[207] prevertebral hematoma compromising the airway,[33,110] perforation of the esophagus,[202] Horner's syndrome indicating damage to the cervical sympathetic nerves,[116] damage to the recurrent laryngeal nerves,[100] spinal cord injury,[148] perilymph fistula,[21,96] thrombosis[221] and aneurysm[106] of a vertebral artery, dissection[115] or strangulation[230] of an internal carotid artery, retinal angiopathy,[101] and anterior spinal artery syndrome.[75,97]

Synopsis

On balance, given the extent to which experiments of different natures have converged to the same conclusion, the structures most likely to be injured in whiplash are the zygapophyseal joints, the intervertebral discs, and the upper cervical ligaments. Injuries of other structures can occur, but the available evidence suggests that these are uncommon.

Table 2. Time of Onset of Symptoms after Whiplash Injury

Source	Number	Proportion of Patients (%) Reporting Onset of Symptoms at Times Shown after Accident				
		< 1 Hr	*< 5 Hr*	*< 12 Hr*	*< 24 Hr*	*> 24 Hr*
208	93	70	9		9	9
104	137	52			20	28
158	61	85	11	2		2
52	137			78	13	9

SYMPTOMATOLOGY

Patients develop symptoms quite soon after a whiplash accident, typically within 24 hours, with neck pain or headache being the cardinal symptoms and the ones noticed soonest. Studies from various parts of the world are in agreement on this aspect of whiplash symptomatology (Table 2).

Although some studies do not describe the clinical features of whiplash,[52,149,158,160,167] those that do are reasonably consistent (Table 3). Such variance as does occur pertains only to the associated features reported by a minority of patients. Some authors admit certain of these features, others do not. Consequently, their reported prevalence amongst patients differs from study to study.

The symptoms of whiplash are dominated by pain in the neck and headache. The second most common symptom is pain in the shoulder girdle, followed by paresthesiae and weakness in the upper limbs. Less common and irregularly reported are symptoms of dizziness, visual disturbances, and tinnitus. Other similar symptoms, such as unsteadiness, have been recorded by some investigators,[83,178] but have not attracted the explicit attention of others.

Table 3. Proportion of Patients with Particular Clinical Features of Whiplash

Symptom	Proportion of Patients (%) Reporting Symptoms						
	Acute				*Chronic*		
Neck pain	89	90	92	88	79	74	100
Headache	26		57	54	89	33	88
Shoulder pain	37	80	49	40	50		
Paresthesiae		50	15		25	45	68
Weakness							68
Dizziness		62	15	23			53
Visual problems				9	54	2	42
Tinnitus		30	4	4	7	14	
Memory or concentration impairment		26					71
Back pain		42	39		39	42	
Number	102	320	117	93	28	43	68
Source	141	65	178	104	83	209	131

Absent entries indicate that the study in question did not consider the particular symptom.

Although understated in Table 3, disturbances of memory and/or concentration are common amongst patients with whiplash, but the literature concerned with these symptoms focuses explicitly on them, and does not provide comparative figures on their incidence relative to other symptoms. Also conspicuous in Table 3 is the number of studies that record back pain as a symptom of whiplash, and the proportion of patients reporting it.

Neck Pain

The literature is reasonably consistent with respect to descriptions of the neck pain of whiplash.[8,34,40,85,86,108,114,141,158,160,166,167,193] Typically, the pain is perceived over the back of the neck and is either dull and aching in quality, and exacerbated by movement of the neck; it may be sharp in quality when exacerbated. Frequently, there is associated neck stiffness or restricted movement. Pain may radiate to the head, shoulder, arm, or interscapular region. These patterns of somatic referred pain do not necessarily indicate what structure is the primary source of pain, but rather, suggest the segmental level mediating the nociception.[24] No studies in the literature discriminate between the features of acute and chronic neck pain.

Conspicuously absent from the literature are any studies correlating neck pain and pathology. The relationship between most of the pathological entities described above and the patients' symptoms remains circumstantial. The investigation of whiplash injuries has typically consisted of increasingly elaborate imaging techniques—plain radiographs being followed by specialized views, tomography, computerized tomography, and even MRI. However, none of these investigations has ever been calibrated against a gold standard of known painful pathology and hence their utility in determining the cause of neck pain in whiplash injury remains unknown.

The most logical approach to investigating neck pain following whiplash injury is to provoke or eliminate the pain by stimulating or anesthetizing structures suspected of being symptomatic. Through addressing the pain itself, this approach allows the source of pain to be identified, even in the absence of imaging abnormalities, and also provides the necessary gold standard against which putatively diagnostic morphological abnormalities can be correlated.

Techniques that anesthetize the cervical zygapophyseal joints have been developed,[6,28,29] refined,[11] validated,[13,129] and applied systematically to patients with chronic neck pain after whiplash injury.[6,14,129,130,131] They involve local anesthetic blocks of either the joint itself or the nerves that innervate it. Studies have confirmed that these techniques are target-specific,[11] and by using several blocks of the same joint, with either contrasting local anesthetic agents or inactive placebos, controls can be introduced that avoid the problem of false positive blocks.[13,129] When applied to a population of patients with chronic neck pain following whiplash injury, they have revealed a prevalence of cervical zygapophyseal joint pain of over 50%.[5,13,131]

The only regularly used provocation test for neck pain is provocation discography, in which a disc is punctured by a needle and distended by injecting contrast medium. A positive result occurs when the procedure reproduces the patient's usual pain, implicating that disc as the source of pain. The response can occasionally be confirmed by injecting local anesthetic in an attempt to abolish the pain.[183,200] However, no studies have demonstrated the diagnostic or therapeutic utility of discography in the context of whiplash. Moreover, the reliability of discography has been called into question by the observation that in a significant proportion of patients, pain reproduced by discography can be completely eliminated by subsequent zygapophyseal joint blocks at that level.[27] Since zygapophyseal joint blocks do not have any effect on pain perception from the disc, these observations must indicate that discograms are liable to false-positive interpretations, wrongly incriminating the disc as a cause of pain, when the true source lies in the zygapophyseal joint. It seems that in some patients, provocation discography appears positive when other structures innervated by the same segmental nerves sensitize that segment to noxious stimulation.[27] These concerns do not pertain to anesthetic block procedures because the segment is not mechanically stressed, and only those structures affected by the anesthetic are incriminated by a positive response. On the basis of current evidence, discograms should only be considered as truly positive if zygapophyseal joint blocks at that level are negative (i.e., no pain relief).

Headache

After neck pain, headache is the most frequently reported complaint following whiplash injury[8,19,72,108,141,172,193] and in some series constitutes the principal symptom.[34,85] The pain is typically reported to be occipital or suboccipital, radiating anteriorly into the temporal or orbital regions. Some authors have suggested that the headache results from concussion,[40,86] but provide no convincing evidence in support of this proposition. In some circles, the headache is assumed to be cervical in origin.

In neuroanatomical terms, afferents of the upper three cervical nerves (C1–C3) terminate in the cervical portion of the trigeminal nucleus (forming the trigemino-cervical nucleus), so that any pain arising in the distribution of these spinal nerves can be referred to the territory of the trigeminal nerve.[25] Since the ophthalmic division of the trigeminal nucleus projects most caudally, pain originating from the upper cervical structures is likely to be referred to the orbital and temporal regions. Therefore, it is possible to explain the presence of suboccipital headache through injury to one of the upper cervical structures with orbital or temporal radiation indicating referral via the trigemino-cervical nucleus.

There are no noninvasive means of accurately diagnosing the structure involved in the production of cervical headache.[25,26] At best, it has been shown that in patients whose predominant complaint after whiplash is headache, and who have tenderness over the C2–3 zygapophyseal joint, the likelihood of their pain stemming from the C2–3 zygapophyseal joint is 65%.[130] However, pain from the lateral atlantoaxial joint is also perceived in the occipital or suboccipital region,[57,58,68,146] as is pain from the atlanto-occipital joint,[57,58] and would appear to be clinically indistinguishable from C2–3 zygapophyseal joint pain. Other candidate structures that may be responsible for cervical headache following whiplash injury are the transverse and alar ligaments and the median atlantoaxial joint.[26]

The only means currently available of validly pinpointing a cervical source of headache are controlled diagnostic blocks of putatively painful joints. Techniques are available for selectively anesthetizing the lateral atlantoaxial and atlanto-occipital joints,[38,57,58,146] but these have not been systematically applied to any sample of patients with headache after whiplash. Consequently, the prevalence of headache stemming from these joints is not known. Only the C2–3 zygapophyseal joint has been systematically studied.[28,130] Among whiplash patients as a whole, the prevalence of pain stemming from the C2–3 joint is 27%. Among those patients in whom headache is the predominant complaint, the prevalence is 53%.[130]

Anesthetic blocks of the greater occipital nerve (GON) have been used in highly selected post-whiplash patients as a preoperative assessment where greater occipital decompression was being contemplated.[140] This study selected 15 patients with chronic intractable headache out of 272 whose characteristics were not described. All patients had temporary but gratifying pain relief from a mixture of lignocaine and dexamethasone injected into the region of the GON. However, these blocks were not controlled and it is not evident from the paper how many other patients had poor responses to blocks of the GON, so that any sense of the utility of this investigation is lost. Moreover, of the 13 patients who had exploration and decompression of the GON, none achieved complete pain relief. At the final follow-up (whose duration was not stated), eight of the 13 patients rated their maximum pain intensity as ≥ 50% of their preoperative pain. These data fail to substantiate any diagnostic utility for GON blocks in the management of whiplash and indicate an uncertain therapeutic utility, even for highly selected patients.

In addition to cervical causes of headache, intracranial causes such as hemorrhage or other concurrent injury should be considered, but in the chronic setting it seems likely that the majority of chronic whiplash headache will be cervical in origin.

Visual Disturbances

After whiplash, patients often complain of visual disturbances, such as blurred vision or difficulty reading. Blurred vision has been ascribed to errors of accommodation, but without objective evidence.[85,109] Pathophysiological explanations for these visual disturbances have been only tentative or speculative, and include concepts such as impaction of the ventral aspect of the midbrain against the clivus,[109] damage to the vertebral artery,[136] or damage to the cervical sympathetic trunk.[54,136]

Although injuries to the vertebral artery have been described in animal[227] and post mortem studies,[213] such damage should produce diverse neurologic signs. However, neurologic examination of patients with objective evidence of oculomotor defects and complaints of visual disturbance failed to reveal any abnormalities.[103] It is very unlikely that a single, discrete ischemic lesion could affect only those brainstem nuclei responsible for accommodation and focusing, without affecting long tracts, cerebellar connections or other cranial nerve nuclei to produce neurologic signs.

Being an anterior structure in the neck, the cervical sympathetic trunk would certainly be liable to stretch or rupture by hyperextension of the neck, and indeed such damage has been produced experimentally in monkeys.[136] Interruption of the sympathetic trunk, however, would manifest as Horner's syndrome, a condition described far less frequently than visual disturbance alone.[116,195] Blurred vision, on the other hand, without signs of sympathoplegia, cannot be explained on the basis of traumatic sympathectomy, and therefore demands another explanation.

A plausible mechanism that has been advanced to link neck pain and eye symptoms involves the ciliospinal reflex.[23] In this reflex, a noxious stimulus to the skin of the face or neck evokes dilation of the ipsilateral pupil.[222] In more general terms, a painful stimulus delivered to the cutaneous territory of the upper cervical nerves evokes an efferent sympathetic discharge to the eye. Given this background, blurred vision could be explained if two assumptions hold true. The first is that, like cutaneous afferents, deep nociceptive cervical afferents can evoke sympathetic reflexes to the eye. The second is that sympathetic stimulation can flatten the ocular lens.[154] Hypothetically, therefore, blurred vision could be construed as due to inappropriate accommodative power produced by sympathetic activity evoked by cervical pain.

There is a greater body of evidence pertaining to visual disturbances of another kind, in which visual pursuit or tracking is affected, rather than accommodation. A powerful, controlled study has demonstrated objective abnormalities of oculomotor function in patients with chronic neck pain following whiplash injury.[103] Velocity, accuracy, and pattern of eye movements were objectively measured in three groups of patients. The first group had chronic neck pain and stiffness following whiplash injury, the second group comprised individuals who were asymptomatic following whiplash and the third were healthy volunteers. The results showed no differences between the healthy and asymptomatic groups, but significant oculomotor impairment in the chronically symptomatic patients. The same group has followed up these observations with a prospective study that demonstrated persistence of pathological abnormalities of oculomotor function in patients with whiplash injury over 15 months of observation.[102] They conclude that these abnormalities are likely to relate to pathological proprioception from the neck.

Others have conducted similar studies using a variety of tasks, including driving,[88] reading, and following targets.[89,90] In all instances patients with whiplash differed significantly from control subjects matched for age, gender and occupation. Having controlled also for pain, medication, and depression, the investigators were drawn to the conclusion that a disturbed postural control system leading to the disturbance of eye movements was the most likely primary cause of disability. Reduced attention capacity was considered a secondary mediating factor.

Dizziness

Sensations of disequilibrium or dizziness, often in association with other auditory or vestibular symptoms, have been reported in many series of whiplash injuries.[34,40,65,86,158,160,166,167] Typically, these complaints have occurred in the absence of clinically apparent vestibular or neurologic dysfunction. Interest in this phenomenon has stimulated a number of reports using electronystagmography (ENG) as a means of objectively verifying patients' complaints.[43,46,165,186,215-218] These studies have all been of patients referred to specialized ENT units because of symptoms, and have all lacked clearly defined control groups. Nevertheless, they have demonstrated that between 54% and 67% of patients complaining of dizziness after whiplash injury have abnormal ENG studies, most commonly on rotatory testing. Canal paresis and other caloric test abnormalities were also noted in many of these patients.[46,165,215,216,218] Fischer et al.[73] observed increased vestibular hyper-reactivity—often combined with hyperventilation—in a group of referred patients, but provided no controls. Indeed, control observations are mentioned in only two studies. Oosterveld et al.[164] reported that ENG studies were significantly abnormal in whiplash patients when compared to a control group of normal individuals, but no details of the controls were provided. In contrast, when testing only for neck torsion nystagmus, Calseyde et al.[39] found no difference in the frequency of abnormalities between 916 consecutive medicolegal cases and 137 healthy asymptomatic controls undergoing routine clinical assessment for pilot training. The frequency of nystagmus following neck torsion was 11% in both groups. The characteristics and mode of injury of the cases were not described and it is not clear whether the cases were even symptomatic. Furthermore, the frequency of ENG abnormalities is considerably lower than that reported by any of the aforementioned studies. This may reflect a peculiarity of the test used but is more likely due to the population studied. On balance, the data indicate that symptomatic patients frequently have objective evidence of vestibular dysfunction on ENG testing, suggesting either central or peripheral injury.

One study has reassessed patients with proven ENG abnormalities after 12 months.[164] Only a subset of the original cohort was examined and the selection criteria for this group were not given. Nevertheless, less than 5% of the patients demonstrated any improvement over 12 months.

The exact mechanism by which dizziness occurs following whiplash injury remains speculative. It has been argued that vertebral artery injury or irritation may compromise vertebral artery flow, but, as discussed above, such a mechanism would be expected to produce distinctive neurologic signs and symptoms related to ischemia or infarction of the brainstem or cerebellum. More subtle disturbances of balance and equilibrium may result from interference with postural reflexes that have cervical afferents.[50] Anesthetizing the neck muscles of animals and humans results in ataxia and/or nystagmus,[16,22,51,111,112] indicating that important proprioceptive information arises from these structures. It is conceivable that disturbance of this output may result from pain or spasm following damage to these muscles or related structures. Such a proposition is further supported by experimental work on 44 patients with whiplash injury.[105] In this study, deep cervical muscle tone, as measured by EMG, was increased by the administration of isoproterenol, a β-sympathetic agonist. Vestibular function deteriorated and symptoms worsened in 8 of 13 patients. Conversely, when propranolol, a β-sympathetic blocker, was administered, cervical muscle tone decreased, vestibular function improved and symptoms of vertigo improved. Blocking or stimulating α-sympathetic receptors made no difference to either muscle tone or vestibular signs and symptoms.

These data provide a plausible mechanistic explanation for patients with unsteadiness after whiplash. Reliable empiric evidence for subtle abnormalities of postural control has emerged from a study which assessed the ability of patients with whiplash injury to reproduce their head position.[133] Eleven patients with pain or restricted neck movements more than three months after a whiplash injury, were compared with 11 age- and sex-matched controls with no history of injury or symptoms. The whiplash group were significantly less able to reproduce a particular angle of cervical rotation or correctly identify the neutral position of cervical rotation. This suggests a significant proprioceptive defect, similar to that observed in peripheral articular ligamentous injury. It is unclear exactly what symptoms would arise from such a defect, and the symptoms suffered by the whiplash group in this study were not described. However, it would seem reasonable to assume that a disturbance of proprioception could lead to a sense of unsteadiness or dizziness, without causing overt vertigo or nystagmus. An objective defect in postural control in whiplash patients has been detected in another controlled study.[185] Twenty-nine patients with a history of dizziness attributed to either a minor head injury or whiplash were studied using a force plate under different sensory configurations and compared to 51 asymptomatic controls. Increased sway was noted in the injury group, and this was exacerbated in situations where inaccurate visual cues were provided. However, the conclusions of this study are limited by the absence of any information on how many of the injured group had whiplash rather than primary head injury.

Direct damage to the vestibular apparatus has also been proposed as a cause of dizziness following whiplash injuries. Perilymph fistulas of both the round and oval windows have been found in patients with vertigo and disequilibrium.[43,96] A detailed analysis of patients with perilymph fistulae has indicated that such patients may experience a wide range of vestibular and even cognitive symptoms, including poor concentration, poor visual tracking, disorientation in visually complex situations, and clumsiness.[96] To the casual observer, such symptoms may easily be dismissed as inexplicable or may even be attributed to neuroticism or malingering. However, a high index of suspicion and careful assessment may reveal an important and potentially curable lesion.

Concentration, Cognition, and Memory Disturbances

The development of cognitive impairment following minor head injury or whiplash is not widely appreciated in the general community.[7] Patients are therefore unlikely to disclose symptoms reflecting cognitive difficulties, fearing that they may be ascribed to neurotic anxiety, exaggeration, or malingering. Nevertheless, patients with whiplash injuries often, if not commonly, report features suggestive of cognitive impairment, such as disturbed concentration and impaired memory. In different series, such features have been reported by 21%,[174] 34%,[182] 57%,[178] or 71%[131] of patients. To what these features might be ascribed has been a matter of contention.

In theory, impaired cognitive function may be caused by any of many primary factors,[175] such as those listed and grouped in Table 4. Of these, birth trauma is not of relevance to whiplash unless the patient presents a lifelong

Table 4.   The Possible Causes of Cognitive Impairment

Congenital	Acquired				Neurotic
Group A	*Group B*	*Group C*	*Group D*	*Group E*	*Group F*
Birth trauma	Depression	Organic brain damage	Neck pain	Alcohol	"Functional overlay"
	Schizophrenia		Headache	Sedatives	Malingering
			Fatigue	Analgesics	Feigned
			Lack of sleep		

Adapted from Radanov BP, Dvorak J: Impaired cognitive functioning after whiplash injury of the cervical spine. Spine 21:392–397, 1996.

past history of cognitive impairment, nor are the group B disorders unless and until overt psychiatric disease is manifest.

In the context of whiplash, the possibilities lie in groups C, D, E, and F. In the past, viewpoints have been polarized between group C and group F. Some investigators have claimed that impaired cognitive function in whiplash patients indicates that they have suffered brain damage as a result of the accident.[122,124,219,231] In support, they cite the results of experiments in which animals subjected to whiplash injury exhibit behaviors suggestive of concussion or evidence of brain damage at post mortem.[189,228] At the other extreme, assessors unable to find evidence of brain damage in patients have preferred to ascribe the features of alleged cognitive impairment to neurosis or "functional overlay," or to interpret them as factitious or the behavior of frauds or malingerers.[8,40,72,86,93,107,166]

A recent review, however, highlighted the difficulties with the previous literature.[175] Previous studies have been conducted retrospectively and on highly selected patients, sometimes involving only small numbers of patients, and often without corroboration of impaired cognitive function by formal testing. Furthermore, this review urged that whiplash be defined as only a neck injury and that patients who reported loss of consciousness should be excluded. The authors argued that loss of consciousness is indicative of head injury and that, therefore, patients who suffer whiplash but also lose consciousness should not be regarded as simply suffering from whiplash injury. This distinction governs the conclusions that can be drawn from the available literature.

Pure Whiplash

The most extensive and rigorous data on cognitive function after whiplash comes from a series of studies in which patients who suffered loss of consciousness or amnesia were specifically excluded. This action permits an evaluation of the extent to which cognitive impairment is found among patients who suffer a pure whiplash injury.

Early after injury, such patients do not, on the average, subjectively feel cognitively impaired,[174] yet paradoxically on objective testing they score somewhat below normal limits on a variety of tests. Later, patients who become asymptomatic are not impaired on formal testing, nor do they feel impaired upon self-evaluation. However, patients who remain symptomatic at 6 months subjectively feel impaired but objective testing does not corroborate this. On formal testing they perform, on the average, no differently from asymptomatic patients.[174] After one year, symptomatic patients show a tendency towards worsening performance on objective testing, with some 50% scoring in the abnormal range, but this difference is not statistically significant if corrected for age and use of medication.[178]

These data demonstrate that, on the average, whiplash patients do not develop cognitive impairment. Observations of apparent cognitive impairment must be corrected for the side effects of medication.[153]

Another study compared the cognitive function of a group of whiplash patients (again with no history of loss of consciousness), a group of patients with mild head injury, and a group of patients with chronic pain but no head injury or whiplash injury.[211] That study found that all three groups performed slightly below normal standards, but enigmatically the patients with mild head injury did not differ in performance from those with whiplash, but neither did those with chronic pain. The enigma is that if mild head injury, rather than whiplash, caused cognitive impairments, the patients with head injury should have performed worse, but they did not. One resolution of this enigma is that the psychometric tests used were insufficiently sensitive to detect significant difference in performance. An alternative resolution is that patients with mild head injury are only minimally affected, but so too are whiplash patients.

More captivating is the similarity between patients with whiplash and those with chronic pain. This suggests that the slight cognitive impairment exhibited by both groups is not due to brain injury but is secondary to their suffering from persistent pain. Indeed, the authors were drawn to that conclusion,[211] as have others,[153] but they also raised concern about malingering. They drew attention to the availability of psychometric tests in this regard which have been used in the assessment of compensable head injury, although not in whiplash.[18]

One component of cognitive function is attentional processing. Patients will feel cognitive impairment if they cannot maintain attention to a task. Upon formal testing, the singular correlate that has emerged for impaired attentional processing is headache.[56,176,177] Those patients who suffer headache have greater difficulties maintaining attention. Impairment of attentional processing, therefore, is not a sign of brain injury, but a feature secondary to head pain.

Head Injury

Although purists would prefer people who lose consciousness *not* to be classified as having a whiplash injury,[175] few others have bothered to be so discriminating. Instead, patients who develop neck pain after whiplash but also suffer loss of consciousness have been indiscriminately grouped among patients with whiplash injury. As result it is possible that some patients, loosely defined as having suffered whiplash, may indeed also have suffered head injury, and it may be that such a subgroup of patients accounts for the reputation of whiplash being a possible cause of cognitive impairment. If selected and tested, such patients might exhibit abnormalities of a nature or of a magnitude different from those exhibited by patients with whiplash injury only.

In that regard, a small sample of selected patients in one study exhibited deficits in attention, concentration, and memory when compared to a carefully matched control group of healthy volunteers.[122] On the other hand, a similar study found no difference between whiplash patients and those with similar somatic symptoms but no history of whiplash injury.[159] These differences are not irreconcilable, for although they refute a relationship between cognitive deficit and brain injury, they are concordant with cognitive deficits being secondary to chronic pain.[11]

Brain Damage

Several investigators have sought to detect evidence of organic brain damage using medical investigations. Several studies have failed to detect evidence of brain damage on MRI of patients with whiplash.[70,182,231] It remains possible, however, that subtle, but clinically important injuries may be beyond the resolution of MRI. EEG studies have yielded conflicting and confounded results. One study found EEG abnormalities in 50% of patients with whiplash, compared to 1% of controls.[219] Another study, however, failed to corroborate this result.[113] A Japanese study found that whiplash patients and head injury patients had similar sensitivity to activation of EEG by megimide.[124] A review of this material, however, points out that the studies were inadequately controlled for intensity of pain, depression, anxiety, and the effects of medication.[197]

Intriguingly, however, a recent study reported differences detectable by single photon emission computed tomography (SPECT).[164] Ten patients with persistent concentration and memory disturbances, 1–4 years after whiplash injury, exhibited significantly decreased cerebral perfusion over the parieto-occipital lobes, when compared with 11 healthy, normal volunteers. However, while suggesting a possible tool for future investigations, this study was incomplete in that it did not provide any psychometric data, and it did not provide comparisons with patients with identical symptoms other that putative cognitive impairment.

Weakness

Where weakness occurs in recognized myotomal distributions, and is accompanied by consistent reflex and sensory signs, a diagnosis of nerve root involvement can be made and the patient investigated and treated accordingly. Far more puzzling, and more common, are complaints of subjective weakness, heaviness, or fatigue in the upper limbs that are unaccompanied by clear-cut abnormalities on clinical examination. The inconsistency between symptoms and signs has been attributed to malingering or hysteria,[15] but there is evidence that sensations of heaviness in the limbs have an organic, neurophysiological basis and can be caused by pain.

The sensation of heaviness has been assessed in patients with both pathological and experimentally induced muscle weakness.[82] The pathologically weak group contained stroke patients with pure unilateral motor defects. The experimentally weakened group had one arm partially curarized. Both of these groups perceived a given weight as heavier with the weak arm compared to the normal, contralateral arm. Sensation was normal in the arm so that the impression of heaviness arose through an appreciation of the amount of effort required to lift the weight.[82] Further, elegant experiments have shown that painful cutaneous stimulation can reduce the maximum effort that can be applied by a muscle group through reflex inhibition of muscle contraction, a phenomenon that is independent of voluntary control.[5] Together, these studies show that noxious stimulation can inhibit motor power, and the resultant need for increased "central effort" for a given task is perceived as heaviness or weakness.

In clinical settings, reflex inhibition of the quadriceps muscle has been noted in patients with joint or muscle pain, and also in patients with no pain but with previous joint injury.[187] Furthermore, treatment of chronic knee pain in patients with objectively verified quadriceps inhibition has been shown to reduce inhibition.[206]

In the context of whiplash injury, those patients with chronic neck pain may well develop reflex inhibition of those muscle systems that act on, or in conjunction with, the neck. This would include those muscles of the upper limb which are contracted during lifting. To overcome this inhibition, more central effort is required, resulting in a sensation of increased heaviness or weakness. In addition, where arm pain is present, either through nerve root involvement or as somatic referred pain from the neck, the arm muscles may be inhibited directly, again producing a sensation of heaviness.

Paresthesiae

Sensations of tingling and numbness in the hands, particularly of the ulnar two fingers, have been reported in both prospective and retrospective series.[34,86,108,158,167,193] In the presence of muscle weakness, reflex changes, and objective abnormalities on sensory testing, these symptoms can be attributed to nerve root compression and may be appropriately investigated using well established algorithms.[47] More commonly, however, symptoms are intermittent and are not associated with overt neurologic signs.[158,167] It is this latter group that constitutes a diagnostic problem and whose symptoms demand an adequate explanation.

One of the most plausible theories is that the paresthesiae may be due to thoracic outlet syndrome arising from compression of the lower cords of the brachial plexus as they pass between the scalenus anterior muscle and the scalenus medius muscle, and under the clavicle. In a referral-based series of 35 patients with posttraumatic neck pain and arm symptoms, 30 had objective evidence of slowed nerve conduction across the thoracic outlet on nerve conduction studies.[41] The mean conduction velocity in this group was 55 meters per second compared with 72 meters per second in an asymptomatic control group. Where the symptoms were unilateral, conduction velocities were slower in the symptomatic arm. No formal statistical analysis of these data was performed. In a later study by the same author, clinical tests in conjunction with electrodiagnostic studies suggested a diagnosis of thoracic outlet syndrome in 31% of patients referred to a private neurology practice for evaluation of symptoms following whiplash injury.[42] Notwithstanding any reservations about the electrodiagnostic technique, the former study, by virtue of providing control observations, provides evidence in support of a real abnormality of ulnar nerve conduction in patients with arm symptoms following whiplash injury. The latter study is limited in that it is a retrospective review of referred patients, but the mere fact that a substantial proportion of patients had features suggestive of thoracic outlet syndrome would indicate that this is not a rare phenomenon and is worthy of further, more formal study. Exactly how this syndrome develops remains speculative, but reflex spasm of the scalene muscles, due to pain from other structures in the neck, might compress the lower cords of the brachial plexus and account for an intermittent and at times subclinical impairment of ulnar nerve function.

There is evidence that other pathological processes may affect the brachial plexus after whiplash injury. Recent anecdotal reports of two patients with persistent arm and hand symptoms describe the operative finding of "massive fibrosis" in and around the brachial plexus.[34] These observations invite further research and provide hypotheses for consideration in individual patients.

Back Pain

Although back pain has been reported in several studies as a common feature of whiplash (see Table 3), there are no robust data on the cause or mechanism of this symptom. Given its prevalence amongst whiplash patients, but also its prevalence in the community at large, this symptom is in urgent need of concerted study. Without data, it cannot be ascertained whether back pain is a legitimate symptom of whiplash or a specious, opportunistic complaint.

NATURAL HISTORY AND PROGNOSIS

The most important requirement of any study of prognosis is that an inception cohort is assembled at the outset.[55] It is unacceptable to start with a group of patients who enter the study simply because they are accessible to followup. Furthermore, the sample should be representative of those patients with the condition of interest. Among published studies of whiplash injuries, the most representative samples available (i.e., least affected by possible sampling bias) are derived from hospital-based studies. Applying these simple but vital criteria requires that, in determining the prognosis or natural history of whiplash injury, most series should be discarded from further consideration,* including some purporting to address the very question of prognosis.[95,108]

The longest follow-up has been that of a cohort of 61 patients first seen between 1977 and 1980 at the Bristol Royal Infirmary. These patients have been the subjects of reports of their status at 2, 10.8, and 15 years after initial injury.[83,158,204] The reports have described the proportion of patients fully recovered at each time interval and the proportion continuing to suffer different grades of continuing symptoms. However, these reports are confounded by the small size of the original sample, a substantial loss to follow-up, and the proclivity of the authors to report proportions based on surviving patients, as opposed to proportions of the inception cohort. Nevertheless, they are perhaps the most often quoted studies on this issue. Accordingly, it is appropriate to review the data but with statistical adjustments using a sensitivity analysis and

---

* refs. 8–10,19,54,64,65,72,85,93,98,114,135–139,157,166,172,193,205.

Table 5. Long-term Outcome of Whiplash Patients

| | Best-case Analysis as Proportions of Surviving Patients | | | | | | | | |
| | 2 Years | | | 10.8 Years | | | 15 Years | | |
Symptoms	N	%	95% CI	N	%	95% CI	N	%	95% CI
None	20	34	24–46	5	12	2–22	12	30	16–44
Mild				21	39	24–54	11	28	14–42
	27	47	34–60						
Intrusive				12	28	15–41	13	33	18–48
Severe	11	19	9–29	5	12	2–22	4	10	1–19
Lost to follow-up	3			18			40		
Surviving sample	58	43	40						

| | Worst-case Analysis as Proportions of Original Patients | | | | | | | | |
| | 2 Years | | | 10.8 Years | | | 15 Years | | |
Symptoms	N	%	95% CI	N	%	95% CI	N	%	95% CI
None	20	33	21–35	5	8	1–15	12	20	10–30
Mild				21	34	23–45	11	18	8–28
	27	44	32–56						
Intrusive				12	20	7–33	13	21	11–32
Severe	11	18	8–28	5	8	0–18	4	7	1–13
Unallocated	3	5	0–10	18	30	23–37	21	34	23–45

An original cohort of 61 patients with neck pain after whiplash was analyzed using a best-case analysis based on the authors' reported proportions of a diminishing sample size, and a worst-case analysis in which the proportions have been based on the original sample. Although the patients with symptoms that were not severe were classified as having mild or intrusive symptoms at 10.8 and 15 years, such a distinction was not made at 2 years. Mild symptoms were defined as tolerable, occasional symptoms that did not interfere with activities of daily living. Intrusive symptoms were ones that did interfere with daily activities. Severe symptoms were ones that were not tolerable and which disrupted work and other activities. Based on the data by Norris and Watt,[165] Gargan and Bannister,[83] and Squires et al.[204]

employing confidence intervals to take account of the sample size (Table 5). This indicates that some 19% of patients remain with severe symptoms at two years, diminishing to 12% and 10% by 10.8 years and 15 years, respectively. The confidence limits, however, indicate that, in other samples, these figures could be as low as 9%, 2%, and 1%, respectively, or as high as 29%, 22%, and 19%. The "worst-case" figures indicate a similar diminishing proportion of patients with severe symptoms, although the proportions themselves are somewhat smaller.

With respect to the proportion of patients fully recovered, an irregularity occurs. At 10.8 years, only 12% of patients were without symptoms, as opposed to 34% at 2 years and 30% at 15 years. The confidence intervals of these proportions, however, overlap; so, the apparent difference may be an aberration of small sample size. Nonetheless, the published reports do state that of the patients described in Table 4, seven improved their status between 10.8 years and 15 years, but 11 explicitly deteriorated. Therefore, the natural history of whiplash is not stable.

A larger series, with no losses to follow-up, but followed only for 2 years to date, paints a somewhat more optimistic picture (Fig. 3).[178] Over a 2-year period, the proportion of patients fully recovered steadily increases to 82%. The

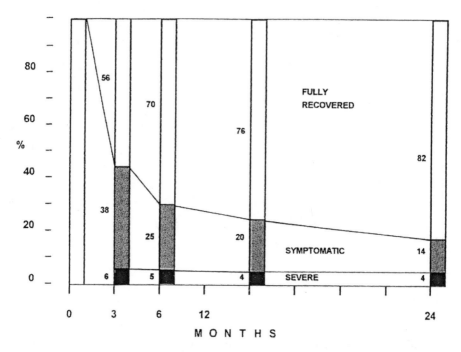

Figure 3. The evolution of symptoms of patients with neck pain after whiplash. (Based on Radanov BP, Sturzenegger M, Di Stefano G: Long-term outcome after whiplash injury: A 2-year follow-up considering features of injury mechanism and somatic, radiologic, and psychosocial findings. Medicine 74:281–297, 1995.)

proportion of patients with severe symptoms at onset is relatively small, but fewer of these patients recover. As a result, the proportion of patients with severe symptoms remains relatively consent, dropping from 6% to 4%. The proportion of patients otherwise symptomatic declines steadily as more patients recover.

The rate of recovery after whiplash injury has been explored in four studies.[84,141,160,178] All indicate that the majority of patients destined to recover will do so in the first two to three months after injury. The rate of recovery then slows dramatically to become asymptotic, with no further changes in symptoms after 2 years.

Prevalence

In light of this natural history and given the frequency of motor vehicle accidents, it follows that at any one time, there must be a measurable number, or prevalence, of patients with chronic symptoms attributable to motor vehicle accidents and whiplash injury. A coarse estimate can be calculated from incidence rates, the natural history of the condition, and the age of the affected population. Such a calculation determined that one could expect in a population a prevalence of about 1% with chronic pain and 0.4% with severe pain as a result of whiplash injury.[12] These figures may seem paltry, but they are well in excess of the estimated prevalence in the community of disorders such as epilepsy. On the other hand, their minitude renders them hard to detect in population surveys. For a study to detect a proportion as small as 1% with 95% confidence intervals of less than 1% would need to sample over 381 people. To detect a proportion of 0.4% with similar precision would require in excess of 956 subjects.

Such considerations pertain to a recent study, in Lithuania, that has been used uncritically and mistakenly to argue that chronic neck pain after whiplash does not occur in communities without a compensation system. That study[192] surveyed 202 accident victims and 202 matched controls, and reported that the prevalence of neck pain and headache was similar in both samples. Of the 202 accident victims, only 31 reported developing acute symptoms of neck pain as a result of the accident, but none of these individuals developed chronic, disabling symptoms. Notwithstanding that the questionnaire instrument itself had not been validated, one could accept these results. However, any deeper inferences or conclusions are limited by the precision of the point estimates derived from the study. The data show that 0 out of 31 subjects developed chronic disabling symptoms. The 95% confidence limits of this proportion are 0–10%. Therefore, finding no patients with chronic symptoms in this sample is nonetheless consistent with a rate of chronicity of up to 10%,[132] which embraces the range of values determined in other studies (see above). In other words, the Lithuanian study suggests that the risk of neck pain after a motor vehicle accident (of any description) is low, about 10–20%, but it cannot be construed to show that chronic neck does not ensue in patients who sustain a neck injury in that accident.

A Model Based on the Natural History

Viewed simplistically, the outcome for an individual patient is dichotomous; either the neck pain will resolve in the first few months or it will persist indefinitely. The pathology affecting those with chronic pain is currently unknown, but in considering the known responses of various tissues to injury it is possible to formulate a model to help explain these observations.

Tears of muscles and ligaments, as described above, would cause pain. Analogous with injuries to these tissues elsewhere in the body, and being vascular structures, they would be expected to heal over several weeks with scar formation and loss of pain. Such a pattern would be consistent with those patients who quickly recover after whiplash injury. Minor, occult fractures would also follow this pattern with painless function following healing after six to eight weeks. On the other hand, injuries to the zygapophyseal joints or intervertebral discs would be expected to have a different prognosis. Discs are avascular, and tears to the anulus fibrosus or separation of the disc from the adjacent vertebral body are unlikely to heal, and therefore constitute an anatomical substrate for pain.[31] Injuries to the zygapophyseal joint or the underlying bone may disrupt the congruity of the joint surfaces, producing a painful, posttraumatic osteoarthritis. Alternatively, hemarthrosis or injury to the intra-articular structures may lead to a chronic, posttraumatic synovitis with ongoing pain and joint damage. Therefore, patients with injuries to the discs or joints may be expected to have prolonged pain with little chance of healing or spontaneous recovery. This model would be consistent with surveys that have shown that most patients with chronic posttraumatic neck pain had symptoms arising from the zygapophyseal joint[131] or disc.[5]

FACTORS INFLUENCING PROGNOSIS

Any study aiming to determine those factors which predict the outlook for an individual patient should be prospective and include sufficient numbers of patients to allow powerful statistical techniques, such as regression analysis, to be applied and therefore enable the "risk of chronicity" to be calculated. The only study meeting these requirements has shown that increasing age, injury-related cognitive impairment, and the severity of the initial neck pain were predictive of persistent symptoms at 6 months.[173] A subsequent report[179] identified the following, in rank order, as the leading predictors of poor outcome: impaired neck movement, previous history of headache, history of head trauma, age, initial pain intensity, initial headache intensity, and abnormal scores on tests that measured nervousness, neuroticism, and focused attention.

In other studies, objective neurologic signs, degenerative changes on x-ray, and thoracolumbar pain have been found to be associated with, but not necessarily predictive of, a poor prognosis.[141,155,158,223] Since degenerative changes occur more frequently with increasing age,[81] it is possible that age is a confounding variable in the relationship between degenerative changes and a poor prognosis following whiplash. In other words, older people do worse after whiplash injury and coincidentally have degenerative changes. Multivariate analyses show this to be the case.[104,179] When corrected for age, degenerative changes disappear as a risk factor.

LITIGATION NEUROSIS

In vivid contrast to the abundant evidence in support of painful, organic lesions in whiplash patients there is little more than speculation and anecdote to suggest that the symptoms are due to "litigation neurosis." Nonetheless, some authors maintain that exaggerated complaints of pain and injury are made in order to secure financial gain.[9,14,91,107,157] However, competent follow-up studies of whiplash patients report that the likelihood of chronicity of symptoms following whiplash injury is independent of litigation.[141,158,167] Formal study of litigation or compensation neurosis unearths little evidence in support of the concept, but reveals a plethora of reports demonstrating that compensation patients are no different to noncompensation patients.[150–153]

An important and unique study comparing the symptoms of patients who had settled compensation claims with those who had yet to do so revealed that current litigants had more complaints of pain than nonlitigants, but had similar functional impairment.[210] Important confounders such as the duration of symptoms were controlled for. The authors concluded that patients pursuing litigation were more likely to be under stress, aggravating their pain, and would also be keen on convincing a skeptical medical and legal profession of the veracity of their symptoms.

Close scrutiny of the early reports proffered in support of the concept of malingering reveals disturbing methodological flaws, unacceptable by contemporary standards. Miller's original report of patients with "accident neurosis" comprised descriptive data on 50 patients assessed for head injury at a major referral center.[156] After settlement, 41 of 45 employed patients returned to work. However, these patients were a small subset who displayed "gross neurotic symptoms" and who had been selected from more than 4000 patients, constituting a prevalence of only 1%. It is impossible to draw any generally applicable, externally valid conclusions from such biased sampling. Gotten's study of whiplash patients after settlement of compensation reports that 88% of patients showed recovery after settlement and over half had no residual symptoms.[93] The study concluded that there was great difficulty in evaluating whiplash patients due to the complicating factor of monetary compensation, and that the injury was being used as a "lever for personal gain." However, this study was conducted with an invalidated questionnaire administered by a single individual. Only 100 of 219 potential subjects were able to be contacted, a response rate of only 45%. No control group was included so that the effect of the natural tendency of many patients to improve spontaneously in the first few months after injury was not considered. Finally, many of the conclusions are based on the anecdotes and opinions of the "interrogator" administering the questionnaire. In the light of these methodological defects, the conclusions drawn from the study cannot be sustained.

Some authors have maintained that preexisting personality traits or psychiatric problems create or contribute to somatic symptoms after whiplash injury.[21,91,92,107] It has even been advanced that "traumatic neurosis" occurs in neurotics who have "been looking for a trauma and have now found one".[92] However, these hypotheses have been refuted by a Swiss study.[67,173] This prospective, observational study involved 78 consecutive whiplash patients. All were assessed, using standard tests, for psychosocial stress, negative affectivity, and personality traits soon after suffering a whiplash injury. None of these factors were found to be predictive of the persistence of symptoms at 6 months. A more recent study has consolidated these findings, finding that personality traits and psychiatric symptoms measured a mean of 1.7 days after a whiplash injury did not predict the presence of symptoms at 6 months.[32] The only study detracting from this view considered whether initial emotional responses to the injury predicted pain at 4 weeks.[59] This is far too premature in the normal course of whiplash injuries to determine whether the patients will develop chronic symptoms.[84]

Therefore, there is no real evidence that either malingering for financial gain or preexisting psychosocial factors contribute in any significant way to the natural history of whiplash injury. The unavoidable conclusion is that the majority of whiplash injuries result in real organic lesions in genuine patients.

CONCLUSION

Much of the skepticism and cynicism that has been applied to patients suffering from whiplash can be traced or ascribed to lack of knowledge about the mechanisms of injury, the possible lesions, and the mechanisms of symptoms. There is now an abundant body of information that dispels many past concerns. The mechanisms of injury has now been demonstrated in normal volunteers. Those mechanisms are consistent with the now extensive literature on lesions found at post mortem, at surgery, and by specialized medical imaging.

The natural history of whiplash is benign, with more than 80% of patients recovering, but some 10% of patients continue to suffer severe symptoms. However, the symptoms of whiplash defy conventional clinical examination and conventional investigations. To a physician using conventional techniques, the patient will appear to have nothing wrong, other than a complaint of pain, and perhaps other symptoms. But that reflects more the lack of validity of clinical examination and conventional imaging than the absence of a cause for symptoms. Studies using invasive techniques have been able to pinpoint the source of pain in the majority of patients with chronic neck pain or headache. Other techniques have been developed but have not yet been systematically applied in the investigation of the remainder of patients. Vague symptoms, such as visual disturbance and dizziness, that are difficult to corroborate by conventional examination have proven to have objective correlates when assessed in specialized laboratories. Formal, prospective studies have dispelled the myth that these patients suffer from premorbid personality problems or suffer a compensation neurosis.

References

1. Abel MS: Moderately severe whiplash injuries of the cervical spine and their roentgenologic diagnosis. Clin Orthop 12:189–208, 1958.
2. Abel MS: Occult traumatic lesions of the cervical vertebrae. Crit Rev Clin Radiol Nucl Med 6:469–553, 1975.
3. Abel MS: The radiology of chronic neck pain: Sequelae of occult traumatic lesions. Crit Rev Diagn Imag 20:27–78, 1982.
4. Amevo B, Worth D, Bogduk N: Instantaneous axes of rotation of the typical cervical motion segments: A study in normal volunteers. Clin Biomech 6:111–117, 1991.
5. Aniss AM, Gandevia SC, Milne RJ: Changes in perceived heaviness and motor commands produced by cutaneous reflexes in man. J Physiol 397:113–126, 1988.
6. Aprill C, Bogduk N: The prevalence of cervical zygapophyseal joint pain: A first approximation. Spine 17:744–747, 1992.
7. Aubrey JB, Dobbs AR, Rule BG: Laypersons' knowledge about the sequelae of minor head injury and whiplash. J Neurol Neurosurg Psychiatry 52:842–846, 1989.
8. Balla JI: The late whiplash syndrome. Aust N Z J Surg 50:610–614, 1980.
9. Balla JI: The late whiplash syndrome: A study of an illness in Australia and Singapore. Cult Med Psychiatry 6:191–210, 1982.
10. Balla JI, Karnaghan J: Whiplash headache. Clin Exp Neurol 23:179–182, 1987.
11. Barnsley L, Bogduk N: Medial branch blocks are specific for the diagnosis of cervical zygapophysial joint pain. Regional Anesth 18:343–350, 1993.
12. Barnsley L, Lord S, Bogduk N: Whiplash injuries. Pain 58:283–307, 1994.
13. Barnsley L, Lord SM, Bogduk N: Comparative local anaesthetic blocks in the diagnosis of cervical zygapophysial joint pain. Pain 55:99–106, 1993.
14. Barnsley L, Lord SM, Wallis BJ, Bogduk N: The prevalence of chronic cervical zygapophysial joint pain after whiplash. Spine 20:20–26, 1995.
15. Berry H: Psychological aspects of chronic neck pain following hyperextension-flexion strains of the neck. In Morley TP (ed): Current Controversies in Neurosurgery. Philadelphia, WB Saunders, 1976, pp 51–60.
16. Biemond A, de Jong JMBV: On cervical nystagmus and related disorders. Brain 92:437–458, 1969.
17. Billig HE Jr: The mechanism of whiplash injuries. Int Rec Med 169:3–7, 1956.
18. Binder LM: Assessment of malingering after mild head trauma with the Portland Digit Recognition Test. J Clin Exp Neuropsychol 15:170–182, 1993.
19. Binet EF, Moro JJ, Marangola JP, et al: Cervical spine tomography in trauma. Spine 2:163–172, 1977.
20. Bingham R: Whiplash injuries. Med Trial Tech Q 14:69–80, 1968.
21. Blinder M: The abuse of psychiatric disability determinations. Med Trial Tech Q 25:84–91, 1978.

22. Bogduk N: Local anaesthetic blocks of the second cervical ganglion: A technique with application in occipital headache. Cephalalgia 1:41–50, 1981.
23. Bogduk N: The anatomy and pathophysiology of whiplash. Clin Biomech 1:92–101, 1986.
24. Bogduk N: Innervation and pain patterns in the cervical spine. Clin Phys Ther 17:1–13, 1988.
25. Bogduk N: Anatomy and physiology of headache. Biomed Pharmacother 49:435–445, 1995.
26. Bogduk N: Headache and the neck. In Goadsby PJ, Silberstein SD (eds): Headache. Boston, Butterworth-Heinemann, 1997, pp 369–381.
27. Bogduk N, Aprill C: On the nature of neck pain, discography and cervical zygapophysial joint pain. Pain 54:213–217, 1993.
28. Bogduk N, Marsland A: On the concept of third occipital headache. J Neurol Neurosurg Psychiatry 49:775–780, 1986.
29. Bogduk N, Marsland A: The cervical zygapophysial joints as a source of neck pain. Spine 13:610–617, 1988.
30. Bogduk N, Simons DG: Trigger points and cervical zygapophysial joint pain. In Merskey H (ed): Progress in Fibromyalgia and Myofascial Pain. Amsterdam, Elsevier, 1993, pp 267–273.
31. Bogduk N, Windsor M, Inglis A: The innervation of the cervical intervertebral discs. Spine 13:2–8, 1988.
32. Borchgrevink GE, Stiles TC, Borchgrevink PC, et al: Personality profile among symptomatic and recovered patients with neck sprain injury, measured by MCMI-I acutely and 6 months after car accidents. J Psychosom Res 42:357–367, 1997.
33. Biby L, Santora AH: Prevertebral hematoma secondary to whiplash injury necessitating emergency intubation. Anesth Analg 70:112–114, 1990.
34. Bring G, Westman G: Chronic posttraumatic syndrome after whiplash injury: A pilot study of 22 patients. Scand J Prim Health Care 9:135–141, 1991.
35. Brooke RI, Lapointe HJ: Temporomandibular joint disorders following whiplash. Spine State Art Rev 7:443–454, 1993.
36. Bucholz RW, Burkhead WZ, Graham W, et al: Occult cervical spine injuries in fatal traffic accidents. J Trauma 119:768–771, 1979.
37. Buonocore E, Hartman JT, Nelson CL: Cineradiograms of cervical spine in diagnosis of soft tissue injuries. JAMA 198:143–147, 1966.
38. Busch E, Wilson PR: Atlanto-occipital and atlanto-axial injections in the treatment of headache and neck pain. Reg Anesth 14(Suppl 2):45, 1989.
39. Calseyde P, Ampe W, Depondt M: ENG and the cervical syndrome neck torsion nystagmus. Adv Otorhinolaryngol 22:119–124, 1977.
40. Cammack KV: Whiplash injuries to the neck. Am J Surg 93:663–666, 1957.
41. Capistrant TD: Thoracic outlet syndrome in whiplash injury. Ann Surg 185:175–178, 1977.
42. Capistrant TD: Thoracic outlet syndrome in cervical strain injury. Minn Med 69:13–17, 1986.
43. Chester JB Jr: Whiplash, postural control, and the inner ear. Spine 16:716–720, 1991.
44. Clark CR, Igram CM, el Khoury GY, et al: Radiographic evaluation of cervical spine injuries. Spine 13:742–747, 1988.
45. Clemens HJ, Burow K: Experimental investigation on injury mechanisms of cervical spine at frontal and rear-frontal vehicle impacts. Proceedings of the 16th STAPP Car Crash Conference. Warrendale, PA, Society of Automotive Engineers, 1972, pp 76–104.
46. Compere WEJ: Electronystagmographic findings in patients with "whiplash" injuries. Laryngoscope 78:1226–1233, 1968.
47. Cooper C: Cervical root irritation. In Klippel J, Dieppe P (eds): Rheumatology, 2nd ed. London, Mosby, 1997.
48. Craig JB, Hodgson BF: Superior facet fractures of the axis vertebra. Spine 16:875–877, 1991.
49. Davis SJ, Teresi LM, Bradley WGJ, et al: Cervical spine hyperextension injuries: MR findings. Radiology 180:245–251, 1991.
50. de Jong JMBV, Bles W: Cervical dizziness and ataxia. In Bies W, Brandt T (eds): Disorders of posture and gait. Amsterdam, Elsevier, 1986, pp 185–205.
51. de Jong PTVM, de Jong JMBV, Cohen B, et al: Ataxia and nystagmus caused by injection of local anaesthetic in the neck. Ann Neurol 1:240–246, 1977.
52. Deans GT, Magalliard JN, Kerr M, et al: Neck pain: A major cause of disability following car accidents. Injury 18:10–12, 1987.
53. Deng YC: Anthropomorphic dummy neck modeling and injury considerations. Accid Anal Prev 21:85–100, 1989.
54. DePalma AF, Subin DK: Study of the cervical syndrome. Clin Orthop 38:135–142, 1965.
55. Department of clinical epidemiology and biostatistics: How to read clinical journals: III. How to learn the clinical course and prognosis of disease. Can Med Assoc J 124:869–872, 1981.

56. Di Stefano G, Radanov BP: Course of attention and memory after common whiplash: A two-year prospective study with age, education and gender pair-matched patients. Acta Neurol Scand 91:346–352, 1995.
57. Dreyfuss P: Atlanto-occipital and lateral atlantoaxial joint injections. In Lennard TA (ed): Physiatric Procedures in Clinical Practice. Philadelphia, Hanley & Belfus, 1995, pp 227–237.
58. Dreyfuss P, Michaelsen M, Fletcher D: Atlanto-occipital and lateral atlanto-axial joint pain patterns. Spine 19:1125–1131, 1994.
59. Drottning M, Staff PH, Levin L, et al: Acute emotional response to common whiplash predicts subsequent pain complaints. Nord J Psychiatry 49:293–299, 1995.
60. Dvorak J, Hayek J, Zehnder R: CT-functional diagnostics of the rotatory instability of the upper cervical spine. Part 2: An evaluation on healthy adults and patients with suspected instability. Spine 12:726–731, 1987.
61. Dvorak J, Panjabi MM: Functional anatomy of the alar ligaments. Spine 12:183–189, 1987.
62. Dvorak J, Panjabi MM, Gerber M, et al: CT-functional diagnostics of the rotatory instability of upper cervical spine. 1: An experimental study on cadavers. Spine 12:197–205, 1987.
63. Dvorak J, Schneider E, Saldinger P, et al: Biomechanics of the craniocervical region: The alar and transverse ligaments. J Orthop Res 6:452–461, 1988.
64. Dvorak J, Valach L, Schmid S: Injuries of the cervical spine in Switzerland. Orthopade 16:2–12, 1987.
65. Dvorak J, Valach L, Schmid ST: Cervical spine injuries in Switzerland. J Manual Med 4:7–16, 1989.
66. Dworkin SF, Truelove EL, Bonica JJ, Sola A: Facial and head pain caused by myofascial and temporomandibular disorders. In JJ Bonica (ed): The Management of Pain, 2nd ed. Philadelphia, Lea & Febiger, 1990, pp 727–745.
67. Editorial: Neck injury and the mind. Lancet 338:728–729, 1991.
68. Ehni GE, Benner B: Occipital neuralgia and the C1–2 arthrosis syndrome. J Neurosurg 61:961–965, 1984.
69. Epstein JB: Temporomandibular disorders, facial pain and headache following motor vehicle accidents. J Can Dent Assoc 58:488–495, 1992.
70. Ettlin TM, Kischka U, Reichmann S, et al: Cerebral symptoms after whiplash injury of the neck: A prospective clinical and neuropsychological study of whiplash injury. J Neurol Neurosurg Psychiatry 55:943–948, 1992.
71. Evans RW: Some observations on whiplash injuries. Neurol Clin 10:975–997, 1992.
72. Farbman AA: Neck sprain: Associated factors. JAMA 223:1010–1015, 1973.
73. Fischer AJ, Huygen PL, Folgering HT, et al: Vestibular hyperreactivity and hyperventilation after whiplash injury. Neurol Sci 132:35–43, 1995.
74. Fletcher G, Haughton VM, Khang-Cheng Ho, et al: Age-related changes in the cervical facet joints: Studies with cryomicrotomy, MR, and CT. Am J Neuroradiol 11:27–30, 1990.
75. Foo D, Rossier AB, Cochran TP: Complete sensory and motor recovery from anterior spinal artery syndrome after sprain of the cervical spine: A case report. Eur Neurol 23:119–123, 1984.
76. Forret-Bruno JY, Tarrière C, Le Coz JY, et al: Risk of cervical lesions in real-world and simulated collisions. Proceedings of the 34th STAPP Car Crash Conference. Warrendale, PA, Society of Automotive Engineers, 1990, pp 373–390.
77. Foust DR, Chaffin DB, Snyder RG, et al: Cervical range of motion and dynamic response and strength of cervical muscles. Proceedings of the 17th STAPP Car Crash Conference. Warrendale, PA, Society of Automotive Engineers, 1973, pp 285–308.
78. Frankel VH: Temporomandibular joint pain syndrome following deceleration injury to the cervical spine. Bull Hosp Jt Dis 26:47–51, 1965.
79. Frankel VH: Pathomechanics of whiplash injuries to the neck. In Morley TP (ed): Current Controversies in Neurosurgery. Philadelphia, WB Saunders, 1976, pp 39–50.
80. Fricton JR: Myofascial pain and whiplash. Spine State Art Rev 7:403–422, 1993.
81. Friedenberg ZB, Miller WT: Degenerative disc disease of the cervical spine: A comparative study of symptomatic and asymptomatic patients. J Bone Joint Surg 45A:1171–1178, 1963.
82. Gandevia SC, McCloskey DI: Sensations of heaviness. Brain 100:345–354, 1977.
83. Gargan MF, Bannister GC: Long-term prognosis of soft-tissue injuries of the neck. J Bone Joint Surg 72B:901–903, 1990.
84. Gargan MF, Bannister GC: The rate of recovery following whiplash injury. Eur Spine J 3:162–164, 1994.
85. Gates EM, Benjamin DJ: Studies in cervical trauma. 2: Cervical fractures. Int Surg 48:368–375, 1967.

86. Gay JR, Abbott KH: Common whiplash injuries of the neck. JAMA 152:1698–1704, 1953.
87. Gershon-Cohen J, Budin E, Glauser F: Whiplash fractures of cervicodorsal spinous processes: Resemblance to shoveller's fracture. JAMA 155:560–561, 1954.
88. Gimse R, Bjorgen IA, Straume A: Driving skills after whiplash. Scand J Psychol 38:165–170, 1997.
89. Gimse R, Tjell C, Bjorgen IA, Saunte C: Disturbed eye movements after whiplash due to injury to the posture control system. J Clin Exp Neuropsychol 18:178–186, 1996.
90. Gimse R, Bjorgen IA, Tjell C, et al: Reduced cognitive functions in a group of whiplash patients with demonstrated disturbances in the posture control system. J Clin Exp Neuropsychol 19:1–12, 1997.
91. Gorman W: The alleged whiplash "injury." Ariz Med 31:411–413, 1974.
92. Gorman WF: "Whiplash" fictive or factual. Bull Am Acad Psychiatry Law 7:245–248, 1979.
93. Gotten N: Survey of 100 cases of whiplash injury after settlement of litigation. JAMA 162:865–867, 1956.
94. Grauer JN, Panjabi MM, Cholewicki J, et al: Whiplash produces an S-shaped curvature of the neck with hyperextension at lower levels. Spine 22:2489–2494, 1997.
95. Greenfield J, Ilfeld FW: Acute cervical strain: Evaluation and short-term prognostic factors. Clin Orthop 122:196–200, 1977.
96. Grimm RJ, Hemenway WG, Lebray PR, et al: The perilymph fistula syndrome defined in mild head trauma. Acta Otolaryngol 464(Suppl):1–40, 1989.
97. Grinker RR, Guy CC: Sprain of the cervical spine causing thrombosis of the anterior spinal artery. JAMA 88:1140–1142, 1927.
98. Gukelberger M: The uncomplicated post-traumatic cervical syndrome. Scand J Rehabil Med 4:150–153, 1972.
99. Heise AP, Laskin DM, Gervin AS: Incidence of temporomandibular joint symptoms following whiplash injury. J Oral Maxillofac Surg 50:825–828, 1992.
100. Helliwell M, Robertson JC, Todd GB, Lobb M: Bilateral vocal cord paralysis due to whiplash injury. BMJ 288:1876–1877, 1984.
101. Haslett RS, Duvall-Young J, McGalliard JN: Traumatic retinal angiopathy and seat belts: Pathogenesis of whiplash injury. Eye 8:615–617, 1994,
102. Hildingsson C, Wenngren B, Toolanen G: Eye motility dysfunction after soft-tissue injury of the cervical spine. Acta Orthop Scand 64:129–132, 1993.
103. Hildingsson C, Wenngren BI, Bring G, et al: Oculomotor problems after cervical spine injury. Acta Orthop Scand 60:513–516, 1989.
104. Hildingson C, Toolanen G: Outcome after soft tissue injury of the cervical spine: A prospective study of 93 car-accident victims. Acta Orthop Scand 61:357–359, 1990.
105. Hinoki M, Niki H: Neurological studies on the role of the sympathetic nervous system in the formation of traumatic vertigo of cervical origin. Acta Otolaryngol 330(Suppl):185–196, 1975.
106. Hinse P, Thie A, Lachenmayer L: Dissection of the extracranial vertebral artery: Report of four cases and review of the literature. J Neurol Neurosurg Psychiatry 54:863–869, 1991.
107. Hodge JR: The whiplash neurosis. Psychosomatics 12:245–249, 1971.
108. Hohl M: Soft-tissue injuries of the neck in automobile accidents: Factors influencing prognosis. J Bone Joint Surg 56A:1675–1682, 1974.
109. Horwich H, Kasner D: The effect of whiplash injuries on ocular functions. South Med J 55:69–71, 1962.
110. Howcroft AJ, Jenkins DH: Potentially fatal asphyxia following a minor injury of the cervical spine. J Bone Joint Surg 59B:93–94, 1977.
111. Igarashi M, Alford BR, Watanabe T, et al: Role of neck proprioceptors in the maintenance of dynamic body equilibrium in the squirrel monkey. Laryngoscope 79:1713–1727, 1969.
112. Igarashi M, Miyata H, Alford BR, et al: Nystagmus after experimental cervical lesions. Laryngoscope 82:1609–1621, 1972.
113. Jacome DE: EEG in whiplash: A reappraisal. Clin Electroencephalogr 18:41–45, 1987.
114. Janes JM, Hooshmand H: Severe extension-flexion injuries of the cervical spine. Mayo Clin Proc 40:353–368, 1965.
115. Janjua KJ, Goswami V, Sagar G: Whiplash injury associated with acute bilateral internal carotid arterial dissection. J Trauma 40:456–458, 1996.
116. Jeffreys E: Disorders of the Cervical Spine, 2nd ed. Oxford, Butterworth-Heinemann, 1993, pp 105–112.
117. Jónsson H Jr, Bring G, Rauschning W, et al: Hidden cervical spine injuries in traffic accident victims with skull fractures. J Spinal Disord 4:251–263, 1991.

118. Kaneoka K, Ono K, Inami S, et al: Human cervical spine kinematics during whiplash loading. Proceedings of the International Conference on New Frontiers in Biomechanical Engineering, Tokyo, 1997, pp 265–268.
119. Kaneoka K, Ono L, Inami S, Hayashi K: The mechanism of zygapophysial joint injury in rear-end motor vehicle collisions. J Jap Spine Res Soc 8:244, 1997.
120. Kaneoka K, Ono L, Inami S, Hayashi K: Abnormal segmental motion of the cervical spine during whiplash loading. J Jap Orthop Assoc 71:S1680, 1997.
121. Keller RH: Traumatic displacement of the cartilagenous vertebral rim: A sign of intervertebral disc prolapse. Radiology 110:21–24, 1974.
122. Kischka U, Ettlin T, Heim S, et al: Cerebral symptoms following whiplash injury. Eur Neurol 31:136–140, 1991.
123. Kolbinson DA, Epstein JB, Burgess JA: Temporomandibular disorders, headaches, and neck pain following motor vehicle accidents and the effect of litigation: Review of the literature. J Orofacial Pain 10:101–125, 1996.
124. Koshino K, Tanaka M, Kubota S, et al: Activated irregular spike and wave complex in traumatic cervical syndrome. No To Shinkei 24:49–55, 1972.
125. Kupperman A: Whiplash and disc derangement. J Oral Maxillofac Surg 46:519–519, 1988.
126. La Rocca H: Acceleration injuries of the neck. Clin Neurosurg 25:209–217, 1978.
127. Lee C, Woodring JH: Sagittally oriented fractures of the lateral masses of the cervical vertebra. J Trauma 31:1638–1643, 1991.
128. Levine AM, Edwards CC: Traumatic lesions of the occipitoatlantoaxial complex. Clin Orthop 239:53–68, 1989.
129. Lord SM, Barnsley L, Bogduk N: The utility of comparative local anesthetic blocks versus placebo-controlled blocks for the diagnosis of cervical zygapophysial joint pain. Clin J Pain 11:208–213, 1995.
130. Lord SM, Barnsley L, Wallis BJ, et al: Third occipital headache: A prevalence study. J Neurol Neurosurg Psychiatry 57:1187–1190, 1994.
131. Lord SM, Barnsley L, Wallis BJ, et al: Chronic cervical zygapophysial joint pain after whiplash: A placebo-controlled prevalence study. Spine 21:1737–1745, 1996.
132. Lord SM, McDonald GJ: Commentary on Schrader H et al: "Natural evolution of late whiplash syndrome outside the medicolegal context." Pain Med J 3:40–43, 1997.
133. Loudon JK, Ruhl M, Field E: Ability to reproduce head position after whiplash injury. Spine 22:865–868, 1997.
134. Lysell E: The pattern of motion in the cervical spine. In Hirsch C, Zotterman Y (eds): Cervical Pain. Oxford, Pergamon Press, 1972, pp 53–58.
135. MacNab I: Acceleration injuries of the cervical spine. J Bone Joint Surg 46A:1797–1799, 1964.
136. MacNab I: Whiplash injuries of the neck. Manit Med Rev 46:172–174, 1966.
137. MacNab I: Acceleration-extension injuries of the cervical spine. Symposium on the Spine. St. Louis, Mosby, 1969, pp 10–17.
138. MacNab I: The "whiplash syndrome." Orthop Clin North Am 2:389–403, 1971.
139. MacNab I: The whiplash syndrome. Clin Neurosurg 232–241, 1973.
140. Magnusson T, Ragnarsson T, Bjornsson A: Occipital nerve release in patients with whiplash trauma and occipital neuralgia. Headache 36:32–36, 1996.
141. Maimaris C, Barnes MR, Allen MJ: "Whiplash injuries" of the neck: A retrospective study. Injury 19:393–396, 1988.
142. Mankin HJ: Clinical features of osteoarthritis. In Kelley WN, Harris ED, Ruddy S, et al (eds): Textbook of Rheumatology, 3rd ed. Philadelphia, WB Saunders, 1989, pp 1480–1500.
143. Martino F, Ettore GC, Cafaro E, et al: L'ecographia musculo-tendinea nei traumi distorvi acuti del collo. Radiol Med Torino 83:211–215, 1992.
144. Matsushita T, Sato, TB, Hirabayashi K, et al: X-ray study of the human neck motion due to head inertia loading. Proceedings of the 38th STAPP Car Crash Conference. Warrendale, PA, Society for Automotive Engineers, 1994, pp 55–64.
145. McConnell W E, Howard RP, Guzman HM, et al: Analysis of human test subject kinematic responses to low velocity rear end impacts. Proceedings of the 37th STAPP Car Crash Conference. Warrendale, PA, Society for Automotive Engineers, 1993, pp 21–30.
146. McCormick C: Arthrography of the atlanto-axial (C1–C2) joints: Techniques and results. J Intervent Radiol 2:9–13, 1987.
147. McKenzie JA, Williams JF: The dynamic behaviour of the head and cervical spine during "whiplash." J Biomech 4:477–490, 1971.
148. McMillan BS, Silver JR: Extension injuries of the cervical spine resulting in tetraplegia. Injury 18:224–233, 1987.

149. McNamara RM, O'Brien MC, Davidheiser S: Posttraumatic neck pain: A prospective and follow-up study. Ann Emerg Med 17:906–911, 1988.
150. Mendelson G: Not "cured by a verdict." Effect of legal settlement on compensation claimants. Med J Aust 2:132–134, 1982.
151. Mendelson G: Follow-up studies of personal injury litigants. Int J Law Psychiatry 7:179–188, 1984.
152. Mendelson G: Compensation and chronic pain. Pain 48:121–123, 1992.
153. Merskey H: Psychiatry and the cervical sprain syndrome. Can Med Assoc J 130:1119–1121, 1984.
154. Middleton JM: Opthalmic aspects of whiplash injuries. Int Rec Med 169:19–20, 1956.
155. Miles KA, Maimaris C, Finlay D, et al: The incidence and prognostic significance of radiological abnormalities in soft tissue injuries to the cervical spine. Skeletal Radiol 17:493–496, 1988.
156. Miller H: Accident neurosis. BMJ 1:919–925, 1961.
157. Mills H, Horne G: Whiplash—manmade disease? N Z Med J 99:373–374, 1986.
158. Norris SH, Watt I: The prognosis of neck injuries resulting from rear-end vehicle collisions. J Bone Joint Surg 65B:608–611, 1983.
159. Olsnes BT: Neurobehavioral findings in whiplash patients with long-lasting symptoms. Acta Neurol Scand 80:584–588, 1989.
160. Olsson I, Bunketorp O, Carlsson G, et al: An in-depth study of neck injuries in rear end collisions. Bron, France, Proceedings of the IRCOBI Conference, 1990, pp 269–280.
161. Ommaya AK, Faas F, Yarnell P: Whiplash injury and brain damage: An experimental study. JAMA 204:285–289, 1968.
162. Ommaya AK, Yarnell P: Subdural haematoma after whiplash injury. Lancet 2:237–239, 1969.
163. Oosterveld WJ, Kortschot HW, Kingma GG, et al: Electronystagmographic findings following cervical whiplash injuries. Acta Otolaryngol 111:201–205, 1991.
164. Otte A, Ettlin T, Fierz L, et al: Parieto-occipital hypoperfusion in late whiplash syndrome: First quantitative SPET study using technetium 99m bicisate (ECD). Europ J Nucl Med 23:72–74, 1996.
165. Pang LQ: The otological aspects of whiplash injuries. Laryngoscope 81:1381–1387, 1971.
166. Pearce JM: Whiplash injury: A reappraisal. J Neurol Neurosurg Psychiatry 52:1329–1331, 1989.
167. Pennie B, Agambar L: Patterns of injury and recovery in whiplash. Injury 22:57–59, 1991.
168. Penning L: Prevertebral hematoma in cervical spine injury: Incidence and etiolgic significance. Am J Roentgenol 136:553–561, 1981.
169. Penning L: Differences in anatomy, motion development and aging in the upper and lower cervical disk segments. Clin Biomech 3:37–47, 1991.
170. Pettersson K, Hildingsson C, Toolanen G, et al: MRI and neurology in acute whiplash trauma: No correlation in prospective examination of 39 cases. Acta Orthop Scand 65:525–528, 1994.
171. Pietrobono R, Allen WB, Walker HR: Cervical strain with residual occipital neuritis. J Int Coll Surg 28:293–295, 1957.
172. Probert TCS, Weisenfeld D, Reade PC: Temporomandibular pain dysfunction disorder resulting from road traffic accidents—an Australian study. Int J Oral Maxillofac Surg 23:338–341, 1994.
173. Radanov BP, Di Stefano G, Schnidrig A, et al: Role of psychosocial stress in recovery from common whiplash. Lancet 338:712–715, 1991.
174. Radanov BP, Di Stefano G, Schnidrig A, et al: Cognitive functioning after common whiplash: A controlled follow-up study. Arch Neurol 50:87–91, 1993.
175. Radanov BP, Dvorak J: Impaired cognitive functioning after whiplash injury of the cervical spine. Spine 21:392–397, 1996.
176. Radanov BP, Dvorak J, Valach L: Cognitive deficits in patients after soft tissue injury of the cervical spine. Spine 17:127–131, 1992.
177. Radanov BP, Hirlinger I, Di Stefano G, et al: Attentional processing in cervical spine syndromes. Acta Neurol Scand 85:358–362, 1992.
178. Radanov BP, Sturzenegger M, Di Stefano G: Long-term outcome after whiplash injury: A 2-year follow-up considering features of injury mechanism and somatic, radiologic, and psychosocial findings. Medicine 74:281–297, 1995.
179. Radanov BP, Sturzenneger M: Predicting recovery from common whiplash. Eur Neurol 36:48–51, 1996.
180. Rauschning W: Anatomy of the normal and traumatized spine: In Sances A, Thomas DJ, Ewing CL, et al (eds): Mechanisms of Head and Spine Trauma. Deer Park, NY, Aloray, 1986, pp 531–563.
181. Rauschning W, McAfee PC, Jónsson H Jr: Pathoanatomical and surgical findings in cervical spinal injuries. J Spinal Disord 2:213–221, 1989.

182. Ronnen HR, de Korte PJ, Brink PRG, et al: Acute whiplash injury: Is there a role for MRI imaging? A prospective study of 100 patients. Radiology 201:93–96, 1996.
183. Roth DA: Cervical analgesic discography: A new test for the definitive diagnosis of the painful disk syndrome. JAMA 235:1713–1714, 1976.
184. Roydhouse RH: Whiplash and temporomandibular dysfunction. Lancet 1:1394–1395, 1973.
185. Rubin AM, Woolley SM, Dailey VM, et al: Postural stability following mild head or whiplash injuries. Am J Otol 16:216–221, 1995.
186. Rubin W: Whiplash with vestibular involvement. Arch Otolaryngol 97:85–87, 1973.
187. Rutherford OM, Jones DA, Newham DJ: Clinical and experimental application of the percutaneous twitch superimposition technique for the study of human muscle activation. J Neurol Neurosurg Psychiatry 49:1288–1291, 1986.
188. Saldinger P, Dvorak J, Rahn B, et al: Histology of the alar and transverse ligaments. Spine 15:257–261, 1990.
189. Sano K, Nakamura N, Hirakawa K, et al: Correlative studies of dynamics and pathology in whiplash and head injuries. Scand J Rehabil Med 4:47–54, 1972.
190. Schneider LW, Foust DR, Bowman BM, et al: Biomechanical properties of the human neck in lateral flexion. Proceedings of the 19th STAPP Car Crash Conference. Warrendale, PA, Society of Automotive Engineers, 1975, pp 453–485.
191. Schonstrom N, Twomey L, Taylor J: The lateral atlanto-axial joints and their synovial folds: An in vitro study of soft tissue injuries and fractures. Trauma 35:886–892, 1993.
192. Schraeder H, Obelieniene D, Bovim G, et al: Natural evolution of late whiplash syndrome outside the medicolegal context. Lancet 347:1207–1211, 1996.
193. Schutt CH, Dohan FC: Neck injury to women in auto accidents: A metropolitan plague. JAMA 206:2689–2692, 1968.
194. Seletz E: Whiplash injuries: Neurophysiological basis for pain and methods used for rehabilitation. JAMA 168:1750–1755, 1958.
195. Seletz E: Trauma and the cervical portion of the spine. J Int Coll Surg 40:47–62, 1963.
196. Severy DM, Mathewson JH, Bechtol CO: Controlled automobile rear-end collisions: An investigation of related engineering and medical phenomena. Can Serv Med J 11:727–759, 1955.
197. Shapiro AP, Teasell RW, Steenhuis R: Mild traumatic brain injury following whiplash. Spine State Art Rev 7:455–470, 1993.
198. Shmueli G, Herold ZH: Prevertebral shadow in cervical trauma. Isr J Med Sci 16:698–700, 1980.
199. Signoret F, Feron JM, Bonfait H, et al: Fractured odontoid with fractured superior articular process of the axis. J Bone Joint Surg 68B:182–184, 1986.
200. Simmons EH, Segil CM: An evaluation of discography in the localization of symptomatic levels in discogenic disease of the spine. Clin Orthop 108:57–69, 1975.
201. Smith GR, Beckly DE, Abel MS: Articular mass fracture: A neglected cause of posttraumatic neck pain? Clin Radiol 27:335–340, 1976.
202. Spenler CW, Benfield JR: Esophageal disruption from blunt and penetrating external trauma. Arch Surg 111:663–667, 1976.
203. Spitzer WO, Skovron ML, Salmi LR, et al: Scientific monograph of the Quebec Task Force on Whiplash-associated Disorders: Redefining "whiplash" and its management. Spine 20(Suppl 8):1S–73S, 1995.
204. Squires B, Gargan MF, Bannister GC: Soft tissue injuries of the cervical spine: 15-year follow-up. J Bone Joint Surg 78B:955–957, 1996.
205. States JD, Korn MW, Masengill JB: The enigma of whiplash injury. NY State J Med 70:2971–2978, 1970.
206. Stokes M, Young A: The contribution of reflex inhibition to arthrogenous muscle weakness. Clin Sci 67:7–14, 1984.
207. Stroobants J, Fidler L, Storms JL, et al: High cervical pain and impairment of skull mobility as the only symptoms of an occipital condyle fracture. J Neurosurg 81:137–138, 1994.
208. Sturzenegger M, Di Stefano G, Radanov B, Schnidring A: Presenting symptoms and signs after whiplash injury: The influence of accident mechanisms. Neurology 44:688–693, 1994.
209. Sturzenegger M, Radanov BP, Di Stefano G: The effect of accident mechanisms and initial findings on the long-term course of whiplash injury. J Neurol 242:443–449, 1995.
210. Swartzman LC, Teasell RW, Shapiro AP, et al: The effect of litigation status on adjustment to whiplash injury. Spine 21:53–58, 1996.
211. Taylor AE, Cox CA, Mailis A: Persistent neuropsychological deficits following whiplash: Evidence for chronic mild traumatic brain injury. Arch Phys Med Rehabil 77:529–535, 1996.
212. Taylor JR, Kakulas BA: Neck injuries. Lancet 338:1343–1343, 1991.

213. Taylor JR, Twomey LT: Acute injuries to cervical joints: An autopsy study of neck sprain. Spine 9:1115–1122, 1993.
214. Teasell RW, Shapiro AP, Mailis A: Medical management of whiplash injuries: An overview. Spine State Art Rev 7:481–500, 1993.
215. Toglia JU: Vesticular and medicolegal aspects of closed cranio-cervical trauma. Scand J Rehabil Med 4:126–132, 1972.
216. Toglia JU: Acute flexion-extension injury of the neck: Electronystagmographic study of 309 patients. Neurology 26:808–814, 1976.
217. Toglia JU, Rosenberg PE, Ronis ML: Vestibular and audiological aspects of whiplash injury and head trauma. J Forensic Sci 14:219–226, 1969.
218. Toglia JU, Rosenberg PE, Ronis ML: Posttraumatic dizziness: Vestibular, audiologic, and medicolegal aspects. Arch Otolaryngol 92:485–492, 1970.
219. Torres F, Shapiro SK: Electroencephalograms in whiplash injury. Arch Neurol 5:28–35, 1961.
220. Travell J, Simons DG: Myofascial Pain and Dysfunction: The Trigger Point Manual. Baltimore, Williams & Wilkins, 1983.
221. Viktrup L, Knudsen GM, Hansen SH: Delayed onset of basilar thrombotic embolus after whiplash injury. Stroke 26:2194–2196, 1995.
222. Walton JN: Brain's Diseases of the Nervous System, 8th ed. Oxford, Oxford University Press, 1977, p 91.
223. Watkinson A, Gargan MF, Bannister GC: Prognostic factors in soft tissue injuries of the cervical spine. Injury 22:307–309, 1991.
224. Weinberg S, Lapointe H: Cervical extension-flexion injury (whiplash) and internal derangement of the temporomandibular joint. J Oral Maxillofac Surg 45:653–656, 1987.
225. Weir DC: Roentgenographic signs of cervical injury. Clin Orthop 109:9–17, 1975.
226. Wickstrom J, Martinez JL, Johnston D, et al: Acceleration-deceleration injuries of the cervical spine in animals. In Severy DM (ed): Proceedings of the 7th STAPP Car Crash Conference. Springfield, IL, Charles C Thomas, 1965, pp 284–301.
227. Wickstrom J, Martinez JL, Rodriguez R Jr: The cervical sprain syndrome: Experimental acceleration injuries to the head and neck. In Selzer ML, Gikas PW, Huelke DF (eds): The Prevention of Highway Injury. Ann Arbor, MI, Highway Safety Research Institute, 1967, pp 182–187.
228. Wolfe F, Simons DG, Fricton J, et al: The fibromyalgia and myofascial pain syndromes: A preliminary study of tender points and trigger points in persons with fibromyalgia, myofascial pain and no disease. J Rheumatol 19:944–951, 1992.
229. Woodring JH, Goldstein SJ: Fractures of the articular processes of the cervical spine. Am J Roentgenol 139:341–344, 1982.
230. Wosazek GE, Balzer K: Strangulation of the internal carotid artery by the hypoglossal nerve. J Trauma 30:332–335, 1990.
231. Yarnell PR, Rossie GV: Minor whiplash head injury with major debilitation. Brain Inj 2:255–258, 1988.
232. Yetkin Z, Osborn AG, Giles DS, et al: Uncovertebral and facet joint dislocations in cervical articular pillar fractures: CT evaluation. Am J Neuroradiol 6:633–637, 1985.

5

Whiplash-Associated Disorders: Prognosis After Injury

Andrea J. Boon, M.D., and Jay Smith, M.D.

Whiplash-related hyperextension-hyperflexion injuries of the cervical spine continue to challenge the medicolegal system and society in general. Crowe originally introduced "whiplash" in 1928 to describe a specific motion of the head and neck resulting from a rear-end automobile accident, although the term "whiplash" is now used much more broadly in a medicolegal context.[11] Whiplash-associated injuries can result from all types of motor vehicle accidents (MVAs), but the typical mechanism involves rear-end collision with neck hyperextension.[12,33,44] Macnab and others have reported that the rear-end collision hyperextension mechanism is significantly more likely to result in chronic soft tissue symptoms than flexion and lateral flexion injuries.[34] Pathological findings noted by White et al support an anterior-to-posterior transmission of force with progressive disruption of anatomic structures from front to back.[73] Injuries include muscular strains (sternocleidomastoid, longus colli, scalene), retropharyngeal hematoma, intraesophogeal hemorrhage, cervical sympathetic chain traction, and disruption of the anterior longitudinal ligament, disc, or facet capsule. Seat belts do not appear to be protective, and many studies indicate that mandatory seat belt laws have possibly increased the incidence of whiplash-associated disorders (WADs).[12,17,28,61]

Initially, 30% to 62% of people seen in a hospital after an MVA will complain of neck pain and related symptoms; an additional 35% may have delayed symptom onset of 12 to 48 hours.[12,36,44,54,64] Initial complaints may include neck pain, headache, interscapular pain, visual disturbances, dizziness, weakness, paresthesias, and concentration and memory disturbances.[27,36] Even in the absence of litigation or compensation, up to 50% of patients chronically report neck or back pain, shoulder pain, headaches, or sleep disturbance, and more than 30% report visual disturbances, concentration loss, anxiety, fatigue, or depression.[19,22,27,35,52,58] Given the high prevalence of MVAs and chronic symptoms, it is important for clinicians to understand the anticipated clinical outcome of patients with WADs.[61] The following review summarizes studies pertaining to prognosis in WADs. Specific discussions regarding temporal course of recovery, development of cervical spondylosis, and litigation follow.

PROGNOSIS AND FACTORS ASSOCIATED WITH OUTCOME

Multiple studies have attempted to determine the "natural history" of patients with WADs and delineate early prognostic factors. Most are limited by retrospective design, selection and follow-up bias, heterogeneity of injury mechanism, small patient numbers, incomplete follow-up and data collection, lack of consistent injury definitions or standard measures of outcome, and outcome biases due to sociocultural differences or insurance and compensation schemes.[12,22,27,33,36,44,53,58] Few prospective studies have considered premorbid state despite the fact that high rates of chronic neck pain have been reported in both the general population and a representative population of working society.[7,37] Nonetheless, examination of the literature to date is warranted because it represents our current knowledge base regarding prognosis after WADs. Table 1 summarizes major outcome studies that are discussed throughout the text. For purposes of the following discussion, the Quebec Task Force grading system is used to describe differing severities of WADs.[61]

Radanov and colleagues published several studies from a prospective cohort of 117 primary care referral patients aged 19 to 51 years (mean 31) initially evaluated within 7 days of injury and followed for 2 years.[51-53,63] The authors investigated the significance of patient history, initial psychosocial and somatic factors, radiographic findings, and features of injury mechanism in the recovery from WADs. These studies provide the most detailed contemporary analyses of whiplash patients. The recovery rate was 56% at 3 months, 70% at 6 months, 76% at 1 year, and 88% at 2 years. Factors statistically associated with poorer prognosis included older age (mean 35 vs 30 years), pretraumatic migraine headaches, rotated or inclined head position at time of impact, more severe initial neck and head pain ratings, a wide variety of subjective complaints (eg, fatigue, blurry vision, anxiety, sleep disturbance), radicular symptoms, radiographic spondylosis, and early patient concerns with respect to the possibility of disability or long-lasting symptoms. In this study, vocation, symptom onset interval, and psychosocial stress did not correlate with prognosis.

The same group later applied a logistic regression analysis to develop a predictive model for prognosis at 1 year. In this analysis, continued significant symptoms at 1 year were associated with impaired neck movement, inclined or rotated head position at impact, unpreparedness for trauma, the car being stationary when hit, pretraumatic headache, head trauma, older age, initial neck pain severity, initial headache severity, nervousness score, neuroticism score, and impaired focused attention.[51,63] The model accurately predicted outcome in 96% of the 117 patients in the primary care group. In addition, the same model successfully predicted outcome in 88% of 16 patients aged 25 to 51 years (mean 33) referred from an insurance company, of whom 56% had complete recovery at 1 year.

Based on data collected from these studies, Radanov et al concluded that poor outcome after whiplash injury is primarily related to factors associated directly or indirectly with the severity of the initial injury. Interestingly, comparisons revealed no statistically significant differences in symptomatic disabled versus symptomatic nondisabled subjects at 2 years of follow-up. Consequently, symptom persistence but not disability can be predicted based on early examination.

Hildingsson and Toolanen performed a prospective study of 93 consecutive patients presenting to an emergency department.[24] Eighty-eight patients were available for final follow-up, with an average follow-up of 2 years. A total of 42% recovered completely, 15% had only minor discomfort, and 43% had discomfort

Table 1. Outcome Studies in Whiplash

Author	Year	Study Type	Patients	Follow-up	Recovery*	Symptoms†	Prognostic of Ultimate Outcome‡
Hohl	1974	Retrospective	146	5 y	57	43	Upper extremity symptoms, female, severity, treatment type, x-ray§
Deans	1987	Retrospective	85	18 mo	64	36	Rear impact, seat belt
Maimaris	1988	Retrospective	102	2 y	66	34	Occipital headache, referred symptoms, rear and front collision, interscapular pain, neurologic abnormality, x-ray
Miles	1988	Retrospective	73	2 y	71	29	X-ray
McKinney	1989	Prospective	167	2 y	62	38	Specific prognostic factors not studied
Hildingsson	1990	Prospective	88	2 y	57	43	X-ray: see page 80, last paragraph
Gargan‖	1990	Prospective	43	11 y	60	40	Neurologic abnormality, range of motion loss, older age, x-ray
Watkinson‖	1991	Retrospective	35	11 y	65	35	Extracervical symptoms
Pennie	1991	Prospective	144	5 mo	86	14	Specific prognostic factors not studied
Parmar	1993	Retrospective	100	3 y	82	18	Onset of symptoms <12 hours, history of neck pain
Jonsson	1994	Prospective	50	5 y	68	32	Specific prognostic factors not studied
Suissa: Quebec Task Force¶	1995	Retrospective	2810	>5 y	99	1	Female, older age, number of dependents, marital status, severity, collision type, no seat belt
Radanov	1996	Prospective	117	2 y	76	24#	Multiple: see page 80
Mayou	1996	Prospective	57	1 year	51	49	Female passenger, immediate neck pain
Obelieniene	1999	Prospective	210	1 year	9	4**	Specific prognostic factors not studied
Bonk	2000	Prospective	97	12 wk	84	16	Treatment type: see page 84, paragraph 4
Brison	2000	Prospective	336	6 mo	65	35	Female, older age
Parthani	2000	Prospective	180	6 mo	98	2	

* Percent of patients in recovery implies complete recovery or minimal nondisabling symptoms.

† Percent of patients with continued symptoms implies clinically significant symptoms of a moderate or severe nature.

‡ Factors associated with poor outcome.

§ See section on cervical spondylosis for full discussion of x-ray findings and prognosis.

‖ Gargan and Bannister review of Norris and Watt cohort at mean of 10.8 years and reexamined by Watkinson, Gargan, and Bannister in 1991. Data presented are from the 1990 review.

¶ "Recovery" defined by duration of compensation.

\# Symptomatic not divided by severity: "many subjectively mild."

** Not statistically different from age-matched controls.

that precluded a return to work. The authors were unable to determine any positive prognostic factors from the 17 they studied but did conclude that rear-impact mechanism, initial symptoms, reversal of cervical lordosis, or degenerative spondylosis on cervical spine films were not prognostic of final outcome within this study population.

Norris and Watt reported on a series of 61 patients aged 19 to 76 years (mean 37) evaluated in an emergency department within 7 days postinjury and divided into 3 clinical groups for follow-up: 27 patients with grade I WAD and mean follow-up of 20 months (group 1), 24 patients with grade II WAD and mean follow-up of 24 months (group 2), and 10 symptomatic patients with grade III WAD and mean follow-up of 25 months (group 3).[44] Common complaints at presentation and follow-up were neck pain, headaches, and paresthesias. Dizziness, weakness, and auditory or visual symptoms were less common and reported predominantly in group 3. Delayed symptom onset occurred in 20% to 25% of patients. At follow-up, patients in group 3 were more likely to have lost more time from work and report continued neck pain compared with group 1 patients. Only 10% of group 3 patients were pain-free, compared with 19% of group 2 and 56% of group 3 patients. Overall, neurologic deficits (ie, group 3), restricted neck motion, and abnormal cervical curves on radiographs were statistically correlated with persistent symptoms.

Gargan and Bannister later reviewed 43 patients (5 of 61 had died; 13 of 61 were lost to follow-up) from the Norris and Watt cohort at 8 to 12 years (mean 11) postinjury.[19] Sixty percent had complete recovery or mild symptoms not interfering with work or leisure activity, 28% reported moderate "intrusive" symptoms requiring activity modification and intermittent treatment, and 12% reported severe or disabling symptoms accompanied by job loss, continued treatment, or repeated medical consultation. The most common residual symptoms were neck pain (74%), paresthesias (45%), low back pain (42%), and headaches (33%). The mean age of patients with recovery or mild symptoms was significantly below that of patients with severe, disabling symptoms.

Watkinson et al later reevaluated 35 of the 61 patients from the Norris and Watt cohort who were available for follow-up (mean 11 years post-MVA) and whose original radiographs were available for review.[19,44,70] Fourteen percent had recovered completely; however, no patient initially presenting with extracervical symptoms had a complete recovery. Squires et al evaluated 40 patients who had participated in Norris and Watt's original study at a mean of 15.5 years postinjury. Subjects were evaluated for range of motion, neurologic deficit, pain, and psychological disturbance. Seventy percent of patients still had symptoms 15 years after injury (10% were disabled by their symptoms), and only 5% of patients aged over 40 at the time of injury were symptom-free.[62]

In a study of the natural history of WADs, Parmar and Raymakers reviewed the medicolegal reports of 204 patients involved in rear-end accidents resulting in neck injuries.[47] All patients were a minimum of 3 years postinjury and were seeking compensation. The authors clinically and radiographically examined 100 (64%) of the 144 patients who could be located, at an average of 8 years (range 3-20) postinjury. Fifty percent reported having had moderate or severe pain at 8 months, decreasing to 22% at 2 years. At the minimum 3-year follow-up, 82% were completely pain-free or had minimal, nondisabling symptoms, and 18% continued to have significant symptoms. Those followed longer than 3 years showed little change from that point on. Pain lasted longer in patients who were older (>45 years), were front-seat passengers, experienced symptoms in less than 12 hours, reported preexisting neck symptoms, or exhibited spondylosis on initial radiographs. Multivariate analysis indicated that only a history of neck pain was independently correlated with prolonged recovery. The extent of final recovery, however, correlated only with the temporal onset of symptoms: patients experiencing symptoms after 12 hours postinjury had a statistically better outcome. This latter finding supported previous reports by Macnab, Norris and Watt, and Deans.[12,33,44]

Hohl reviewed 146 of 534 patients (mean age 29 years) seen in "walk-in" orthopedic office practices a minimum of 5 years post-MVA.[27] All patients had sustained soft tissue cervical injuries without preexisting radiographic spondylosis. Complete symptomatic recovery occurred in 57%, whereas 37% reported moderate and 6% reported severe neck symptoms. Upper extremity numbness or pain, female sex, hospitalization (as index of injury severity), use of collar immobilization for more than 12 weeks, use of home traction, need to resume physical therapy more than once for symptom recurrence, and single segment motion restriction on cervical films were associated with poor recovery. Property damage amount was not correlated with recovery. The study design was subject to selection and follow-up biases.

Jonsson et al reported 5-year follow-up on 50 patients with WADs evaluated at 5 years by an independent examiner.[28] Fifty-two percent reported no pain at 6 weeks postinjury. At 5 years, 68% reported no or minimal nondisabling symptoms, whereas 32% still had significant symptoms. Between the 6-week and 5-year follow-up, 20% of patients with continued neck and/or radicular pain had surgical intervention. Specific prognostic factors were not examined.

Brison et al followed 383 subjects who presented to an emergency department after having been involved in a rear-end MVA. Sixty-one percent of subjects reported some form of WAD at initial interview. Fifty-one percent continued to report symptoms at 1 month from injury, 37% at 5 months, and 34% to 36% at 6 to 24 months postinjury. Female gender and older age were associated with an increased incidence of WADs at 6 months.[8]

Maimaris et al evaluated 102 of 120 patients aged 17 to 72 years (mean 37) with WADs at 18 to 30 months postinjury.[36] Sixty-six percent were asymptomatic and 34% continued to have symptoms of neck pain or stiffness, shoulder pain, or headaches. Compared with the asymptomatic group, patients in the symptomatic group were statistically more likely to have been involved in combination rear and front collisions and to have abnormal neurologic examinations (33% vs 10%), settled/unsettled insurance claims (57% vs 18%), preexisting cervical spondylosis, and occipital headaches, interscapular pain, or referred symptoms.

Deans et al completed a questionnaire and telephone follow-up of 137 subjects 1 to 2 years (mean 18 months) after evaluation in the Royal Victoria Hospital following MVA.[12] Only 85 subjects (62%) reported any pain related to the injury anytime postinjury. Of this group, 36% still complained of symptoms at follow-up, and 6% of those had continuous symptoms. A rear-impact mechanism and use of seat belt were statistically correlated with continued symptoms.

McKinney completed a questionnaire follow-up of 167 (68%) of 247 consecutive patients (mean age 31 years) seen within 48 hours of whiplash-type injury, some of whom received advice or formal physiotherapy.[40] At a minimum 2-year follow-up, 38% of patients still had some symptoms. Of the 104 patients who had recovered, 60% recovered at 3 months, 90% at 6 months, and 97% within 9 months postinjury. Specific prognostic variables were not studied.

In contrast to the studies outlined above, which show WADs to be prolonged and disabling in many cases, several recent prospective studies from outside the United States have suggested that symptoms after whiplash injury are short-lived and nondisabling. In a study out of Lithuania, Obelieniene et al prospectively identified 210 patients from consecutive rear-end collisions in which police reports were filed, as well as 210 sex- and age-matched asymptomatic controls.[45] Questionnaires were sent out immediately after the accident, with follow-up questionnaires at 2 and 12 months postaccident. Controls filled out an initial questionnaire, with a follow-up questionnaire at 12 months. The response rate was > 75% in both groups to the initial questionnaires and > 90% to follow-up questionnaires. In this cohort, acute neck pain or headache never persisted longer than 3 weeks, and at 2- and 12-month follow-up, accident victims had no greater incidence of neck pain or headache than their age-matched controls.

This study was a follow-up to an earlier study out of Lithuania that found similar results but was criticized because data were gathered retrospectively and subject to recall bias.[57] Both of these studies were based solely on response to questionnaires and therefore did not include any objective clinical data; nor was the severity of injury graded, making direct comparison with other studies more difficult. The excellent outcomes may have in part reflected the study population, which differed from most WAD studies in that patients with very mild injuries, who never presented for medical evaluation, were included.

A prospective randomized study in Germany compared 97 whiplash victims (grade I or grade II) with 50 normal controls.[4] In the injured group, subjects were assigned to either active therapy or to soft collar and rest. Six weeks after injury, symptom prevalence between the active therapy group and the control group did not differ significantly, and by 12 weeks there were no significant differences between either injury group and controls. This would suggest that in this culture WADs show recovery in less than 3 months.

Parthani et al prospectively studied 180 patients with grade I or II WADs who presented to an emergency department in Greece within 2 days of injury.[48] Subjects were followed for 6 months, and outcome variables included headache, neck pain, shoulder or arm pain, and dizziness. Ninety percent of patients had resolution of symptoms at 4 weeks from injury, and 99% were back to baseline by 6 months.

These studies suggest that there may be significant cultural differences in recovery rates from WADs. Both Germany and Greece are similar to other Western countries in that there are advanced health care systems, insurance disability coverage, and the possibility of litigation for personal injury if one is concerned about potential injury. Parthani et al postulated that the cultural expectation of chronic pain following an acute neck sprain represents a critical factor.[48] Without this, there is no motivation to seek extensive therapy or compensation. Symptom amplification may also contribute; not only must the patient view his symptoms as not benign, but there must be an audience before which to repeatedly focus and report pain. Prolonged therapy and repeated medical appointments to establish injury may contribute to symptom persistence. In cultures where the acute injury is viewed as benign, people return to work within days and neither the patient nor the health care provider sees the need for these other measures.

Other studies that support a more benign outcome after whiplash injury include a short-term prospective study by Pennie and Agambar, who followed a 151-patient cohort originally treated for WADs in two accident/emergency departments. At a maximum 5-month follow-up of 144 patients, 86% had recovered completely, 12% were improved but still symptomatic, and 2% had no improvement. Specific prognostic factors were not investigated.

Satoh et al retrospectively studied 6167 Japanese patients presenting to an emergency department with WADs, normal neurologic examination, and no evidence of bony injury on plain radiographs.[55] Those who presented for ongoing treatment at 1.5, 3, and 6 months were compared with those who discontinued medical treatment. At 6 months of follow-up, 11% of victims were still receiving medical care. Female gender, use of emergency vehicle transportation, and early complaint of symptoms were correlated with persistence of symptoms.

As part of the Quebec Task Force on Whiplash-Associated Disorders monograph, Suissa et al reported outcome in 2810 subjects receiving compensation for WADs.[61,64] The authors used duration of compensation postinjury as the end point, stating that this roughly correlated to the time out of work (if employed) or the time the subject could not carry out his or her usual activities. The rate of recovery as defined in the study (ie, termination of compensation) was approximately 20% in 1 week, 50% in 1 month, 64% in 2 months, 87% in 6 months, and 97% in 12 months. At the final follow-up of more than 5 years, less than 1% of subjects were still receiving compensation. Female gender, older age, increased number of dependents, married/cohabitant status, multiple injuries, greater collision severity, vehicle other than a car or taxi, collisions other than rear-end ones, and nonuse of seat belt were associated with longer periods of compensation. This study has been criticized as having significant selection bias and criticized because no data were gathered regarding symptoms and functional impairment.[15]

The role of iatrogenic injury in delayed recovery from WADs has not been well studied. It seems clear that extended use of soft cervical collars in WADs can prolong symptoms.[4,41] However, the outcome associated with injection therapy (both soft tissue trigger point injections and axial injections such as cervical epidural steroid or facet joint injections), manipulation, or cervical spine surgery (decompression, discectomy, or fusion) is unknown. In addition, most studies do not control for these potentially confounding variables.

In summary, studies on WAD prognosis suggest general trends in recovery despite varied methodologies. Considering Table 1, approximately 75%±15% of patients will have no or minimal symptoms within 1 to 2 years post-MVA, while chronic symptoms develop in 25%±15%.[2,3] Approximately 10% may develop constant, severe pain.[19,27,70] There do appear to be significant cultural differences in recovery rates, for reasons that are not entirely clear.[4,45,48,57] Many variables have been inconsistently associated with a poor prognosis for recovery, but only Radanov et al have developed a predictive model.[51-54,63] These authors concluded that prognosis can be predicted based on factors primarily related directly or indirectly to the severity of injury. In general, most of the studies discussed would support this hypothesis, although further predictive models should be developed and validated for more practical clinical applications. Multiple studies associate older age and female sex with poor outcome, but only the former demographic variable was predictive as reported by Radanov et al.[19,51-54,63,64]

PSYCHOLOGICAL ASPECTS OF WHIPLASH-ASSOCIATED DISORDER

It has been suggested that emotional aspects are an integral part of the whiplash-related injury and are not necessarily related to preexisting psychological disease.[20,32,39] Shapiro and Merskey found no substantive data implicating psychological symptoms as a primary cause of persistent symptoms but suggested that psychological disturbances are more likely secondary to a chronic pain state.[42,59,69] No single personality trait has been associated with chronicity.[51-53] Gargan et al found that patients were psychologically normal at the time of injury but if symptoms persisted for 3 months they developed psychological disturbance (as measured by an abnormal General Health Questionnaire score).[18] The follow-up study by Squires et al showed an abnormal psychological profile in symptomatic patients after 15 years, suggesting that this is both reactive to physical pain and persistent.[62]

Mayou and Bryant completed a follow-up study of 74 consecutive patients aged 18 to 70 years diagnosed with posttraumatic neck injury in an emergency/accident center.[39] Follow-up was obtained for 63 and 57 patients at 3 months and 1 year, respectively. Common initial symptoms at injury included neck pain and motion restriction, upper back and shoulder pain, and headaches. At 1 year, 49% of patients had some persistent neck symptoms "although many were subjectively mild." In this study, approximately 25% of patients were rated as having a poor social outcome (disrupted quality of life: work, leisure, social relationships, family) at 3 months to 1 year postinjury. Poor social outcomes correlated strongly with preexisting psychological problems and emotional distress shortly after the injury. Physical outcome was statistically correlated only with immediate complaints of neck pain after the accident and being a female passenger. The authors concluded that psychosocial variables were important determinants of social disability and psychological outcome, similar to other musculoskeletal and chronic pain conditions.

In a retrospective review of 136 individuals seen for independent medical examination, Farbman reported that age, sex, race, marital status, hospitalization, habits, radiographic findings, and car damage did not correlate with symptom duration after MVA.[14] The author did report that "strong emotional factors" such as nervousness, pressure at work, caring for invalid relatives, and recent death of a relative were most strongly associated with prolonged symptoms. Also, extensive medical history (serious injury, chronic illness, or surgery), prolonged and frequent treatments (especially including traction, manipulation, and collar), and litigation correlated with longer symptom duration. Patients with multiple factors typically exhibited longer duration of symptoms. The data should be viewed with caution because this was not a specific analysis of treatment efficacy and most of the data were collected based on record review and patient recall.

Galasko et al found that "nervousness" among WAD patients at the time of injury or 6 months later was associated with a worse outcome at 48 months, with only 60% recovered, compared with 86%, independent of the severity of the original injury.[17] Similarly, Smed looked at 28 patients with grade III WAD and evaluated them prospectively with clinical and neuropsychological testing at 1 month and 7 months after injury. Patients reporting stressful life events at the time of but unrelated to the injury had a worse outcome.[60] Karlsborg et al prospectively followed a cohort of 34 patients with WADs (88% were grade III). Twenty-nine percent were symptom-free at 7 months. The presence of stress, at the time of but unrelated to the accident, did correlate with a higher rate of complaints at 7-month follow-up.[29]

In summary, it appears that psychological distress unrelated to the injury, but at the time of or shortly after injury, is associated with a poorer prognosis.[17,29,60] Patients with ongoing physical symptoms develop an abnormal psychological profile, which appears to be both reactive to physical pain and persistent.[18,42,59,69]

TEMPORAL COURSE OF RECOVERY

Understanding the anticipated temporal course of recovery for patients with WADs provides a foundation for counseling patients and involved parties, rational pursuit of further diagnostic evaluation and treatment, determination of maximum medical improvement, and more timely resolution of compensation claims. Although few studies have reported serially collected data regarding recovery rates, studies by McKinney, Jonsson, Pennie and Agambar, Parmar and Raymakers, and Radanov et al do allow formulation of some generalizations.[28,40,47,49,51-54] Within 1 year, 52% to 97% of patients who will eventually recover will demonstrate clinically significant recovery. By 2 years, an additional 12% to 26% of patients will recover.[47,51-54] Parmar and Raymakers reported the only serially collected data in the interval of 2 to 3 years postinjury.[47] In this single study, an additional 17% of patients of the group that recovered exhibited significant clinical recovery. Olivegren et al reevaluated a group of 22 patients at an average of 3 years after whiplash injury and compared the patients with a group of age- and sex-matched controls. In comparison to 1 year postinjury, they had improved in terms of both mental well-being and pain intensity, although they had not yet reached the level of healthy controls.[46]

The actual percentages of recovery over time must be considered imprecise due to methodologic shortcomings, inconsistencies among studies, and overall paucity of research. In addition, the recovery percentages are strongly influenced by a ceiling effect imposed by study duration. Nonetheless, the data do reflect an initial period of rapid recovery, followed by a period of slower recovery. A plateau in the extent of recovery probably occurs between 1 and 2 years postinjury. This is supported by the lack of significant differences in outcome between short-term (up to 2 years) and long-term (8 to 10 years) follow-up studies in Table 1.[19,22,27,58]

In summary, the recovery course in WADs parallels that of many musculoskeletal injuries.[3,23] Most patients who will eventually exhibit clinically significant recovery will typically do so during the first year, particularly during the first 3 to 6 months postinjury.[3,39] A smaller, though not insignificant, percentage of patients will recover between 1 and 2 years. Consequently, although each case must be considered individually, an interval of 2 years postinjury appears to be a reasonable time in which to make a medicolegal decision.[47]

WHIPLASH AND LITIGATION

Litigation is extremely common after whiplash-related injuries, with many studies reporting litigation proceedings in more than 50% of cases.[10,14,44,49,58,72] Prolonged or incomplete recovery from whiplash-related injuries has been repeatedly linked to the litigation process. These hypotheses have been based primarily on previous studies reporting that up to 88% of patients with WADs will improve after settlement of litigation.[22] This situation has nurtured the development of terms such as "compensation neurosis" and "accident neurosis."

In fact, multiple studies have failed to document an association between timing of compensation and symptom resolution.[13,27,33,34,44,47,58] Macnab reported that only 55% of 266 patients with severe injuries referred for specialty evaluation recovered after settlement.[33,34] In studies by both Hohl and by Norris and Watt, there was no indication that absence or settlement of litigation influenced long-term outcome.[27,44] Norris and Watt reported that patients with more severe injuries (including objective findings) were statistically more likely to file claims.[44] Because severity was graded within 7 days postinjury, this difference was hypothesized to reflect injury severity because insufficient time would have passed to develop "compensation neurosis." There was no statistical improvement in symptoms after settlement of litigation: 39% improved, 56% remained the same, and 5% worsened (all in the most severely symptomatic group). Gargan and Bannister's 8- to 12-year evaluation of the same group found that patients with more severe initial injuries continued to have more symptoms.[19] The authors of these studies concluded that settlement of litigation did not lead to significant symptom resolution or improvement.

Gore et al reported 10-year follow-up on 205 patients with neck pain (not all necessarily WAD), 58 (28%) of whom had filed personal injury claims.[21] Patients with more severe symptoms initially also tended to have more symptoms at follow-up regardless of the status of litigation. These findings were supported by Maimaris et al, who also proposed that a higher frequency of insurance claims in patients with continued symptoms likely reflected the severity of the injury.[36] In this study, approximately 50% of patients with symptoms more than 18 months had continued to have symptoms after completion of litigation. Pennie and Agambar also found no statistically significant difference in recovery between claimants and nonclaimants despite the fact that 81% of the 144 patients were claiming compensation.[49]

In 1993, Shapiro and Roth provided an excellent review of the effects of litigation on recovery from whiplash.[59] The authors concluded that the findings correlating litigation with outcome were equivocal and dependent in a large part on patient population and outcome criteria. For example, litigation appears to affect return to work in workers' compensation cases but not in other types of insurance claims.[65,66] The reader is referred to this review for an in-depth discussion. Since that time, several additional related studies have been reported.

Parmar and Raymakers reported that 91 of their 100 patients had settled their legal claims at a minimum 3-year follow-up: 58 were pain-free at the time of settlement, with a third of the remaining 33 patients demonstrating some improvement within 3 months after settlement.[47] Because most patients actually improved prior to settlement and only a third improved after settlement, the authors concluded that the timing of litigation was not associated with symptom improvement.

Schofferman and Wasserman completed a prospective, longitudinal, uncontrolled, descriptive study of 37 litigant patients aged 15 to 63 years treated for neck pain or low back pain after MVA but prior to settlement of litigation.[56] All patients were initially referred for specialty treatment a mean of 15 weeks post-MVA; none were involved in workers' compensation claims. After a mean 29 weeks of treatment, the authors reported significant improvements in pain and function scores and a reduction in medication use. Thirty-eight (97%) had returned to work. No patients had settled their claims during the study period. The authors concluded that a significant number of patients may improve despite litigation and that litigation status does not significantly impact outcome.

Recently, Mayou and Bryan reported no difference in any aspect of 1-year outcome between the two-thirds of patients who were claimants and those who were not.[39] In this study, the authors stated that it was "very obvious that the difficulties associated with legal proceeding were a cause of considerable worry, anger, and frustration which may have contributed to determining symptomatic and quality of life outcome."

In comparison to the studies discussed above, the literature concluding that litigation status is a major determinant of outcome in WADs is scarce.[14,22,26,30,56,59] Obelieniene et al published a prospective study of 210 Lithuanian subjects involved in rear-end collisions as identified in accident reports.[45] In Lithuania, there is no formal compensation system for injury and "little awareness about the potentially disabling consequences of whiplash." Subjects were contacted 1 week, 2 months, and 1 year post-MVA and asked about neck pain, headache, and low back pain. Responses were compared with an age- and sex-matched control group. None of the 210 MVA subjects stated that they had persistent or disabling symptoms caused by the car accident, and the authors found no significant differences between subjects and controls at any end point. The authors concluded that chronic symptoms after MVA may be related more to expectation of disability, family history, and attribution of preexisting conditions or symptoms to the accident rather than pathoanatomic injury. Other studies outside the medicolegal context, in Greece and Germany, have reported similar, excellent outcomes, with full recovery within weeks to months.[4,48]

In a large study by Cassidy et al in Saskatchewan, Canada, the incidence of injury claims decreased significantly when the law was changed from a tort compensation system for traffic injuries, which included payments for pain and suffering, to a no-fault system, which did not include such payments.[9] In addition to claim incidence decreasing by 28%, the median time to claim closure was reduced by more than 200 days. Pain intensity, level of physical functioning, and presence or absence of depressive symptoms were strongly associated with time to claim closure in both systems.[9]

In an often-quoted study, Gotten reported that 88% of 100 litigant patients with neck sprain "recovered" after settlement of litigation.[22] However, 46% still had some persistent symptoms (34% minor and 12% significant), and 3% of the total group continued to lose some work time after settlement of litigation. This study has been criticized due to significant design flaws, including lack of controls and incomplete follow-up.[30,56] Farbman reported a longer duration of symptoms in patients referred for independent medical examination who had retained a lawyer, but Farbman could not establish a direct causal relationship between litigation and poor outcome because of incomplete data.[14]

Gargan and Bannister did report that the amount of compensation and the time required to reach settlement correlated with symptom severity at long-term outcome a mean of 11 years postinjury.[19] However, the authors hypothesized that more severely injured individuals were involved in cases with larger settlements and more prolonged litigation. Several authors have correlated continued symptoms with protracted legal proceedings.[19,22,27] In Hohl's study, 50 (34%) of 146 patients were involved in litigation. At 5-year follow-up, 83% of those whose claims were settled in the first 6 months recovered, whereas only 38% of those whose claims were settled after 18 months were asymptomatic at follow-up, a statistically significant difference.[27] Hohl hypothesized that patients required to maintain the sick role may be more likely to have persistent symptoms.

Litigation is often a slow, laborious process. Settlements are prolonged, trials frequently postponed, and patients often continue to receive repeated evaluations and treatments throughout the pretrial process.[14,19,44] Average times to claims settlement have exceeded 2 years in some studies.[44] During this time, patients with continued symptoms may develop significant psychological disturbances independent of litigation status. Patients with chronic (>6 months), symptomatic WADs exhibit an increased prevalence of depression compared with head-injured subjects and a greater prevalence of anxiety, depression, and exaggerated pain responses compared with controls.[31] These findings are similar to those reported for chronic pain patients in general. Taylor et al compared 15 whiplash patients with 10 patients with moderate to severe head injury and 24 patients with chronic pain with neuropsychological testing.[67] The significant finding was less depression and pain in the head injury patients compared with the whiplash and chronic pain patients, who showed no difference. Whiplash injury patients with chronic pain also exhibited a characteristic psychological profile on the SCL-90R, similar to patients with rheumatoid arthritis and organic low back pain.[69] Uninformed, asymptomatic subjects were unable to "fake" this profile in a later study.[68]

Swartzman et al retrospectively examined the effect of civil litigation on pain and disability reports in whiplash patients.[65] Questionnaires were obtained from 41 current litigants and 21 post-litigants. Litigants reported more pain even after controlling for time since the accident and initial injury severity. Demographic characteristics, employment status, and psychological distress did not differ between groups. The authors proposed that litigation does not affect pain-related disability or psychological distress and that the stress of litigation itself may be important in explaining differences in reports of pain between current versus past litigants.

In summary, financial gain may not automatically result in symptom resolution, and there is no consistent evidence that monetary gain significantly affects outcome.[2] Many patients improve prior to settlement of litigation, and a significant number remain symptomatic after settlement. Several studies suggest that patients with more severe injuries are more likely to file compensation claims and have continued symptoms irrespective of the litigation status. These same patients with continued symptoms may develop a chronic pain state, and the stress and anxiety of the litigation process itself may complicate their situation. Early settlement, if feasible, may shorten the duration of symptoms and simplify treatment.[14,27] Improvement after litigation may not necessarily represent "compensation neurosis" but may reflect improvement in the stress and anxiety involved in the litigation process itself.[42]

WHIPLASH AND CERVICAL SPONDYLOSIS

Initial radiographic findings in whiplash-related injury may be minimal. The prognostic significance of preexisting or subsequent radiographic cervical spondylosis has been the subject of multiple studies. Many contain methodologic flaws previously discussed. In addition, most lack control groups, analysis for confounding variables, or consistent radiographic criteria to assess the presence or extent of "preexisting" spondylosis. Radiographic spondylosis is not rare in the age groups typically affected by WADs. Friedenberg and Miller reported radiographic spondylosis in up to 6% of asymptomatic 30- to 40-year-olds, with the prevalence increasing rapidly in older groups.[16] Furthermore, cervical curves are influenced by patient positioning, and up to 20% of normal controls may exhibit loss of cervical lordosis or kyphosis.[1,6,71]

Shortly after whiplash-related injury, Hohl reported prevalence of 35% for straight cervical curves and 9% for multisegment reversed cervical curves.[27] Both a sharp cervical lordotic reversal and single segment motion restriction on early flexion-extension films correlated with the development of radiographic spondylosis at 5-year follow-up. Thirty-nine percent of subjects demonstrated new radiographic spondylosis at that time. Changes were significantly more common in individuals who were older at the time of the initial injury (mean 31 vs 29 years). Hohl, however, reported no difference in outcome comparing those with versus without new spondylosis postinjury. Only single segment motion restriction seen on early flexion-extension views correlated with poor recovery. Although reports vary regarding an increased frequency of "new" spondylosis over controls postinjury, several recent reports generally support Hohl's hypothesis that the presence or development of spondylosis does not significantly predict outcome.[28,47,49]

In comparison, several researchers have associated poor clinical outcomes with spondylosis, reporting a higher prevalence of spondylosis in patients with continued symptoms.[36,44,53,70] It is certainly theoretically possible that symptoms from a previously asymptomatic cervical spondylosis are precipitated by trauma and are responsible for the continuing pain. It is generally accepted, for example, that a previously asymptomatic hip or knee with long-standing radiographic degenerative changes can become painful after an apparently minor injury. It seems reasonable to presume that a similar outcome can occur with so-called soft tissue strains to the cervical spine. Watkinson et al reported that

87% of patients with spondylosis on initial radiographs reported continued symptoms, compared with only 20% of patients with normal initial radiographs.[70] In this study, only 35 patients were reviewed, patients were generally older, and statistical controls for confounding variables were not discussed.

Maimaris et al reported a higher frequency of spondylotic changes on initial radiographs in individuals with persistent symptoms (51% vs 12%).[36] However, patients with persisting symptoms were an average of 9 years older at the time of initial injury. Radanov et al also reported a higher frequency of initial radiographic spondylosis comparing symptomatic (43%) and asymptomatic (19%) patients at 2 years.[53] Similar to the study of Maimaris et al, patients with persistent symptoms were also statistically significantly older. In further multiple regression analysis, radiographic changes were not found to independently predict prognosis at 1 year.[51,63] Bonucelli et al looked at MRI of the cervical spine in a group of 33 patients with persistent symptoms more than 6 months postinjury. Patients with abnormal MRI were more symptomatic, and the most common abnormality noted was preexistent spondylosis (58%).[5]

Miles et al reviewed radiographs in 73 patients aged 17 to 73 years (mean 37) with whiplash-related injuries and without osseous injury.[43] Approximately two-thirds had abnormal initial radiographs: 21% with spondylotic changes and 37% with acute angulation. Only spondylotic changes were statistically correlated to outcome. Prevertebral soft tissue swelling had little prognostic significance. Of note, 33% of the 15 patients with initial spondylosis had abnormal neurologic examinations. Neurologic findings are thought to represent an independent poor prognostic factor and may confound the results.[19,44] Furthermore, no patient younger than 35 years had initial spondylosis, suggesting a possible age-confounding effect. These factors were not specifically addressed in the study.

Watkinson et al and Norris and Watt reported that patients with the most severe injuries (motion loss and abnormal neurologic examinations) were more likely to exhibit abnormal x-rays than patients with less severe injuries.[44,70] Patients with grade III WAD were statistically more likely to have "abnormal curve patterns" than those with grades I or II WADs. Although patients with more severe injuries had a higher incidence of spondylosis and the authors suggest preexisting spondylosis is prognostic, no formal statistical analysis was presented. Norris and Watt demonstrated preexisting spondylosis in 27%, increasing to 67% after 10 years.

Pettersson et al measured radiographic sagittal canal diameter on 48 consecutive patients with acute whiplash-related injuries and reevaluated these patients 12 months postinjury.[50] The canal diameter was significantly smaller in patients with persistent symptoms. Pettersson et al hypothesized that smaller canal diameters may predispose to chronic symptoms after whiplash injuries. This finding is in some disagreement with that of Pennie and Agambar, who reported that spinal canal diameter was not related specifically to neurologic symptoms or signs postinjury; however, the studies are not directly comparable.[49] Interestingly, Pettersson et al found that females exhibited significantly smaller diameters than males, possibly supporting previous reports that females often exhibit more (although not necessarily statistically significant) symptoms after whiplash-related injuries.[12,27]

Many other factors have been studied in the radiographs of patients with WADs without osseous injury. The presence of congenital anomalous formations may be associated with an increased potential for incomplete recovery.[25] In addition, at least two studies have documented a gradual loss of cervical motion on follow-up flexion-extension views, suggesting possible residua of soft tissue injury.[28,70] This finding may be partially aging-related and was not associated with poor outcome in one study.[70] Changes in cervical curves have been mentioned previously. Hohl reported an association between a sharp curve reversal and subsequent spondylosis development but no effect on final outcome.[27] This finding was supported by Miles et al and Maimaris et al, who failed to find a significant association between curve reversal and prognosis, but not by Norris and Watt as discussed above.[36,43,44,70]

Matsumoto et al prospectively evaluated cervical curvature in 488 patients with acute whiplash injury and compared these with 495 asymptomatic healthy volunteers. They found no significant difference in the frequency of nonlordotic cervical curvature and local angular kyphosis between the two groups.[38]

In summary, the prognostic significance of radiographic findings in the absence of fracture or gross instability is unclear. Several studies have reported that the presence or development of spondylosis is not predictive of outcome.[24,27,28,47,49] Studies reporting associations between spondylosis and persistent symptoms are often confounded by lack of control for age or injury severity.[36,43,70] Spondylosis was not a predictive factor in the model proposed by Radanov et al.[51-54] A deeply lordotic or flat cervical curve is a normal variant and not necessarily predictive of outcome.[27,36,38] There are insufficient data to predict outcome based on cervical spondylosis independent of age and injury severity factors. Single segment motion restriction, small canal diameter, and congenital abnormalities may be associated with poor outcome, but this awaits further prospective confirmation.

CONCLUSIONS

Symptoms after whiplash-type injuries are common. Most patients will recover within the first weeks to months postinjury, with little clinically significant recovery occurring after 1 to 2 years postinjury. Some patients with WADs never completely recover, with 25%±15% experiencing ongoing symptoms, approximately a third of which may be severe or constant. Despite associations of multiple factors with outcome, our ability to predict outcome in individual patients remains limited and deserves further study. Injury severity appears to be important but often difficult to quantify. Preexisting spondylosis does not appear to predict outcome independent of age and injury severity. The relationship between litigation proceedings and outcome is complex. However, it is important for clinicians to understand that ongoing litigation does not necessarily preclude meaningful recovery.

References

1. Babcock JL: Cervical spine injuries. Diagnosis and classification. Arch Surg 111:646–651, 1976.
2. Barnsley L, Lord S, Bogduk N: Whiplash injury. Pain 58:283–307, 1994.
3. Bogduk N: Post whiplash syndrome. Aust Fam Physician 23:2303–2307, 1994.
4. Bonk AD, Ferrari R, Giebel GD, et al: Prospective, randomized, controlled study of activity versus collar, and the natural history for whiplash injury, in Germany. J Muscle Pain 8:123–132, 2000.

5. Bonuccelli U, Pavese N, Lucetti C, et al: Late whiplash syndrome: a clinical and magnetic resonance imaging study. Funct Neurol 14:219–225, 1999.
6. Borden AR, Rechtman A, Gershon-Cohen J: The normal cervical lordosis. Radiology 74:806–809, 1960.
7. Bovim G, Schrader H, Sand T: Neck pain in the general population. Spine 19:1307–1309, 1994.
8. Brison R, Hartling L, Pickett W: A prospective study of acceleration-extension injuries following rear-end motor vehicle collisions. J Muscle Pain 8:97–113, 2000.
9. Cassidy JD, Carroll LJ, Cote P, et al: Effect of eliminating compensation for pain and suffering on the outcome of insurance claims for whiplash injury [see comments]. N Engl J Med 342:1179–1186, 2000.
10. Cole ES: Psychiatric aspects of compensable injury. Med J Aust 2:93–100, 1970.
11. Crowe H: Whiplash injuries of the cervical spine. In Proceedings of the Section of Insurance Negligence and Compensation Law. Chicago, American Bar Association, 1958, pp 176–184.
12. Deans GT, Magalliard JN, Kerr M, Rutherford WH: Neck sprain—a major cause of disability following car accidents. Injury 18:10–12, 1987.
13. DePalma AF, Subin DK: Study of the cervical syndrome. Clin Orthop 38:135–142, 1965.
14. Farbman AA: Neck sprain. Associated factors. JAMA 223:1010–1015, 1973.
15. Freeman MD, Croft AC, Rossignol AM: "Whiplash associated disorders: redefining whiplash and its management" by the Quebec Task Force. A critical evaluation. Spine 23:1043–1049, 1998.
16. Friedenberg ZM, Miller W: Degenerative changes in the cervical spine: a comparative study of asymptomatic and symptomatic patients. J Bone Joint Surg Am 45:1171–1178, 1963.
17. Galasko CSB, Murray PA, Pitcher M: Prevalence and long-term disability following whiplash-associated disorder. J Muscle Pain 8:15–27, 2000.
18. Gargan M, Bannister G, Main C, Hollis S: The behavioural response to whiplash injury. J Bone Joint Surg Br 79:523–526, 1997.
19. Gargan MF, Bannister GC: Long-term prognosis of soft-tissue injuries of the neck. J Bone Joint Surg Br 72:901–903, 1990.
20. Gay JA, Abott K: Common whiplash injuries of the neck. JAMA 152:1698, 1953.
21. Gore DR, Sepic SB, Gardner GM, Murray MP: Neck pain: a long-term follow-up of 205 patients. Spine 12:1–5, 1987.
22. Gotten N: Survey of 100 cases of whiplash injury after settlement of litigation. JAMA 162:865–867, 1956.
23. Greenfield J, Ilfeld FW: Acute cervical strain. Evaluation and short term prognostic factors. Clin Orthop 122:196–200, 1977.
24. Hildingsson C, Toolanen G: Outcome after soft-tissue injury of the cervical spine. A prospective study of 93 car-accident victims. Acta Orthop Scand 61:357–359, 1990.
25. Hirsch S, Hirsch P, Hiramoto H: Whiplash syndrome: fact or fiction. Orthop Clin North Am 19:791–795, 1988.
26. Hirschfeld AB, Behan R: The accident process. JAMA 186:193–199, 1963.
27. Hohl M: Soft-tissue injuries of the neck in automobile accidents. Factors influencing prognosis. J Bone Joint Surg Am 56:1675–1682, 1974.
28. Jonsson H Jr, Cesarini K, Sahlstedt B, Rauschning W: Findings and outcome in whiplash-type neck distortions. Spine 19:2733–2743, 1994.
29. Karlsborg M, Smed A, Jespersen H, et al: A prospective study of 39 patients with whiplash injury. Acta Neurol Scand 95:65–72, 1997.
30. LaBan M: Whiplash: its evaluation and treatment. Phys Med Rehabil State Art Rev 4:293–307, 1990.
31. Lee J, Giles K, Drummond PD: Psychological disturbances and an exaggerated response to pain in patients with whiplash injury. J Psychosom. Res 37:105–110, 1993.
32. Leopold R, Dillon H: Psychiatric considerations in whiplash injuries of the neck. Pa Med 63:385–389, 1960.
33. Macnab I: Acceleration injuries of the cervical spine. J Bone Joint Surg 46:1797–1799, 1964.
34. Macnab I: The whiplash syndrome. Orthop Clin North Am. 2:389–403, 1971.
35. Magnusson T: Extracervical symptoms after whiplash trauma. Cephalalgia 14:223-227; discussion 181–182, 1994.
36. Maimaris C, Barnes MR, Allen MJ: 'Whiplash injuries' of the neck: a retrospective study. Injury 19:393–396, 1988.
37. Marshall PD, O'Connor M, Hodgkinson JP: The perceived relationship between neck symptoms and precedent injury. Injury 26:17–19, 1995.
38. Matsumoto M, Fujimura Y, Suzuki N: Cervical curvature in acute whiplash injuries: prospective comparative study with asymptomatic subjects. Injury 29:775–778, 1998.

39. Mayou R, Bryant B: Outcome of 'whiplash' neck injury. Injury 27:617-623, 1996.
40. McKinney LA: Early mobilisation and outcome in acute sprains of the neck. Br Med J 299:1006–1008, 1989.
41. Mealy K, Brennan H, Fenelon GCC: Early mobilization of acute whiplash injuries. Br Med J 292:656–657, 1986.
42. Merskey H: Psychiatry and the cervical sprain syndrome. Can Med Assoc J 130:1119–1121, 1984.
43. Miles KA, Maimaris C, Finlay D, Barnes MR: The incidence and prognostic significance of radiological abnormalities in soft tissue injuries to the cervical spine. Skeletal Radiol 17:493–496, 1988.
44. Norris SH, Watt I: The prognosis of neck injuries resulting from rear-end vehicle collisions. J Bone Joint Surg Br 65:608–611, 1983.
45. Obelieniene D, Schrader H, Bovim G, et al: Pain after whiplash: a prospective controlled inception cohort study. J Neurol Neurosurg Psychiatry 66:279–283, 1999.
46. Olivegren H, Jerkvall N, Hagstrom Y, Carlsson J: The long-term prognosis of whiplash-associated disorders (WAD). Eur Spine J 8:366–370, 1999.
47. Parmar HV, Raymakers R: Neck injuries from rear impact road traffic accidents: prognosis in persons seeking compensation. Injury 24:75–78, 1993.
48. Partheni M, Constantoyannis C, Ferrari R, et al: A prospective cohort study of the outcome of acute whiplash injury in Greece. Clin Exp Rheumatol 18:67–70, 2000.
49. Pennie B, Agambar L: Patterns of injury and recovery in whiplash. Injury 22:57–59, 1991.
50. Pettersson K, Karrholm J, Toolanen G, Hildingsson C: Decreased width of the spinal canal in patients with chronic symptoms after whiplash injury. Spine 20:1664–1667, 1995.
51. Radanov BP, Sturzenegger M: Predicting recovery from common whiplash. Eur Neurol 36:48–51, 1996.
52. Radanov BP, Sturzenegger M, De Stefano G, Schnidrig A: Relationship between early somatic, radiological, cognitive and psychosocial findings and outcome during a one-year follow-up in 117 patients suffering from common whiplash. Br J Rheumatol 33:442–448, 1994.
53. Radanov BP, Sturzenegger M, Di Stefano G: Long-term outcome after whiplash injury. A 2-year follow-up considering features of injury mechanism and somatic, radiologic, and psychosocial findings. Medicine 74:281–297, 1995.
54. Radanov BP, Sturzenegger M, Di Stefano G, et al: Factors influencing recovery from headache after common whiplash. Br Med J 307:652–655, 1993.
55. Satoh S, Naito S, Konishi T, et al: An examination of reasons for prolonged treatment in Japanese patients with whiplash injuries. J Muscle Pain 5:71–84, 1997.
56. Schofferman J, Wasserman S: Successful treatment of low back pain and neck pain after a motor vehicle accident despite litigation. Spine 19:1007–1010, 1994.
57. Schrader H, Obelieniene D, Bovim G, et al: Natural evolution of late whiplash syndrome outside the medicolegal context. Lancet 347:1207–1211, 1996.
58. Schutt CH, Dohan FC: Neck injury to women in auto accidents. A metropolitan plague. JAMA 206:2689–2692, 1968.
59. Shapiro A, Roth R: The effect of litigation on recovery from whiplash. Spine State Art Rev 7:531–556, 1993.
60. Smed A: Cognitive function and distress after common whiplash injury. Acta Neurol Scand 95:73–80, 1997.
61. Spitzer WO, Skovron ML, Salmi LR, et al: Scientific monograph of the Quebec Task Force on Whiplash-Associated Disorders: redefining "whiplash" and its management. Spine 20(suppl):1S–73S, 1995.
62. Squires B, Gargan MF, Bannister GC: Soft-tissue injuries of the cervical spine. 15-year follow-up. J Bone Joint Surg Br 78 6:955–957, 1996.
63. Sturzenegger M, Radanov BP, Di Stefano G: The effect of accident mechanisms and initial findings on the long-term course of whiplash injury. J Neurol 242:443–449, 1995.
64. Suissa S, Harder S, Veilleux M: The Quebec whiplash-associated disorders cohort study. Spine 20(suppl):12S–20S, 1995.
65. Swartzman LC, Teasell RW, Shapiro AP, McDermid AJ: The effect of litigation status on adjustment to whiplash injury. Spine 21:53–58, 1996.
66. Talo S, Hendler N, Brodie J: Effects of active and completed litigation on treatment results: workers' compensation patients compared with other litigation patients. J Occup Med 31:265–269, 1989.
67. Taylor AE, Cox CA, Mailis A: Persistent neuropsychological deficits following whiplash: evidence for chronic mild traumatic brain injury? Arch Phys Med Rehabil 77:529–535, 1996.

68. Wallis BJ, Bogduk N: Faking a profile: can naive subjects simulate whiplash responses? Pain 66:223–227, 1996.
69. Wallis BJ, Lord SM, Barnsley L, Bogduk N: Pain and psychologic symptoms of Australian patients with whiplash. Spine 21:804–810, 1996.
70. Watkinson A, Gargan MF, Bannister GC: Prognostic factors in soft tissue injuries of the cervical spine. Injury 22:2307–309, 1991.
71. Weir DC: Roentgenographic signs of cervical injury. Clin Orthop 109:9–17, 1975.
72. Weiss HD, Stern BJ, Goldberg J: Post-traumatic migraine: chronic migraine precipitated by minor head or neck trauma. Headache 31:451–456, 1991.
73. White AA III, Johnson RM, Panjabi MM, Southwick WO: Biomechanical analysis of clinical stability in the cervical spine. Clin Orthop 109:85–96, 1975.

6

New Concepts in Head Restraint Technology in the Prevention of Whiplash Injury

Ronald P. Dellanno, D.C.

In the mid 1950s, padded head restraints added to the top of car seats were proposed to reduce injuries incurred during rear-end collisions. The work of Macnab[7] and Mertz and Patrick[8] suggested that the primary mechanism of injury in rear-end impacts was hyperextension of the head on the cervical spine. This theory was accepted and acted upon. The National Highway Traffic Safety Administration made it a requirement for all cars made in the United States to have head restraints. Federal Motor Vehicle Safety Standard 202 made this official in 1969, and it has remained unchanged.

In the mid 1990s, several automotive manufacturers attempted to develop more efficient designs that are higher and closer to the back of the head. This was done to prevent hyperextension of the head and neck and to conform to what was believed to be a good head restraint position. However, in an accident analysis study[9] conducted by the Transport Research Laboratory, Berkshire, United Kingdom, and the University of Manchester, Hope Hospital, Manchester, United Kingdom, the benefits of good head restraint positioning could not be clearly demonstrated. The data in rear-end collisions, where the benefits of a well-positioned head restraint should have been clear, indicated that a larger distance from head to restraint was associated with lower disability. This study suggests that other injury mechanisms are at work during whiplash.

TWO FAULTY PREMISES REGARDING WHIPLASH INJURY EVALUATION

Two faulty premises currently exist regarding evaluation of rear-end, low-speed collisions. The first faulty premise is that the Hybrid III Dummy series are biofedelic. They simply do not have humanlike flexibility; nor do they posses the most often injured anatomy: zygapophyseal joints, discs, paraspinal muscles, and ligaments.[10]

The second faulty premise is that whiplash injury is caused by a typical hyperextension movement of the head and neck. In the normal extension movement, the head rotates on the vertebra below C1, C1 rotates over the instantaneous axis of rotation[6] of C2, and then C2 rotates on the C3 instantaneous axis of rotation, and so on until the entire cervical spine completes its full extension motion. In rear-end collisions, this pattern of extension motion does not occur; rather, a completely unnatural motion is observed when high-speed x-ray is used to observe human aberrant spinal kinematic motion. Matshushita6 observed axial loading from thoracic spine[4] straightening, causing impaction of the cervical facet plates above and, then, hyperextension of the lower cervical vertebrae rotating and compressing each vertebra from under the vertebra above. This is initiated by the seat back, which is sweeping the lower portion of the neck under the upper portion of the neck. This results in an abnormal double harmonic curve in the cervical spine often referred to as the dreaded "S" curve.[3] (see Fig. 3A).

WHIPLASH TESTING PROTOCOL

The currently available methods of evaluating rear-end impact injury include human volunteers, cadavers, finite-element modeling, and Hybrid III dummies. The least reliable modality appears to be the Hybrid III Dummy series. The disadvantage of Hybrid III Dummy testing is that the dummies were designed for front- and side-impact collisions but not rear-end impact. They also are especially poor at detecting changes in low-speed crashes because of their rigid construction. (Fig. 1). Lastly, they lack human anatomic analogs such as discs, ligaments, zygapophyseal joints, cervical lordosis, and the sensors to measure potential injury in these structures.[10] Unfortunately, these Hybrid III dummies are currently the primary testing tools the automotive industry uses to evaluate whiplash injury.

Cadavers, when observed under high-speed cineradiography, will reveal data on global kinematic behavior and localized joint data from surgically implanted sensors. Unfortunately, cadaver availability is always a constraint in this type of testing. Cadavers also have degenerative joint disease and overall poor tissue compliance that skews the accuracy because consistent detailed data are dependent on healthy tissue specimens.

Human volunteers provide real-life evidence of global kinematics of whiplash injury and follow-up assessment. Occupant awareness can marginally skew the data because in rear-end collisions passengers are usually unaware of impending impact. This testing method has obvious ethical concerns but is perhaps the most reliable.

Finite-element model rear-end crash simulation offers several significant advantages in the evaluation of whiplash potential. Humanlike anatomy is

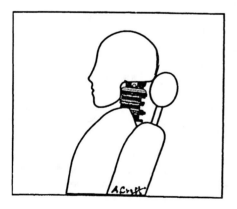

Figure 1. The Hybrid III dummy has no facet joints, discs, ligaments, muscles, or cervical lordosis. (Adapted from Croft A, Foreman S: Whiplash Injuries: The Cervical Acceleration/Deceleration Syndrome, 2nd ed. Baltimore, Williams & Wilkins, 1995.)

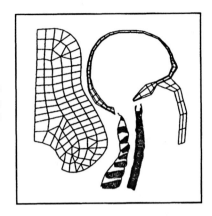

Figure 2. The Wayne State University Finite Element Model of the human neck features the complete anatomy as well as sensors to measure forces of whiplash at each vertebra.

programmed into the model. This includes the zygapophyseal joints, discs, paraspinal ligaments, muscles, normal cervical lordosis, and the sensors to evaluate each segment of the cervical spine. It is relatively cost-effective versus the other testing modalities and provides consistent test parameters, yielding force data at each vertebral unit (Fig. 2).

In summary, all testing methods have advantages and disadvantages. Using them in combination and applying what is learned in conjunction with the clinical scenarios encountered in practice will enhance the overall understanding of this phenomenon. This will ultimately be useful in the development of technologies that mitigate the tissue damage associated with whiplash injuries.

PATHOPHYSIOLOGY OF WHIPLASH INJURY: NEW CONCEPTS

Lord et al[5] contributed to the understanding of injury mechanism by identifying the zygapophyseal joint as the source of pain in 54% of patients with chronic neck pain after whiplash injury. With the zygapophyseal joint identified as the primary injury site, the next development was observation of what happened to these cervical joints during the rear-end impact event on human volunteers. This was accomplished with cineradiography. Kaneoka et al[4] observed significant aberration in motion during rear-end impact, resulting in facet plate collision and impingement. Increased shear force and extension motion to the lower cervical vertebra was observed while the upper portion of the cervical spine followed the head into flexion, giving the formation of an "S" curve (Fig. 3A). The transition area of the S curve was at the level of C4, C5, and C6, the most common injury sites observed in a whiplash victim in postaccident x-ray analysis[1] (Fig. 3B).

PREVENTION OF WHIPLASH IN REAR-END COLLISIONS

Many variables can influence the forces to the spine that can cause injury: the size of the vehicles, the size of the occupants, and the speeds of the vehicles. Attempting to prevent whiplash injury thus can be a daunting task. However, reducing the global movement of the entire spine and the relative movement of each vertebra would seem to be the most practical approach in the prevention of injury to the spine. To accomplish this, all spinal curves should be supported and decelerated at as close to a zero delta velocity as possible. This

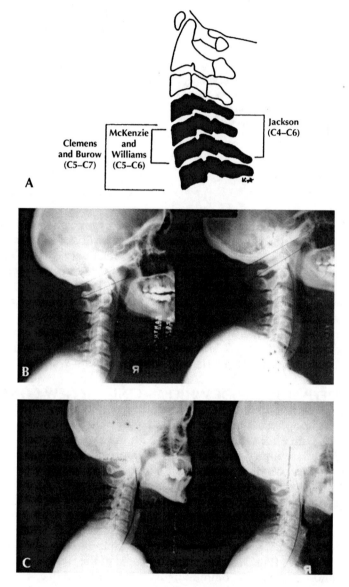

Figure 3.　**A,** Most researchers have found that the lower cervical spine sustains the greatest amount of damage in the acceleration/deceleration injury. (Adapted from Croft A, Foreman S: Whiplash Injuries: The Cervical Acceleration/Deceleration Syndrome, 2nd ed. Baltimore, Willims & Wilkins 1995.) **B,** The left x-ray was taken after a rear-end collision; note the S curve. The right x-ray shows correction into lordosis. Vehicle headrests that only provide head support are not designed to support the neck during impact. **C,** The left x-ray is that of a 51-year-old woman who was in a rear-end collision 4 years previously; note loss of the lordotic curve. The patient suffered chronic neck pain and headache after the accident. The right x-ray shows correction of the S-shaped spine. The S-shape of the cervical spine is observed via high-speed x-ray of the human spine during rear-end impact. This patient's headrest had no neck support.

would require support systems within head-neck restraints and seats that are contoured to the spine to reduce the spinal straightening observed during rear-end impact.[6]

Additionally, the head-neck restraint and seat back should have complementary dampening characteristics so that simultaneous deceleration of the head, neck, thoracic, and lumbopelvic areas can be achieved.

These two components (head-neck restraint and seat back contour) make up the entire sitting apparatus and are the last line of defense against external intrusion forces. In combination they offer occupants the maximum protection in the interior of the vehicle. A system[2] has been developed with a plastically deforming crush zone behind a stiff pectin wall that supports the thoracic spine in combination with an anatomically supportive head-neck restraint. Protection of the thoracic spine is considered important because flattening is observed in conjunction with cervical spine straightening and may be a significant factor in initiating cervical whiplash injury. In this seating system, the stiff concave pectin wall acts as a dome that protects the thoracic kyphosis, and the crush zone material behind it acts to absorb energy that will disperse impact forces and reduce the injury potential. The crush zone material also dampens the impact to the cervical spine as the thoracic kyphosis presses into the seat back. This allows the head and neck to decelerate with the thoracic spine and reduce injury caused by relative differences in head-neck–thoracic spine velocities (Fig. 4).

A SAFER HEAD-NECK RESTRAINT SYSTEM

A good restraint system should prevent excessive head and neck kinematics during rear-end collisions. The head-neck restraint should be high enough to

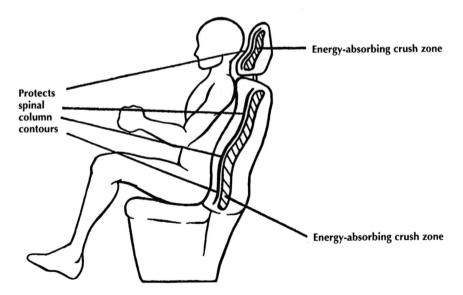

Figure 4. As the thoracic spine presses into the seat back, the head and neck move rearward and are supported by the contoured head-neck restraint.

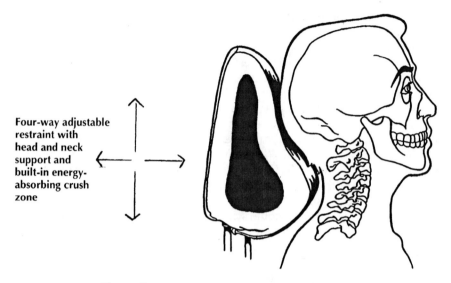

Figure 5. Apparatus for preventing whiplash.

prevent the head of the occupant from accelerating over the top of the restraint and close enough to the back of the head and neck to prevent an excessive hyperextension and shear. A head restraint should have a neck contour to enable support of the cervical lordosis; hence the new term *head-neck restraint* (Fig. 5). The neck support was developed to prevent the cervical zygapophyseal joints from excessive stress by reducing the straightening of the cervical lordosis that occurs during rear-end collisions.[4,6]

This hypothesis has been supported by test simulations using the Wayne State University human neck model[11] to compare the performance of a contoured head-neck restraint with a standard head restraint system. These simulations were done with the restraint systems in both full up and full down positions. This means the restraint was vertically adjusted in its lowest and highest positions. The contoured head-neck restraint system reduced capsular ligament stretch and intervertebral disc shear load significantly better at all cervical levels (Table l).

A restraint system should have enough adjustability to accommodate a broad range of occupant sizes and should lock in place. The evolution of a head restraint to a head-neck restraint system should result in an improvement in mitigation of injuries from rear-end collisions.

Table 1A.   Rear-End Crash Simulations*

Forces on Neck Joints	Cervigard Contoured Restraint Vs. Standard Head Restraint
Facet capsular ligament stretch	Much better
Intervertebral disc shear load	Better
Intervertebral disc axial load	As good

* Wayne State University Finite Element Model of the human neck.

Table IB. Facet Joint Peak Force

Joint	Standard Down	Standard Up	Cervigard Down	Cervigard Up
	(kN)	(kN)	(kN)	(kN)
C2-C3	0.287	0.302	0.160	0.070
C3-C4	0.289	0.328	0.160	0.061
C4-C5	0.293	0.339	0.163	0.117
C5-c6	0.291	0.291	0.291	0.243
C6-C7	0.673	0.673	0.673	0.621
C7-TI	0.617	0.617	0.617	0.565

CONCLUSION

Future developments in reducing whiplash injuries should focus on a cooperative effort between clinical researchers, treating physicians, and automotive engineers. All aspects of this substantial health hazard need to be fully explored. The bridge between engineering efforts and human anatomy and physiology requires a thorough perspective to resolve this difficult problem.

References

1. Croft A, Foreman S: Whiplash Injuries: The Cervical Acceleration/Deceleration Syndrome, 2nd ed. Baltimore, Williams & Wilkins, 1995.
2. Dellanno RP: U.S. patent No. 5,580,124: issued December 3, 1996; U.S. patent No. 5,769,489: issued June 23, 1998.
3. Grauer JN, Panjabi MM, Cholewicki J, et al: Whiplash produces an S-shaped curvature of the neck with hyperextension at lower levels. Spine 22:2489–2494, 1997.
4. Kaneoka K, Ono K, Inami S, Hayashi K: Motion analysis of cervical vertebrae during whiplash loading. Spine 24:763–776, 1999.
5. Lord S, Barnsley L, Bogduk N: Cervical zygapophyseal joint pain in whiplash. Spine 20:20–25, 1995.
6. Matsushita T, Sato TB, Hirabayashi K, et al: X-ray study of the human neck motion due to head inertia loading. Proceedings of the 38th Stapp Car Crash Conference. Society of Automotive Engineers, Warrendale, PA, 1994; paper No. 942208.
7. Macnab I: Whiplash injuries of the neck. Proceedings of the Annual Meeting of the American Association of Automotive Medicine 11-15 AAAM, Lake Bluff, IL, 1965.
8. Mertz HJ, Patrick LM: Investigation of the kinematics and kinetics of whiplash. Society of Automotive Engineers, Warrendale, PA, 1967; SAE technical paper 670919.
9. Mintin R: Accident Analysis and Prevention 32 (177-185). Pergamon, Transport Research Laboratory, Crowthorne, Berkshire, United Kingdom, 2000.
10. Steffan H, Dippel CH, Muser MH, et al: Comparison of head-neck kinematics during rear end impact between standard Hybrid III, rid neck, volunteers and PMTO's. International Research Council on Biokinetics of Impact, Bron, France, 1995; paper No. 1995-13-0018.
11. Yang, King H Zhu, Fuchun. Luan, Feng, Zhao, Longmao,Begement, Paul C: Development of a finite element model of the human neck. 42nd Strapp Car Crash Conference. Tempe, AZ, 1998; SAE No. 983157.

7

The Clinical Picture
of Whiplash Injuries

*Robert W. Teasell, M.D., FRCPC,
and Allan P. Shapiro, Ph.D.*

Whiplash injuries remain a significant public health problem throughout the developed industrialized world. In many countries, states, and provinces, this problem has had significant socioeconomic consequences leading to controversial management strategies aimed primarily at cost containment or limiting the economic consequences. The scientific literature has recently coalesced around two themes: one aimed at justifying the above strategy and the second focused on determining the pathophysiology of chronic whiplash.

The Quebec Task Force (QTF)[85] adopted the following definition of whiplash: "Whiplash is an acceleration-deceleration mechanism of energy transfer to the neck. It may result from rear-end or side-impact motor vehicle collisions, but can also occur during diving or other mishaps. The impact may result in bony or soft tissue injuries (whiplash injuries), which in turn may lead to a variety of clinical manifestations."[85] Typically, the injured individual is the occupant of a stationary vehicle that is struck from behind,[7,21,29,43,56,65] although injury frequently occurs following side-on and head-on collisions.[21]

INCIDENCE AND NATURAL HISTORY
The incidence of claims for whiplash is 1 to 6 per 1,000 population per year,[5,15] with the variance being most easily explainable by the criteria for making a claim and the ease in doing so. Not all victims of motor vehicle accidents develop symptoms, and most symptomatic patients do not become chronic. After acute injury, most patients rapidly recover; some 80% of those who seek help are asymptomatic by 12 months.[78] After 12 months, only 15–20% of patients remain symptomatic, and only about 5% are severely affected. The latter, however, constitute the major burden to insurance companies and to health care resources, and most treatment strategies attempt to reduce this latter number.

A critical element of the debate regarding pathophysiology revolves around the normal anticipated time for musculoligamentous healing to occur. The QTF noted: "Apart from anatomic studies, much of the scientific understanding of soft tissue injury and healing is derived from animal models, and there is little information on the normal recuperation period. In the animal model of soft tissue healing, there is a brief period (less than 72 hours) of acute inflammation and reaction, followed by a period of repair and regeneration (approximately 72 hours to up to 6 weeks), and finally by a period of remodeling and rematuration that can last up to 1 year."[85] As mentioned earlier, the applicability of these animal studies to humans becomes suspect when one considers common musculoskeletal sports injuries involving the rotator cuff or internal derangement of the knee. Although these injuries usually heal rapidly, some persist and, in the case of many professional athletes, may be career-ending despite access to first-rate medical care. Despite this evidence that not all soft tissue injuries heal, curiously the persistence of pain in a certain percentage of patients with whiplash injuries has remained a source of controversy, although this debate rarely occurs outside medicolegal disputes.

Barnsley et al[5] have argued that whiplash patients can be roughly divided into two groups: those who recover rapidly and those whose symptoms persist indefinitely. This type of pattern is not unlike that seen following a knee and ankle sprain, where most of the injuries heal rapidly while a small but significant number continue to have persistent pain that may necessitate surgical intervention or be intractable to treatment. The same authors note: "Tears of muscles and ligaments...would cause pain. Analogous with injuries to these tissues elsewhere in the body, and being vascular structures, they would be expected to heal over several weeks with scar formation and loss of pain. Such a pattern would be consistent with those patients who quickly recover after whiplash injury."[5] However, there remains a group with chronic symptoms, and only recently has this group been more carefully studied with regard to pathophysiology.

Importantly, the point at which patients enter a study designed to look at the natural history of whiplash will greatly influence the outcome. Some studies[85] have tried unsuccessfully to use insurance claims as a proxy for incidence, although this has obvious limitations. Table 1 provides a conservative estimate of the natural history of whiplash based on two studies,[77,82] beginning with collisions for which it has been estimated that one in four or five collisions results in some initial neck pain. In the Lithuanian study by Schrader et al,[82] based upon a retrospective questionnaire, this number was only 15%, likely a result of the timing of the questionnaire and the fact that virtually all of the individuals who were in the cars and answered the questionnaire were men, which would be anticipated to produce a lower percentage. Using retrospective questionnaires, Schrader et al[82] looked at individuals involved in rear-end collisions and then determined whether they had been injured. Only 15% had initial neck

Table 1.   Estimated Number of Patients with Initial and Continuing
Symptomatology After a Motor Vehicle Collision*[77,82]

Neck Pain After Collision	Estimated No. Patients
Initially	200–250
1 wk	60–75
3 mo	26–34
6 mo	19–24
1 y	15–19
2 y	11–14
Total Collisions	1,000

* Usually a rear-end collision

Table 2. Studies of Whiplash Natural History

Authors and Location	Study Population and Study Methods	Outcomes Measured	Results
Hildingsson and Toolanen,[41] Sweden	Prospective study. Whiplash patients attending an acute orthopedic clinic.	Continuing pain.	30% recovered by 3 mo, 52% by 1 y, and 38% by 2 y. Selection bias a concern.
Gargan and Bannister,[32] Britain	Prospective study. Whiplash patients attending an emergency department.	Continuing pain.	42% reportedly asymptomatic at 2-y follow-up while 57% reported symptoms not interfering with work. ? selection bias.
Radanov et al,[77] Switzerland	Prospective study. 164 whiplash patients referred to the study by family doctors and carefully evaluated within 10 d of the injury; 27 did not meet study criteria and 20 dropped out at 6 mo; 117 subjects (74 women and 43 men) completed the study at 1 y.	Continuing pain and return to work.	56% reported asymptomatic at 3 mo, 69% at 6 mo, 76% at 1 y, 82% at 2 y. 96% had returned to work at 2 y. Selection bias a concern.
QTF cohort study,[85] Quebec, Canada	Retrospective study. Cohort of 2,810 subjects who submitted claims of injury to SAAQ with no previous history of motor vehicle accident–related injury. Excluded patients who did not have adequate police records, suffered other injuries, or suffered "recurrences" of symptoms.	Recovery defined as no longer receiving insurance payments.	Cumulative "recovery" rates were 22% within 1 wk, 53% within 4 wk, 64% within 60 d, 87% by 6 mo, 87% by 6 mo, and 97% by 1 y. When recurrences are added (they were excluded from the data set) the recovery rate at 1 y may only be 90%. Did not measure symptomatic recovery but simply when individuals were no longer receiving compensation payments (presumably because they were deemed able to return to work).
Schraeder et al,[82] Lithuania	Retrospective study. Police accident records used to identify 202 individuals involved in rear-end collisions 1-3 y previously. Compared to randomly selected age- and sex-matched population control. Patients sent a retrospective questionnaire. Because the study had too many men, 30 female passengers were specifically recruited for the study.	Neck/back pain, head-headache memory/concentration problems initially and at 1 y.	31 of the 202 accident subjects who responded to the questionnaire reported initial pain; only 9 reported pain persisting a week or more. No patients had chronic disabling symptoms (95% CI, 0%-10%). Male to female ratio was 4:1. Two accident subjects and three controls controls reported long-term symptoms. Male to female ratio is very high in study, which did not have sufficient power to draw any conclusions. Questionnaire instrument has yet to be validated.

(Table continued on next page.)

Table 2. Studies of Whiplash Natural History *(Continued)*

Authors and Location	Study Population and Study Methods	Outcomes Measured	Results
Cassidy et al,[15] Saskatchewan, Canada	Prospective study. Comparison of all Saskatchewan whiplash claims 6 mo before the introduction of no-fault and for 12 mo after. Patients filled out a base-line questionnaire and 6 wk and 4, 8, and 12 mo after the collision.	Measured number of days to claim closure. Intensity of neck, head, and other pain. Health-rated quality of life and depression.	7,462 claimants met criteria for whiplash injuries. 28% reduction in claims under no-fault. The median time to claim closure during tort was 433 d to 194 and 203 d during the two 6-mo no-fault periods. The intensity of neck pain, the level of physical functioning, and the presence or absence of depressive symptoms strongly associated with time to claim closure. Claim closure was defined differently for tort and no-fault groups. Study was unblinded, potentially biasing outcome. 28% of study reopenings excluded from study.

pain, as mentioned above. Although more than 200 subjects were studied, the actual number with initial whiplash pain was only 31 and, at 1 week, only 9. In contrast, Radanov et al[77] studied 117 patients with pain who were studied prospectively from 1 week after injury, on average. These differences must be taken into account when comparing these two studies; the one study[77] has the statistical power to support its conclusions while the other[82] does not.

PREVALENCE OF WHIPLASH

Barnsley et al[5] have noted that based upon the incidence and natural history of whiplash it is possible to determine the prevalence of whiplash injuries in the population. It was determined that the prevalence would be 1% with chronic whiplash pain and 0.4% with severe chronic pain as a result of a whiplash injury.[3] To detect such a small percentage with acceptable confidence limits would mean sampling about 1,000 individuals.[5] Barnsley et al also noted: "The longest follow-up has been that of a cohort of 61 patients first seen between 1977 and 1980 at the Bristol Royal Infirmary. These patients have been the subjects of reports of their status at 2, 10.8 and 15 years after initial injury.[31,69,86] Some 19% of patients remain with severe symptoms at 2 years, diminishing to 12% and 10% by 10.8 years and 15 years, respectively. The confidence limits, however, indicate that, in other samples, these figures could be as low as 9%, 2% and 1%, respectively, or as high as 29%, 22%, and 19%."[5]

PHYSICAL FACTORS AS PREDICTORS OF CHRONIC SYMPTOMATOLOGY

Further evidence supporting a physical basis for chronic whiplash pain comes from a prospective study that suggests "physical" but not "psychological" factors predict nonresolution of whiplash pain. In a prospective study of

Table 3. Review of Cohort Studies of Whiplash Patients

Time Since Motor Vehicle Accident	QTF: Spitzer et al[85]*	Gargan and Bannister[32]†	Radanov et al[78]†	Hildingsson et al[41]†
3 mo	70%	30%	56%	—
6 mo	87%	—	69%	—
1 y	97%	52%	76%	—
2 y	—	38%	82% 96%‡	42% 57%‡

* Claim no longer compensated.
† Asymptomatic.
‡ Not interfering with work.

whiplash mentioned above, 117 patients were recruited through family physicians in Switzerland; 164 consecutive patients were referred, 27 did not meet study criteria, and 20 dropped out at 6 months.[77] The remaining 117 patients underwent neurologic evaluation and a semistructured interview and completed various self-report questionnaires including ratings of mood, cognitive function, and personality inventories within 10 days (mean 7.4 days) of injury. A total of 31% of patients remained symptomatic at 6 months. There were no significant differences between symptomatic and asymptomatic patients on baseline assessment of premorbid psychiatric history or neuroticism.

However, symptomatic patients did report higher pain levels and more cognitive difficulties at baseline. The authors argued that these differences reflected the severity of the initial injury. The fact that both pain and cognitive function are sensitive to emotional factors may limit the conclusiveness of these results, but the authors also showed that personality factors, as measured by the Freiburg personality inventory, did not correlate with the initial complaint of pain. At 1-year follow-up, these same researchers[88] reported that 24% of the study subjects were still symptomatic. Baseline factors differentiating symptomatic from asymptomatic subjects were as follows: rotated or inclined head position at impact, unpreparedness at time of impact, the car being stationary when hit, and initial intensity of neck pain and headache. The same authors had previously demonstrated that a rotated or inclined head position and unpreparedness at time of impact was predictive of more severe acute (at 1 week) injury as evidenced by a higher frequency of multiple symptoms and radicular involvement, more signs of cervical strain, and more severe headaches. Psychological and personality traits were still not predictive of the failure of symptoms to resolve at 1 year postinjury. The authors concluded that "accident mechanisms and initial findings suggestive of more severe injury were significantly related to long-term persistence of symptoms after a whiplash injury."[87,88]

ATTEMPTS TO DISCOUNT CHRONIC WHIPLASH

Whiplash injuries remain a common problem despite more than half a century of studies designed to discount "whiplash" injuries. Freeman et al[30] reported on no less than 20 studies-found through a literature search-attempting to discredit whiplash. The articles ranged from literature reviews to cohort studies. They were either designed a priori as a refutation of whiplash syndrome or were conducted for another purpose but made statements by extrapolation that refuted the validity of whiplash. The articles were divided primarily between biomedical studies, editorials, and engineering studies.[30] All 20 articles were found to have significant methodologic flaws relative to their proclamations regarding the validity of whiplash syndrome. These flaws were great enough to cast doubts on the theoretical basis for the stated link between the study results and the conclusions of the study in regard to the validity of whiplash.[30] The flaws most often found were inadequate study size, nonrepresentative study samples, nonrepresentative study samples, nonrepresentative crash conditions (for crash tests), and inappropriate study design. The authors concluded from the review that there was no epidemiologic scientific basis in the literature for the following statements: Whiplash injuries do not lead to chronic pain; rear-impact collisions that do not result in vehicle damage cannot cause injury; and whiplash trauma is biomechanically comparable with the common movements of daily living. All these conclusions were found to be lacking in adequate support or overtly refuted.[30]

Two recent studies, the QTF cohort study[85] and the Lithuanian study,[82] are of particular interest because they suggest that chronic whiplash syndrome is either rare or a consequence of the availability of compensation. A third, the Saskatchewan insurance study of tort and no-fault cases,[15] suggested that both the incidence of whiplash injury claims and the rate of recovery were strongly and negatively influenced by the availability of compensation for pain and suffering. These three studies have been used to downplay the importance of whiplash injuries, emphasize the generally positive natural course of whiplash, and suggest that limiting compensation will reduce chronicity and hasten recovery. Given their influential nature, we critically examine each.

The Quebec Task Force Cohort Study

In an attempt to determine the natural history of whiplash-associated disorders, a retrospective cohort study was conducted of 4,757 subjects who submitted claims in 1987 to the Quebec provincial (single-payer) insurance plan. Of these, 1,745 claimants were excluded because of lack of a police collision report, leaving 3,014 cases. This cohort study reported a remarkable recovery rate of 97.1% after 1 year.[40,85] However, some methodologic issues remain that need to be addressed before one can accept such a conclusion.

Defining Recovery as No Longer Receiving Compensation

Although it has been assumed that recovery denotes a resolution of symptoms or even a return to work, the QTF did not use symptom relief or even return to work as indicators of "recovery." Rather, the QTF appears to have measured recovery by the insurer's decision that individuals no longer needed to be compensated. This criterion omitted cases in which individuals were not successful in returning to work. Certainly the high number of reported and accepted "recurrences" suggested that the process was inadequate. It also stated as recovered those individuals who may have reduced their work hours or changed their type of work (modifications). It was telling that only 19 (0.4%)of the total 4,757 whiplash claimants were assigned to a rehabilitation program by the provincial no-fault insurer. Defining recovery as discontinuance of insurance benefits significantly overestimated the return to work and the resolution of symptomatology in whiplash and other musculoskeletal injuries.[18,90]

Failure to Include Recurrences

Of the 3,014 cases initially studied, 204 subjects were excluded from the final data analysis because they had suffered a "recurrence." Although it was not entirely clear what a recurrence was, the QTF defined these as "the recurrence of symptoms of collision-related injuries" that were "found to have occurred in 204, or 6.8% of the study subjects." These recurrences were not due to further collisions. They were in patients who were deemed at one point to have recovered but continued to complain of symptoms to such a significant degree that their files were reopened and compensation renewed. These 204 patients were remarkably left out of the final analysis. The recurrences were in all likelihood unresolved whiplash injuries in patients who were initially deemed by the provincial no-fault insurer to have recovered but who complained of continuing symptoms to the point that they were allowed back into the system. If these were added to the 81 subjects who had been receiving compensation throughout the first year, at the end of 1 year as many as 285 claimants were still receiving compensation for their whiplash injuries. This represented 285 of 3,014 claimants, or 9.5%, even when the very liberal criterion for recovery was used (ie, discontinuance of insurance payments), and was a far cry from the 2.9% suggested by the QTF.

Overoptimistic Estimation of Whiplash Recovery

The QTF, using very liberal criteria for recovery and failing to include "recurrences," also ignored its own literature. In a critique of the QTF, Freeman et al[30] observed that "in a table labeled 'Prevalence of symptoms at follow-up,' the QTF enumerated the four studies on prognosis that were accepted for review, along with their findings, which were as follows: Norris and Watt[69] reported that 66% of their cohort had neck pain at an average of 2 years postinjury,[69] Radanov et al[74] reported that 27% of their cohort were symptomatic 6 months post-crash,[76] and in a study 2 years later,[76] reported that 27% of their cohort had headaches 6 months post-crash[76]; and Hildingsson and Toolanen[41] reported that 44% of their cohort symptomatic at an average of 2 years post-crash.[41] Yet, based on its literature review and cohort study, the QTF concluded that whiplash-associated disorders are usually self-limiting, inaccurately summarizing the results of its own literature review and case-series study."[30]

QTF Consensus Guidelines

After 3 years of deliberations by the QTF, the evidence was found to be sparse and generally of unacceptable quality. Accordingly, for many aspects of its mandate, the QTF was forced to invoke expert opinion to make recommendations in areas in which the literature was weak. The danger of such consensus guidelines is that they give the false impression of being built on a foundation of scientific truth or facts because they followed an exhaustive best-evidence evaluation of interventions, which in fact found little acceptable scientific evidence upon which to base guidelines.

The consensus guidelines are even more suspect when one considers that they were in part guided by the cohort study's conclusions regarding the natural history of whiplash injuries. The resultant classification scheme, WAD 0-IV, is an arbitrary one because there is little or no supporting evidence apart from the cohort study's conclusions. It presumed that one could determine the natural history based on the early physical examination-this despite the fact that reliability or the degree of interobserver agreement for examination of the cervical spine is generally regarded as poor and validity has never been established. The optimistic recovery rates are undoubtedly based on the cohort study, which was overoptimistic. As such, the arbitrary guidelines of the QTF on WAD, if used to guide the management of whiplash, are likely to create a false expectation that whiplash patients, as an aggregate, should do far better than they actually do.

The Lithuanian Study

Schrader et al[82] used police accident records from a city in Lithuania to identify 202 individuals whose cars were rear-ended in automobile collisions 1 to 3 (average 21.7 months) years earlier. They compared these subjects to a nonaccident control group selected randomly from the population register and found no statistically significant differences between groups in the incidence of neck/back pain, headache, or memory/concentration difficulties. They concluded that "the late whiplash syndrome has little validity" and argued that reports of chronic whiplash in other countries are likely due to the existence of a medicolegal context that compensates whiplash injury: In Lithuania few drivers are covered by automobile insurance. However, the gender ratio was four males to one female, and then only when the study was modified and unblinded to bring in 30 female passengers. This would likely result in and of itself in a significantly lower incidence of chronic pain and disability. Only 31 of the 202 accident subject in the Lithuanian study actually reported an acute injury and, of these, only 9 reported that their pain lasted 1 week or more. A prospective study of acute whiplash injury from Switzerland[77] of subjects who had pain at initial intake that was, on average, 1 week postinjury found that 24% continued to report symptoms at 2-year follow-up. Indeed, the Lithuanian study reported that three more subjects in the accident group reported chronic neck pain relative to the nonaccident group, a difference that, given the small sample, could not have reached (and did not reach) statistical significance.

The Saskatchewan Insurance Tort versus No-Fault Insurance Study

A study by Cassidy et al[15] was entitled "Effect of eliminating compensation for pain and suffering on the outcome of insurance claims for whiplash injury." In the abstract, the authors conclude: "The elimination of compensation for pain and suffering is associated with a decreased incidence and improved prognosis of whiplash injury." As we will see, the same methodologic errors in the QTF cohort study are repeated in this study despite the fact that it is a prospective study and the chief editor of the QTF is the primary author of this paper.

Number of Claims is Not Incidence

Cassidy et al purported to want to compare patients under the tort system just before the introduction of no-fault and those under no-fault in a provincially run insurance system for automobiles. According to the authors,[15] "Under the tort system, persons injured in motor vehicle collisions could sue for pain and suffering, and the number and cost of claims were escalating. With the change to a no-fault system, payments for pain and suffering-and therefore most court actions-were eliminated, and medical and income-replacement benefits were increased." Therefore, under the no-fault plan, whiplash victims could no longer seek compensation for pain and suffering and were eligible only for medical care above that provided by the provincial health plan and for replacement of lost wages. Given that the amount of compensation available was substantially less and that individuals who were previously not employed-or who were able to remain employed postinjury-would not be eligible for compensation, one would anticipate that the number of claims to the government no-fault insurance plan would drop. In fact, that is what happened. However, tort claims can be filed for up to 2 years in most jurisdictions, while no-fault claims must be filed shortly after the injury. It would be anticipated that in the last 6 months before the introduction of no-fault there would be a surge in claims by people attempting to file before the deadline. Therefore, in this study it is not even certain that the number of claims was actually high, because the time when the claim was filed determined into what group the patient was entered as opposed to when the injury actually occurred.

Claim Closure as a Proxy for Recovery

The principal outcome measure in this study was claim closure, which was reported to be a proxy for recovery. The evidence that claim closure is an adequate proxy for recovery appears to be speculative, but there is some good evidence that it is not a good proxy with regard to return to work.[18] Moreover, under tort claim, closure occurred when a settlement was reached and signed off by the insurer and the injured party. This is much different than claim closure under the no-fault system in which the individual is deemed to have recovered when the insurer has simply discontinued payments. Not only is claim closure a limited proxy for recovery, but there appears to be evidence that claim closure may have been determined by different mechanisms under the tort and the no-fault system. Under the tort system, an agreed-to settlement among all of the parties represented claim closure while, under no-fault, discontinuance of payments represented claim closure. This alone could account for the discrepancy in claim closure between the tort and no-fault systems.

Failure to Include Recurrences and Missing Data

Even more disturbing is failure to include recurrences. This was a problem with the QTF study, in which recurrences were removed from the data set, giving an overly optimistic picture of whiplash recovery. Failure to include these recurrences was one of the principal criticisms of the QTF cohort study.

Recurrences were an immense problem in this study. Of the 7,462 individuals who entered the study, 2,064 of the claims were reopened after claim closure. This included 22% of the tort cases and 32% of the no-fault cases. Remarkably, particularly given that this is a prospective study, the recurrences were not included in the time-to-event analyses. The reason given was, "Because of uncertainty about the reasons for reopening 2,064 claims and the lack of information about the first closure date, these claims were not included in the time-to-event analysis." In other words, individuals whose claims were reopened, presumably because they were symptomatic, were simply removed from the claim closure comparison between the two groups. To not have included these data in a prospective study in which this is the main end point is either a remarkable oversight or a procedure of breathless audacity. Fully 28% of those patients who finally made it into the study were excluded for this reason, and these individuals are those most likely to have more chronic symptomatology. Remarkably, first closure data are only missing for the 2,064 recurrences and for none of the 5,398 nonrecurrences. Despite the fact the authors claim they do not have these data, they fortunately can provide us with quite detailed data on how long the claim was reopened, which in turn support their conclusions as presented.

The authors also report that for the 2,064 recurrences, 37% of those were only 1-day reopenings, presumably for administrative purposes, usually to pay a bill and hardly a reason to exclude these patients from the study data. The median time for recurrent claims was 12 days, which is somewhat remarkable when one considers that 37% were only open for 1 day. The nature of the tort system is that when claims are settled they cannot be reopened if the individual was still complaining of pain or even developed new symptoms. In contrast, no-fault claims that are closed, as we have already seen, are considered closed when the insurer is no longer making payments to the whiplash victim. Therefore, it stands to reason that most of the 669 recurrences associated with the tort group but not included in the natural history were short recurrences (ie, 1 day). The longer recurrences would be primarily in the no-fault group (1,395) and would tend to be patients who would have longer lasting or permanent symptoms.

Summary

Recent attempts to discredit whiplash patients, particularly those with chronic whiplash injuries, appear to have irredeemable flaws despite being published in good journals. It begs the question as to why a clinical condition, well recognized for more than a century and in virtually every country where it has been studied, would be subjected to this flawed and highly biased scrutiny. It is even more surprising when one considers the consistency of the clinical picture that we describe next.

THE CLINICAL SYNDROME

The clinical syndrome of whiplash is dominated by head, neck, and upper thoracic pain and often is associated with a variety of poorly explained symptoms, such as dizziness, tinnitus, and blurred vision. The symptom complex is remarkably consistent from patient to patient and across various language and cultures and is frequently complicated by psychological sequelae, such as anger, anxiety, depression, and concerns over litigation or compensation. In their cohort study, the QTF[85] found the highest incidence of whiplash claims among the 20- to 24-year age group, although recovery was more delayed the older the patient.

A delay in onset of symptoms of several hours following impact is characteristic of whiplash injuries.[22,25,28] Most patients feel little or no pain for the first few minutes following injury, after which symptoms gradually intensify over the next few days. In the first few hours, findings on examination are generally minimal.[44] After several hours, limitation of neck motion, tightness, muscle spasm or swelling, and tenderness of both anterior and posterior cervical structures become apparent.[44,97] This delay is likely due to the time required for traumatic edema and hemorrhage to occur in injured soft tissues.[50,58]

Neck Pain

Patients with whiplash injuries invariably complain of an achy discomfort in the posterior cervical region radiating out over the trapezius muscles and shoulders, down to the interscapular region, up into the occiput, or down the arms. This pain is often associated with burning and stiffness, with the latter typically being most apparent in the morning. Initially, there is marked restricted range of motion of the cervical spine, which may be associated with palpable muscle spasm and localized paraspinal tenderness. Range of motion is often restricted by pain, with extension more often limited than forward flexion.

Local Tenderness and Referred Pain

Local tenderness and pain in the cervical and thoracic region with symptoms referred distally are two characteristic features of whiplash injuries. The etiology of this pain/tenderness and referral of symptoms remains enigmatic; one possible explanation is myofascial pain. Myofascial pain remains a poorly understood clinical entity characterized by trigger points, self-sustaining hyperirritable foci of tenderness reportedly located within a taut band of skeletal muscle, and its associated fascia.[93] Compressing this hyperirritable focus is locally painful and often gives rise to characteristic tenderness, referred pain, and even autonomic phenomena.[93] Myofascial pain as a medical disorder has been questioned by a variety of authors because of a lack of known pathophysiology.[10]

Cervical Facet Joint and Discogenic Injuries

Experiments on normal volunteers indicate the most likely sites of injury and their mechanism.[53] During the early phase of a rear-end collision, the trunk is forced upward towards the head, and the cervical spine undergoes a sigmoid deformation. During this motion, at about 100 msec after impact, the lower cervical vertebrae undergo extension but without translation. This motion causes the vertebral bodies to separate anteriorly and the zygapophyseal joints to impact posteriorly. The lesions likely to result from such motion are tears of the anterior anulus fibrosus and fractures or contusions of the zygapophyseal joints.[9,53] These are the same lesions discovered postmortem in victims of fatal motor vehicle accidents.[51,52,89]

Epidemiologic studies using double-blind, controlled diagnostic blocks have shown that injury to the zygapophyseal joint is the single most common basis for chronic neck pain after whiplash.[4,61] It accounts for at least 50% of cases and up to 80% of patients involved in high-speed collisions.[37] The segmental levels most commonly affected are C2-C3 and C5-C6. Of patients with chronic headache as the dominant complaint after whiplash, the source of pain can be traced to the C2-C3 zygapophyseal joints in some 53% of cases.[61]

Two Australian studies[4,61] have provided the evidence for implicating the cervical facet joint as a potential source of chronic pain following whiplash trauma. In these blinded studies, 50 and 68 consecutively referred patients with chronic neck pain after whiplash injury were assessed by means of controlled diagnostic blocks of cervical zygapophyseal joints. Each joint was separately anesthetized with short-acting (lignocaine) or long-acting (bupivacaine) local anesthetics via injections to the medial branches of the dorsal nerve rami. A total of 54% (27 of 50) and 60% (41 of 68) of these chronic whiplash patients experienced pain relief from injections concordant with the expected duration of the anesthetic. In the second study,[61] control saline blocks were also used.

Recently, the same investigators,[62] using radiofrequency neurotomy of the medial branches of the dorsal cervical rami, effectively denervated the affected facet joint, achieving virtually complete relief of chronic whiplash pain in patients with a median pain duration of 34 months. In this randomized, double-blind clinical trial, 7 of 12 patients receiving the active treatment obtained pain relief in excess of 6 months. Only one of 12 patients in the sham surgical placebo control group was pain-free. In a subsequent paper summarizing their work to date, these authors[66] reported that a second neurotomy was successful in reeliminating pain in eight of nine patients in whom pain had eventually returned after the first successful radiofrequency neurotomy. These demonstrations of facet joint involvement in chronic whiplash pain are consistent with postmortem studies of motor vehicle accident victims, which have shown that zygapophyseal joint injuries are common.[51]

Zygapophyseal joint pain is the only basis for chronic neck pain after whiplash that has been subjected to proper scientific scrutiny.[5,63,64] However, it cannot be firmly diagnosed by physical examination only or by the common imaging methods. The diagnosis relied on fluoroscopically guided, controlled diagnostic blocks of the painful joint. No techniques of comparable validity have been developed for diagnosing pain stemming from discs, ligaments, or muscles. Accordingly, the prevalence of pain from these latter sources is not known.[9]

Taylor and Twomey[89] provided suggestive evidence of physical pathology when they compared autopsies of the cervical spine of 16 subjects who died of major trauma with 16 age-matched subjects who died of natural causes. Lesions attributable to antemortem trauma were found in 15 of the 16 subjects who died of major trauma. All 15 demonstrated linear clefts within the cartilage plate in one or more cervical discs (average three discs affected). "This was a continuous split between the tissue planes of the cartilage plate and annulus. Other lesions included six traumatic disc ruptures with posterior herniation, 10 lesions involving annular bruising (blood within the outer annulus) and 21 examples of soft tissue damage to the synovial joints." These latter facet joint injuries consisted mostly of hemarthroses, presumably from small capsular or synovial tears. These were most frequently found in spines in which there was a probable flexion injury. Occult damage to bone or cartilage of facet joints was uncommon when compared with disc damage. These findings were in marked contrast to control subjects, in whom only two small defects in the cartilage plates near the vertebral body were found. The same authors provided evidence that deep rim lesions of the disc anulus, as evidenced in the posttrauma victims, often did not heal and were associated with early disc degeneration at that level. The forces experienced at the cervical spine in individuals killed by trauma are likely of greater magnitude than in simple whiplash trauma, thus limiting the applicability of this study. However, these findings illustrate that motor vehicle accident-associated lesions of the cervical spine that are not observable with standard radiographic techniques may not heal.[89]

Radiologic Investigations

Radiologic studies of the cervical spine taken at the time of the accident are generally unremarkable or reveal evidence of preexisting degenerative changes. The most commonly reported abnormal x-ray finding is straightening of the normal cervical lordotic curve.[43] However, Hohl[45] noted that straightening of the cervical spine was not necessarily indicative of a pathological condition[13,43,73] and can be regarded as a normal variant. Rarely, x-rays may reveal evidence of bony injury such as posterior joint crush fractures or minimal subluxation,[65] but x-rays as a rule are nondiagnostic.[26,42] Computed tomography and magnetic resonance imaging should be reserved for cases in which cervical disc protrusion or spinal cord injury are suspected, but studies to date using magnetic resonance imaging have revealed nothing but age-related changes consistent with the prevalence in asymptomatic people.[11,80] Radionucleotide bone scanning is warranted only when there is significant clinical suspicion of an undiagnosed fracture.[45]

Headaches

Headaches are common symptoms following whiplash injury and are the characteristic clincial sequelae of a C2-C3 facet joint injury. Within 24 hours of the accident, many patients complain of diffuse neck and head pain. The headache may be limited to the occipital area or may spread to the vertex, temporofrontal, and retroorbital areas.[84] The pain may be a dull pressure or a squeezing sensation and may include pounding and throbbing (migrainous) components.[2,84] Muscle contraction and vascular headaches often are present simultaneously (posttraumatic mixed headache). Patients may experience concomitant nausea, vomiting, and photophobia. The frequency of these various forms of headache in whiplash is not known. However, the incidence of unspecified headache in a retrospective analysis of 320 cases referred for medicolegal assessment was 55%.[99] Lord et al[60] note that 53% of patients with chronic headache as the dominant complaint can have their pain traced to the C2-C3 zygapophyseal joints.

Visual Disturbances, Dizziness, and Tinnitus

Whiplash patients may complain of intermittent blurring of vision.[46,56,65] Blurring of vision by itself is not believed to have diagnostic significance unless associated with damage to the cervical sympathetic trunk, which is regarded as rare. Complaints of dizziness or vertigo-like symptoms are common following whiplash injuries.[72] Several theories have been postulated to explain these features, including vertebral artery insufficiency, inner ear damage, injury to the cervical sympathetic chain, and an impaired neck-righting reflex.[7,91] The "reflex," or "neuromuscular," theory proposes that interference with normal signals coming from the upper cervical joints, muscles, or nerves to the inner ear produces a feeling of ataxia.[23,65] The entire concept of chronic vertigo arising from the cervical region has been questioned because of the relatively small cervical afferent input to the vestibular nuclei and the capacity of the system for making adjustments.[1,28]

Tinnitus or difficulties with auditory acuity are frequently reported in association with whiplash injuries.[17,58,65] Tinnitus may theoretically be due to vertebral artery insufficiency, injury to the cervical sympathetic chain, or inner ear damage.[7,67] Tinnitus alone does not appear to have prognostic significance,[65] although anecdotally we have noted it to be common with more severe injuries. Additional auditory complaints include decreased hearing and loudness recruitment.[36,58]

Arm Pain and Paresthesias

Arm pain and paresthesias are frequently reported following whiplash injury. Historically, these symptoms have been attributed to cervical nerve root compression and disc herniation.[33] However, modern imaging techniques have shown that disc herniations attributable to whiplash injuries are uncommon and of uncertain significance. Moreover, objective neurologic tests such as nerve conduction and needle electromyographic studies are invariably normal. Arm pain has been attributed to the thoracic outlet syndrome with intermittent or transient compression of the brachial plexus.[14] However, objective evidence of a pathophysiologic cause for thoracic outlet syndrome remains elusive, leading some authors to doubt its existence.[68,98] One of the greatest concerns about attributing symptoms to thoracic outlet syndrome is that it may lead to surgical interventions of dubious efficacy.[16]

Memory and Concentration Problems

Many patients with chronic whiplash pain complain of memory and concentration difficulties. A number of researchers have argued that these difficulties are a consequence of a mild traumatic brain injury sustained as a consequence of a violent hyperflexion and hyperextension of the neck.[6,55,70,75,100] This has been postulated to occur on vehicular impact because the skull presumably accelerates faster than the brain and subsequently impacts with the brain as it rotates backward and accelerates forward. Mild traumatic brain injury has been postulated to occur even though loss of consciousness and posttraumatic amnesia are rare, factors considered by some authorities to be very important diagnostic criteria for mild traumatic brain injury.[39,54,57] Although some laboratory studies using nonhuman primates indicate brain damage can occur in simulated hyperextension-flexion or acceleration injuries without loss of consciousness,[24,59,71,96] the anatomy of nonhuman primates is markedly different from that of humans. This renders animal data suggestive but in need of confirmatory human research.

A review of research in humans finds little or no evidence for enduring brain injury after whiplash.[79,83] There is no conclusive evidence of neuropathological abnormalities after whiplash. A number of studies have reported electroencephalography abnormalities suggestive of brain injury in patients with whiplash; however, the reported incidence of these abnormalities ranges from 4% to 46%.[35,48,92] Although all of these electroencephalography studies suffer from methodologic problems, the study reporting the highest incidence of electroencephalography abnormalities (46%) is particularly flawed.[92] Neuropsychological assessment is thought to be more sensitive for detecting mild brain injury, and a number of studies report poorer performance on neuropsychological measures of concentration and memory in groups of chronic whiplash patients 1 or more years after injury.[55,70,75,100] Patients in these studies are usually recruited from specialty clinics and typically represent a selected sample with long-standing complaints of disabling pain, emotional distress, and cognitive difficulties. These studies have failed to control for the documented effects of pain, medications, depression, anxiety, and arousal on cognitive functioning.[79,83]

The effect of emotions and medications on cognitive functioning is well documented[19,49]; more recently, studies have documented the deleterious effect of pain on attentional processes and task performance.[20] In addition, studies of patients with mild traumatic brain injuries suggest that difficulties in cognitive functioning, as assessed by neuropsychological testing, normalize by 3 months after injury.[34,38,47,81] Given this information, one need not postulate a traumatic brain injury to account for persisting cognitive problems in samples of chronic whiplash patients.[83] The two prospective studies assessing neuropsychological functioning within a week of injury failed to use adequate control groups.[27,76] The only prospective study to follow an unselected sample of patients with whiplash found no evidence of cognitive deficits 6 months after injury.[76] Accordingly, a definitive prospective study of acute cognitive deficits related to mild traumatic brain injury that adequately controls for pain and emotional functioning has yet to be performed.

Psychological Distress

Psychological distress is common after whiplash.[9] However, psychosocial factors do not cause neck pain and are not predictive of chronicity.[12,74,77,79,94]

In a study discussed earlier, Radanov et al[77] studied whiplash patients referred by family doctors for purposes of the study. Of 164 consecutive patients referred, 117 (74 women) qualified for a completed study that went on for 1 year. Within 10 days of injury, these patients underwent a neurologic evaluation, a semistructured interview, self-rating of patients' well-being and subjective cognitive ability, and personality traits, including neuroticism, nervousness, aggressiveness, passivity, and depression. The mean time between the accident and baseline examination was 7.4 days (SD 4.2). Patients who were symptomatic and asymptomatic at 6 months had scored within the normal range at baseline on personality scales (using the Freiburg personality inventory) with no difference between the groups on any scale. The results indicated that "(1) the disposition of patients (personality traits) does not primarily influence the course of recovery from common whiplash; (2) psychological and cognitive problems of patients with common whiplash may rather be seen as correlates of somatic symptoms; and (3) injury-related psychological and cognitive difficulties can initiate a vicious circle, which may explain the secondary neurotic reaction..."[77] The authors concluded that based upon their prospectively conducted study there was little evidence that psychological problems, unrelated to the trauma, predicted who would recover from whiplash injuries.

Australian researchers[95] convincingly demonstrated that the psychological distress often evident in chronic whiplash patients is a consequence of the pain and appears to have no etiologic significance. As part of their protocol for treating zygapophyseal joint pain using radiofrequency neurotomy, they administered the SCL-90 both before and after treatment. The typical SCL-90 profile pretreatment showed clinically significant elevations of the somatization, depression, and obsessive-compulsive scales. Notably, elevations on the somatization scale reflect somatic complaints that can be organic or psychological in origin. Successful relief of pain following neurotomy resulted in significant reduction of elevated scale scores to levels consistent with nonclinical ("normal") populations. When the pain eventually returned, the SCL-90 scales again became elevated. Moreover, after a second neurotomy successfully reeliminated the pain, the elevated SCL-90 scale scores once again decreased to normal levels.

CONCLUSIONS

Whiplash injuries are common, and most get better with time. Physical indicators and not psychological factors are predictive of recovery. Recent studies that cast doubt on the legitimacy of chronic whiplash injuries have had serious methodologic flaws that cast doubt on the conclusions. The clinical picture of whiplash injuries has many characteristic features.

References

1. Balch RW: Dizziness, Hearing Loss and Tinnitus: The Essentials of Neurology. Philadelphia, FA Davis, 1984.
2. Balla JI, Moraitis S: Knights in armour. A follow-up study of injuries after legal settlement. Med J Aust 2:355–361, 1970.
3. Barnsley L, Lord SM, Wallis BJ, Bogduk N: Lack of effect of intraarticular corticosteroids for chronic pain in the cervical zygapophyseal joints. N Engl J Med 330;1047–1050, 1994.
4. Barnsley L, Lord SM, Wallis BJ, Bogduk N: The prevalence of chronic cervical zygapophysial joint pain after whiplash. Spine 20:20–25, 1995.
5. Barnsley L, Lord S, Bogduk N: The pathophysiology of whiplash. Spine 12:209–242, 1998.
6. Berstad JR, Baerum B, Lochen EA, et al: Whiplash: chronic organic brain syndrome without hydrocephalus ex vacuo. Acta Neurol Scand 51:268–284, 1975.
7. Bogduk N: The anatomy and pathophysiology of whiplash. Clin Biomech 1:92–101, 1986.
8. Bogduk N, Lord SM: Cervical zygapophysial joint pain. Neurosurg Q 8:107–117, 1998.
9. Bogduk N, Teasell R: Whiplash injuries: the evidence for an organic etiology. Arch Neurol 57:590–591, 2000.

10. Bohr T: Fibromyalgia syndrome and myofascial pain syndrome. Do they exist? Neurol Clin 13:365–384, 1995.
11. Borchgrevink GE, Smevik O, Nordby A, et al: MRI imaging and radiography of patients with cervical hyperextension-flexion injuries after car accidents. Acta Radiol 36:425–428, 1995.
12. Borchgrevink GE, Stiles TC, Borchgrevink PC, Lereim I: Personality profile among sympto-matic and recovered patients with neck sprain injury, measured by MCMI-I acutely and 6 months after car accidents. J Psychosom Res 42:357–367, 1997.
13. Borden AGB, Rechtman AM, Gershom-Cohen J: The normal cervical lordosis. Radiology 74:806, 1960.
14. Capistrant TD: Thoracic outlet syndrome in whiplash injury. Ann Surg 185:175–178, 1977.
15. Cassidy JD, Carroll LJ, Cote P, et al: Effect of eliminating compensation for pain and suffer-ing on the outcome of insurance claims for whiplash injury. N Engl J Med 342:1179–1186, 2000.
16. Cherington M, Happer I, Machanic B, Parry L: Surgery for thoracic outlet syndrome may be hazardous to your health. Muscle Nerve 9:632–634, 1986.
17. Chrisman OD, Gervais RF: Otologic manifestations of the cervical syndrome. Clin Orthop 24:34–39, 1962.
18. Corey DT, Koepfler LE, Etlin D, Day IH: A limited functional restoration program for injured workers: a randomized trial. J Occup Rehabil 6:239–249, 1996.
19. Coyne JC, Gotlib IH: The role of cognition in depression: a critical appraisal. Psychol Bull 39:593–597, 1983.
20. Crombez G, Eccleston C, Baeynes F, Eelen P: Habituation and the interference of pain with task performance. Pain 70:149–154, 1997.
21. Deans GT: Incidence and duration of neck pain among patients injured in car accidents. Br Med J (Clin Res Ed) 292:94–95, 1986.
22. Deans GT, McGailliard JN, Kerr M, Rutherford WH: Neck pain-a major cause of disability fol-lowing car accidents. Injury 18:10–12, 1987.
23. DeJong PTVM, DeJong JMBV, Cohen B, Jongkees LBW: Ataxia and nystagmus induced by in-jection of local anaesthetics in the neck. Ann Neurol 1:240–246, 1977.
24. Domer FR, Lin YK, Chadron KB, Krieger KW: Effect of hyperextension-hyperflexion (whip-lash) on the function of the blood brain barrier of rhesus monkeys. Exp Neurol 63:304–310, 1979.
25. Dunsker SB: Hyperextension and hyperflexion injuries of the cervical spine. In Youmans JR (ed): Neurological Surgery, 2nd ed. Philadelphia, WB Saunders, 1982, pp 2332–2343.
26. Ellertsson AB, Sigurjonsson K, Thorsteinsson T: Clinical and radiographic study of 100 cases of whiplash injury. Acta Neurol Scand 5(suppl 67):269, 1978.
27. Ettlin TM, Kischka U, Reichmann S, et al: Cerebral symptoms after whiplash injury of the neck: a prospective clinical and neuropsychological study of whiplash injury. J Neurol Neurosurg Psychiatry 55:943–948, 1992.
28. Evans RW: Some observations on whiplash injuries. Neurol Clin 10:975–995, 1992.
29. Frankel VH: Pathomechanics of whiplash injuries to the neck. In Morley TP (ed): Current Controversies in Neurosurgery. Philadelphia, WB Saunders, 1976, pp 39–50.
30. Freeman MD, Croft AC, Rossignol AM, et al: A review and methodologic critique of the litera-ture refuting whiplash syndrome. Spine 24:86–98, 1999.
31. Gargan MS, Bannister GC: Long-term prognosis of soft tissue injuries of the neck. J Bone Joint Surg Br 72:901–903, 1990.
32. Gargan MF, Bannister GC: The rate of recovery following whiplash injury. Eur Spine J 3:162–164, 1994.
33. Gay JR, Abbott KH: Common whiplash injuries of the neck. JAMA 152:1698–1704, 1953.
34. Gentilini M, Nichelli P, Schoenhuber R, et al: Neuropsychological evaluation of minor head injury. J Neurol Neurosurg Psychiatry 48:137–140, 1985.
35. Gibbs FA: Objective evidence of brain disorder in cases of whiplash injury. Clin Electro-encephalogr 2:107–110, 1971.
36. Gibson JW: Cervical syndromes: use of a comfortable cervical collar as an adjunct in their management. South Med J 67:205–208, 1974.
37. Gibson T, Bogduk N, Macpherson J, McIntosh A: The accident characteristics of whiplash as-sociated chronic neck pain. J Musculoskel Pain. In press.
38. Gronwall D: Cumulative and persisting effects of concussion on attention and cognition. In Levin HS, Eisenberg HM, Benton AI (eds): Mild Head Injury. New York, Oxford University Press, 1989.
39. Gronwall D: Minor head injury. Neuropsychology 5:253–266, 1991.

40. Harder S, Veilleux M, Suissa S: The effect of socio-demographic and crash-related factors in the prognosis of whiplash. J Clin Epidemiol 51:377–384, 1998.
41. Hildingsson C, Toolanen G: Outcome after soft tissue injury of the cervical spine: a prospective study of 93 car-accident victims. Acta Orthop Scand 61:357–359, 1990.
42. Hoffman JR, Schringer DL, Mower W, et al: Low-risk criteria for cervical-spine radiography in blunt trauma: a prospective study. Am Emerg Med 21:1454–1460, 1992.
43. Hohl M: Soft tissue injuries of the neck in automobile accidents: factors influencing prognosis. J Bone Joint Surg Am 56:1675–1682, 1974.
44. Hohl M: Soft tissue injuries of the neck. Clin Orthop 109:42–49, 1975.
45. Hohl M: Soft tissue neck injuries. In The Cervical Spine Research Society Editorial Committee (ed): The Cervical Spine, 2nd ed. Philadelphia, JB Lippincott, 1989, pp 436–441.
46. Horwich H, Kasner D: The effect of whiplash injuries on ocular functions. South Med J 55:69–71, 1962.
47. Huggenholtz H, Stuss DT, Stethem LL, Richard MT: How long does it take to recover from a mild concussion? J Neurosurg 22:853–858, 1988.
48. Jacome DE: EEG in whiplash: a reappraisal. Clin Electroencephalogr 18:41–45, 1987.
49. Jamison RN, Brocco TS, Parris WL: The influence of problems with concentration and memory on emotional distress and daily activities in chronic pain patients. Int J Psychiatry Med 18:183–191, 1988.
50. Jeffreys E: Disorders of the Cervical Spine. London, Butterworths, 1980.
51. Jonsson H Jr, Bring G, Ranschning W, Sahlstedt B: Hidden cervical spine injuries in traffic accident victims with skull fractures. J Spinal Disord 4:251–263, 1991.
52. Jonsson H, Cesarini K, Sahlstedt B, Rauschering W: Findings and outcomes in whiplash-type neck distortions. Spine 19:2733–2743, 1994.
53. Kaneoka K, Ono K, Inami S, Hayashi K: Motion analysis of cervical vertebrae during whiplash loading. Spine 24:763–769, 1999; discussion 770).
54. Kay T, Newman B, Carallo M, et al: Towards a neuropsychological model of functional disability after mild traumatic brain injury. Neuropsychology 6:371–384, 1992.
55. Kischka U, Ettlin TH, Heim S, Schmid G: Cerebral symptoms following whiplash injury. Eur Neurol 31:136–140, 1991.
56. LaRocca H: Acceleration injuries of the neck. Clin Neurosurg 25:205–217, 1978.
57. Levin HS, Eisenberg HM, Benton AL (eds): Mild Head Injury. New York, Oxford Press, 1989.
58. Lieberman JS: Cervical soft tissue injuries and cervical disc disease. In Principles of Physical Medicine and Rehabilitation in the Musculoskeletal Diseases. New York, Grune & Stratton, 1986, pp 263–286.
59. Lin K, Chandran KB, Heath RG, et al: Subcortical EEG changes in rhesus monkeys following experimental hyperextension-hyperflexion (whiplash). Spine 9:329–338, 1984.
60. Lord SM, Barnsley L, Wallis BJ, et al: Third occipital headache: a prevalence study. J Neurol Neurosurg Psychiatry 57:1187–1190, 1994.
61. Lord SM, Barnsley L, Wallis BJ, Bogduk N: Chronic cervical zygapophysial joint pain after whiplash. A placebo-controlled prevalence study. Spine 21:1737–1745, 1996.
62. Lord SM, Barnsley L, Wallis BJ, McDonald GJ, Bogduk N: Percutaneous radio-frequency neurotomy for chronic cervical zygapophyseal-joint pain. N Engl J Med 335:1721–1726, 1996.
63. Lord SM, Barnsley L, Bogduk N: Cervical zygapophyseal joint pain in whiplash injuries. Spine 12:301–344, 1998.
64. Lord SM, McDonald GJ, Bogduk N: Percutaneous radiofrequency neurotomy of the cervical medial branches: a validated treatment for cervical zygapophysial joint pain. Neurosurg Q 8:288–308, 1998.
65. Macnab I: Acceleration extension injuries of the cervical spine. In Rothman RH, Simeone FA (eds): The Spine, 2nd ed. Philadelphia, WB Saunders, 1982, pp 647–660.
66. McDonald G, Lord SM, Bogduk N: Long-term follow-up of cervical radiofrequency neurotomy for chronic neck pain. Neurosurgery 45:61–67, 1999.
67. Medical News: Animals riding in carts show effects of "whiplash" injury. JAMA 194:40–41, 1965.
68. Nelson DA: Thoracic outlet syndrome and dysfunction of the temporomandibular joint: proved pathology or pseudosyndromes? Perspect Biol Med 33:567–576, 1990.
69. Norris SH, Watt I: The prognosis of neck injuries resulting from rear-end vehicle collisions. J Bone Joint Surg Br 65:608–611, 1983.
70. Olsnes BT: Neurobehavioral findings in whiplash patients with longstanding symptoms. Acta Neurol Scand 80:584–588, 1989.
71. Ommaya AK, Faas F, Yarnell P: Whiplash and brain damage. JAMA 204:285–289, 1968.

72. Oosterveld WJ, Kortschot HW, Kingma GG, et al: Electronystagmographic findings following cervical whiplash injuries. Acta Otolaryngol 111:201–205, 1991.
73. Rachtman AM, Borden AGB, Gershon-Cohen J: The lordotic curve of the cervical spine. Clin Orthop 20:208, 1961.
74. Radanov BP, DiStefano G, Schnidrig A, et al: Role of psychosocial stress in recovery from common whiplash. Lancet 338:712–715, 1991.
75. Radanov BP, DiStefano GD, Schnidrig A, et al: Cognitive functioning after common whiplash. A controlled follow-up study. Arch Neurol 50:87–91, 1993.
76. Radanov BP, Dvorak J, Valach L: Cognitive deficits in patients after soft tissue injury of the cervical spine. Spine 17:127–131, 1992.
77. Radanov BP, Sturzenegger M, DeStefano G, Schnidrig A: Relationship between early somatic, radiological, cognitive and psychosocial findings and outcome during a one-year follow-up in 117 patients suffering from common whiplash. Br J Rheumatol 33:442–448, 1994.
78. Radanov BP, Sturzenegger M, DiStefano G: Long-term outcome after whiplash injury: a 2-year follow-up considering features of injury mechanism and somatic, radiologic, and psychosocial findings. Medicine 74:281–297, 1995.
79. Radanov BP, Dvorak J: Impaired cognitive functioning after whiplash injury of the cervical spine. Spine 21:393–397, 1996.
80. Ronnen HR, de Korte PJ, Brink PRG, et al: Acute whiplash injury: is there a role for MR imaging? A prospective study of 100 patients. Radiology 201:93–96, 1996.
81. Ruff RM, Levin HS, Mattis S, et al: Recovery of memory after head injury. A three centre study. In Levin HS, Eisenberg HM, Benton AL (eds): Mild Head Injury. New York, Oxford University Press, 1989, pp 176–188.
82. Schrader H, Obelieniene D, Bovim G, et al: Natural evolution of the late whiplash syndrome outside the medical legal context. Lancet 347:1207–1211, 1996.
83. Shapiro AP, Teasell RW, Steenhuis R: Mild traumatic brain injury following whiplash. Spine 7(3):455–470, 1993.
84. Speed WG: Psychiatric aspects of post-traumatic headaches. In Adler CS, et al (eds): Psychiatric Aspects of Headache. Baltimore, Williams & Wilkins, 1987, pp 210–216.
85. Spitzer WO, Skovron ML, Salmi LR, et al: Scientific monograph of the Quebec Task Force on Whiplash-Associated Disorders: redefining "whiplash" and its management. Spine 20(8 suppl):1S–73S, 1995.
86. Squires B, Gargan MF, Bannister GC: Soft tissue injuries of the cervical spine: 15-year follow-up. J Bone Joint Surg Br 788:955–957, 1996.
87. Sturzenegger M, DiStefano G, Radanov BP, Schnidrig A: Presenting symptoms and signs after whiplash injury. The influence of accident mechanisms. Neurology 44:688–693, 1994.
88. Sturzenegger M, Radanov BP, DiStefano G: The effect of accident mechanisms and initial findings on the long-term course of whiplash injury. J Neurol 242:443–449, 1995.
89. Taylor JR, Twomey LT: Acute injuries to cervical joints: an autopsy study of neck sprain. Spine 9:1115–1122, 1993.
90. Teasell RW, Shapiro AP: Whiplash injuries: an update. Pain Res Manage 3:81–90, 1998.
91. Toglia JV: Acute flexion-extension injury of the neck. Electronystagmographic study of 309 patients. Neurology 26:808–814, 1976.
92. Torres F, Shapiro SK: Electroencephalograms in whiplash injury. Arch Neurol 5:28–35, 1961.
93. Travell J, Simons DG: Myofascial Pain and Dysfunction: The Trigger Point Manual. Baltimore, Williams & Wilkins, 1983.
94. Wallis BJ, Lord SM, Barnsley L, Bogduk N: Pain and psychological symptoms of Australian patients with whiplash. Spine 21:804-810, 1996.
95. Wallis BJ, Lord SM, Bogduk N: Resolution of psychological distress of whiplash patients following treatment by radiofrequency neurotomy: a randomized, double-blind, placebo-controlled trial. Pain 73:15–22, 1997.
96. Wickstrom JK, LaRocca H: Management of patients with cervical spine and head injuries from acceleration forces. Curr Pract Orthop Surg 6:83, 1975.
97. Wickstrom JK, Martinez JL, Rodriguez R, et al: Hyperextension and hyperflexion injuries to the head and neck of primates. In Gurdijian ES, Thomas LM (eds): Neckache and Backache. Springfield, IL, Charles C Thomas, 1970, pp 108–119.
98. Wilbourn AJ: The thoracic outlet syndrome is overdiagnosed. Arch Neurol 47:328–330, 1990.
99. Wiley AM, Lloyd J, Evans JG, et al: Musculoskeletal sequelae of whiplash injuries. Advocates Q 7:65–73, 1986.
100. Yarnell PR, Rossie GV: Minor whiplash head injury with major debilitation. Brain Inj 2:255–258, 1988.

8

Whiplash-Related Headache

Paul R. McCrory, M.B.B.S., Ph.D.

Whiplash injury and the associated symptom complex that accompanies such injuries excite debate in both the medical and lay press. The argument as to whether the symptoms are physical or psychological in origin is the central point at issue.[1] The concern that is often raised as to the effect of litigation or compensation on either the existence or persistence of symptoms causes a great deal of skepticism among clinicians. This chapter examines the evidence for the most common postwhiplash symptom complex: headache.

DEFINITIONS
Whiplash may be defined as an acceleration-deceleration or hyperextension-hyperflexion mechanism of impulsive energy transfer to the cervical spine without direct head contact. Whiplash causes cervical soft tissue injury or damage to the zygapophyseal joints or their surrounding structures. Chronic or late whiplash syndrome refers to persistent symptoms present more than 6 months after the accident.

This mechanism of injury is typically seen in rear-end or, to a lesser degree, side-on impact in motor vehicle crashes. Interestingly, the injury is seen in the occupants of the struck vehicle rather than the vehicle that is impacting from behind.[2] This emphasizes that it is the hyperextension-hyperflexion mechanism and not flexion-extension that produces the injurious force.

HISTORICAL NOTE
The medical origin of the term "whiplash" is obscure. The term is attributed to an American orthopedic surgeon who apparently coined the term in a lecture in 1928, although the term was not in widespread use until the 1950s.[3,4] It is likely that the sorts of "whiplash" injuries caused by cervical acceleration-deceleration mechanisms may have been initially recognized in naval air pilots following World War I when attempting catapult-assisted takeoff from aircraft carriers.

In the 1950s, as the number of motor vehicle whiplash injuries steadily climbed, a number of researchers began to explore the biomechanical mechanisms behind these injuries. In some studies, the cause of the injury was felt to be cervical flexion.[5] In 1955, Severy et al studied rear-end collisions in considerable detail and correctly identified the sequence of hyperextension followed by flexion of the neck. In rear-end collisions, they noted that the incidence of whiplash injuries also decreased as impact severity increased.[6]

Although head, neck, and upper limb pain and radicular symptoms arising from structural injuries to the neck have long been recognized, there is concern in some circles where similar symptoms are attributed to cervical "dysfunction" postinjury.[7-9] In such situations, the dysfunction described is one of joint or segmental movement with clinical signs that may be subtle or subjective in nature. Not surprisingly, opinion remains divided as to the veracity of such claims.[1,8,9]

CLINICAL SYMPTOMS

Following a whiplash or cervical acceleration-deceleration injury, a variety of symptoms may be encountered. In some cases, these symptoms reflect structural injury and compromise of neurologic structures.

In other cases, a constellation of cognitive, somatic, psychological, and other phenomena may occur. For such symptoms, an organic or structural basis is not clear.[10] Such symptoms may include headaches; dizziness; paresthesia; weakness; cognitive, somatic, and visual symptoms; and psychological sequelae (such as memory, attention, and concentration impairment; nervousness and irritability; sleep disturbances; fatigability; depression; and personality change).[11,12]

Following a motor vehicle accident, almost two-thirds of patients report acute neck pain or headache.[13] Most of the symptoms commence within 6 hours of the accident. Acute neck pain in this setting typically is due to myofascial cervical sprain.[2]

Headache is a common symptom in this setting and is occipitally located in 46%, generalized in 34%, and in other locations in 20%.[14] Whiplash trauma can also injure the temporomandibular joint and cause jaw pain often associated with headache.[15] Headache may also be referred from the C2-C3 facet joint that is innervated by the third occipital nerve; hence, the so-called "third occipital headache."[16] Injury to the C2-C3 facet joint can result in pain complaints in the upper cervical region extending at least onto the occiput and at times toward the ear, vertex, forehead, or eye. Using third occipital nerve blocks to diagnose the condition, the prevalence of this type of headache among patients with persistent headaches after whiplash injury has been reported as 38–50%.[17,18]

With regard to the other somatic, behavioral, psychological, and cognitive symptoms seen following whiplash injury, one study reported vertigo in 50%, "floating" sensations in 35%, tinnitus in 14%, and hearing impairment in 5%.[19] Similarly, paresthesias are commonly reported symptoms, occurring in one-third of patients.[20] There are also many similarities between chronic whiplash symptoms and the symptoms reported in the postconcussion syndrome seen following head injury.[21,22]

CLINICAL HISTORY AND EXAMINATION

Typically, a patient with a whiplash-related headache describes a motor vehicle accident (or other cervical acceleration-deceleration injury) following which his symptoms commenced. Headache may be present on awakening in the morning or may begin after coming home from work, lasting several hours. Later the pain can become continuous but even then manifests diurnal variations in intensity. The distribution affects one or both sides of the head, less frequently the forehead. Starting in the neck or the occiput, the pain sweeps forward over the parietal region to the temple or forehead, or it travels in the opposite direction. Some patients indicate a line accurately outlining the origin of the temporalis muscles, others the anterior fibers of that muscle at the temple; however, neck pain can be referred to the forehead, extend over the entire hemicranium, or be bilateral. Heat, such as when showering, gives temporary relief, and cold accentuates the regional pain. Neck movement influences the pain arising from that region, and neck crepitus may be present. Neck pain often extends along the upper fibbers of the trapezius muscle to one or both shoulders. Corroborative evidence for organic pain origin derives from the response to analgesics: partial or total relief commencing in less than an hour, lasting for 3 to 4 hours, or until the pain recurs later or the next day.

Physical examination reveals local unilateral or bilateral cervical muscle tenderness and discomfort or crepitus on neck movements, especially restricted on lateral flexion. Formal neurologic examination is usually normal, although subjective sensory symptoms may be reported.

When assessing such patients, the history and examination must be thorough and comprehensive—not restricted to just the head and neck. Thus, system review may reveal other joint involvement, especially ligamentous hypermobility. The past history as well as the occupational and social history are also important.

EPIDEMIOLOGY

In the United States in 1997, there were 13.8 million motor vehicle accidents, including 3.9 million rear-end collisions.[23] Although the precise number of whiplash injuries remains speculative, research from other countries suggests that approximately 35% of drivers involved in rear-end collisions suffer whiplash injuries.[24] Rear-end collisions are responsible for about 85% of all whiplash injuries, and whiplash injuries typically occur in occupants of the vehicle that was struck.[2,6,13] For reasons that are not entirely clear, women have persistent neck pain and headache more often than men do, especially in the 20- to 40-year-old age group, by a ratio of 7:3.[14,25]

ETIOLOGY

Although it is generally felt that both the early and late symptoms following whiplash injury may have a physical basis, concerns have been raised as to the confounding effects of social, personality, and cultural factors.

An interesting and important study was performed in Lithuania, where the authors retrospectively examined symptoms after rear-end motor vehicle crashes. In Lithuania, few people are covered by motor vehicle insurance. Chronic headaches were no more common in accident victims than in controls. The authors concluded that expectation of disability, a family history, and attribution of preexisting symptoms to the trauma may be important determinants for those who develop chronic symptoms.[26,27] Similarly, when the compensation system in Saskatchewan, Canada, was changed to a no-fault system without payments for pain and suffering, the number of claims decreased by about 25%.[28] These studies suggest the close interplay between organic and nonorganic factors in the genesis of such symptoms.

THE PATHOPHYSIOLOGY OF WHIPLASH HEADACHE

Many animal studies have demonstrated structural cervical damage from whiplash injuries, including soft tissue damage, disc injuries, nerve root injury, and cervical cord contusions.[29] Human studies demonstrate ligamentous ruptures, vertebral end-plate avulsion and fracture, acute cervical disc herniations, and prevertebral fluid collections.[30,31] That structural injury can occur in this setting is not in doubt but, rather, the origin of the various symptoms remains controversial.

Evidence of pain referred from the neck to the head can be derived only from human experiments. Kellgren injected 0.1 mL of 6% saline into suboccipital muscles, provoking "pain felt deeply in the head described as 'headache.'"[32] Studies by Cyriax and, later, Fredriksen were more precise: Injecting 4% saline close to the occipital insertion of the muscles produced a band of pain encircling half the head, the pain reaching maximal intensity in the temple and forehead over the eye. Injections 1 to 2 inches below the occiput induced pain extending up the back of the head to the vertex, but after lower injections pain was limited to the upper end of the cervical muscles.[7,33] Evidence for the route of transmission of the pain derives from observations by Kerr, who stimulated C1 nerve rootlets in patients undergoing surgery with local anesthesia, provoking pain in the orbit, forehead, or the vertex and parietal regions.[34]

DIAGNOSTIC WORKUP FOR WHIPLASH-RELATED HEADACHE
In the patient with headache following whiplash injury, it is prudent to perform neuroimaging to exclude a structural injury. No evidence-based guidelines exist upon which to base such recommendations. Cerebral and cervical magnetic resonance is recommended. A cervical computed tomography myelogram scan may be helpful if magnetic resonance imaging cannot be performed for technical reasons or if the study demonstrates equivocal findings.

Although no published studies in whiplash injury are available to guide the clinician as to which patients are likely to have a positive imaging study, the migraine and headache literature has some useful parallels. The indications and usefulness of neurodiagnostic studies for headache specifically have been recently reviewed.[35] The pickup rate for significant neuropathological injury is between 1% and 3% in patients with posttraumatic headache. It was also noted that the typical headaches found in life-threatening conditions were nonspecific in nature. A high index of suspicion needs to be retained in the setting of posttraumatic headache along with a low threshold for obtaining neuroimaging studies.

Recent reports suggest that cerebral "hypoperfusion" may occur after whiplash injuries. This finding has been invoked to explain some of the protean symptoms associated with the whiplash syndrome outside of headache. In one study, positron emission tomography (PET) and single photon emission computed tomography (SPECT) evidence of parietooccipital hypometabolism was reported.[36,37] However, in another study of patients with chronic whiplash symptoms, no correlations were found between regional perfusion or metabolism in any brain area on SPECT or PET studies and the scores of divided attention or working memory.[38] Because of such conflicting results and the nonspecific nature of the findings, PET and SPECT imaging should not be used as diagnostic tools in the routine evaluation of patients with whiplash syndrome. Of note, SPECT imaging is a nonquantitative measure of metabolic function and blood flow, and many "abnormalities" are often noted even in normal subjects.

PROGNOSIS OF WHIPLASH-RELATED HEADACHE

Studies on the prognosis of whiplash injuries are difficult to compare because of methodologic differences, including selection criteria of patients, prospective and retrospective designs, patient attrition rates, duration of follow-up, and treatments used.[11,39,40]

Studies have shown that headache may persist for long periods after injury.[41-43] In these studies, 57% of patients reported headache at 1 week, 35% at 3 months, 21% at 12 months, and 15% at 24 months. This suggests that few patients remain significantly troubled by persistent symptoms. Interestingly, psychosocial factors, negative affectivity, and personality traits were not significant in predicting the duration of symptoms.[43]

MANAGEMENT OF WHIPLASH-RELATED HEADACHES

Whether symptoms are caused by neurologic injury or psychological factors, most patients are genuinely distressed by the pain and require medical treatment. Despite this, there are few prospective controlled studies of treatment for any of the whiplash-related symptoms.[44]

Where cervical injury or dysfunction occurs, standard physical therapeutic modalities are recommended in the first instance. This may include modalities such as biofeedback, massage, joint mobilization, trigger point injections, and acupuncture. Although these treatment modalities are generally considered conservative in nature, no evidence-based guidelines have been published in this area upon which clinicians can base their treatment decisions.

The treatment of pain arising from facet joint injury is being increasingly studied. A controlled prospective study showed a lack of effect of intra-articular corticosteroid injections in the cervical facet joints for chronic pain after whiplash injuries.[39,45] Percutaneous radiofrequency neurotomy and lower cervical medial branch neurotomy should be used cautiously for the treatment of chronic facet joint pain and should be considered only where the origin of the pain is clearly documented by local anesthetic blocks.[17,46]

Whiplash-related headaches are generally treated in the same fashion as primary headache syndromes. Importantly, analgesic-rebound headache can complicate a posttraumatic headache disorder, and this condition may need specific consideration in overall patient management.[47]

With regard to headache symptoms, routine treatment often consists of pain medications and nonsteroidal anti-inflammatory medications. Some patients with greater occipital neuralgia benefit from nerve blocks.[48,49] For persistent complaints, cyclic antidepressants amitriptyline, nortriptyline, maprotiline, and doxepin are the agents most often prescribed. Fluoxetine is less effective, but patients often prefer this agent because of the absence of significant weight gain, sedation, and anticholinergic adverse effects. The value of other serotonin-specific reuptake inhibitors is uncertain, but they may be as effective as tricyclic agents but with fewer adverse effects.[50-52] The monoamine oxidase inhibitors are highly effective and may help patients who have not responded to other agents. The chronic frequent use of opiates, benzodiazepines, barbiturates, and carisprodol should be sparingly recommended because of the potential for dependency. Clearly, adequately controlled prospective studies of current treatments and more effective treatments for chronic pain are greatly needed.

CONCLUSION

Postwhiplash headache is a common occurrence following cervical trauma, particularly as seen in motor vehicle accidents. Surprisingly, it is more common with low-velocity crashes than with more severe impacts. Although the pathophysiology and classification of this condition remain controversial, patients may be treated with the same spectrum of medication and nonpharmacologic strategies that are used in primary headache disorders. Despite these advances, one-third of patients experience headache at 3 months postinjury and one-fifth at 12 months. Clinicians need to be aware of this entity and its management strategies.

References

1. Alexander MP: In the pursuit of proof of brain damage after whiplash injury [editorial; comment]. Neurology 51:336–340, 1998.
2. Deans G, McGalliard J, Kerr M, Rutherford W: Neck sprain-a major cause of disability following car accidents. Injury 18:10–12, 1987.
3. Crowe H: A new diagnostic sign in neck injuries. Calif Med 100:12–13, 1964.
4. Davis A: Injuries of the cervical spine. JAMA 127:149–156, 1945.
5. Gay J, Abbott K: Common whiplash injuries of the neck. JAMA 152:1698–1704, 1953.
6. Severy D, Mathewson J, Bechtol C: Controlled automobile rear-end collisions, an investigation of related engineering medical phenomena. Can Serv Med J 11:727–759, 1955.
7. Cyriax J: Rheumatic headache. Br Med J 2:1367–1368, 1938.
8. Pearce J: Cervicogenic headache—a personal view. Cephalgia 15:463–470, 1995.
9. Pearce J: Post-traumatic syndrome and whiplash injuries. In Kennard C (ed): Recent Advances in Clinical Neurology. New York, Churchill Livingstone, 1995, pp 133–150.
10. Evans R: Some observations on whiplash injuries. Neurol Clin 10:975–997, 1992.
11. Evans R: Whiplash injuries. In Evans R (ed): Neurology and Trauma. Philadelphia, WB Saunders, 1996, pp 439–457.
12. Evans R: Whiplash around the world. Headache 35:262–263, 1995.
13. Deans G, McGalliard J, Rutherford W: Incidence and duration of neck pain among patients injured in car accidents. Br Med J 292:94–95, 1986.
14. Balla J, Karnaghan J: Whiplash headache. Clin Exp Neurol 23:179–182, 1987.
15. Brooke R, LaPointe H: Temporomandibular joint disorders following whiplash. Spine State Art Rev 7:443–454, 1993.
16. Bogduk N, Marsland A: On the concept of third occipital headache. J Neurol Neurosurg Psychiatry 49:775–780, 1986.
17. Lord S, Barnsley L, Wallis B, Bogduk N: Chronic cervical zygapophysial joint pain after whiplash. A placebo-controlled prevalence study. Spine 21:1737–1745, 1996.
18. Lord S, Barnsley L, Wallis B, Bogduk N: Third occipital headache: a prevalence study. J Neurol Neurosurg Psychiatry 57:1187–1190, 1994.
19. Oosterveld W, Kortschot H, Kingma G: Electronystagmographic findings following cervical whiplash injuries. Acta Otolaryngol 111:201–205, 1991.
20. Norris S, Watt I: The prognosis of neck injuries resulting from rear-end vehicle collision. J Bone Joint Surg Br 65:608–611, 1983.
21. Evans R: The postconcussion syndrome and the sequelae of mild head injury. Neurol Clin 10:815–847, 1992.
22. Kischka U, Ettlin T, Heim S: Cerebral symptoms following whiplash injury. Eur Neurol 31:136–140, 1991.
23. National Safety Council: Accident Facts. Itasca, IL, National Safety Council (US), 1996.
24. Dolinis A: Risk factors for 'whiplash' in drivers: a cohort study of rear-end traffic crashes. Injury 28:173–179, 1997.
25. Balla J: The late whiplash syndrome. Aust N Z J Surg 50:610–614, 1980.
26. Schrader H, Obelieniene D, Bovim G: Natural evolution of late whiplash syndrome outside the medicolegal context. Lancet 347:1207–1211, 1996.
27. Obelieniene D, Schrader H, Bovin G: Pain after whiplash: a prospective controlled inception cohort study. J Neurol Neurosurg Psychiatry 66:279–283, 1999.
28. Cassidy J, Carroll L, Cotye P: Effect of eliminating compensation for pain and suffering on the outcome of insurance claims for whiplash injury. N Engl J Med 342:1179–1186, 2000.

29. Ommaya AK, Faas F, Yarnell P: Whiplash injury and brain damage: an experimental study. J Am Med Assoc 204:285–289, 1968.
30. Taylor J, Kakulas B: Neck injuries. Lancet 338:1343, 1991.
31. Taylor J, Twomey L: Acute injuries to cervical joints. An autopsy study of neck sprain. Spine 18:1115–1122, 1993.
32. Kellgren J: Observations on referred pain arising from muscles. Clin Sci 3:175–190, 1938.
33. Fredriksen T, Horval H, Sjaastad O: "Cervicogenic headache": clinical manifestations. Cephalalgia 7:147–160, 1987.
34. Kerr P: A mechanism to account for headache in cases of posterior-fossa tumors. J Neurosurg 18:605–609, 1961.
35. Evans R: Diagnostic testing for the evaluation of headaches. Neurol Clin 14:1–26, 1996.
36. Otte A, Ettlin T, Nitzsche E: PET and SPECT in whiplash syndrome: a new approach to a forgotten brain. J Neurol Neurosurg Psychiatry 63:368–372, 1997.
37. Otte A, Mueller-Brand J, Fierz L: Brain SPECT findings in late whiplash syndrome. Lancet 345:1513–1514, 1995.
38. Radanov B, Bicik I, Dvorak J: Relation between neuropsychological and neuroimaging findings in patients with late whiplash syndrome. J Neurol Neurosurg Psychiatry 66:485–499, 1999.
39. Barnsley L, Lord S, Wallis B, Bogduk N: Lack of effect of intraarticular corticosteroids for chronic pain in the cervical zygapophyseal joints. N Engl J Med 330:1047–1050, 1994.
40. Barnsley L, Lord S, Bogduk N: Whiplash injury. Pain 58:283–307, 1994.
41. Radanov B, Di Stefano G, Schnidrig A, Sturzenegger M: Common whiplash: psychosomatic or somatopsychic? J Neurol Neurosurg Psychiatry 57:486–490, 1994.
42. Radanov B, Sturzenegger M, Di Stefano G: Long-term outcome after whiplash injury. A 2-year follow-up considering features of injury mechanism and somatic, radiologic, and psychosocial findings. Medicine 74:281–297, 1995.
43. Radanov B, Di Stefano G, Schnidrig A, Ballinari P: Role of psychosocial stress in recovery from common whiplash. Lancet 338:712–715, 1991.
44. Spitzer WO, Skovron ML, Salmi LR, et al: Scientific monograph of the Quebec Task Force on Whiplash-Associated Disorders: redefining "whiplash" and its management. Spine 20(suppl 8):1S–73S, 1995.
45. Barnsley L, Lord S, Wallis B, Bogduk N: Chronic cervical zygapophyseal joint pain: a prospective prevalence study. Br J Rheumatol 32(suppl 2):52, 1993.
46. Lord S, Barnsley L, Bogduk N: Percutaneous radiofrequency neurotomy in the treatment of cervical zygapophysial joint pain: a caution. Neurosurgery 36:732–739, 1995.
47. Warner J, Fenichel G: Chronic post-traumatic headache often a myth? Neurology 46:915–916, 1996.
48. Sjaastad O, Fredriksen T, Pfaffenrath V: Cervicogenic headache: diagnostic criteria. Headache 30:725–726, 1990.
49. Anthony M: Headache and the greater occipital nerve. Clin Neurol Neurosurg 94:297–301, 1992.
50. Packard R: Posttraumatic headache—permanency and relationship to legal settlement. Headache 32:496–500, 1992.
51. Packard R, Ham L: Post-traumatic headache. J Neuropsych Clin Neurosci 6:229–236, 1994.
52. Packard RC: Epidemiology and pathogenesis of posttraumatic headache. J Head Trauma Rehabil 14:9–21, 1999.

9

Mandibular Whiplash

Gary M. Heir, DMD

The dynamic forces incurred by an individual in an acceleration-deceleration accident can extend beyond the cervical spine during the extension and flexion that ensues. In the same manner that hyperextension of the cranium on the cervical spine can cause injury to the supporting structures of the occipitocervical articulation, hyperextension of or direct trauma to the temporomandibular articulation has been thought to result in injury and dysfunction of this complex joint and its associated musculoskeletal system.

Controversy exists as to the mechanisms of injury. Questions arise concerning how indirect trauma, hyperextension of the mandible, occurs and how it results in a temporomandibular disorder (TMD). Clinical experience tells us that this is the case; however, some research argues that the forces acting on the temporomandibular joint (TMJ) during a traumatic event such as a motor vehicle accident are less than or equal to the forces brought to bear on the TMJ during normal mastication and therefore cannot be injurious. It may be argued that there are biological variables that cannot be accounted for in laboratory models such as the stature of the patient, the position of the head at the moment of impact, protective equipment in the vehicle, and the patient's awareness of the impending accident.

This chapter discusses TMJ anatomy, function, proposed mechanisms of injury, diagnosis, and treatment.

A TEMPOROMANDIBULAR DISORDER DEFINED

TMDs are defined as clinical problems that involve the masticatory musculature, the TMJs and associated structures, or both. Articular disorders of the TMJ often coexist with masticatory muscle pain. Articular disorders of the TMJs include disc displacement disorders, arthritic or degenerative changes, and neoplasm.[1] TMD is considered the most common musculoskeletal disorder causing orofacial pain. Pain can arise from the muscles of mastication or can be referred to the orofacial region from cervical or shoulder structures. Myogenous pain occurs more frequently than articular disorders.[1]

ANATOMY

The craniomandibular articulation of the TMJ is within the glenoid or temporomandibular fossa of the skull. The fossa is located in the temporal bones bilaterally just anterior to the external auditory meatus. The TMJ fossa is more of a depression in the base of the skull in which the mandibular condyle functions.

The mandibular condyle is an elliptical structure capable of a wide range of anterior and lateral movements. Interposed between the condyle and fossa is a

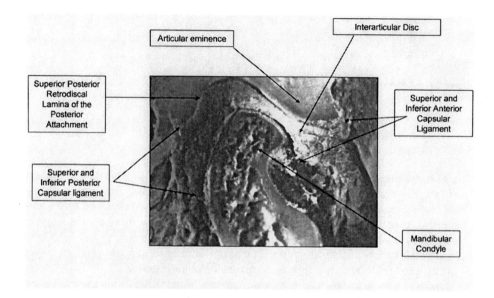

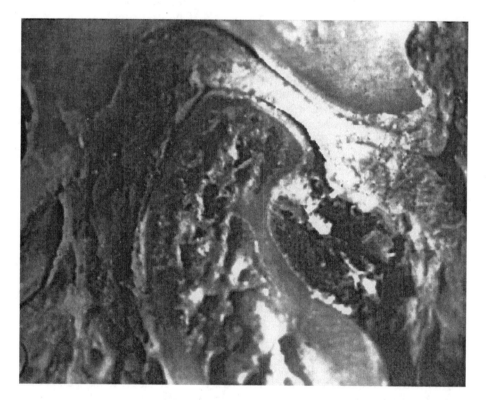

Compliments of Peter Neff, D.D.S.

Figure 1. Major components of the temporomandibular joint, sagittal view.

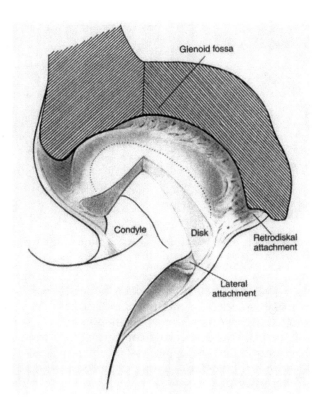

Figure 2. An anterior view of the mandibular condyle with the disc partly removed demonstrates the elliptical shape of this structure. (From Mongini F: Headache and Facial Pain. New York, Thieme, 1999; with permission.)

fibrocartilaginous disc, which is attached to the mandibular condyle by lateral and medial collateral ligaments and also blends into the capsule anteriorly. Posteriorly, the disc attaches to more complex retrodiscal tissues. The disc and its circumferential attachments separate the joint into an upper and lower joint space. The disc-condyle complex and mandibular fossa are enclosed within a capsular ligament that is lined by synovial tissue, with collateral ligaments blending into the capsule. The TMJ lateral ligament complex arises from the articular eminence and attaches to the posterior aspect of the neck of the condyle. The lateral ligament complex functions to limit lateral movement.

NORMAL BIOMECHANICS

The TMJ is a ginglymoarthrodial joint that is capable of both rotational and translocational movements. The lateral and medial discal collateral ligaments allow for rotational movement of the condyle on the inferior surface of the disc. The superior surface of the disc translates or slides along the posterior aspect of the articular eminence during function.

Biomechanically, the TMJ has significant mobility. The mandibular condyle freely rotates on the inferior surface of the interarticular disc, and the disc-condyle

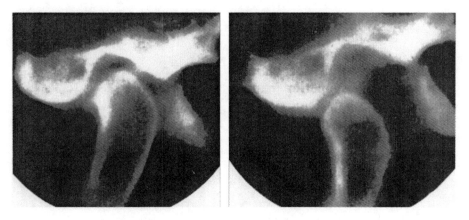

Figure 3. Tomographic imaging of normal translation of the temporomandibular joint. **A,** Closed mouth position; **B,** Open mouth position

complex moves within the fossa and translates unimpeded along the posterior slope of the articular eminence. In addition, limited lateral movements are also possible. During all of these movements the interarticular disc is always positioned between the fossa/eminence and condyle by the action of the superior lateral pterygoid muscle and the uppermost elastic properties of the posterior attachment known as the posterior, superior retrodiscal lamina of the retrodiscal tissue. Translation of the condyle occurs as a result of the action of the inferior lateral pterygoid muscle acting in concert with other mandibular depressors located in the anterior structures of the infrahyoid and suprahyoid musculature.

ABNORMAL BIOMECHANICS
Smooth and coordinated opening and closing, in the absence of pain or joint sounds, characterize normal function of the TMJs. The cardinal signs of a TMD therefore include any or all of these findings: limited or irregular jaw movements, discomfort, or sound emanating from the joint during function.

Impediments to normal joint movement can be extracapsular or intracapsular. Extracapsular conditions affecting joint movements are typically caused by muscle dysfunction. In addition, myofascial pain, myositis, myalgia, and muscle contracture can limit mandibular depression and result in discomfort. Myofascial trigger points of the masticatory musculature can refer pain to the TMJ.[20] Care must be taken during the history and physical examination to clearly define the source of the problem. Primary intracapsular pathofunctional disorders include anterior disc displacement with and without reduction. Anterior disc displacement is characterized by a partially displaced disc anterior or anteromedially. Chronic anterior disc displacement may occur for a variety of reasons. Chronic discal displacements may be adaptive changes that occur within the joint as a result of functional demands. An anterior disc displacement with reduction is characterized by joint sounds during function that occur at variable positions during mandibular movement. Soft tissue imaging such as magnetic resonance imaging (MRI) may reveal a displaced disc that improves its position during jaw opening. Hard

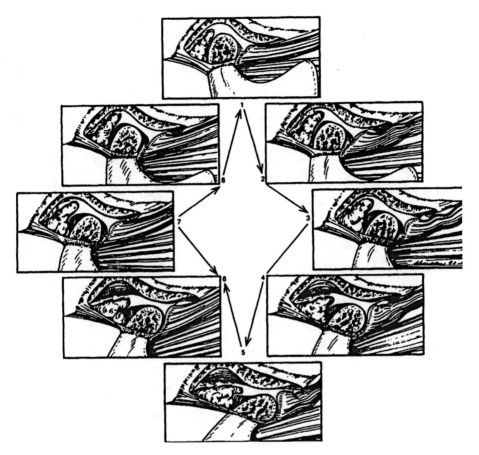

Figure 4. Normal rotational and translatory movement of the temporomandibular joint. (From Okeson JP: Orofacial Pain: Guidelines for Assessment, Diagnosis, and Management, 3rd ed. Carol Stream, IL, Quintessence Books, 1996; with permission.)

tissue imaging shows an absence of degenerative changes, although there may be adaptive remodeling of the articular surfaces. Disc displacement with reduction is also accompanied by pain with joint movement and deviation of the mandible during opening that coincides with a click as the displaced disc returns to normal. There is no restriction of mandibular movement despite the possibility of an episodic and momentary catch of jaw movement. An abnormal disc-condyle relationship is characteristic of disc displacement with reduction.[1]

Disc displacement without reduction can be chronic but may present as an acute problem as well. Anterior disc displacement with reduction may evolve to nonreducing disc displacements. Direct or indirect mandibular trauma may result in a nonreducing disc displacement in such a patient who is predisposed by a preexisting anterior disc displacement with reduction.

Anterior disc displacement without reduction is the state in which the anteriorly displaced disc is maintained in this position throughout translation. This is often referred to as a "closed lock." Essentially, the disc no longer allows the

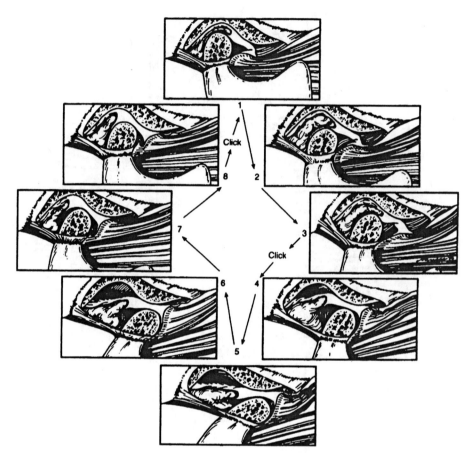

Figure 5. Disc displacement *with* reduction of the temporomandibular joint. (From Okeson JP: Orofacial Pain: Guidelines for Assessment, Diagnosis, and Management, 3rd ed. Carol Stream, IL, Quintessence Books, 1996; with permission.)

condyle to translate along the articular eminence. Deformation of the disc, or damage to the posterior attachment, causes the disc to get caught or interfere with condylar movement.[1]

A patient with disc displacement without reduction may have had a history of clicking during mandibular movement but, typically, a nonreducing disc displacement occurs in the absence of joint sounds. Soft tissue imaging reveals a displaced disc that does not improve its position during jaw opening. Hard tissue imaging may show degenerative changes. An acute "closed lock" or nonreducing anterior disc displacement is of sudden onset, with nearly immediate limited mouth opening of less than 35 mm. The mandible deflects to the affected side, and there is limited lateral movement to the opposite side. Soft tissue imaging reveals the displaced disc, while hard tissue imaging may be normal.[1]

A chronic anterior disc displacement without reduction or chronic closed lock typically includes a history of a sudden onset of limited mouth opening more than 4 months in the past. Soft tissue imaging demonstrates the displaced disc without reduction. There are typically no extensive arthritic or degenerative changes.[1]

Another posttraumatic condition affecting mandibular and TMJ function is intracapsular adhesions. As previously described, the TMJ functions within a capsular ligament. This ligament is of varying degrees of toughness, with the strongest portion at the medial aspect of the superior joint space. The superior, anterior TMJ capsular ligament is a very fragile tissue (see Fig. 1). A hypertranslation of the condyle during an acceleration-deceleration event could traumatically encroach on this structure during a subluxation of the condyle. If injured, bleeding may occur into the superior joint space, resulting in its organization into fibrous bands known as adhesions. These intracapsular adhesions can prevent normal translation of the disc and, while giving the appearance and history of a chronic disc displacement without reduction, are actually attributable to fixation of the disc to the roof of the fossa.

In contrast to hypermobility caused by disc interference or muscle contraction is the chronic subluxation seen when, due to laxity in the supporting ligaments, the mandibular condyle translates beyond the articular eminence. This subluxation of the condyle will result in a soft click or thud as the condyle passes beyond the articular eminence at maximum opening.

Aside from the mechanical dysfunction caused by trauma or injury to the TMJ is the inflammatory process that normally accompanies trauma. Inflammation of the joint capsule, capsulitis, or inflammation of the joint lining, synovitis, can also result in pain with jaw movement. The retrodiscal tissue is highly innervated and richly vascularized. Trauma to the retrodiscal tissue, as might occur with a blow to the jaw driving the condyle upward and backward, can impart a direct trauma to this tissue that results in swelling and pain. Theoretically, traumatic hypertranslation as described in a mandibular whiplash can also impart trauma to the retrodiscal tissue by overstretch of this attachment. Pain within the joint may result in secondary muscle splinting or protective guarding of the joints that may have a delayed onset of limited mandibular range of motion and pain. Inflammatory mediators within the inflamed joint may perpetuate pain and dysfunction. Synovial fluid, which may be diminished in quality and or quantity, will also compromise nutrition of the articular surfaces and lubrication of the joints.

MECHANISMS OF INJURY

A causal relationship among motor vehicle accidents, acceleration-decleration injuries, and TMD has been postulated. Debate continues as to whether adequate trauma can be imparted to precipitate an internal derangement of the TMJ or injury to the masticatory musculature.

A review of the early literature finds that mandibular whiplash was reported in motor vehicle accidents as one of the most common injuries associated with the cervical strain of whiplash injuries. The onset of TMJ pain and dysfunction associated with such injuries was reported as occurring in some cases weeks and months after the trauma. It was further reported that such injuries had a degree of permanency.[13]

Later studies using MRI as a means for diagnosing injuries to the temporomandibular joints contend that following whiplash trauma there is no significant

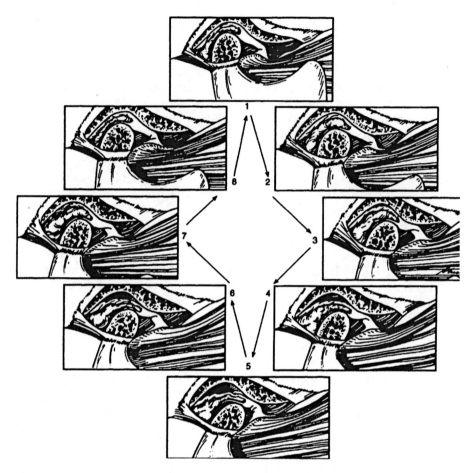

Figure 6.   Disc displacement *without* reduction of the temporomandibular joint. (From Okeson JP: Orofacial Pain: Guidelines for Assessment, Diagnosis, and Management, 3rd ed. Carol Stream, IL, Quintessence Books, 1996; with permission.)

increase in the incidence of internal derangement, joint effusion, or other TMJ injuries.[2] This study compared 60 patients with symptoms of neck pain following a motor vehicle accident involving a rear-end collision with 53 healthy volunteers in a control group. The incidence of complaints of joint pain in the posttrauma group was 5%.

Despite this and similar studies, clinicians treating TMD have long suspected a relationship between the onset of symptoms and a whiplash-type event. Of a group of 28 patients who presented for arthrographic analysis following a whiplash injury, 22 of 25 were diagnosed with internal derangement of the TMJ.[21] However, there was no control group in this clinical series, and the preaccident status of the subjects was not established.

A study in which 40 consecutive patients with a cervical whiplash injury were examined and compared with 40 matched controls found that signs and symptoms of a TMD were high in both groups. However, joint sounds, pain during mandibular function, and restricted opening were found more frequently in the posttrauma group than in the controls. Joint sounds and mandibular deviation during opening were equally reported in the patient and control groups. Of interest is the fact that more of the symptomatic posttrauma patients were willing to seek treatment for their symptoms than were symptomatic individuals in the control population.[11]

Other literature suggests that TMD symptomatology following whiplash injuries is not an independent condition caused solely by the motor vehicle accident but is the "expression of an insidious and progressive pre-existing (preaccident) disease entity."[15] This literature suggests the presence of a pretrauma inflammatory condition that would have predisposed the individual toward having a TMD.

A survey of postarthroscopy TMJ patients compared their symptoms to those of other TMD patient populations. This survey concluded that symptoms of a TMD following whiplash trauma differed from complaints reported by patients with nontraumatic or insidious onset TMD.[18]

The most commonly accepted proposed mechanisms for mandibular whiplash describe a dynamic posterior rotation of the cranium, most typically as a result of a rear-end motor vehicle accident. This theory further suggests that during the rapid extension and flexion of the head on the cranium the anterior cervical musculature connecting the mandible and chest does not have time to relax. As a result, these muscles maintain the mandible in a stable position relative to the neck and chest as the cranium rapidly rotates posteriorly. This theory contends that the mandibular condyles subluxate and are then forcefully pushed posteriorly as the head moves rapidly forward and backward, resulting in disc displacement and intracapsular injury. The consequence of this movement is a sprain of the capsular ligaments, overstretching of the posterior attachment, and injury to the retrodiscal tissue. The ensuing pain and dysfunction is pathognomonic for a TMD.

Direct trauma is readily accepted as a prime etiology for pain and dysfunction of the TMJ. It cannot be argued that a blow to the chin or trauma to the side of the face involving the mandible is capable of causing a variety of injuries of the TMJ. Possible injuries include fractures, damage to the disc, stretching of ligaments, capsular injuries, bleeding into the joint space, inflammation, and swelling. Generally the patient will report immediate pain or dysfunction.

Controversy exists when considering indirect mandibular trauma and its relationship to the formation of a TMD. The focus of indirect trauma of the TMJ seems more on damage to or displacement of the interarticular disc, its attachments, and the concomitant dysfunction that cause discal displacement. The question remains: Are the forces exerted on the TMJ during an extension-flexion injury of such magnitude that they could result in the absence of direct trauma? The literature seems equally strong on both sides of the argument. There is no clear answer.

The premise that traumatic mouth opening is due to the contraction of the mandibular depressor muscles that anchor the mandible during the rapid posterior rotation of the head has not been clearly demonstrated. Surface electromyographic values were recorded on six subjects who assumed various craniocervical positions from neutral to extension. Relative contraction of the

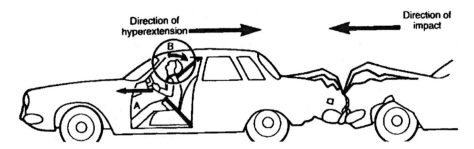

Figure 7. During a rear-end collision the torso is simultaneously driven forward as the cranium and cervical spine are hyperextended backward. (From Goldman J: Soft tissue trauma. In Kaplan A, Assail L (eds): Temporomandibular Disorders: Diagnosis and Treatment. Philadelphia, WB Saunders, 1991, pp 190–223; with permission.)

anterior cervical musculature was determined. The distance between maxillary and mandibular incisors was also measured, and it was found that the incisors were never separated by more than 2.6 mm during neutral, medium, and maximum extension of the neck. There was no evidence of a continual or induced voluntary or involuntary depressor force that would or could anchor the mandible in a position of traumatic mouth opening.[14] Unfortunately, the dynamic forces encountered by an individual in a motor vehicle accident cannot be reproduced in the laboratory setting, and the biological variables discussed earlier cannot be taken into account.

One explanation for accepting the premise that myofascial structures can be injured when stretched beyond their physiologic capacity is provided in a description of the "jolt syndrome." In the words of the author, "Myofascial structures can be made painful without injury when stretched into the supraphysiologic realm or suddenly, reflexly contracted as might occur when 'jolted' during a motor vehicle collision. Forced muscle lengthening (against the resistance of contracted muscles), perhaps similar to eccentric contraction, may be followed by immediate or delayed onset of muscle pain."[6] This same mechanism may play a role in anchoring the mandible during the cervical extension seen in whiplash.

Overall, the literature appears weak in regard to TMD. In a dynamic study of linear and angular force-time histories experienced at the TMJ, it was demonstrated that linear and rotational forces generated at the TMJ in low-energy rear-end impacts did not cause injury. However, the sample size was small and there was no evidence of follow-up with these subjects regarding TMJ symptoms. Furthermore, one can only speculate as to the subject's response to an anticipated impact when compared with a spontaneous motor vehicle accident.[9] The patient's position in the vehicle, the speed of impact, the proper or improper adjustment of the headrest, the use of restraints, and the deployment of air bags all most be taken into account when assessing the potential for injury (J. Mannheimer, personal communication, March 2001).

Despite the equivocal data, clinical evidence supports a relationship among whiplash, orofacial pain, nd TMD. Alternative mechanisms for post-whiplash and TMJ pain and dysfunction have been suggested. Myofascial pain, cervical muscle pain, and referred pain disorders are all potential contributory factors and may lead to abnormal jaw posturing. It is suggested that acquired jaw imbalance can result in symptoms of a TMD.[12]

Additional studies support damage of the TMJ as a common finding in motor vehicle accidents. The relationship between cervical whiplash and TMJ injuries was documented in 87 consecutive motor vehicle accident cervical whiplash patients who presented with a temporomandibular disorder but who had not sustained a direct trauma to the face, head, or mandible and had no prior history of a TMD. This study found a high percentage of TMJ abnormalities related to indirect trauma and cervical injuries. Findings include a disc displacement with and without reduction, joint effusion, inflammation, and edema. This study demonstrated a clear relationship between cervical whiplash and TMJ injuries.[7]

Another study attempted to determine if abnormalities of the TMJ were associated with cervical hyperextension-hyperflexion injuries. In this study, 33 consecutive symptomatic post–motor vehicle accident patients with no direct trauma to the jaw, mouth, head, or face and no prior history of TMJ dysfunction

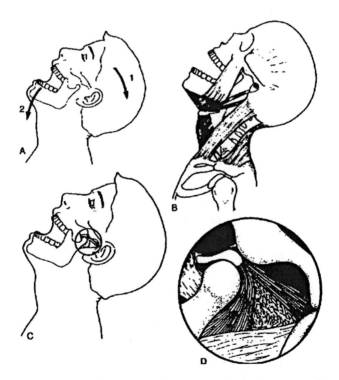

Figure 8. **A,** During the hyperextension component of a rear-end collision, the mandible tends to lag behind as the cranium goes into hyperextension. **B,** The submandibular musculature tends to anchor the mandible as the cranium hyperextends. **C** and **D,** The hyperextension of the cranium produces a condylar hypertranslation, resulting in a significant stretch on the posterior discal attachment. (From Goldman J: Soft tissue trauma. In Kaplan A, Assail L (eds): Temporomandibular Disorders: Diagnosis and Treatment. Philadelphia, WB Saunders, 1991, pp 190–223; with permission.)

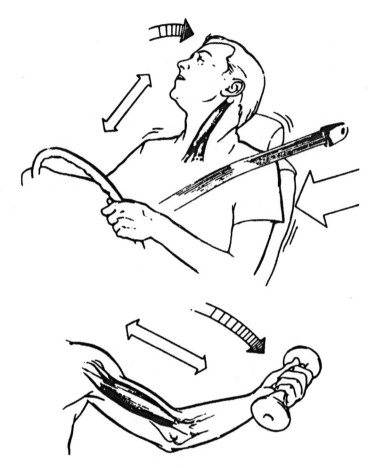

Figure 9. Muscle lengthening against resistance: eccentric contraction. (From Schenck RC (ed): Athletic Training and Sports Medicine. American Academy of Orthopaedic Surgeons, Chicago, 1984; with permission.)

underwent MRI. This study also demonstrated a high incidence of disc displacement with or without reduction as well as joint effusions.[16] However, the lack of controls in this study makes this somewhat speculative.

A review of the literature found few, if any, reliable studies on any psychological instrument capable of determining what psychological traits may be predictors of the TMD. However, a well-designed study of more than 700 subjects demonstrated that trauma patients did not differ from nontrauma patients in initial symptom levels or in levels of symptoms. Stress and psychological dysfunction were predictive of higher initial symptom perception levels but were not significantly related to treatment outcomes. It appears from these data that psychological variables have no impact on treatment outcome in regard to TMD.[17]

Beyond actual damage to the TMJ is the concept of traumatic brain injury. There are implications that TMD might be somehow related to the postconcussion headache syndrome or to psychological effects posttrauma.[4,8]

A discussion of whiplash would not be complete without some mention of litigation. A study that reviewed motor vehicle accidents, whiplash, and TMD found that many patients recovered from accident-related symptoms of TMD prior to settlement of any legal claims. Most patients who were not successfully treated continued with symptoms even after settlement. In fact, this study found that there was no significant differences in symptoms or treatment outcomes in litigating or nonlitigating patients.[10]

MANAGEMENT

Diagnosis

The goal of any treatment regimen regarding injury to or dysfunction of a joint is the restoration of function and decrease in pain. The TMJ is no different from any other joint in that regard.

Regardless of the etiology, pain, dysfunction movements, and sounds due to degenerative changes in the articular surfaces characterize a TMD. Although trauma may have been the precipitating event leading to the onset of the patient's complaints, there may be perpetuating factors that result in lengthier and less productive treatment if not recognized and eliminated. Therefore, the first goal in implementing a well-defined management program relies on the identification of contributing factors. This should include addressing physical, emotional, and psychological factors.

A comprehensive evaluation must include a detailed history including:

1. The chief complaint
2. The history of the present illness, including description of any trauma
3. The patient's medical and dental histories
   a. Has this individual ever been treated for a similar problem?
   b. What were the results of that treatment?
4. The findings of the clinical examination
   a. An evaluation of the muscles of mastication and the supporting muscles of the neck and shoulders
   b. The conditions found within the oral cavity that might be contributing to the patient's pain complaints, ie, an evaluation of the soft tissues, periodontium, and teeth
   c. Myofunctional and/or parafunctional habits
   d. Mandibular range of motion measurements
   e. An analysis of the occlusion
5. A summary of the radiologic findings.

Diagnostic Imaging

TMDs often involve displacement or dislocation of the interarticular disc and arthritic changes of the bony components of the joint. These alterations from normal anatomy and function may result from various causes, including trauma. It is an accepted standard of practice to include some form of diagnostic imaging in a TMJ evaluation to aid in arriving at a diagnosis. Various methods of radiologic imaging are available.

The most readily available diagnostic radiograph found in the dental office is the panoramic radiograph. This study is often all that is necessary to identify fracture, gross arthritic changes, or hard tissue abnormalities such as tumor or bone cysts.

The next most common radiographic study, one that is also easily done in a dental office, is the transcranial view. Performed with standard dental x-ray equipment, this study normally includes views of each condyle in the open, closed, and rest position. Transcranials provide more information concerning contours of bony elements. Transcranial radiographs are often inappropriately used to determine condylar position in the fossa: This determination is not possible from this type of study. As with the panoramic radiograph, this study may be useful in ruling out gross arthritic changes as well as fracture. While more detail is offered in the transcranial radiographs, the information provided is similar to that seen in the panoramic radiograph.

Tomography also offers an evaluation of only the osseous structures. It is a more accurate study in that it can focus on "cuts" only several millimeters thick. This ability enables a tomographic study to evaluate a TMJ like a loaf of bread, evaluating one slice at a time. Greater detail of the articular surfaces is rendered. More accurate information regarding condylar displacement and arthritic changes is also possible.

While transcranials and tomographic studies are acceptable for evaluating the hard tissues of the temporomandibular joints, they do not demonstrate the

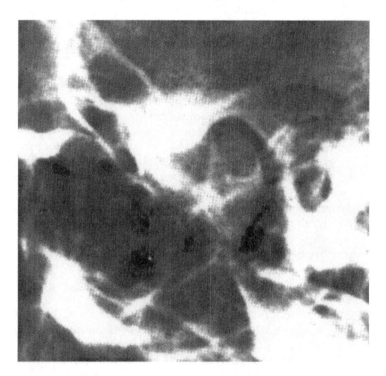

Figure 10.   Transcranial view of the TMJ.

interarticular disc. One of the objectives of conservative TMJ therapy is to reduce, or return, the disc to its normal position in relation to the mandibular condyle. Often, conservative therapy fails to achieve this goal. In such a case, it is important to determine the locations of the disc.

Various imaging techniques may be used to determine the position of the interarticular disc. Arthrography is an excellent method of imaging the disc position. It is performed by injecting a small amount of radiopaque material into the inferior or, in some cases, the inferior and superior joint compartments. The radiopaque solution outlines the disc. This procedure, which may be combined with videofluoroscopy, provides a great deal of information. The problem with this test is that it can be quite uncomfortable for the patient, requires a certain degree of expertise on the part of the radiologist, and exposes the patient to a great deal of radiation. This test is now performed infrequently.

Noninvasive imaging studies include the computed tomography (CT) scan and MRI. CT has the capacity to image not only the hard, bony tissues, but soft tissues as well. Through computerized analysis of the x-ray signal, soft tissues such as the TMJ disc may be observed. This procedure has been demonstrated to be fairly accurate in its depiction of disc position although often lacking in detail. On the negative side is the fact that with this test, as well as with arthrography, the patient is exposed to a good deal of radiation.

MRI represents the gold standard of diagnostic imaging technology. It does not use radiation at all. The image is produced by computer analysis of the signals emitted by the oscillation of water molecules of the water-containing soft tissues. These signals are produced by placing the patient into a strong magnetic field. MRI does not visualize bone; it can only image water-containing structures. The detail of soft tissues that an MRI study can reveal is often quite remarkable. Not only can MRI visualize the TMJ interarticular disc, often in more detail than the former studies, but it can also demonstrate scar tissue and inflammation of soft tissues. In addition, the muscles of mastication can be imaged. There are no adverse effects. The test is noninvasive and provides a maximum amount of information with the smallest risk.[3,5,19] There is no discomfort to the patient. Currently, the only drawback is the cost. MRI is the most expensive test of the three.

In a case in which a treating doctor feels it necessary to determine the position of a suspected disc displacement or is required to confirm a diagnosis of intracapsular adhesions, arthrography, CT, or MRI might be considered appropriate. Conversely, these imaging studies should not be done routinely for every patient or as an initial diagnostic test. While transcranial studies or tomography may be considered as initial diagnostic tests, utilization of the more sophisticated imaging examinations should be restricted only to those cases when indicated. The attending doctor should justify their need based on clinical symptoms of acute disc dislocation or less than successful conservative therapy where surgery may be considered.

Adjunctive Diagnostic Testing

The diagnosis of a TMD is best made via a meticulous history and clinical evaluation. The use of adjunctive testing should be secondary to a well-taken history and thorough clinical examination. These tests should be used judiciously.

The type of adjunctive diagnostic testing to be employed should be individualized for the specific patient. Their consideration should depend upon the potential for adding any information necessary for determining a diagnosis and treatment plan and, also, their cost-effectiveness.

TREATMENT
Treatment for TMD is consistent with that for any other musculoskeletal disorder. Because TMDs are often self-limiting, aggressive or nonreversible therapy such as surgery, extensive dental treatment, and orthodontia should be avoided.

Appropriate conservative management may include behavior modification, physical therapy, jaw exercises, intraoral orthopedic appliances, and medications. All modalities may not be appropriate or necessary in all cases, and treatment must be specific and consistent with the patient's complaints, clinical findings, and diagnoses.

In limited cases, surgical intervention may be necessary. Surgical intervention must be based upon clearly defined criteria of intracapsular pathologic conditions or anatomic derangement. The American Association of Oral and Maxillofacial Surgeons has adapted strict indications for the performance of TMJ meniscus surgery:

1. Documentation of TMJ disc derangement and that it is a major source of the patient's pain and/or dysfunction.
2. The pain and/or dysfunction are of such a magnitude as to constitute a disability to the patient.
3. Failure of nonsurgical therapy to resolve the problem.

Psychological or emotional conflicts can be an integral component in TMD and chronic pain behavior. Referral to a mental health professional such as a psychologist or psychiatrist for psychotherapeutic intervention in conjunction with reversible physical treatment modalities may be indicated for chronic TMD.

CONCLUSIONS
There is no clear consensus as to the role of indirect trauma or mandibular whiplash in the formation of a TMD. Despite this, dentists, physical therapists, and physicians have observed TMD in patients with acceleration-deceleration or extension-flexion injuries to the neck. Although the literature is equivocal as to the mechanism of injury, numerous patients present with similar symptoms and clinical findings following whiplash-type traumas. Arguments for or against various theories on this problem have filled volumes, but no clear consensus exists. What we do know is that TMDs include a variety of musculoskeletal problems that affect mandibular function. dysfunction of the TMJs and associated structures can be a source of often debilitating headache and orofacial pain. While science waits for a more specific answer as to the cause, the clinician must be ready to make an accurate assessment of these disorders and be prepared to institute effective and appropriate treatment based on a comprehensive evaluation and accurate diagnosis to resolve the patient's pain and dysfunction.

Acknowledgment

The author expresses appreciation to Dra. Cibele Nasri for her invaluable assistance in the preparation of this manuscript.

References

1. Orofacial Pain: Guidelines for Assessment, Diagnosis, and Management, 3rd ed. Carol Stream, IL, Quintessence Books, 1996.
2. Bergman H, Andersson F, Isberg A: Incidence of temporomandibular joint changes after whiplash trauma: a prospective study using Mr imaging. Am J Roentgenol 171:1237–1243, 1998.
3. Cholitgul W, Nishiyama H, Sasai T, et al: Clinical and magnetic resonance imaging findings in temporomandibular joint disc displacement. Dentomaxillofac Radiol 26:183–188, 1997.
4. Duckro PN, Chibnall JT, Greenberg MS, et al: Prevalence of temporomandibular dysfunction in chronic post-traumatic headache patients. Headache Q 8:228–233, 1997.
5. Eberhard D, Bantleon HP, Steger W: Functional magnetic resonance imaging of temporomandibular joint disorders. Eur J Orthod 22:489–497, 2000.
6. Elson LM: The jolt syndrome. Pain Manage Nov/Dec:317–326, 1990.
7. Garcia R Jr, Arrington JA: The relationship between cervical whiplash and temporomandibular joint injuries: an MRI study. Cranio 14:233, 1996.
8. Goldberg MB, Mock D, Ichise M, et al: Neuropsychologic deficits and clinical features of post-traumatic temporomandibular joint disorders. J Orofac Pain 10:126–140, 1996.
9. Howard RP, Bowles AP, Guzman HM, Krenrich SW: Head, neck, and mandible dynamics generated by 'whiplash.' Accid Anal Prev 30:525–534, 1998.
10. Kolbinson DA, Epstein JB, Burgess JA: Temporomandibular disorders, headaches, and neck pain following motor vehicle accidents and the effect of litigation: review of the literature. J Orofac Pain 10:101–125, 1996.
11. Kronn E: The incidence of TMJ dysfunction in patients who have suffered a cervical whiplash injury following a traffic accident [published erratum appears in J Orofac Pain 7:234, 1993]. J Orofac Pain 7:209–213, 1993.
12. Lader E: Cervical trauma as a factor in the development of TMJ dysfunction and facial pain. J Craniomandibular Pract 1:85–90, 1983.
13. Mannheimer J, Attanasio R, Cinotti WR, Pertes R: Cervical strain and mandibular whiplash: effects upon the craniomandibular apparatus. Clin Prev Dent 11:29–32, 1989.
14. McKay DC, Christensen LV: Electrognathographic and electromyographic observations on jaw depression during neck extension. J Oral Rehabil 26:865–876, 1999.
15. McKay DC, Christensen LV: Whiplash injuries of the temporomandibular joint in motor vehicle accidents: speculations and facts. J Oral Rehabil 25:731–746, 1998.
16. Pressman BD, Shellock FG, Schames J, Schames M: MR imaging of temporomandibular joint abnormalities associated with cervical hyperextension/hyperflexion (whiplash) injuries. J Magn Reson Imaging 2:569–574, 1992.
17. Steed PA: Etiological factors and temporomandibular treatment outcomes: the effects of trauma and psychological dysfunction. Funct Orthod 14:17–20, 1997.
18. Steigerwald DP, Verne WV, Young D: A retrospective evaluation of the impact of temporomandibular joint arthroscopy on the symptoms of headache, neck pain, shoulder pain, dizziness, and tinnitus. Cranio 14:46–54, 1996.
19. Toyama M, Kurita K, Koga K, Rivera G: Magnetic resonance arthrography of the temporomandibular joint. J Oral Maxillofac Surg 58:978–983, 2000, discussion 984.
20. Travel IJ, Simons D, Simons L: The Myofascial Trigger Point Manual. Philadelphia, Lippincott Williams & Wilkins, 1999.
21. Weinberg S, Lapointe H: Cervical extension-flexion injury (whiplash) and internal derangement of the temporomandibular joint. J Oral Maxillofac Surg 45:653–656, 1987.

10

Whiplash-Induced Cervical Facet Joint Syndrome

David W. Chow, M.D., and Curtis W. Slipman, M.D.

Facet (zygapophyseal) joints were first suggested by Goldthwait in 1911 to serve as a major source of back pain.[1] Crowe was the first to describe whiplash as a cause of neck pain in 1928.[2] The concept that zygapophyseal joints could be a source of back pain was demonstrated in 1938 by Steindler and Luck,[3] who injected local anesthetic percutaneously into the assumed area of the zygapophyseal joint to relieve pain. Since then, much literature has been published describing zygapophyseal joint pathology[4-27] precipitating axial with or without extremity pain.

ANATOMY AND BIOMECHANICS

Paired superior and inferior articular processes project from each pedicle-lamina junction. (Fig. 1). The superior articular processes of each vertebra articulate with the inferior articular processes of the next higher vertebra to form hyaline cartilage–covered synovial facet joints. The type and amount of motion that occurs between contiguous vertebrae is largely determined by the facing direction of their facet joints. The zygapophyseal joints are true synovial joints with hyaline cartilage, synovial lining, and a joint capsule that encloses the joint space. Mechanoreceptors and nociceptors richly innervate each cervical zygapophyseal joint. The facet joint capsule for the subatlantoaxial zygapophyseal joints are generally sufficiently lax to permit gliding movements of the facet joints in planes compatible with their facing direction (Fig. 2).[28] This aforementioned zygapophyseal joint laxity predisposes the capsule to rupture in hyperflexion injuries (Fig. 3). The atlantooccipital (AO) and atlantoaxial (AA) joints are not true facet joints. True joints extend from the C2-C3 to the C7-T1 levels.

The capsule of the AO joint is thicker laterally, resisting lateral bending to the opposite side. A posterior and anterior AO membrane extends from the foramen magnum to the posterosuperior and anterosuperior arch of the atlas, respectively. The posterior AO membrane is thinner than its anterior counterpart and thus has less ability to resist flexion. The apical and alar ligaments extend from the tip of the dens to the foramen magnum. The transverse axis around which flexion-extension occurs passes though these ligaments just above the dens. As a result, they have little effect on flexion and extension. The tectorial membrane is the upper broadened end of the posterior longitudinal ligament, and it assists in resisting the extremes of both flexion and extension.

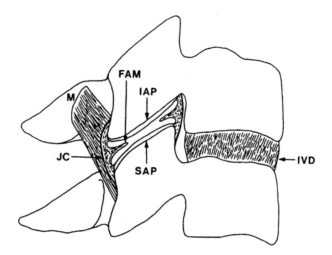

Figure 1. Sketch of a typical cervical motion segment highlighting the structures of the zygapophyseal joint. IAP, inferior articular process; SAP, superior articular process; JC, joint capsule; FAM, fibroadipose meniscoid; M, multifidus muscle; IVD, intervertebral disc. (From Lord SM, Barnsley L, Bogduk N: Cervical zygapophyseal joint pain in whiplash injuries. Spine State Art Rev 12(2):301–322, 1998; with permission.)

The superior articular processes of C1 are concave and ovoid and are directed upward and inward for the reception of the occipital condyles. The inferior articular facet joints are almost circular and slightly concave. They face downward and slightly medially and backward, articulating with the superior articular facet joints on the axis. Flexion and extension motion of the AO joint is approximately 13 degrees. Lateral bending motion averages 8 degrees, with rotational motion being negligible.

The AA joint articulates at three locations, creating a medial atlantodental and two lateral AA joints. Several restraining ligaments extend from the atlas to the axis, while others extend from the axis to the foramen magnum. The medial AA joint is a dual pivot joint between the dens and the anterior arch of the atlas

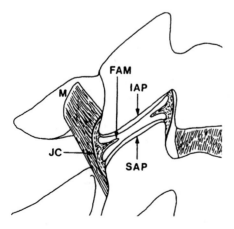

Figure 2. Tracing of a C4–5 motion segment demonstrating rotation of C4 relative to C5. The inferior articular process of C4 follows the arc of the circle which runs tangentially to the joint surface and whose center lies at the instantaneous axis of rotation of that segment. (From Lord SM, Barnsley L, Bogduk N: Cervical zygapophyseal joint pain in whiplash injuries. Spine State Art Rev 12(2):301–322, 1998; with permission.)

Figure 3 Hypothetical mechanism of injury to the zygapophyseal joints during flexion. A, the face of the inferior articular process may be driven against the upper edge of the superior articular process resulting in either subchondral fractures (*a*) or fractures of the superior articular process (*b*). B, excessive flexion may sprain or tear the joint capsule. (From Lord SM, Barnsley L, Bogduk N: Cervical zygapophyseal joint pain in whiplash injuries. Spine State Art Rev 12(2): 301–322, 1998; with permission.)

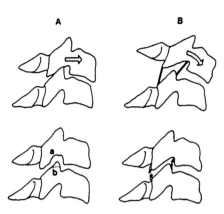

anteriorly and the transverse atlantal ligament posteriorly.[28] The lateral AA joints are formed between the inferior articular facets of the atlas and the superior articular facets of the axis. They have a thin, loose capsule that permits rather free motion. The C2 vertebra is unlike others in the cervical spine. The superior pair of facets are anterior in position to the inferior pair. Axial rotation of the AA joint averages 47 degrees and is limited by the lateral AA facet joint capsule and the opposite alar ligament. The AA joint accounts for 50% of the total rotation of the cervical spine, primarily occurring within the initial 45 degrees of cervical spine rotation emanating from the neutral position.[4] There are 10 degrees of total flexion and extension at the AA joint, with a negligible amount of lateral bending. From the axis distally, the superior articular processes of the zygapophyseal joints are oriented posteriorly and superiorly at 45 degrees from the horizontal plane. The superior articular processes form the inferior portion of the cervical zygapophyseal joints. The inferior articular processes from the vertebral body above are oriented anteriorly and inferiorly at 45 degrees from the horizontal plane.

Although the C3-C7 zygapophyseal joints are obliquely placed between the horizontal and coronal plane, they are the most horizontally oriented regional facet joints. Flexion and extension are greatest at the C5-C6 and C6-C7 interspaces, where they amount to 17 degrees and 16 degrees, respectively.[29] Lateral bending and rotation of the five lower cervical zygapophyseal joints tend to be most extensive at the C3-C4 and C4-C5 levels, averaging 11 to 12 degrees.[30]

FACET JOINT INNERVATION

Innervation to the zygapophyseal joints varies depending on the cervical level. The C2-C3 zygapophyseal joint is innervated by the superficial medial branch of the C3 dorsal ramus, also called the third occipital nerve. The third occipital nerve continues to course around the lower one-third and dorsal surface of the C2-C3 joint, finally investing in the joint capsule.

The cervical zygapophyseal joints C3-C4 to C7-T1 are innervated by the medial branches of the dorsal rami from the level above and below the joint.[31] This has important implications because medial branch blocks and radiofrequency ablations need to be performed at two different levels to anesthetize or denervate the joint.

PATHOANATOMY

Multiple structures in the cervical spine may be injured from a whiplash injury.[5,32-37] These structures include the cervical zygapophyseal joint, nerve root, disc, and ligaments. Likewise, one or more zygapophyseal joints could be implicated in chronic neck pain and headaches after an inciting traumatic event such as whiplash. Clinical and experimental studies of whiplash injuries in animals and humans have revealed tears of the zygapophyseal joint capsules, hemarthroses, and fractures of the articular cartilage and subchondral bone.[5,6,32-37] Macnab, using an experimental whiplash model with anesthetized monkeys, demonstrated injuries to the cervical zygapophyseal joints.[36,37] In a detailed autopsy study of trauma victims, Taylor demonstrated capsular or synovial tears and hemarthroses of the zygapophyseal joints.[33,34] Therefore, in assessing subjects after a whiplash event, the treating physician should be cognizant of the pathoanatomy that may result from this injury.

HISTORY AND EXAMINATION

A detailed history and neuromuscular examination should be performed on any patient presenting after a whiplash injury. Details of the accident and neck position at the time of the accident are important. However, clinical history provides no pathognomonic findings to distinguish zygapophyseal joint–mediated pain from other sources of axial pain.[6] Cole et al[7] outlined four potentially important but not diagnostic clinical findings of zygapophyseal joint pain: (1) site of maximal tenderness, (2) concordant pain on provocative segmental testing, (3) "articular restriction" and local soft tissue changes such as increased muscle tone, and (4) pain in recognized zygapophyseal joint referral zones.[8] The physical examination should include a standard neurologic examination with provocative maneuvers and assessment of range of motion. Examinations findings of increased focal suboccipital pain with 45 degrees of cervical flexion and sequential rotation may suggest pain emanating from the C1-C2 joint.[9,10]

One may suspect cervical facet joint syndrome (CFJS) when there is focal tenderness following palpation of an isolated cervical zygapophyseal joint or when the patient is able to point to the painful area corresponding to the distribution of pain reported for a particular zygapophyseal joint.[11] Despite these suggestions, there have been no well-designed studies that have demonstrated any clinical examination findings that are diagnostic for CFJS.

IMAGING

With the exception of zygapophyseal joint fracture or subluxation, injury to a cervical zygapophyseal joint cannot be detected by routine imaging studies (Fig. 4). Single photon emission computed tomography, as opposed to planar bone scintigraphy, provides a three-dimensional view of the cervical spine that helps to localize the location of the lesion.[38] Nuclear imaging may demonstrate increased tracer uptake if there is an abnormality within the zygapophyseal joint. However, it cannot discriminate whether this abnormality is symptomatic.

DIAGNOSTIC INJECTIONS AND PAIN REFERRAL PATTERNS

If a patient remains symptomatic after a reasonable course of nonoperative treatment, a consideration may then be given toward diagnostic injection

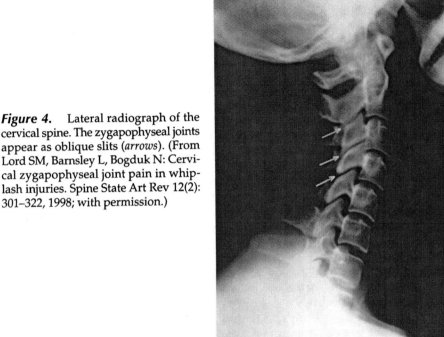

Figure 4. Lateral radiograph of the cervical spine. The zygapophyseal joints appear as oblique slits (*arrows*). (From Lord SM, Barnsley L, Bogduk N: Cervical zygapophyseal joint pain in whiplash injuries. Spine State Art Rev 12(2): 301–322, 1998; with permission.)

techniques.[39,40] Disorders of the cervical zygapophyseal joints can be a source of neck pain and headaches. Bogduk[12] investigated and identified the value of local anesthetic blockade of the third occipital nerve to diagnose cervicogenic headaches emanating from the C2-C3 zygapophyseal joint. In addition, Bogduk and Marsland[6] demonstrated the utility of diagnostic cervical medial branch and zygapophyseal joint blocks in the assessment of neck and head pain. Interestingly, symptoms of neck pain and headache most frequently stemmed from the C2-C3 zygapophyseal joint, while neck pain and shoulder pain commonly involved the C5-C6 joint. Pain maps were constructed from the areas from which patients obtained symptom relief.

Dwyer et al[8] constructed pain referral patterns, dynatomal maps, of the cervical facet joints in normal volunteers by distending the joint capsule with fluoroscopically guided injections of contrast. It was demonstrated that reasonably distinct patterns of pain referral were associated with specific joints. These results were similar to those obtained by Bogduk[6] in 1988. A follow-up study by April et al[13] assessed the accuracy of the constructed pain charts in predicting the segmental location of symptomatic joints in patients with cervical zygapophyseal joint pain. A separate sequence of pain maps was developed from this study. Dreyfuss et al[9,10] demonstrated that the AO and AA joints can also be a source of pain. Pain maps of the AO and AA joints were constructed using information gleaned from asymptomatic volunteers. (See next chapter for a description of the mechanism of somatic pain referral.)

The reliability of local anesthetic blockade of the zygapophyseal joints has been investigated.[6,15-17] Barnsley established the validity of cervical medial branch blocks for detecting symptomatic zygapophyseal joints.[15] It was demonstrated that slow injection of an aliquot of 0.5 mL of local anesthetic will not randomly disperse to inadvertently anesthetize structures other than the target medial branch. To further enhance the accuracy of zygapophyseal joint blocks, comparative injections using short- and long-acting local anesthetics were assessed and demonstrated to be a valid diagnostic technique in the identification of painful zygapophyseal joints.[16] It should be noted that this technique is inferior to placebo-controlled injections.[16,17] A false-positive rate of 27% has been reported for single, uncontrolled diagnostic cervical zygapophyseal joint injections.[18]

Headaches are a commonly associated complaint in patients with chronic neck pain after a whiplash event, reportedly occurring with a frequency as high as 66% in this patient population.[5,39,40] Lord et al,[19] in a placebo-controlled study, reported the prevalence of chronic cervical zygapophyseal joint pain after whiplash to be 60%. A triple-block paradigm was used. Patients with dominant headache were first screened by using comparative local anesthetic injections of the C2-C3 zygapophyseal joint (Fig. 5). Those who did not experience pain relief with the initial injections and those with dominant neck pain underwent placebo-controlled local anesthetic blocks. Two different local anesthetics and a placebo injection of normal saline were administered randomly and under double-blinded conditions. A positive diagnosis was made if the patient's symptoms were completely and reproducibly relieved by each local anesthetic but not by the placebo injection. Among the patients with a chief complaint of chronic headaches after whiplash, up to 50% have demonstrated a painful C2-

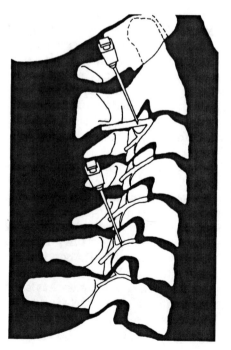

Figure 5. Diagram of a lateral radiograph showing the target points for a third occipital nerve block and a cervical medial branch block. The target points for a third occipital nerve block lie over the midpoint of the lateral projection of the C2–3 zygapophyseal joint (upper needle). The target point for a medial branch block lies at the centroid of the relevant articular pillar, proximal to the origin of the articular branches (lower needle). (From Lord SM, Barnsley L, Bogduk N: Cervical zygapophyseal joint pain in whiplash injuries. Spine State Art Rev 12(2): 301–322, 1998; with permission.)

C3 joint. Whiplash-induced lower neck pain emanating from a zygapophyseal joint was most common at C5-C6. Bogduk and Aprill[20] investigated the prevalence of traumatically induced disc pain and zygapophyseal joint pain with provocative discography and diagnostic cervical zygapophyseal joint injections. A symptomatic disc and zygapophyseal joint in the same segment was found in 41% of patients. Symptomatic zygapophyseal joints with asymptomatic discs occurred in 23% of cases.

TREATMENT

CFJS is sometimes difficult to diagnose and treat. The main reasons for treatment failure lie in incomplete assessment of the underlying problems that surround this condition. The initial strategy should be to control pain through appropriate use of nonsteroidal anti-inflammatory agents in combination with muscle relaxants. In the event that pain is incompletely treated with these medications, consideration may be given toward the use of appropriate opiate medications to allow the necessary pain control so that a physical therapy program can be initiated. A comprehensive treatment program should address strength, flexibility, posture, and ergonomics. The treating provider also must have a clear understanding of the barriers to treatment, including psychosocial issues.

All patients referred for physical therapy must have a clear understanding of their home exercise program, and the treating physician must review and upgrade the program to ensure compliance and achievement of treatment goals. In combination with a physical therapy program, joint mobilization and manipulation may provide additional results. Manipulation and mobilization have been advocated for the treatment of cervical facet syndrome.

While most individuals treated with this comprehensive approach will significantly improve, a few may require further diagnostic testing and treatment. The remainder of this chapter details injection strategies for patients who may remain symptomatic.

Therapeutic Injections

Zygapophyseal joint injections may be appropriate in individuals who, despite appropriate pharmacologic and nonpharmacologic intervention, remain symptomatic. The injections are performed under fluoroscopic control to ensure that medication is delivered intraarticularly. Barnsley reported a lack of effect of intraarticular corticosteroids in more than 50% of patients for chronic whiplash-induced cervical zygapophyseal joint pain syndrome leading to neck pain.[22] This study used one outcome measure, the visual analog scale (VAS), and evaluated the efficacy of one intraarticular steroid injection per joint. Subjects pursued unrestricted activities, including physical therapy, after injection. In our experience, fluoroscopically guided therapeutic intraarticular steroid injections have been efficacious in the treatment of CFJS.

Slipman et al[23,24] demonstrated good to excellent results in 61% of patients treated with intraarticular steroids who experienced constant daily unremitting headaches emanating from the C2-C3 facet joint subsequent to a whiplash injury. In that study, the average duration of symptoms was 3 years and no patient obtained any relief with any analgesics prior to the injections. The average follow-up period after therapeutic injections was 19 months, with a minimum follow-up period of 12 months. Multiple outcome measures were used. In that patient population, 61% had improvement following injections such that fewer than three headaches were experienced each week; 50% had improvement such that fewer than three headaches were experienced each month. Furthermore, these headaches were relieved within 20 minutes of ingestion of an oral analgesic that had been previously ineffective. There was a reduction of 2.7 points in the average VAS pain score at follow-up compared with initial presentation. This change in VAS pain score was statistically and clinically significant.[25]

Additionally, work status was assessed. Full-time work employment status improved from 17% preinjection to 56% at postinjection follow-up. The initial third of the study population working either part time or limited duty returned to full-time work status without restrictions following treatment. Therapeutic intraarticular C2-C3 zygapophyseal joint injections provided significant improvements in lifestyle and functional ability in a challenging patient population with whiplash-induced chronic daily unremitting headaches unresponsive to conservative treatments.

Radiofrequency Neurotomy

Lord et al[26] reported the efficacy of percutaneous radiofrequency neurotomy in a double-blind, placebo-controlled trial for patients with neck pain due to CFJS. All patients had been diagnosed with CFJS by double-blind, placebo-controlled local anesthetic injections. The control treatment consisted of the radiofrequency neurotomy procedure except that the radiofrequency current was not turned on. The median time that elapsed before the pain returned to at least 50% of the preneurotomy level in the active-treatment group was 9 months versus 1 week in the sham control group. McDonald et al[27] demonstrated the long-term efficacy of cervical radiofrequency neurotomy for chronic neck pain. Complete relief of pain was obtained in 71% of patients after an initial procedure. The median duration of relief after a successful procedure was 422 days. In addition, it was demonstrated that repeat radiofrequency ablation can reinstate the same pain relief if pain returns after a successful initial procedure. Radiofrequency neurotomies were performed from C3-C4 to the C6-C7 levels.

Radiofrequency neurotomies of the AO, AA, and the C2-C3 zygapophyseal joints were not investigated in this study. There is currently no technique for radiofrequency neurotomies of the AO or AA joints. Radiofrequency neurotomy of the C2-C3 zygapophyseal joint may not have been studied because of the adverse effect of suboccipital hypoesthesia from the third occipital nerve. We have successfully employed radiofrequency neurotomy to the C2-C3 zygapophyseal joint.

In our experience, patients who have had this procedure are satisfied with their symptom relief and are not distressed by suboccipital hypoesthesia.

Surgery

Surgery may consist of an open facet joint denervation procedure or fusion of that cervical segment. Prior studies have not advocated open neurectomy because of poor success rates of 40% or less and the risk of neuroma formation. In our experience, a few patients with CFJS confirmed with diagnostic cervical zygapophyseal joint injections and who had failed radiofrequency neurotomy had good results with surgical zygapophyseal joint denervation. A well-designed prospective study is needed to investigate these surgical techniques and their outcomes for CFJS confirmed with diagnostic cervical zygapophyseal joint blocks.

SUMMARY

Cervical zygapophyseal joint pain is a common phenomenon after whiplash injury. This condition can be difficult to diagnose based on the history and physical examination, and a strong clinical suspicion is necessary. An understanding of the anatomy, pathophysiology, and biomechanics of the zygopophysial joint is necessary to properly assess these complex joints. A comprehensive treatment program is necessary to improve outcomes that should include strength, flexibility, and posture in combination with mobilization and manipulation. Proper pain control needs to be emphasized because this surely can impact on whiplash patients' ability to undergo therapy. Various injection procedures may be used in those individuals who fail pharmacologic and nonpharmacologic treatment.

Acknowledgment

The authors wish to thank William S. Whyte, II, MD, for his assistance in preparation of this chapter.

References

1. Goldthwait JE: The lumbosacral articulation: an explanation of many cases of "lumbago, sciatica and paraplegia." Boston Med Surg J 164:356–372, 1911.
2. Crowe HE: Injuries to the cervical spine. Presented at the meeting of the Western Orthopaedic Association, San Francisco, 1928.
3. Steindler A, Luck JV: Differential diagnosis of pain in the low back: allocation of the source of pain by procaine hydrochloride method. JAMA 110:106–113, 1938.
4. Aprill C, Bogduk N: The prevalence of cervical zygapophyseal joint pain—a first approximation. Spine 17:744–747, 1992.
5. Barnsley L, Lord SM, Wallis BJ, Bogduk N: Chronic cervical zygapophysial joint pain after whiplash: a prospective prevalence study. Spine 20:20–26, 1995.
6. Bogduk N, Marsland A: The cervical zygapophysial joints as a source of neck pain. Spine 13:610–617, 1988.
7. Cole AJ, Dreyer SJ, Dreyfuss P, Stratton SA: Zygapophyseal (facet) joint pain: a functional approach. In Soft Tissue Injuries: Diagnosis and Treatment. Philadelphia, Hanley and Belfus, 1997, pp 47–64.
8. Dwyer A, Aprill C, Bogduk N: Cervical zygapophyseal joints pain patterns. I: a study in normal volunteers. Spine 15:453–457, 1990.
9. Dreyfuss P, Michaelsen M., Fletcher D: Atlanto-occipital and lateral atlanto-axial joint pain patterns. Spine 19:1125–1131, 1994.
10. Dreyfuss P, Rogers J, Dreyer S, Fletcher D: Atlanto-occipital joint pain. A report of three cases and description of an intra-articular joint block technique. Reg Anesth 19:344–351, 1994.
11. Jull G, Bogduk NK, Marsland A: The accuracy of manual diagnosis for cervical zyagpophysial joint pain syndromes. Med J Aust 148:233–236, 1988.
12. Bogduk N, Marsland A: On the concept of third occipital headache. J Neurol Neurosurg Psychiatry 49:775–780, 1986.
13. Aprill C, Dwyer A, Bogduk N: Cervical zygapophyseal joint pain patterns. II: a clinical evaluation. Spine 15:458–461, 1990.

14. Bovim G, Berg R, Dale LG: Cervicogenic headache: anesthetic blockade of cervical nerves (C2-C5) and facet joint (C2/C3). Pain 49:315–320, 1992.
15. Barnsley L, Bogduk N: Medial branch blocks are specific for the diagnosis of cervical zygapophyseal joint pain. Reg Anesth 18:343–350, 1993.
16. Barnsley L, Lord SM, Bogduk N: Comparative local anesthetic blocks in the diagnosis of cervical zygapophysial joint pain. Pain 55:99–106, 1993.
17. Lord SM, Barnsley L, Bogduk N: The utility of comparative local anesthetic blocks versus placebo-controlled blocks for the diagnosis of cervical zygapophysial joint pain. Clin J Pain 11:208–213, 1995.
18. Barnsley L, Lord SM, Wallis BJ, Bogduk N: False positive rates of cervical zygapophysial joint blocks. Clin J Pain 9:124–9130, 1993.
19. Lord SM, Barnsley L, Wallis BJ, Bogduk N: Chronic cervical zygapophysial joint pain after whiplash: a placebo-controlled prevalence study. Spine 21:1737–1745, 1996.
20. Bogduk N, Aprill C: On the nature of neck pain, discography, and cervical zygapophysial joint blocks. Pain 54:213–217, 1993.
21. Slipman CW, Chow DW, Whyte WS, et al: An evidence-based algorithmic approach to cervical spinal disorders. Crit Rev Phys Rehabil Med. In press.
22. Barnsley L, Lord SM, Wallis BJ, Bogduk N: Lack of effect of intra-articular corticosteroids for chronic cervical zygapophyseal joint pain. N Engl J Med 330:1047–1050, 1994.
23. Slipman CW, Lipetz JS, Plastaras CT, et al: Outcomes of therapeutic zygapophyseal joint injections for headaches emanating from the C2-C3 joint. Am J Phys Med Rehabil 78:1023, 1997.
24. Slipman CW, Lipetz JS, Plastaras CT, et al: Outcomes of therapeutic zygapophyseal joint injections for headaches emanating from the C2-C3 joint. Am J Phys Med Rehabil 80:182–188, 2001.
25. Saal JA, Saal JS: Intradiscal electrothermal treatment for chronic discogenic low back pain. Spine 25:2622–2627, 2000.
26. Lord SM, Barnsley L, Wallis B, et al: Percutaneous radiofrequency neurotomy for chronic cervical zygapophyseal joint pain. N Eng J Med 335:1721–1726, 1996.
27. McDonald GJ, Lord SM, Bogduk N: Long-term follow-up of patients treated with cervical radiofrequency neurotomy for chronic neck pain. Neurosurgery 45:61–67, 1999.
28. White AA, Panjabi MM: Clinical Biomechanics of the Cervical Spine. Philadelphia, JB Lippincott, 1978.
29. Mooney V, Robertson J: Facet joint syndrome. Clin Orthop 115:149–156, 1976.
30. Schneck CD: Functional and clinical anatomy of the spine. Spine State Art Rev 9:525–558, 1995.
31. Bogduk N: The clinical anatomy of the cervical dorsal rami. Spine 7:319–330, 1982.
32. Rauschning W, McAfee PC, Jonsson H Jr: Pathoanatomical and surgical findings in cervical spinal injuries. J Spinal Disord 2:213–222, 1989.
33. Taylor JR, Finch P: Acute injury of the neck: anatomical and pathological basis of pain. Ann Acad Med Singapore 22:187–192, 1993.
34. Taylor JR, Twomey LT: Acute injuries to cervical joints. An autopsy study of neck sprain. Spine 18:1115–1122, 1993.
35. Davis SJ, Teresi LM, Bradley WG Jr, et al: Cervical spine hyperextension injuries: MR findings. Radiology 180:245–251, 1991.
36. Macnab I: Acceleration injuries of the cervical spine. J Bone Joint Surg Am 46:1797–1799, 1964.
37. Macnab I: The "whiplash syndrome." Orthop Clin North Am 2:389–403, 1971.
38. Sarikaya I, et al. The role of single photon emission computed tomography in bone imaging. Semin Nuclear Med 31(1):3–16, 2001.
39. Maimaris C, Barnes MR, Allen MJ: Whiplash injuries of the neck: a retrospective study. Injury 19:393–396, 1988.
40. Norris SH, Watt I: The prognosis of neck injuries resulting from rear-end vehicle collisions. J Bone Joint Surg Br 65:608–611, 1983.

11

Whiplash-Induced Cervical Disc and Radicular Pain

Curtis W. Slipman, M.D., and David W. Chow, M.D.

This chapter reviews the anatomy, pathophysiology, evaluation, and treatment of patients with cervical disc injury following whiplash injury. About 8% to 20% of motor vehicle accidents are rear-end collisions resulting in acceleration hyperextension or whiplash injuries.[1,2] Almost half of the injured patients consult the physician within the first 12 hours and another 40% within the first 3 days.[3] Two-thirds of cases spontaneously resolve, while the remaining third go on to experience chronic cervical pain involving the head, neck, or upper limb.[4] The high-energy accelerative and decelerative forces during cervical hyperextension-flexion may frequently injure the cervical discs or nerve roots.

ANATOMY

There are seven cervical vertebrae and eight cervical nerve roots. The vertebral segments are connected via the zygapophyseal joints, which preclude excessive motion of the cervical spine. The uncovertebral (UV) joints are unique to the cervical spine and are clinically significant. UV joints are jointlike structures located between the uncinate processes of the C3-C6 vertebrae.[5] These joints commonly develop osteoarthritic changes, which can narrow the diameter of the intervertebral foramina. The foramina are widest at C2-C3 and progressively decrease in size to the C6-C7 level. The radicular complex of ganglia, nerve roots, spinal nerve, and surrounding sheath accounts for 20% to 35% of the cross-sectional area of the intervertebral foramina.[6-8] The dorsal root ganglia (DRG) reside either immediately proximal or distal to the midportion of the pedicle. The remainder of the intervertebral foramina is occupied by loose areolar or adipose tissue, Hoffman ligaments, radicular artery, and numerous venous channels that often encircle the nerve roots. The neuroforamina are bordered anteromedially by the UV joint, superiorly and inferiorly by successive pedicles, and medially by the edge of the vertebral end plate and intervertebral disc.

The intervertebral discs are located between the vertebral bodies of C2 through C7. The anterior longitudinal ligament (ALL) and posterior longitudinal ligament (PLL) course over the intervertebral discs and vertebral bodies on the anterior and posterior surfaces, respectively. The ALL, the largest ligament in the cervical spine, originates at the anteroinferior C2 vertebra. It adheres to the midpoint of the vertebral body and is thickest over the disc where it blends with the anulus. One of its major functions is to limit sheer movement between vertebrae in cervical extension. The PLL is a narrower and weaker band than the ALL and runs from the C2 vertebra to the sacrum. It helps prevent hyperflexion of the vertebral column and posterior protrusion of the discs. The dural ligaments of Hoffman attach to the PLL and periosteum of the vertebral body. This attachment occurs where the nerve root exits the dura. More caudal fixation occurs at the intervertebral foramen where the epineural sheath is attached to various structures within the intervertebral foramen.

Each intervertebral disc is composed of an outer anulus fibrosus and an inner nucleus pulposus. Together they function as force dissipaters by transmitting compressive loads throughout various ranges of motion. The nucleus pulposus is a semifluid mass that allows it to be deformed under pressure, transmitting the applied pressure in all directions. However, its volume cannot be compressed. The anulus fibrosus consists of concentrically arranged collagen in sheets called lamellae. The collagen fibers within each lamella lie parallel to one another and measure about 65 degrees from the vertical axis of the spinal column. However, 40% to 50% of lamellae in any given quadrant of the anulus do not form a complete ring around the circumference of the disc.[9] The lamellae of intervertebral discs are thicker anteriorly and laterally, but posteriorly they are thinner and more tightly packed. Each intervertebral disc is covered superiorly and inferiorly by a cartilaginous vertebral end plate. Each end plate covers the nucleus pulposus in its entirety but peripherally fails to traverse the entire extent of the anulus fibrosus. Because the end plate does not span over the ring apophysis of the vertebral body, the most superficial lamellae of the anulus insert directly into the bone of the vertebral body. Unlike the weak attachment between the end plates and vertebral bodies, the bonds—"Sharpey's fibers"—between the end plates and the intervertebral disc are strong. Therefore, certain forms of spinal trauma may wholly tear the end plates from a vertebral body.

The innervation of the intervertebral disc is complex (Fig. 1). There are nociceptive nerve endings in the outer third of the anulus. Rami communicates from the sympathetic chains on either side of the disc help to form anterior, lateral, and posterior longitudinal nerve plexi that surround and innervate the disc. The anterior plexus covers and innervates the ALL while bridging the two sympathetic trunks. The posterior plexus is derived from sinuvertebral nerves and microscopic nerve fibers. Sinuvertebral nerves are recurrent branches of the ventral rami that reenter the intervertebral foramina and innervate the disc and PLL superiorly and at its level of origination. The lateral sides of the disc are innervated by the anterior and post plexus, lateral plexus, sinuvertebral nerve, and gray rami communicates.[9] Normal cervical spine anatomy may be subject to trauma, leading to various cervical spinal disorders including cervical radiculopathy, cervical radicular pain, cervical zygapophyseal joint syndrome, and cervical internal disc disruption (CIDD).

WHIPLASH INJURY BIOMECHANICS

Crowe introduced the term whiplash in 1928.[10] Whiplash involves sudden high-energy forces that cause cervical hyperextension and hyperflexion. These forces are usually generated during a motor vehicle accident. Whiplash syndrome refers to a constellation of signs and symptoms that may occur after cervical hyperextension-flexion. Whiplash syndrome is a descriptive term and not

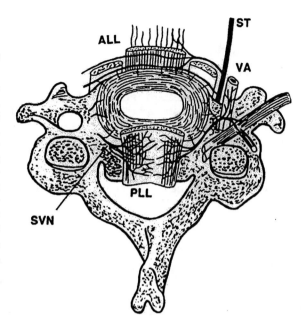

Figure 1. The innervation of the cervical intervertebral disc. ST, cervical sympathetic trunk; ALL, anterior longitudinal ligament; VA, vertebral artery; SVN, cervical sinuvertebral nerve; PLL, posterior longitudinal ligament. (From Bogduk N: Innervation and pain patterns of the cervical spine. In Grant R (ed): Clinics of Physical Therapy: Physical Therapy of the Cervical and Thoracic Spine, 2nd ed. New York, Churchill Livingstone, 1994, pp 65–76; with permission.)

a diagnosis. Hence, whiplash syndrome has good descriptive validity but poor construct validity.[11]

Whiplash injuries may even be caused by low-velocity motor vehicle accidents. Severy demonstrated that a collision at 15 mph can accelerate the head with a force of 10g and result in injury to structures in the cervical spine.[12] Cervical hyperextension injury may be caused by direct anterofacial or craniofacial trauma but is most commonly the result of rear-end collisions. Cervical hyperextension injuries result from inertia of the head when the body accelerates forward after a rear-end impact. This occurs when the trunk of the occupant moves forward in relation to the head by the forward momentum of the seat upright, creating an extension moment and forcing the head backward. When the tone of the anterior cervical muscles is overcome, there is nothing to resist the extension movement of the neck except the ALL and the anterior fibers of the anulus. Hyperextension usually centers on the C5-C6 level and continues until the neck reaches the end of its range of motion or when the occiput strikes the upper back or another structure such as a head restraint.[13] When the car stops accelerating, the head rebounds forward (recoil flexion). This forward movement may be accelerated by contraction of the cervical flexor muscles because of induction of a stretch reflex during the extension phase of movement.

There are numerous variables in a motor vehicle accident that can affect the type and severity of injury sustained by the cervical spine. For example, the presence of a lap belt or whether the person braces himself with his hands on the steering wheel will impact the forces transmitted to the cervical spine.[14] In such instances, forward sliding of the pelvis is prevented, thereby increasing the acceleration extension strain applied to the neck. In high-speed impacts, the force with which the occupant's body strikes the seat tends to break the upright of the front seat. As the car accelerates, the occupant is lying almost horizontally, resulting in traction rather than an extension force, which is ultimately applied to the neck.

Several studies have attempted to identify the mechanism of whiplash injury in the cervical spine. Macnab,[13,14] using an animal experimental trauma model with anesthetized monkeys, found a predominance of anterior element injuries. He demonstrated that cervical hyperextension from accelerative forces may tear anterior cervical muscles and the ALL. Furthermore, rupture of the ALL and intervertebral disc was more common when cervical rotation was combined with extension. Tearing of the ALL was associated with separation of the disc from the end plates of the vertebral body. This disc injury could not be detected on routine radiographs even after several months had passed. In human cadaveric studies, Taylor[15,16] demonstrated linear fissures or rim lesions in the cartilage plates of cervical discs from trauma victims. Traumatic disc ruptures, herniations, anular bruising, and ligamentous injuries were also found. Surgical findings in whiplash-injured humans undergoing an anterior fusion demonstrated disc separation from the vertebral body with blunt dissection.[14] This confirms the disc separation or avulsion as seen in the animal model.

In frontal and side collisions, the neck usually experiences the same type of inertial loading from the head as in rear-end accidents. Penning demonstrated that during the initial phase of these neck-loading situations, the head normally undergoes a horizontal translational displacement relative to the torso.[17,18] This translational motion may be manifested as forward protraction or rearward retraction. The cervical spine is vulnerable to injury from significant mechanical loads when the end range of protraction or retraction is reached. In the upper cervical spine, cervical rotational injuries were most common.[17,18] Svenson reported that the cervical spine initially formed an S-shaped curve and then complete extension using a dummy model.[19] Panjabi confirmed the development of the S-shaped curvature of the cervical spine with lower-level extension and upper-level flexion in an experimental whiplash model with high-speed filming.[20] The initial S-shaped curvature was followed by extension of the entire cervical spine. In contrast to Macnab's findings, this simulated whiplash model did not produce occiput extension beyond the physiologic limits, suggesting that injury may not be solely caused by cervical extension. Other studies have also observed the lack of head hyperextension.[20-22] Furthermore, physiologic ranges of extension were more frequently and consistently exceeded in the lower cervical levels until higher trauma intensities affected the upper levels. Each cervical level may be subjected to various combinations of vertical forces, horizontal shear forces, and bending moments that correspond to certain patterns of reproducible fractures, ligamentous injuries, and soft tissue injuries. Six components of displacement (translations and rotations) and load (forces and moments) have been proposed to describe the biomechanical environment.[23]

PATHOANATOMY

Disc injuries have been implicated during examination, surgery, or at autopsy of patients with acceleration injuries. In a detailed autopsy study of trauma victims, Taylor demonstrated linear clefts in the cartilage plates of cervical discs in

15 of 16 spines.[15,16] These are quite distinct from the UV clefts and central disc fissures that are a normal feature of aging in cervical discs. Posterior disc herniations through a damaged anulus were commonly observed. No comparable lesions were found in control subjects. Age-related UV clefts or fissures extended transversely from the UV joints and medially toward the center of each disc. These fissures were usually situated midway between vertebral end plates and were confined to the posterior half of each cervical disc without involving the cartilage plates. The traumatically induced linear clefts in the cartilage plates ran close and parallel to the end plate and often affected the peripheral portion of the disc near the vertebral rim where the cartilage plate lamellae were continuous with the anular lamellae. In this situation they resembled the rim lesions as described by Vernon-Roberts in lumbar discs.[24] The traumatically induced clefts were usually between the transversely oriented lamellae of the anulus. Anterior rim lesions are from extension injuries caused by anterior distraction at the disc-vertebral junction. They were found between the tissue planes of the cartilage plate and anulus, where they were continuous with each other. Blood was usually present in clefts that extended to the vertebral end plate or outer anulus. In some cases, the cartilage plate was almost completely separated from the disc. Other disc injuries included traumatic disc ruptures with posterior herniation and anular bruising. Disc herniations usually breached the lamellae of the posterior anulus or the cartilage plate near its junction with posterior anulus.

Disc herniations have also breached the PLL or entered the neuroforamina. The anterior spinal column is the initial site of serious hyperextension injury. It consists of the ALL and the anterior two-thirds of the vertebrae. The ALL may be stretched and torn away from the anulus, causing hemorrhage and edema in the prevertebral fascia. The PLL may be torn with recoil flexion. Hyperextension disc injuries include a characteristic separation of the intervertebral disc from the vertebral end plate. This lesion has been described experimentally in monkeys as a result of a whiplash event and has been seen at autopsy in severe hyperextension injuries resulting in humans.[14-16] Macnab also found comparable lesions in eight patients undergoing operation within 2 years of injury and during preoperative discography.[14] Intraoperatively, the disc could be easily separated from the adjacent vertebra at blunt dissection, indicating little or no reattachment of the disc to the vertebra from which it had been avulsed. Evidence of this injury was seen in five of seven patients with anterior column injuries (at more than one level in three patients) and at follow-up 9 months after.

Whiplash can cause injury to the cervical nerve roots or the DRG.[15,16,24] Sudden forces can cause traction injury or bruising to these structures. Compression or irritation of the cervical nerve root or DRG by venous engorgement or hematoma formation from nearby venous plexi has been reported.[15,16] Intraneural DRG hemorrhage has been shown to occur with injury to the dorsal root ganglion.

PATHOPHYSIOLOGY
There are critical external loading conditions and initial head and body positions that determine the vertebral stresses and presence and severity of injury to the cervical disc and nerve root. Accelerative forces cause sudden cervical flexion, extension, rotation, lateral bending, or compression. This creates powerful

shear forces that can cause fissures, ruptures, and herniations of the cervical disc. In severe trauma, discs may be wholly torn from the end plates or the end plates may be separated from the vertebral body. Most frequently, axial compression in combination with flexion or flexion in combination with rotation seems to cause the most severe injuries. Intradiscal pressures are highest with forward flexion. Flexion with rotation exponentially increases shear forces on the disc, creating anular fissures or tears.[25] Shear forces are highest during rotation because the zygapophyseal joints are locked and the longitudinally oriented paraspinal musculature is unable to fully dissipate these forces. Flexion and compression also promotes posterior anular bulging and anular fissures. Flexion, compression, and lateral bending may predispose to posterolateral herniations of the nucleus pulposus through the thin posterolateral lamellae of the anulus fibrosus.

Although rare, acute traumatic cervical disc herniations do occur. One study reported several C3-C4 disc herniations after whiplash, with cranial symptoms responding to anterior discectomy and fusion.[26] Traumatic cervical disc herniations causing radicular pain may occur at any level regardless of injury level or preexisting spondylosis. There is little literature regarding acute disc herniation due to hyperextension injury. This may be because of a lack of epidemiologic studies focusing on traumatic disc herniations or perhaps because disc herniation tends to develop after the acute phase of a hyperextension injury, with radicular symptoms typically occurring after 1 month and spontaneously resolving. In addition, because of the anatomy of the cervical spine, traumatic disc herniations may more frequently cause clinically significant central stenosis, resulting in myelopathy or central cord syndrome rather than radicular pain as occurs in the lumbar spine.

Cervical disc injuries from whiplash frequently involve multiple levels and a transverse tear or "rim lesion" near the anterior vertebral rim.[15,16] Rim lesions in discs are strongly associated with trauma but not with degenerative change. They involve the avascular cartilage plates but often extend into the innervated, vascular outer anulus and sometimes into the highly vascular bony vertebral end plates. The increased frequency of rim lesions in the upper cervical discs compared with the lower discs may be related to the increased translational movement that accompanies flexion and extension at the upper segmental levels. During these motions, the plane of the zygapophyseal joints are closer to the transverse plane of the corresponding disc. Shearing results from the horizontal sliding of one vertebra on another, which accompanies flexion or extension, because of the 45-degree orientation of the cervical zygapophyseal joints.[15] Movement occurs in an arc around an axis located in the vertebra below the moving vertebra. Translation and shearing are greatest in the upper parts of the motion segment. It has been shown that rim lesions produced surgically to a depth of 5 mm in sheep discs did not heal when followed for 18 months.[29] Although the outer third of the anulus has the ability to heal, most rim lesions heal slowly and extend inward with deformation of the anular lamellae and degeneration of the nucleus pulposus. Rim lesions have been shown to predispose the disc to premature degeneration.[14,16,27,28] This may occur by disrupting the normal nutritional flow from the vertebral marrow and outer anulus to the rest of the avascular disc.

Various combinations of vertical forces, horizontal shear forces, and bending moments may cause injury to cervical nerve roots. These forces may cause radicular pain by traction, compression, or direct pressure from a nearby structure. The nerve root, which occupies 25% to 35% of the foraminal space, is vulnerable to compression by pathology from three structures: the zygapophyseal joint, joints of Luschka, and the disc. Cervical nerve roots can be injured from a focal disc protrusion and are also susceptible to significant injury in the absence of more overt trauma to contiguous structures.[29-31] During the extension phase of injury, the nerve root may become entrapped in a transiently narrowed neural foramen.[29,30,32,33] Compression of the nerve roots is dependent on the effective space available within the intervertebral foramen. Foraminal stenosis is a dynamic condition because cervical flexion and extension changes the amount of foraminal constriction. Significant reductions in neuroforaminal diameter, and increases in neuroforaminal pressures have been observed with increasing neck extension.[33-35] Yoo examined changes in neuroforaminal sizes at C5, C6, and C7 levels.[33] He demonstrated a significant decrease in neuroforaminal size with cervical extension and an increase with cervical flexion. Farmer and Wisneski measured pressures within neural foramens using balloon catheters with pressure transducers during ranges of motion.[35] They demonstrated a significant increase in pressure on the C5, C6, and C7 nerves in cervical extension, whereas a significant decrease of pressure was found with moving the arm from the neutral to the abducted position. Decreased pressure with the shoulder abduction relief position may be due to increased opening of the intervertebral foramen or decreased tension on the nerve root from the dural ligaments.

The most common cause of nerve root compression is a focal disc protrusion or hyperostotic foraminal stenosis. Compression of nerve roots is dependent on the space available within the neural foramen, osseoarticular structures surrounding the foramen, and the tethering effects of intraspinal and extraspinal ligamentous structures. Because nerve roots lack a perineurium and have a poorly developed epineurium, they may be more susceptible to compression.[33] Lu demonstrated that the size of the intervertebral foramen is directly related to the height of the intervertebral disc space.[34] A decrease in the height of an intervertebral disc can constrict the intervertebral foramen sufficiently to cause entrapment or compression of the spinal nerve root. Lu revealed that a 1-mm and 3-mm narrowing of the intervertebral disc space corresponded to a reduction of 20% to 30% and 35% to 45% of the foraminal area, respectively.[34] With the collapse of the disc space, there is a reduction of the adjacent intervertebral foraminal area as the inferior zygapophyseal joints of the upper cervical vertebra slide down the superior zygapophyseal joints of the adjacent lower segment and settle. This zygapophyseal joint settling results in foraminal stenosis.[34] Hyperostosis from a posteriorly protruding UV spur into the already compromised foramen contributes to the stenosis.

The nerve root, initially compressed due to cervical extension, may then be subjected to a traction injury as the neck is thrown into a rebound flexion. This direct root trauma likely leads to intraneural vascular congestion and edema. Edema formation in nerve roots has been shown to be particularly pronounced in the setting of rapid compression.[36] These combined insults render the nerve root susceptible to chronic injury and dysfunction. Inflammatory materials such as phospholipase A_2 and synovial cytokines may continue to leak from an adjacent injured disc or zygapophyseal joint, resulting in sustained neural irritation.[37] Intraneural and perineural fibrosis may evolve subsequent to prolonged intraneural edema and chronic exposure to inflammatory substances. Continued mechanical insult may result as adhesions develop between the nerve root and surrounding structures, minimizing root glide within the foramen.

The DRG have been shown to fire repetitively following minimal compression, in the absence of neural irritation, likely demonstrating even greater mechanosensitivity than the nerve root in the setting of chronic injury.[38,39] Injury to the dorsal root ganglion with intraneural DRG hemorrhage has been reported in blunt injuries.[15] Yabuki and Kikuchi reported that the DRG were located proximal to the midportion of the pedicle in 48% of spines at C6 and 27% at C7.[40] An increased incidence of radiculopathy was found in the spines with more proximal DRG. The end stage of these multiple insults and alterations may include a sensitization of the peripheral and central nervous systems, resulting in persistent radicular pain.

The tethering effects of spinal ligaments may play an important role in the pathophysiology of nerve root trauma and cervical radicular pain. Spencer reported that tensile forces can be generated on the exiting nerve root from attachments of the dural ligaments of Hoffman to the PLL and the periosteum of the vertebral body.[41,42] This attachment occurs just at the level where the nerve root exits the dura. More caudal fixation is noted to occur at the intervertebral foramen where the epineural sheath is attached to various structures within the intervertebral foramen. A disc placing pressure on the nerve root may exert compressive as well as tensile force via ligamentous attachments. Spencer demonstrated increased pressures at the contact point between the bulging disc and nerve root.[43] Consequently, tensile forces on the ligaments that attach the nerve root to surrounding structures can play an important role in whiplash injuries.

PAIN REFERRAL

Understanding radicular pain referral patterns is important. However, other cervical structures such as the anulus of the intervertebral disc, PLL, and zygapophyseal joint may cause somatic referral of pain into the limb or extremity.[44-47] Kellegren[44,45] was the first to investigate the pain referral patterns of nonneural structures by using hypertonic saline to stimulate periosteum, fascia, tendon, and muscle. He hypothesized that the mechanism of pain referral was a central nervous system phenomenon because anesthetizing the peripheral nerve distal to the site of stimulation did not diminish the distally referred pain. Von Luschka[48] in 1850 reported that nociceptive fibers supplying the anulus fibrosus and PLL are connected to the central nervous system via the sinuvertebral nerve. This type of pain referral, previously referred to as *sclerotomal*, has been termed *somatic* and occurs when a mesodermal structure such as a ligament, joint capsule, intervertebral disc anulus, or periosteum is stimulated, leading to symptoms that are referred into another mesodermal tissue structure of similar embryonic origin. It is via this mechanism that internal disc disruption syndrome and zygapophyseal joint syndrome create upper limb symptoms. It is assumed that somatic referral has a biomechanical or biochemical basis. Biomechanical or biochemical irritation of nonneural structures may provoke nociceptive nerve fibers via mechanical compression or an inflammatory process and cause pain referral.

Equally important is understanding the distinction between radiculopathy, radiculitis, and radicular pain. Radicular pain refers to pain that radiates in a specific cervical nerve root distribution. Patients frequently describe classic dermatomal symptoms. Patients with pain that is not typical of a dermatomal distribution may still have radicular pain. If further testing demonstrates the nerve root as the offending source, the patient is describing a cervical dynatomal pattern.[49] Radiculopathy is defined as radicular pain with concurrent myotomal deficits or reflex change or a positive electromyography study. Therefore, all patients with radiculopathy have an objective neurologic effect, and most experience radicular pain. Not all patients with radicular pain have a radiculopathy. In this latter clinical scenario, the diagnosis of radicular pain is made with a positive diagnostic selective nerve root block. Patients with radiculitis will only have symptoms of radicular pain and without evidence of radiculopathy. In this subset of patients with radiculitis, an inflammatory basis elicits the radicular pain, while other patients with radicular pain do not have an inflammatory component. Examples of such cases include patients who have radicular pain consequent to intraneural or epidural fibrosis.

OBTAINING THE HISTORY

Collect precise details of the accident. Besides the speed and type of accident, neck position at the time of the accident is important. Another significant point is whether the accident occurred unexpectedly or expectedly. This may aid in determining neck muscle tone or cervical spine position at the time of the accident. The patient's medical history prior to the accident as related to absence from work and necessity of treatment should be noted. Several studies have described a relatively poor prognosis for whiplash patients presenting with initial upper limb pain and sensory disturbances.[4,50–52] These studies related outcomes to presenting symptomatology; patients were not provided a specific diagnosis. Radanov has reported that increased severity of injury, premorbid history of headaches or radiologic degenerative changes, and radicular deficits are indicators of poor prognosis.[53–56]

The most frequent complaints after a whiplash injury were neck symptoms and headaches.[1,50,53] Shoulder and upper limb symptoms, disturbance of consciousness, and dizziness were also common. The Quebec Task Force on Whiplash-Associated Disorders has classified the signs and symptoms into four grades according to the clinical presentation.[1] In general, most patients with radicular pain usually present with arm pain greater than neck pain, with or without motor weakness, reflex change, or paresthesias. Those with discogenic-mediated pain usually have greater neck than arm pain. Upper limb pain that is somatically referred from the disc is usually in a nondynatomal distribution, which may be symmetric bilaterally. In addition, psychosocial symptoms or neuropsychological deficits were found to be common in whiplash patients receiving disability pensions. Depression, decreased confidence, loss of vitality, lack of concentration, and sleep disturbances were the most common neuropsychological deficits.

EXAMINATION AND PROVOCATIVE MANEUVERS

During the physical examination, passive and active range of motion of the cervical spine should be assessed. Evaluation of cervical rotation out of flexion and extension is important in assessing the function of the upper and lower cervical spine. Segmental manual examination may be helpful to identify the most painful segment of the cervical spine. Myotomal or dermatomal deficits and/or a depressed muscle stretch reflex suggest cervical nerve root injury. The reliability of certain manual examination tests has been investigated. Good reliability was obtained in the cervical compression and axial manual traction tests. Fair reliability was obtained in muscle strength testing and in the estimation of the range of motion, and poor reliability was obtained for manual palpation.[57] Poor standardization of examination procedures and changes in the patients' attention were considered the main factors affecting reliability.

Provocative maneuvers such as Spurling's test, nerve tension, or root traction may be used. Spurling's test involves cervical extension, rotation, and lateral bending to the affected side with axial compression applied to the top of the head for up to 1 minute. The test is positive if there is a reproduction or increase in the usual radicular symptoms. Yoo's study appears to confirm that Spurling's maneuver dynamically narrows the neural foramen.[33] The brachial plexus tension test was first described by Elvey.[58] The test attempts to place tension on the upper cervical nerve roots of the brachial plexus. Reproduction of symptoms suggests that there is a cervical origin. In addition, nerve root relief maneuvers may be performed. One of the most commonly used maneuvers is the shoulder abduction relief test. A positive test occurs when there is improvement of symptoms when placing the painful arm in the abducted position with the palm of the hand resting on the head. Relief of radicular pain with abduction of the shoulder is thought to be due to increased opening of the intervertebral foramen or decreased tension on the nerve root.[35] Good interexaminer reliability of Spurling's maneuver, axial manual traction, and the shoulder abduction test has been demonstrated. In a subsequent study, Viikari-Juntura revealed that these clinical tests had a high specificity but a low sensitivity for detecting cervical nerve root lesions.[59] Despite the low sensitivity, these clinical tests are considered valuable tools in the clinical examination of a patient with radicular pain.

Other provocative maneuvers include Lhermitte's sign and Adson's test. Lhermitte's sign is present if electric-like pain or shock sensations shoot down the spine when the neck is flexed briskly. The sign was first described in multiple sclerosis patients and is indicative of a spinal cord disorder but may be present in some patients with central cervical stenosis. The mechanism is thought to be due to traction on the neural elements. Adson's maneuver tests for neurovascular compromise due to a thoracic outlet problem from a cervical rib, trauma, or a tight scalenus anterior medius muscle. The symptomatic arm is placed in extension and lateral rotation. The radial pulse is monitored as the patient takes a deep breath and turns the head toward the ipsilateral side. The presence of subclavian artery compression is confirmed if there is a marked diminution or absence of the radial pulse. This test is sensitive but not specific, resulting in many false positive findings.

DIFFERENTIAL DIAGNOSIS

Entities that may mimic a cervical spinal disorder include primary shoulder pathology, brachial plexopathy, thoracic outlet syndrome, entrapment neuropathy, myofascial pain syndrome, and medical diseases. Shoulder pain may be due to a primary shoulder entity, such as rotator cuff tendinitis/bursitis, bicipital tendinitis, adhesive capsulitis, acromioclavicular or glenohumeral joint dysfunction, or a rotator cuff tear. Dermatomal or myotomal deficits and an electrodiagnostic examination will aid in the diagnosis of brachial plexopathy, entrapment neuropathy, and other peripheral nerve pathologies. Provocative maneuvers and magnetic resonance imaging (MRI) of the thoracic inlet and brachial plexus are also helpful. Likewise, one must be cognizant of cervical radicular pain masquerading as a primary shoulder disorder. Medical entities such as infection, tumor, and cardiovascular diseases should be included in the differential diagnosis. Myofascial pain syndrome is a diagnosis of exclusion. Other injuries that may occur and may masquerade as cervical radicular or discogenic pain include temporomandibular joint strain, mandibular fracture, vertebral artery stretch causing ischemia, and traction to the sympathetic chain, brachial plexus, or larynx.

When formulating a differential diagnosis, one must be cognizant that a whiplash event may have injured a zygapophyseal joint, intervertebral disc, nerve root, or a combination in the cervical spine. Injury to multiple structures in the cervical spine has been demonstrated in pathoanatomic studies. Segmenting the distribution of pain into quadrants (head, neck, upper back/periscapula, upper arm, and forearm) allows the clinician to organize the differential diagnosis. The relative distribution of pain in these regions affects the judgement of whether the pain is axial or radicular. Axial pain includes central neck pain, occipital headache, and interscapular pain. Radicular pain is most consistent with arm symptoms that are more intense than axial complaints but may include periscapular pain. Symptom laterality and ascertaining whether the chief complaint is axial or radicular help to formulate a probability analysis for each grouping. For example, bilateral symptoms would be more suggestive of somatic referral from CIDD than cervical radicular pain. A chief complaint of upper limb pain in a dermatomal or dynatomal distribution would suggest injury to a cervical nerve root more than somatic referral from CIDD. An evidence-based algorithmic approach to cervical spinal disorders can be helpful in both evaluation and treatment.[60]

DIAGNOSTIC IMAGING

Routine radiographic studies following an acute cervical whiplash injury often fail to demonstrate focal pathology.[61,62] Furthermore, 70% of asymptomatic women and 95% of asymptomatic men have degenerative changes on cervical spine films.[63] Foraminal stenosis caused by disc space collapse has been radiographically demonstrated in 82% of patients with degenerative spondylosis.[64] Cervical flexion and extension radiographs are useful to evaluate for ligamentous subacute instability 1 to 2 weeks after acute trauma.[65]

Cervical myelograms have been shown to demonstrate abnormalities in 21% of lifelong asymptomatic persons.[66]

Cervical disc injuries from whiplash commonly involve a transverse tear or rim lesion near the anterior vertebral rim. They are caused by distraction and shearing during sudden extension. Both the posterior disc and zygapophyseals are compressed, causing disc contusion or herniation, zygapophyseal hemarthrosis, nerve root injury, or fractures of articular processes. Consequently, anular calcification may develop. Cervical extension radiographs may reveal vacuum or lucent clefts and likely represent rim lesions. Nuclear scans may show increased uptake at damaged vertebral end plates or zygapophyseal fractures.

Surgically produced rim lesions are associated with the appearance of marginal osteophytes from 8 months onward. Similar lesions have been described in an MRI study and in Macnab's study.[14,27] Disc splits near the end plate persist for 6 to 18 months or more without healing, and their presence is associated with early disc degeneration.[28]

MRI is indicated in the evaluation of patients with myelopathy, cervical radicular pain, neurologic deficits, soft tissue causes of instability, or cord impingement from ligamentous injuries. It is the most commonly ordered test in the evaluation of degenerative disease of the cervical spine because of its superior depiction of soft tissue anatomy (cervical cord and noncalcified disc herniations). While MRI has a high sensitivity, there are concerns about its clinical specificity. Several studies have demonstrated that a significant percentage of individuals with focal disc protrusions or foraminal stenosis are asymptomatic.[67-70] Boden reported that cervical MRI was interpreted as demonstrating an abnormality in 19% of asymptomatic volunteers.[67] Herniated nucleus pulposus and foraminal stenosis were visualized in 8% and 9%, respectively. The role of MRI in patients without neurologic signs is controversial, but it may be indicated when there is a high risk of instability.

MR findings after cervical spine hyperextension injuries have demonstrated lesions in multiple structures and at multiple levels. In one study, six of seven patients with anterior column injuries had multilevel involvement,[27] including paravertebral muscle tears, tears and ruptures of the ALL, fractures or avulsion of the vertebral end plates, disc separation from vertebral end plates, intervertebral disc tears, herniations, and ruptures. High signal intensity at the interface of the disc and vertebral end plate was seen as late as 9 months after injury. These disc injuries produce characteristic shortening and thickening of the torn anterior anulus with separation of the anulus from the end plate.

Repair of anular rents may be slow and incomplete. Follow-up radiographs 7 years after whiplash showed a higher rate of spondylosis, suggesting disc injury and accelerated degeneration.

The degree of foraminal narrowing and lateral neural encroachment is more difficult to evaluate by MRI. Foraminal encroachment can be assessed in oblique radiographs; however, multiplanar reformatted thin-section computed tomography, especially with contrast enhancement, remains the gold standard test to identify osseous foraminal stenosis.[71]

When evaluating for internal disc disruption and identifying a painful symptomatic disc, provocative discography has been shown to be superior to MRI. Schellhas compared cervical MRI and discography.[72] He demonstrated that MRI often missed significant anular tears and could not reliably identify the source of cervical discogenic pain.

ELECTRODIAGNOSIS

The cervical nerve roots are susceptible to injury from a whiplash event. Nerve root trauma may result in painful neck and limb complaints with or without associated neurologic deficit.[29,30,32,73–75] The specific etiology of such pain has eluded physicians because of the absence of consistent radiologic or neurophysiologic correlates. The diagnostic sensitivity for needle electromyography in detecting radiculopathy has been reported in various studies, ranging from 45% to 94%.[76–83] Furthermore, electromyography abnormalities may persist long after symptomatic recovery. A recent study confirmed that a five-muscle screen including paraspinals identified 90% to 98% of radiculopathies, six muscle screens identified 94% to 99%, and seven muscle screens identified 96% to 100%[84] (see Chapter 17).

DIAGNOSTIC SELECTIVE NERVE ROOT BLOCK

When electromyography does not demonstrate evidence of radiculopathy, a fluoroscopically guided diagnostic cervical selective nerve root block (SNRB) can be used to identify patients whose neck and limb complaints appear to be arising from a whiplash-induced nerve root injury. This requires that a fluoroscopically guided diagnostic SNRB have high sensitivity and specificity. The accuracy of fluoroscopically guided diagnostic cervical SNRB was initially assessed by Kikuchi et al.[85] However, most studies assessing the sensitivity and specificity of fluoroscopically guided diagnostic SNRB were done in the lumbar spine. Because it is generally accepted that the pathomechanism of radicular pain in cervical radiculopathy is no different than that of lumbosacral radicular pain and the anatomy is similar (Fig. 2), prior investigations of the sensitivity and specificity of lumbar fluoroscopically guided diagnostic SNRB are likely

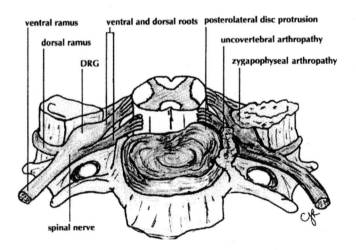

Figure 2. A cervical segment with potential pathologies that may result in cervical radiculopathy.

applicable to the cervical spine. The sensitivity and specificity of fluoroscopically guided diagnostic SNRB has been reported to be 95% to 100%[86,87] and 87% to 100%,[86–91] respectively. Since the advent of spinal MRI and its known high sensitivity, the specificity of a diagnostic SNRB has become the critical issue. Diagnostic SNRB can be particularly useful when a patient has radicular pain and normal or equivocal imaging studies.[92] It is similarly helpful in patients with multilevel abnormalities without corroborative examination findings or electrodiagnostic testing.[93] Although these latter two statements are supported by studies of the lumbar spine, many clinicians believe that they are equally applicable to the cervical spine. This needs to be substantiated by appropriate research.

TREATMENT

Epidemiologic studies have reported that two-thirds of all patients with whiplash injuries were symptom-free by 2 years.[4,50] Of these patients, 88% were symptom-free within 2 months. Consequently, a reasonable course of nonoperative treatment consisting of physical therapy, nonsteroidal anti-inflammatories, relative rest, and activity modifications is recommended as the initial treatment after a whiplash event. For those with cervical radiculopathy, most symptoms will resolve with aggressive nonsurgical treatment.[94] Swezey et al investigated the efficacy of home cervical traction therapy and reported symptomatic relief in 81% of patients with mild to moderately severe (grade 3) cervical spondylosis syndromes.[95] Persson reported that outcomes of physiotherapy, cervical collar, and surgery were no different at 12 months in patients with cervical radicular pain for 3 or more months in duration.[96] Prescribed bed rest is seldom indicated and should always be limited to a short duration. Clinicians should vigorously encourage an aggressive, active therapy program and early return to usual activities.[97] The role of physical therapy following whiplash injuries is described in Chapter 18.

Therapeutic Selective Nerve Root Block

When initial conservative measures fail, therapeutic SNRB can be used in the treatment of symptoms arising from cervical nerve root pathology[94,98]; these disorders may be categorized as traumatic or atraumatic. This may be subdivided into radiculopathy or radicular pain from foraminal stenosis due to focal disc protrusions or spondylosis. Saal[94] demonstrated that many focal cervical disc herniations may be successfully managed with nonsurgical treatment; 83% of the nonoperative treatment group had good to excellent results. Nonsurgical treatment consisted primarily of physiotherapy and spinal injections in patients with atraumatic cervical radiculopathy due to focal disc protrusions. Slipman demonstrated 60% good to excellent results for therapeutic SNRB in the treatment of atraumatic cervical spondylotic radicular pain.[99] However, for traumatically induced cervical radicular pain, the results are poorer. Only a 14% good to excellent outcome of therapeutic SNRB in the treatment of whiplash-induced cervical radicular pain has been noted.[100,101] A 20% success rate was found after therapeutic SNRB in the treatment of traumatically induced cervical spondylotic radicular pain.[102]

The transient symptom relief from therapeutic SNRBs may have resulted from the therapeutic properties of the injected anesthetic agent, corticosteroid, or their combination. In addition to serving as a short-acting anesthetic, lidocaine has demonstrated anti-inflammatory properties, may improve blood flow, and may reduce neural dysfunction in injured nerve roots. Corticosteroids are well known for their anti-inflammatory properties. Relief of radicular pain may also result from the ability of corticosteroids to stabilize neural membranes, thus suppressing ectopic discharges within the sensitized dorsal root ganglion and injured nerve fibers.[103] Additionally, corticosteroids may have a direct anesthetic effect upon small unmyelinated nociceptive C-fibers within irritated neural tissue. These therapeutic effects, though, remain short-lived in the setting of continued chemical or mechanical insult and chronic nerve injury. Prospective clinical trials with a randomly assigned control group are needed to further clarify the role of therapeutic injections in the treatment of this challenging patient population.

Discography

Cervical discography identifies which cervical disc(s) is the source of pain. Typically, patients with CIDD complain mostly of axial pain; however, somatic pain referral symmetrically into the arms and upper extremities is common. Schellhas demonstrated the reliability of cervical discography and its superiority to MRI in identifying painful anular tears.[72] A diagnosis of CIDD is given when a concordant pain response is elicited during filling of an anular fissure with contrast from a nuclear injection. Bogduk investigated the prevalence of traumatically induced disc pain and zygapophyseal joint pain with provocative discography and cervical zygapophyseal joint blocks.[104] Symptomatic discs were demonstrated in 61% of posttraumatic chronic neck pain patients. A symptomatic disc and zygapophyseal joint in the same segment was found in 41% of patients. Symptomatic zygapophyseal joints with asymptomatic discs occurred in 23% of cases, while discs alone were symptomatic in 20%. These observations implicate multiple structure involvement in traumatically induced cervical pain and underscore the importance of a thorough diagnostic work-up to avoid treatment failures. Therefore, the results of discography alone must be interpreted with caution.

Studies have demonstrated the efficacy of cervical discography as an outcome predictor of cervical fusion. Success rates for fusion with discography range from 70% to 90%,[105,106] while those without discography have been as low as 27%[107,108] for symptoms caused by internal disc disruption syndrome. Donner, in a retrospective study, reported a 100% success rate in 37 patients who underwent discography and anterior cervical fusion for traumatically induced cervical symptoms.[109] Discography can be helpful in selected cases in patients with neck and vague proximal extremity pain for which the diagnosis is unclear. A careful stepwise approach has been recommended.[60] In addition, the psychological status may be important when interpreting the results of discography.

Surgery

Surgery is rarely indicated for cervical radiculopathy. Whitecloud demonstrated 70% good to excellent results for cervical fusion with positive discography in patients with traumatically induced neck pain without radicular symptoms.[105] Macnab reported resolution of symptoms in seven of eight patients who underwent discography and required anterior fusion for traumatically induced disc separations from the vertebral end plate.[14] Surgical intervention is most frequently approached via an anterior discectomy with or without interbody fusion. Less frequently, a posterior approach has been used. The results of these surgical procedures have been described in numerous reports in patients with spondylitic and discogenic radiculopathy, with reported success rates ranging from 70% to 96%.[105,106,110–114]

More recently, anterior cervical foraminotomy has been reported to have an equivalent surgical success rate for unilateral radicular pain with more preservation of the cervical disc and motion segments.[115] Jonsson reported good results with anterior discectomy and fusion of eight patients with traumatically induced chronic neck and radicular pain that had large disc protrusions on MRI.[31] Five of these patients had lateral disc herniations on MRI that were found to be sequestered disc fragments lodged behind the uncinate processes. All five patients with severe radicular pain had complete resolution of symptoms after surgery. It is likely that the disc fragment may have exerted pressure or caused an inflammatory process on the traversing nerve roots, dorsal root ganglion, or vessels. Strong conclusions cannot be made from these studies due to the small numbers. It should be clear, however, that few patients with cervical radiculopathy will require surgery.

SUMMARY

Whiplash syndrome refers to a constellation of signs and symptoms that may occur after cervical hyperextension-flexion. It is best viewed as a descriptive term and not a diagnosis. Several studies have related outcomes to presenting symptomatology; however, more studies are needed to determine and relate outcomes to a specific diagnosis. Cervical disc and radicular injuries may frequently occur after a whiplash event. Most patients improve with nonsurgical treatments, including injection procedures, although therapeutic SNRB does not seem to be effective for traumatically induced cervical radicular pain. Surgery is rarely needed but can be effective for patients who have failed nonsurgical measures with appropriate indications.

References

1. Spitzer WO, Skovron MD, Salmi LR, et al: Scientific monograph of the Quebec Task Force on Whiplash-Associated Disorders: redefining "whiplash" and it management. Spine 20(8 suppl):1S–73S, 1995.
2. National Highway Traffic Safety Administration: Traffic Safety Facts 1994: A Compilation of Motor Vehicle Crash Data from the Fatal Accident Reporting System and the General Estimates System. Washington, DC, National Highway Traffic Safety Administration, 1995.
3. Dvorak J, Valach L, Schmid S: [Injuries of the cervical spine in Switzerland.] Orthopade 16:2–12, 1987.
4. Maimaris C, Barnes MR, Allen MJ: Whiplash injuries of the neck: a retrospective study. Injury 19:393–396, 1988.
5. Moore KL, Agur AM: Essential Clinical Anatomy. Baltimore, Williams & Wilkins, 1995.
6. Hoyland JA, Freemont AJ, Jayson MI: Intervertebral foramen venous obstruction. Spine 14:558–568, 1989.
7. Hadley LA: Anatomicroradiographic studies of the spine: changes responsible for certain painful back conditions. N Y State J Med 39:969–974, 1939.

8. Swanberg H: The Intervertebral Foramina in Man. Chicago, Scientific Publishing, 1915.
9. Bogduk N, et al: The innervation of the cervical intervertebral discs. Spine 13:2–8, 1989.
10. Crowe HE: Injuries to the cervical spine. Presented at the meeting of the Western Orthopaedic Association, San Francisco, 1928.
11. Stovner LJ: The nosologic status of the whiplash syndrome: a critical review based on a methodological approach. Spine 21:2735–2746, 1996.
12. Severy DM, et al: Controlled automobile rear-end collisions: an investigation of related engineering and medical phenomena. Can Serv Med J 11:727–759, 1955.
13. Macnab I: Acceleration extension injuries of the cervical spine. In Rothman R (ed): The Spine, 2nd ed. Philadelphia, WB Saunders, 1982, pp 647–660.
14. Macnab I: Acceleration injuries of the cervical spine. J Bone Joint Surg Am 46:1797–1799, 1964.
15. Taylor JR, Finch P: Acute injury of the neck: anatomical and pathological basis of pain. Ann Acad Med Singapore 22:187–192, 1993.
16. Taylor JR, Twomey LT: Acute injuries to cervical joints. An autopsy study of neck sprain. Spine 18:1115–1122, 1993.
17. Penning L: Acceleration injury of the cervical spine by hypertranslation of the head: part 1. Effect of normal translation of the head on the cervical spine motion: a radiological study. Eur Spine J 1:7–12, 1992.
18. Penning L: Acceleration injury of the cervical spine by hypertranslation of the head: part 2. Effect of normal translation of the head on the cervical spine motion: a radiological study. Eur Spine J 1:13–19, 1992.
19. Svensson MY, et al: Pressure effects in the spinal canal during whiplash extension motion: a possible cause of injury to the cervical spinal ganglia. In Proceedings of the 1993 International IRCOBI Conference on the Biomechanics of Impacts. Eindhoven, The Netherlands, 1993, pp 189–200.
20. Panjabi MM, et al: Whiplash trauma injury mechanism: a biomechanical viewpoint. In Gunzburg G (ed): Whiplash Injuries. Philadelphia, Lippincott-Raven, 1998, pp 79–88.
21. Matsushita T, et al: X-ray study of the human neck motion due to head inertia loading. Proceedings of the 38th Stapp Car Crash Conference. Warrendale, PA, Society of Automotive Engineering, 1994, paper no. 942208.
22. McConnell WE, et al: Analysis of human test subject responses to low velocity rear end impacts. Proceedings of the 38th Stapp Car Crash Conference. Warrendale, PA, Society of Automotive Engineering, 1993, paper no. 930889.
23. White AA, Panjabi MM: Clinical Biomechanics of the Spine. Philadelphia, JB Lippincott, 1978.
24. Vernon-Roberts B, Pirie CJ: Degenerative changes in the intervertebral discs of the lumbar spine and their sequelae. Rheumatol Rehabil 16:13–21, 1977.
25. Crowell RR, et al: Mechanisms of injury in the cervical spine: experimental evidence and biochemical modeling. In The Cervical Spine Research Society: The Cervical Spine, 2nd ed. Philadelphia, JB Lippincott, 1989, pp 70–90.
26. Tamura TJ: Cranial symptoms after cervical injury. J Bone Joint Surg Br 71:283–287, 1989.
27. Davis SJ, Teresi LM, Bradley WG Jr, et al: Cervical spine hyperextension injuries: MR findings. Radiology 180:245–251, 1991.
28. Osti OL, Vernon-Roberts B, Fraser RD: Annulus tears and intervertebral disc degeneration: an experimental study using an animal model. Spine 15:762–767, 1990.
29. Gay JR, Abbott KH: Common whiplash injuries to the neck. JAMA 152:1698–1704, 1953.
30. Seletz E: Whiplash injuries. Neurophysiological basis for pain and methods used for rehabilitation. JAMA 168:1750–1755, 1958.
31. Jonsson H, Cesarini K, Sahlstedt B, Rauschning W: Findings and outcome in whiplash type neck distortions. Spine 19:2733–2743, 1994.
32. Cain CM, Ryan GA, Fraser R, et al: Cervical spine injuries in road traffic crashes in south Australia. Aust N Z J Surg 59:15–19, 1989.
33. Yoo JU, Zou D, Edwards WT, et al: Effects of cervical spine motion on neuroforaminal dimension of the human cervical spine. Spine 17:1131–1136, 1992.
34. Lu J, Ebraheim NA, Huntoon M, Haman SP: Cervical intervertebral disc space narrowing and size of intervertebral foramina. Clin Orthop 370:259–264, 2000.
35. Farmer JC, Wisneski RJ: Cervical spine nerve root compression. Spine 19:1850–1855, 1994.
36. Olmarker K, Rydevik B, Holm S: Edema formation in spinal nerve roots induced by experimental graded compression. An experimental study of the pig cauda equina with special reference to differences in effects between rapid and slow onset of compression. Spine 14:569–573, 1989.

37. Hasue M: Pain and the nerve root. An interdisciplinary approach. Spine 18:2053–2058, 1993.
38. Howe JF, Loeser JD, Calvin WH: Mechanosensitivity of dorsal root ganglia and chronically injured axons: a physiological basis for the radicular pain of nerve root compression. Pain 3:25–41, 1977.
39. Weinstein J: Mechanisms of spinal pain: the dorsal root ganglion and its role as a mediator of low back pain. Spine 11:999–1001, 1986.
40. Yabuki S, Kikuchi S: Positions of dorsal root ganglia in the cervical spine. An anatomic and clinical study. Spine 21:1513–1517, 1996.
41. pencer DL, Irwin GS, Miller JR: Anatomy and significance of fixation of the lumbosacral nerve roots in sciatica. Spine 8:672–679, 1983.
42. Spencer DL: The anatomical basis of sciatica secondary to herniated lumbar disc: a review. Neurol Res 21:S33–S36, 1999.
43. Spencer DL, Miller JA, Bertolini JE: The effect of intervertebral disk space narrowing on the contact force between the nerve root and a simulated disk protrusion. Spine 9:422–426, 1984.
44. Kellegren JH: Observations on referred pain arising from muscle. Clin Sci 3:175–190, 1938.
45. Kellegren JH: On the distribution of pain arising from deep somatic structures with charts of segmental pain. Clin Sci 3:35–46, 1939.
46. Keegan JJ, Garrett GD: The segmental distribution of the cutaneous nerves in the limbs of man. Anat Rec 102:409–437, 1948.
47. Kuslich SD, Ahern JW, Garner MD: An in vivo, prospective analysis of tissue sensitivity of lumbar spinal tissues. Presented at the 12th annual meeting of the North American Spine Society, New York, 1997.
48. Von Luschka H: Die Nerven des menschlichen Wirbelkanales. Tubingen, Laupp and Siebeck, 1850.
49. Slipman CW, Plastaras CT, Palmitier RS, et al: Symptom provocation of fluroscopically guided cervical nerve root stimulation: are dynatomal maps identical to dermatomal maps? Spine 23:2235–2242, 1998.
50. Norris SH, Watt I: The prognosis of neck injuries resulting from rear-end vehicle collisions. J Bone Joint Surg Br 65:608–611, 1983.
51. Greenfield J, Ilfield FW: Acute cervical strain. Evaluation and short term prognostic factors. Clin Orthop 122:196–200, 1977.
52. Hohl M: Soft-tissue injuries of the neck in automobile accidents. Factors influencing prognosis. J Bone Joint Surg Am 56:1675–1682, 1974.
53. Radanov BP, di Stefano G, Schnidrig A, Ballinari P: Role of psychosocial stress in recovery from common whiplash. Lancet 338:712–715, 1991.
54. Radanov BP, Hirlinger I, Di Stefano G, Valach L: Attentional processing in cervical spine syndromes. Acta Neurol Scand 85:358–362, 1992.
55. Radanov BP, Sturzenegger M, De Stefano G, Schnidrig A: Relationship between early somatic, radiological, cognitive and psychosocial findings and outcome during one-year follow-up in 117 patients suffering from common whiplash. Br J Rheumatol 33:442–448, 1994.
56. Radanov BP, Sturzenegger M, Di Stefano G, et al: Factors influencing recovery from headache after common whiplash. BMJ 307:652–655, 1993.
57. Viikari-Juntura E: Interexaminer reliability of observations in physical examinations of the neck. Phys Ther 67:1526–1532, 1987.
58. Elvey RL: Brachial plexus tension tests and the pathoanatomical origin of arm pain. In Idczak RM (ed): Biomechanical Aspects of Manipulative Therapy. Carlton, Australia, Lincoln Institute of Health Sciences, 1981.
59. Viikari-Juntura E, Porras M. Laasonen EM: Validity of clinical tests in the diagnosis of root compression in cervical disc disease. Spine 14:253–257, 1989.
60. Slipman CW, Chow DW, Whyte WS, et al: An evidence-based algorithmic approach to cervical spinal disorders. Crit Rev Phys Rehabil Med. In press.
61. Cadoux CG, White JD, Hedberg MD: High-yield roentgenographic criteria for cervical spine injuries. Ann Emerg Med 16:738–742, 1987.
62. Fischer RP: Cervical radiographic evaluation of alert patients following blunt trauma. Ann Emeg Med 13:905–907, 1984.
63. Gore DR, Sepic SB, Gardner GM: Roentgenographic findings of the cervical spine in asymptomatic people. Spine 11:521–524, 1986.
64. Lee C, Woodring JH, Rogers LF, Kim KS: The radiographic distinction of degenerative slippage from traumatic slippage of the cervical spine. Skeletal Radiol 15:439–443, 1986.
65. An HS: Cervical spine trauma. Spine 23:2713–2729, 1998.

66. Hitselberger WE, Witten RM: Abnormal myelograms in asymptomatic patients. J Neurosurg 28:204–206, 1968.
67. Boden SD, Davis DO, Dina TS, et al: Abnormal magnetic resonance scans of the cervical spine in asymptomatic subjects: a prospective investigation. J Bone Joint Surg Am 72:1178–1184, 1990.
68. McRae DL: Asymptomatic intervertebral disc protrusions. Acta Radiol 46:9–27, 1956.
69. Teresi LM, Lufkin RB, Reicher MA, et al: Asymptomatic degenerative disk disease and spondylosis of the cervical spine: MR imaging. Radiology 164:83–88, 1987.
70. Matsumoto M, Fujimura Y, Suzuki N, et al: MRI of cervical intervertebral discs in asymptomatic subjects. J Bone Joint Surg Br 80:19–24, 1998.
71. Yousem DM, Atlas SW, Goldberg HI, Grossman RI: Degenerative narrowing of the cervical spine neural foramina: evaluation with high-resolution 3-DFT gradient echo MR imaging. AJNR Am J Neuroradiol 12:229–236, 1991.
72. Schellhas KP, Smith MD, Gundry CR, Pollei SR: Cervical discogenic pain: prospective correlation of magnetic resonance imaging and discography in asymptomatic subjects and pain sufferers. Spine 21:300–312, 1996.
73. Braaf MM, Rosner S: Whiplash injury of the neck: symptoms, diagnosis, treatment and prognosis. N Y State J Med 58:1501–1507, 1958.
74. Clemens HJ, Burrow K: Experimental investigation on injury mechanism of cervical spine at frontal and rear frontal vehicle impacts. In 16th Stapp Car Crash Conference Proceedings. New York, Society of Automotive Engineers, 1972, pp 96–104.
75. Jonsson H Jr, Bring G, Rauschning W, Sahlstedt B: Hidden cervical spine injuries in traffic accident victims with skull fractures. J Spinal Disord 4:251–263, 1991.
76. Wilbourn AJ, Aminoff MJ: AAEM minimonograph 32: the electrodiagnostic examination in patients with radiculopathies. American Association of Electrodiagnostic Medicine. Muscle Nerve 21:1612–1631, 1998.
77. Levin KH, Maggiano HJ, Wilbourn AJ: Cervical radiculopathies: comparison of surgical and EMG localization of single-root lesions. Neurology 46:1022–1025, 1996.
78. Tullberg T, Svanbor E, Isacsson J, et al: A preoperative and postoperative study of the accuracy and value of electrodiagnosis in patients with lumbosacroal disc herniations. Spine 18:837–842, 1993.
79. Aminoff MJ, Goodin DS, Parry GJ, et al: Electrophysiologic evaluation of lumbosacral radiculopathies: electromyography, late responses, and somatosensory evoked potentials. Neurology 35:1514–1518, 1985.
80. Knutsson B: Comparative value of electromyographic, myelographic and clinical-neurological examinations in diagnosis of lumbar root compression syndrome. Acta Orthop Scand Suppl 49:1–135, 1961.
81. Lajoie WJ: Nerve root compression: correlation of electromyographic, myelographic, and surgical findings. Arch Phys Med Rehabil 53:390–392, 1972.
82. Flax HJ, Berrios R, Rivera D: Electromyography in diagnosis of herniated lumbar disc. Arch Phys Med 45:520–524, 1964.
83. Schoedinger GR: Correlation of standard diagnostic studies with surgically proven lumbar disk rupture. South Med J 80:44–46, 1987.
84. Dillingham TR, Lauder TD, Andary M, et al: Identification of cervical radiculopathies: optimizing the electromyographic screen. Am J Phys Med Rehabil 80:84–91, 2001.
85. Kikuchi S, Macnab I, Moreau P: Localisation of the level of symptomatic cervical disc degeneration. J Bone Joint Surg Br 63:272–277, 1981.
86. Haueisen DC, Smith BS, Myers SR, Pryce ML: The diagnostic accuracy of spinal nerve injection studies. Clin Orthop 198:179–183, 1985.
87. Van Akkerveeken PF: The dignostic value of nerve root sheath infiltration. Acta Orthop Scand 64:61–63, 1993.
88. Dooley JF, McBroom RJ, Taguchi T, Macnab I: Nerve root infiltration in the diagnosis of radicular pain. Spine 19:1125–1131, 1994.
89. Krempen JF, Smith BS: Nerve root injection: a method for evaluating the etiology of sciatica. J Bone Joint Surg Am 56:1435–1444, 1974.
90. Schutz H, Lougheed WM, Wortzman G, Awerbuck BG: Intervertebral nerve-root in the investigation of chronic lumbar disc disease. Can J Surg 16:217–221, 1973.
91. Stanley D, McLaren MI, Euinton HA, Getty CJM: A prospective study of nerve root infiltration in the diagnosis of sciatica: a comparison with radiculography, computed tomography, and operative findings. Spine 6:540–543, 1990.
92. Macnab I: Negative disc exploration: an analysis of the causes of nerve-root involvement in sixty-eight patients. J Bone Joint Surg Am 53:891–903, 1973.

93. Kikuchi S, Hasue M: Combined contrast studies in lumbar spine diseases: myelography (peridurography) and nerve root infiltration. Spine 13:1327–1331, 1988.
94. Saal JS, Saal JA, Yurth EF: Nonoperative management of herniated cervical intervertebral disc with radiculopathy. Spine 21:1877–1883, 1996.
95. Swezey RL, Swezey AM, Warner K: Efficacy of home cervical traction therapy. Am J Phys Med Rehabil 78:30–32, 1999.
96. Persson LC, Carlsson CA, Carlsson JY: Long-lasting cervical radicular pain managed with surgery, physiotherapy, or a cervical collar. Spine 22:751–758, 1997.
97. Malanga G: The diagnosis and treatment of cervical radiculopathy. Med Sci Sports Exerc 29(7 suppl):S236–S245, 1997.
98. Bush K, Hillier S: Outcomes of cervical radiculopathy treated with periradicular/epidural corticosteroid injections: a prospective study with independent clinical review. Eur Spine J 5:319–325, 1996.
99. lipman CW, Lipetz JS, Jackson HB, et al: Therapeutic selective nerve root blocks in the nonsurgical management of atraumatic cervical spondylotic radicular pain. Arch Phys Med Rehabil 81:741–746, 2000.
100. Slipman CW, Plastaras CT, Huston CW, Jackson HB: Outcomes of nerve root blocks for whiplash induced cervical radiculitis. Presented at the 11th annual meeting of the North American Spine Society, 1996.
101. Slipman CW, Lipetz JS, et al: Outcomes of therapeutic selective nerve root blocks for whiplash induced cervical radicular pain. Pain Physician 4: 2001.
102. Slipman CW, Lipetz JS, Jackson HB, et al: Therapeutic selective nerve root blocks in the nonsurgical treatment of cervical spondylotic radicular pain. Arch Phys Med Rehabil 80:1168, 1999.
103. Devor M, Govrin-Lippmann R, Raber P: Corticosteroids suppress ectopic neural discharge originating in experimental neuromas. Pain 22:127–137, 1985.
104. Bogduk N, Aprill C: On the nature of neck pain, discography, and cervical zygapophysial joint blocks. Pain 54:213–217, 1993.
105. Whitecloud TS, Seago RA: Cervical discogenic syndrome: results of operative intervention in patients with positive discography. Spine 12:313–316, 1987.
106. Palit M, Schofferman J, Goldthwaite N, et al: Anterior discectomy and fusion for the management of neck pain. Spine 24:2224–2228,1999.
107. White A III, Southwick WO, Deponte RJ, et al: Relief of pain by anterior cervical fusion for spondylosis. J Bone Joint Surg Am 5:525–534, 1973.
108. Williams JL, Allen MR Jr, Harkess JR: Late results of cervical discectomy and interbody fusion. J Bone Joint Surg Am 50:277–286, 1968.
109. Donner EJ, Pettine KA: The diagnosis and surgical treatment of chronic cervical whiplash disc injuries. In Gunzburg R, Szpalski M (eds): Whiplash Injuries. Philadelphia, Lippincott-Raven, 1998, pp 233–240.
110. Aldrich F: Posterolateral microdiscectomy for cervical monoradiculopathy caused by posterolateral soft cervical disc sequestration. J Neurosurg 72:370–377, 1990.
111. Gore DR, Sepic SB: Anterior cervical fusion for degenerated or protruded discs. A review of 146 patients. Spine 9:667–671, 1984.
112. Grisoli F, Graziani N, Fabrizi AP, et al: Anterior discectomy without fusion for treatment of cervical lateral soft disc extrusion: a follow-up of 120 cases. Neurosurgery 24:853–859, 1989.
113. Herkowitz H, Kurz LT, Overholt DP: Surgical management of cervical soft disc herniation: a comparison between the anterior and posterior approach. Spine 15:1026–1030, 1990.
114. Robertson JT, Johnson SD: Anterior cervical discectomy without fusion: long-term results. Clin Neurosurg 27:440–449, 1980.
115. Johnson PJ, Filler AG, McBride DQ, Batzdorf U: Anterior cervical foraminotomy for unilateral radicular disease. Spine 25:905–909, 2000.

12

Spinal Cord Injury Following Motor Vehicle Accidents

Yong I. Park, M.D., and Steven C. Kirshblum, M.D.

This chapter reviews what is probably the most devastating consequence of cervical trauma following motor vehicle accidents (MVAs): spinal cord injury (SCI). Fortunately, it is a rare event considering that more than 11.2 million MVAs occurred in 1996 alone.[28] Prompt resuscitation, early identification and stabilization of the injury, avoidance of additional neurologic and medical complications, and intensive rehabilitation are necessary to increase chances of recovery. Only recently have pharmacologic agents been shown to improve outcome following SCI.

EPIDEMIOLOGY

MVAs are the most common cause of SCI, accounting for 38.5% of the estimated 11,000 new cases each year.[81] This figure does not include people who die at the scene of the accident, which may be as many as 5000 people.[53] Roughly half of the individuals are the driver, 28% the passenger, and approximately 16% are from motorcycle accidents.

There are an estimated 183,000 to 230,000 people with SCI in the United States today, 80% of whom are male. The mean age at injury, 32.1 years, has risen slowly since 1973 but remains concentrated at the younger end of the age spectrum, with 55% of traumatic SCI occurring in people in the 16- to 30-year-old age group. MVAs are the leading cause of SCI up to age 45, when falls become the leading cause. SCI costs an estimated $2,185,667 over the lifetime of a person injured at the age of 25 years,[81] although this figure varies based upon age at time of injury, neurologic level, and American Spinal Injury Association (ASIA) impairment classification.

SCI is most often seasonal; the incidence increases as daylight hours and the temperature increase. SCI is most common during the summer months (July and August) and on weekend days (40% occur on Saturday and Sunday).[68] The increased incidence of SCI in the summer is due mostly to higher frequencies of diving and other sports and recreational mishaps and increased motor vehicle–related injuries secondary to greater summertime vehicular use.

The cervical region of the spine is most often injured after MVAs,[21] C5 being the most common level of SCI. About half of motor vehicle crashes result in tetraplegia, 32.5% being incomplete and 22.1% complete.[81]

Some studies have noted a higher risk of SCI when the driver is intoxicated[46] or ejected from his vehicle.[83,92] Occupants who do not wear their seat belts are also more likely to incur SCI.[32] Sasso et al. found that 21% of unbelted rear passengers sustained complete cord injuries compared with 9% of belted rear passengers.[76] Rollover accidents are less likely to produce severe injury to the spine as long as the vehicle does not suddenly hit a stationary object, because the energy is dissipated in small amounts each time the vehicle makes contact with the road.

The human body undergoes significant stress in motor vehicle crashes. Peak acceleration of the head of human volunteers reaches 14.5 g when the vehicle is crash-tested at only 9 km/hour.[90] A driver's side airbag can reduce the risk of fatality by 18% when used in conjunction with a lap and shoulder harness.[87] However, airbags have been measured to deploy at speeds more than 100 mph and known to cause injuries to the head, neck, chest, upper extremities, and trunk.[48] If the driver is unrestrained, the airbag inflates up toward the face, and the upper cervical spine is more likely to be damaged. If the body's momentum is unchecked, it continues to move forward and the head strikes the windshield or roof.[30]

ON THE FIELD AND INITIAL MANAGEMENT

Extrication from a motor vehicle can be prolonged and is especially risky in the unconscious patient. About 5% to 10% of unconscious persons will have a cervical spine injury[27]; therefore, in the unconscious victim an SCI is assumed to exist until proven otherwise. One responder should apply manual cervical traction while another responder applies a cervical collar, which must fit snugly. If the patient is found supine, the safest means of immobilization to secure the patient is to log-roll him onto a rigid spine board. The board should extend from the top of the head to the feet. The patient should be strapped to the board at the forehead, thorax, and extremities. The ideal positioning of the spine on the back board is to have the head in neutral alignment with the spine. To achieve this in the adult, an occipital pad may need to be applied. Cervical and head supports attached to the spine board should be used.

During the first seconds after SCI there is release of catecholamines with an initial hypertensive phase. This is followed rapidly by the state of spinal shock, defined as flaccid paralysis and extinction of muscle stretch reflexes below the injury level.[5] The cardiovacular manifestation of spinal shock is neurogenic shock, consisting of hypotension, bradycardia, and hypothermia. Hypothermia is most prominent in extended extrication times. Hypotension is initially managed with intravenous fluids in the field.

The patient should be transported to the nearest trauma facility where a multidisciplinary emergency department team consisting of the trauma or general surgeon, neurosurgeon, orthopedist, physiatrist, anesthesiologist, and trained nursing and respiratory personnel should evaluate the patient. The goals are to normalize the patient's vital signs, prevent hypoxemia and aspiration, establish normal spine alignment, and consider the use of pharmacologic agents thought to limit secondary neuronal cell death.

Hypotension is common in people with a neurologic level of injury at or above T6 because this level of injury leaves most sympathetic outflow from the spinal cord under a state of depressed function. Therefore, there is loss of sympathetically mediated vascular tone and possibly an inability to accelerate the heart rate.[40] The hypotension from neurogenic shock can be differentiated from hypotension secondary to hypovolemic shock by the presence of bradycardia. The parasympathetic influences on heart rate go unopposed in people with a level of injury above T1; thus, heart rates are typically less than 60 per minute. In contrast, tachycardia is present in those with hypovolemic shock, although both can exist together and all sources of potential bleeding must be ruled out.

Treatment of hypotension from spinal shock or hypovolemia involves fluid resuscitation enough to produce adequate urine output (>30 mL/hour). However, in neurogenic shock further fluid administration must proceed judiciously. Loss of sympathetically mediated vasoconstriction and thus an expanded intravascular tree, as well as capillary leak syndrome, place the SCI patient at risk for neurogenic pulmonary edema. Trendelenburg positioning can be used for symptomatic hypotension. For persistent hypotension, the use of vasopressors is preferred over continued fluid administration. Pulmonary artery catheterization (Swan-Ganz catheter) is recommended to give an accurate assessment of the patient's volume status and avoid fluid overload.[88] Arterial blood pressure catheters are needed because keeping mean arterial blood pressure above 85 mm Hg has been associated with enhanced neurologic outcome. Dopamine (2.5-5 mcg/kg/minute) is the vasopressor of choice in the setting of hypotension with bradycardia because it is both an alpha as well as a beta-1 agonist that will directly increase the heart rate. This can be followed by norepinephrine bitartrate (Levophed) if needed (0.01-0.2 mcg/kg/minute) to keep mean arterial blood pressure more than 85 mm Hg.[88] Phenylephrine is a pure alpha agonist, and its use is limited by the potential reflex slowing of heart rate in the setting of an already present bradycardia. The bradycardia itself can be treated with intravenous atropine and pretreatment with atropine prior to any maneuver that may cause further vagal stimulation (such as nasotrachial suctioning). Temporary cardiac pacing as well as permanent pacemakers, although reported, are rarely needed.[27]

Ventilatory assessment is critical for acute SCI patients and should include arterial blood gases with target PaO_2 of 100 mm Hg and $PaCO_2$ of less than 45 mm Hg. Measurement of forced vital capacity in the emergency department will provide the best assessment of inspiratory muscle strength. A vital capacity of less than 1000 mL, or 12–15 cc/kg, indicates an extreme ventilatory defect with impending ventilatory failure and necessitates intubation and mechanical ventilation. A vital capacity of 1000 to 1500 mL is borderline and necessitates careful serial assessment each shift. Patients with levels of injury above T12 may have varying degrees of secretion clearance deficiencies. The higher the level of injury, the worse the deficiency becomes.

A nasogastric tube should be inserted during the initial assessment period to prevent emesis and potential aspiration. A Foley catheter should be inserted for urinary drainage because the bladder demonstrates the same flaccid paralysis as do limb muscles during the period of spinal shock. In addition, an indwelling urinary catheter will allow for an accurate assessment of output.

Neurologic Examination

The most accurate way to neurologically assess a person who has sustained an SCI is by performing a standardized physical examination as endorsed by the International Standards for Neurological and Functional Classification of SCI Patients, also commonly called the ASIA guidelines.[3] These standards provide basic definitions of the most common terms used by clinicians in the assessment of SCI and describe the neurologic examination.

The neurologic examination of the person with SCI has two main components, sensory and motor, with certain required and optional elements. The required elements allow the determination of the sensory, motor, and neurologic levels; determination of the completeness of the injury; as well as help in classifying the impairment. The rectal examination, which tests for voluntary anal contraction and deep anal sensation, is part of the required components of the examination. The information from this neurologic examination can be recorded on a standardized flow sheet that should be included in the medical records.

For the sensory component of the examination there are 28 key dermatomes, each separately tested for pinprick (with a safety pin) and light touch (with a cotton tip applicator) sensation on both sides of the body. A three-point scale (0-2) is used, with the face as the normal control point. For the pinprick examination, the patient must be able to distinguish between the pin (sharp) and dull edge of a disposable safety pin. Absent sensation and the inability to distinguish between the sharp and dull edge of the pin yield a score of 0. A score of 1 (impaired) for pinprick testing is given when the patient can distinguish between the sharp and dull edge of the pin, but the pin is not felt as sharp as on the face. The "impaired" score is also given if the patient reports altered sensation, including hyperesthesia. The score of 2 (normal or intact) is given only if the pin is felt as sharp, in the tested dermatome, as when tested on the face.

For light touch, a cotton tip applicator is used, with 2 (intact) being the same touch sensation as on the face and 1 (impaired) if less than on the face. When testing the digits for dermatomes C6-C8, the dorsal surface of the proximal phalanx should be tested. When testing the chest and abdomen, sensory testing should be performed at the midclavicular line.

It is extremely important to test the S4-S5 dermatome for both pinprick and light touch, because this represents the most caudal aspect of the sacral spinal cord. To test for deep anal sensation, a rectal digital examination is performed. The patient is asked to report any sensory awareness—touch or pressure—with firm pressure of the examiners' digit on the rectal walls. Deep anal sensation is recorded as either present or absent.

If accurate sensory testing in any dermatome cannot be performed, "NT" (not tested) should be recorded, or an alternate location within the dermatome can be tested with notation that an alternate site was used. Optional elements of the ASIA sensory examination are also important and strongly recommended and include proprioception (joint position and vibration) and deep pressure sensations. These can be graded as absent, impaired, or normal.

For the motor examination, the required elements of the ASIA motor examination consist of testing 10 key muscle groups, five in the upper limb (biceps and brachialis, extensor carpi radialis, triceps, flexor digitorum profundus of the third finger, and the abductor digiti mini) and five in the lower limb (iliopsoas, quadriceps, tibialis anterior, extensor hallucis longus, and the gastrocnemius soleus) on each side of the body. Other muscles are also clinically important but are viewed as optional in that they do not contribute to the motor scores or levels.[66] The muscles should be examined in a rostral to caudal sequence, with the patient in the supine position, starting with the elbow flexors (C5 tested muscle) and finishing with the ankle plantar flexors (Sl muscle). The muscles are graded on the standard form, on a six-point scale from 0 to 5.[33] Testing in the supine position, while different from classic teaching for manual muscle testing, is recommended for SCI evaluations to allow for a valid comparison of a patient's scores obtained during the acute period (ie, because of an unstable spine) with those obtained during the rehabilitation and follow-up phases of care.

Voluntary anal contraction is tested as part of the motor examination by sensing contraction of the external anal sphincter around the examiner's finger and graded as either present or absent. It is important not to confuse a reflex contraction of the anal sphincter with voluntary contraction.

The **sensory level** is the most caudal dermatome to have intact (2/2) sensation for both pinprick and light touch on both sides of the body. The **motor level** is defined as the lowest key muscle that has a grade of at least 3, providing the key muscles represented by segments above that level are graded as 5.[3] The **neurologic level** of injury (NLI) is the most caudal level at which both motor and sensory modalities are intact on both sides of the body and should be differentiated from the skeletal level of injury, which is defined as the spinal level at which radiographic examination reveals the greatest vertebral damage. If the motor level is C7 and the sensory level is C8, the overall NLI is C7. Motor and sensory levels are the same in less than 50% of complete injuries, and the motor level may be multiple levels below the sensory level at 1 year postinjury.[60,88]

CLASSIFICATION OF SPINAL CORD INJURY

Many classification systems have been described over the years to describe the extent of the SCI. The ASIA impairment scale[1] replaced the Frankel classification in 1992 and has undergone revisions in 1996[2] and in 2000.[3] These standards were endorsed by the International Medical Society of Paraplegia and thereafter became known as the International Standards for Neurological and Functional Classification of Spinal Cord Injury.[2]

Since 1992, a **complete injury** is defined as the absence of sensory or motor function in the lowest sacral segments, and incomplete injury is defined as preservation of motor function or sensation below the NLI that includes the lowest sacral segments (sacral sparing). Sacral sparing is tested by light touch and pinprick at the anal mucocutaneous junction (S4/S5 dermatome), on both sides, as well as testing voluntary anal contraction and deep anal sensation as part of the rectal examination. If any of these are present (sacral sparing), intact, or impaired, the individual has an **incomplete injury**. According to this definition, a patient with cervical SCI can have sensory and motor function in the trunk or even in the legs, but unless sacral sparing is present the injury must be classified as complete (ASIA-A) with a large zone of partial preservation (see below). When sacral sparing is used early after injury to define incompleteness, motor recovery is significantly more likely to occur than when it is not.[89] The sacral-sparing definition of the completeness of the injury is a more stable definition—because fewer patients convert from incomplete to complete status over time postinjury—and is the basis for changing the definitions from previous definitions. The ASIA impairment scale, similar to the Frankel scale, describes five different severities of SCI.

The **zone of partial preservation** since 1992 is defined as all segments below the NLI with preservation of sensory or motor findings and is used only in complete (ASIA-A) injuries.

Incomplete SCI Syndromes

Different clinical syndromes of SCI are frequently referred to by clinicians and in the literature and include central cord, Brown-Séquard, anterior cord, conus medullaris, and cauda equina syndromes. In general, these syndromes do not accurately describe the extent of the neurologic deficit. However, they are important to define and be aware of.

Central Cord Syndrome: The most common of the incomplete syndromes is central cord syndrome (CCS). CCS is characterized by motor weakness in the upper extremities greater than the lower extremities, in association with sacral sparing. In addition to the motor weakness, other features include bladder dysfunction (usually urinary retention) and varying sensory loss below the level of the lesion. In his original description, Schneider noted that the etiologic factor was hyperextension with simultaneous compression of the cord by anterior osteophytes and posterior impingement caused by buckling of the ligamentum flavum.[77] Although CCS most frequently occurs in older people with cervical spondylosis with hyperextension injuries, the syndrome may occur in people of any age and is associated with other etiologies, predisposing factors, and injury mechanisms.

CCS is commonly believed to result from an injury that primarily affects the center of the spinal cord. Depending on the degree and severity of the lesion, there may be paralysis of both the upper and lower limbs, with relatively more involvement of the upper limbs. This is because of the proposed lamination of the fibers in the corticospinal tract, with the cervical fibers most centrally located in relation to the thoracic, lumbar, and sacral fibers.[38,76] Others have not, however, found this lamination to exist in humans.[47,65] Quencer et al, in a study using magnetic resonance imaging (MRI) and pathological observations, found that CCS is predominantly a white matter peripheral injury and that intramedullary hemorrhage is not a common feature.[72]

CSS generally has a favorable prognosis.[22,62,70,75] The typical pattern of recovery usually occurs earliest and to the greatest extent in the lower extremities, followed by bladder function, upper extremity (proximal) function, and intrinsic hand function. Although multiple initial follow-up reports for CCS confirm a generally good functional prognosis, Penrod et al. noted that the prognosis for functional recovery in acute traumatic CCS should consider the patient's age,[70] with a less optimistic prognosis in older patients relative to younger patients. Specifically, younger patients (less than 50 years of age) were much more successful in becoming independent in ambulation than older patients (97% vs 41%). These numbers are similar to those reported by others.[62] Similar differences were seen between the younger and older patients in independent bladder function (83% vs 29%), independent bowel function (63% vs 24%), and dressing (77% vs 12%).[70] Burns et al also demonstrated that older patients had less functional motor recovery; however, all patients regardless of age who initially were classified as ASIA-D (within 72 hours) were able to ambulate at the time of discharge from inpatient rehabilitation.[22]

Brown-Séquard Syndrome: The initial classic description of spinal hemisection causing ipsilateral hemiplegia and contralateral hemianalgesia is credited to Brown-Séquard in 1846.[20] Brown-Séquard syndrome (BSS) consists of asymmetric paresis with hypalgesia more marked on the less paretic side and accounts for 2% to 4% of all traumatic SCIs.[12,13] Only a limited number of patients have the pure form of BSS, and much more common is Brown-Sequard plus syndrome (BSPS).[20] BSPS refers to a relative ipsilateral hemiplegia with a relative contralateral hemianalgesia. Although BSS has traditionally been associated with knife injuries, stab wounds are rarely the cause of BSPS. A variety of etiologies, including those that result in closed spinal injuries with or without vertebral fractures, may be the cause. Because of the broad range of injury types, BSS does not have a uniform presentation.[75]

Despite the variation in presentation, considerable consistency is found in the prognosis of BSS. Recovery takes place in the ipsilateral proximal extensors and then the distal flexors.[57] Motor recovery of any extremity having a pain or temperature sensory deficit occurs before the opposite extremity, and these patients may expect voluntary motion strength and functional gait recovery by 6 months.

Overall, patients with BSS have a good prognosis for functional outcome. About 75% of patients ambulate independently at discharge from rehabilitation, and nearly 70% perform functional skills and activities of daily living independently.[75] The most important predictor of function is whether the upper or lower limb is the predominant site of weakness. When the upper limb is weaker than the lower limb, patients are more likely to ambulate at discharge. Recovery of bowel and bladder function is also favorable, with continent bladder and bowel function achieved in 89% and 82%, respectively.[75]

Anterior Cord Syndrome: The anterior cord syndrome involves a lesion affecting the anterior two-thirds of the spinal cord while preserving the posterior columns. It may occur with retropulsed disc or bone fragments,[6] direct injury to the anterior spinal cord, or with lesions of the anterior spinal artery, which provides the blood supply to the anterior spinal cord.[25] Lesions of the anterior spinal artery may result from diseases of the aorta, cardiac or aortic surgery, embolism, polyarteritis nodosa, or angioplasty. There is a variable loss of motor as well as pinprick sensation with a relative preservation of light touch, proprioception, and deep-pressure sensation. Usually patients with an anterior cord syndrome have only a 10% to 20% chance of muscle recovery, and even in those with some recovery, there is poor muscle power and coordination.[12]

Conus Medullaris and Cauda Equina Injuries: The conus medullaris, which is the terminal segment of the adult spinal cord, lies at the inferior aspect of the L1 vertebra. The segment above the conus medullaris is called the epiconus, consisting of spinal cord segments L4-S1. Nerve roots then travel, from the conus medullaris caudal, as the cauda equina.

Lesions of the epiconus will affect the lower lumbar roots supplying muscles of the lower part of the leg and foot, with sparing of sacral segments. The bulbocavernosus reflex and micturition reflexes are preserved, representing an upper motor neuron lesion. Spasticity will most likely develop in sacral innervated segments (toe flexors, ankle plantar flexors, and hamstring muscles). Recovery is similar to other upper motor neuron SCIs.

The conus medullaris consists of neural segments S2 and below. Injuries to the conus will present with lower motor neuron deficits of the anal sphincter and bladder due to damage of the anterior horn cells of S2-S4. Bladder and rectal reflexes are diminished or absent, depending on the exact level of the lesion. Motor strength in the legs and feet may remain intact if the nerve roots (L3-S2) are not affected. The lumbar nerve roots may be spared partially or totally in the conus medullaris. This is referred to as "root escape." If the roots are affected as they travel with the sacral cord in the spinal column, this will result in lower motor neuron damage with diminished reflexes. In low conus lesions, the S1 segment is not involved and therefore the ankle jerks are normal, a finding accounting for most instances of failure to make the diagnosis. Due to the small size of the conus medullaris, lesions are more likely to be bilateral than those of the cauda equina. With conus medullaris lesions, recovery is limited.

Injuries below the L1 vertebral level do not cause injury to the spinal cord but, rather, to the cauda equina or nerve roots supplying the lumbar and sacral segments of the skin and muscle groups. This usually produces motor weakness and atrophy of the lower extremities (L2-S2) with bowel and bladder involvement (S2-S4) and areflexia of the ankle and plantar reflexes. Often the patient may have spared sensation in the perineum or lower extremities but have complete paralysis. In cauda injuries there is loss of anal and bulbocavernosus reflexes as well as impotence.

There is consensus that cauda equina injuries have a much better prognosis for recovery than other SCI syndromes. This is most likely due to the fact that the nerve roots are more resilient to injury and because many of the biochemical processes that occur in the spinal cord and produce secondary damage occur to a much less extent in the nerve roots. Progressive recovery may occur over a course of weeks and months.

Separation of cauda equina and conus lesions in clinical practice is difficult, because the clinical features of these lesions overlap. Isolated conus lesions are rare because the roots forming the cauda equina are wrapped around the conus. The conus may be affected by a fracture of L1, whereas a fracture of L2 or lower can impinge on the cauda equina. Sacral fractures as well as fractures of the pelvic ring also frequently damage the cauda equina. Bullet wounds can penetrate the bony structures to traumatize the cauda and conus.

Pain is uncommon in conus lesions but is frequently the presenting complaint in cauda equina lesions. Sensory abnormalities occur in a saddle distribution in conus lesions and, if there is sparing, there is usually dissociated loss with a greater loss of pain and temperature while sparing touch sensation. In cauda equina lesions, sensory loss occurs more in a root distribution and is not dissociated.

BIOMECHANICS AND PATHOPHYSIOLOGY OF SCI

Movement of the spine involves a complex interaction among the bones, joints, ligaments, and soft tissue. Within the normal range of motion, the spinal cord is well protected and adapts to the shape of the spinal canal. The spinal cord lengthens along with the spinal canal during flexion and shortens during extension.[72] However, when extrinsic forces exceed the physiologic tolerances of the anatomic restraints, the spinal cord can be damaged.

Hyperextension of the neck has been classically described as the cause of acceleration-deceleration injury following rear-end collision. Anterior structures such as the ventral neck muscles, soft tissue, and the anterior longitudinal ligament are stretched while the posterior structures such as the posterior longitudinal ligament, interspinous ligament, and dorsal neck muscles are compressed. Marar induced hyperextension injuries to the cervical spine in seven cadavers, causing rupture of the anterior longitudinal ligament, partial dissociation of the posterior longitudinal ligament from the posterior aspect of the vertebrae, and fracture of the lower cervical spine; however, hyperextension did not cause vertebral subluxation and compromise the cord until a posteriorly directed force was also applied.[59]

The amount of damage to the spinal cord depends upon the speed, duration, and amount of deformation of the cord. Kearney et al, in an animal experimental model of SCI, found that the spinal cord could tolerate higher amounts of cord compression as long as it was compressed slowly. At low rates of deformation, the spinal cord could be compressed 60% of its normal anteroposterior diameter before somatosensory potentials were completely lost. At high rates, the spinal cord could tolerate approximately 20% compression.[50] Irrespective of contact velocity, it appears that compression of the cord more than 50% greatly reduces the likelihood of functional recovery.[50]

Raynor and Koplick proposed that the various clinical syndromes seen in traumatic SCI could be explained by stress analysis theory. They theorized that the type of SCI depends on the location and amount of force applied to the spinal cord. When force is applied along a sagittal plane, the bony elements strike the spinal cord along the middle third of each half of the cord. Because the cord is elliptical in shape, most of the shear stress is localized to the center of the spinal cord, with less stress found at the periphery. When the applied force is small, damage is limited to portions of the anterior and posterior horns, causing loss of sensation and weakness at a specific level. With a higher level of applied force, the inner aspects of the lateral corticospinal and lateral spinothalamic tracts are also compromised. A CCS develops because the nerve fibers that lead to the arms are proposed by some to be found more medially. As the applied force is increased again, only the posterior columns are spared from damage, producing a clinical picture consistent with anterior cord syndrome. Finally, if the force is applied obliquely a BSS ensues.[73]

Experimental animal models of traumatic SCI have demonstrated that following cord impact a cascade of events occurs that extends the injury beyond its original site. The initial trauma usually causes hemorrhage in the center of the cord, with little evidence of damage to the nerve tracts in the white matter. However, excitatory amino acids and free radicals are released by damaged cells, which promote cell breakdown that ultimately leads to cell death.[8] Within the first 8 hours, edema develops in the gray matter and then in the white matter.[95] Within 24 hours, erythrocytes leak into the interstitial space through ruptures in capillaries and venules, platelets aggregate around damaged endothelium, and axons swell and accumulate abnormal amounts of organelles, first at the site of the lesion and but then extending rostrally and caudally.[19,24] Within 2 days of injury, central cord necrosis is seen with microcyst formation and demyelination of the surrounding white matter.[95] The ischemic damage is compounded by a fall in blood pressure from neurogenic shock, loss of autoregulation within the spinal cord,[77] vascular spasm, and interstitial edema that occludes blood flow. Upper cervical spine injuries may also occlude the vertebral arteries that supply the spinal cord.[58]

FRACTURES OF THE CERVICAL SPINE FROM MVAs

Occipitocervical Dislocation

Occipitocervical dislocation is almost always fatal although several survivors have been documented in the literature.[64,71] It occurs more often in the pediatric population because of the inherent instability of the cervical spine of children. Stability of the occipitocervical junction is determined by the strength of the craniospinal ligaments. The tectorial membrane prevents forward and vertical translation and hyperextension while the pair of alar ligaments limit vertical translation, lateral bending, and rotation. The mechanism of injury is thought to be a combination of distraction, rotation, and hyperextension.[64] On x-ray, a distance greater than 5 mm in adults and 10 mm in children between the tip of the odontoid and the bastion is considered abnormal. Treatment involves gentle traction to align the spine followed by posterior fusion with bone grafting.[64]

Atlas Fractures

Compressive or lateral tensile loads on the cervical spine can produce fractures of the atlas ring.[9] The classic Jefferson fracture is a four-part fracture of the ring, but two- and three-part fractures occur more commonly. The posterior arch will fracture in isolation if the neck also hyperextends.[92] Jefferson fractures are considered stable and rarely cause SCI because of the tendency of the bony elements to displace away from the spinal canal. The halo vest is the traditional treatment for stable fractures. If the atlas spreads laterally more than 7 mm in the open-mouth view of the x-ray, there is a high probability of an associated transverse ligament rupture making the fracture unstable.[80] Posterior fusion is then required.

Atlantoaxial Subluxation and Dislocation

The atlas may sublux anteriorly, posteriorly, or rotate over the axis when the transverse ligament ruptures. The direction of subluxation is differentiated by the appearance of the lateral masses in comparison to the dens on open-mouth views. An atlas-dens interval greater than 3 mm on the lateral view suggests rupture of the transverse ligament.[4] Treatment consists first of traction. Rotatory deformities may be treated conservatively with a cervical orthotic or halo brace, but anterior or posterior subluxations require posterior cervical fusion.

Fractures of the Axis

Axis fractures occur in 20% of all acute cervical fractures. The most common cause is MVAs.[42] Fractures of the dens may be classified into three types depending on the location of the fracture. A type I fracture is rare and consists of an oblique avulsion of the tip of the dens. A type II fracture is found at the junction of the base of the dens and the second vertebral body. A type III fracture extends from the base of the dens into the vertebral body. The mechanism of injury is horizontal and vertical compression.[92]

A type I fracture is stable and is treated with a hard cervical collar for 3 months. A type III fracture generally heals well with a cervical orthotic, but some have advocated halo immobilization.[26] Type II fractures have a higher rate of nonunion and may require internal fixation. Ziai and Hulbert retrospectively compared surgical versus conservative treatment with a brace and found that all surgical patients had successful fusion and 76% of the patients treated with braces had satisfactory results. Patients older than 65 years had a 50% rate of nonunion when treated with bracing.[97]

Fractures of the bilateral pedicles of C2 with anterior subluxation occur when the head strikes the windshield, inducing hyperextension and axial loading. It is known as a "hangman's fracture" due to the similar appearance following judicial hanging. In his classic article, Effendi et al. differentiated fractures of the ring of the axis by their radiographic appearance and stability.[35] The incidence of associated neurologic damage is low given the large size of the spinal canal in this area. However, the true number may be higher because those who die at the accident scene are not examined. A hard cervical collar is usually sufficient except in cases where there is significant displacement or angulation of the fragments.

Lower Cervical Fractures

Fractures in the lower cervical spine are associated with either flexion or extension loading. A displacement of greater than 3.5 mm or an angulation greater than 11 degrees between two adjacent vertebrae is considered unstable.[4] Compression fractures are usually stable when there is no disruption of the facets or subluxation of the vertebral bodies. The teardrop fracture is a triangular bone fragment at the inferior margin of a vertebral body that often signifies the presence of ligamentous damage and concomitant fractures within the spine. These fractures can occur by either a flexion or extension mechanism.

Burst fractures are most common at the C5 and C6 vertebral bodies and are secondary to axial loading.[4] The spinal cord is compromised when bone fragments are retropulsed into the spinal canal and impinge the thecal contents. Significant ligamentous damage usually accompanies burst fractures, necessitating decompression and fusion of the cervical spine. The anterior approach is recommended and consists of corpectomy and iliac crest bone grafting, followed by use of a plate and screws for stability. Some surgeons prefer to also apply a halo vest for added stability. In compression burst or flexion teardrop fractures, anterior decompression is superior to conservative treatment with a halo vest in terms of neurologic recovery and preventing kyphotic deformity.[51]

Facet Dislocation

Unilateral facet dislocations are the result of a combination of extreme lateral flexion and axial rotation that tears the interspinous ligament and facet capsule.[7] The inferior facet surface of the rostral vertebra rotates anterior to the superior facet surface of the caudal vertebrae. When axial compression is also present the articular process may fracture. In bilateral facet dislocations, a sudden flexion force causes the superior vertebra to slide over the inferior segment. Bilateral facet dislocations occur more frequently than unilateral dislocations and are more commonly associated with a complete injury. Spinal nerves can be impinged within the neural foramina by the subluxed articular process. When the spinal canal diameter is reduced by more than 50%, complete SCI frequently occurs.[10] However, preinjury canal diameter does not seem to affect neurologic outcome after either unilateral or bilateral facet dislocation.[55]

The dislocation should be reduced as soon as possible, especially in the presence of neurologic damage. Typically, closed reduction is attempted with cervical traction. A halo vest may be tried to stabilize a unilateral dislocation in the absence of neurologic compromise. Open reduction is done in the event closed reduction fails, there is an adjacent fracture, pain or neurologic symptoms worsen, or there is a severe preexisting spinal disease.[94]

Facet dislocation is frequently complicated by disc herniation, especially in the presence of SCI.[44,74] For cervical spine injuries, MRI has been recommended prior to attempting closed reduction to identify disc herniation and its potential for neurologic worsening with manipulation.[36] Eismont et al have presented data showing the frequency of acute disc herniation compressing the neural elements ventrally in acute SCI. These authors proposed that an MRI should be obtained prior to the use of traction for fear that cervical traction could cause ascending (worse) neurologic deficit if the bony subluxation was reduced against a ventrally located (herniated disc).[36] On the other hand, Cotler et al published a study in 1993 demonstrating the safety of immediate skeletal traction in awake patients using evoked potentials. In this study, 24 patients treated this way demonstrated no neurologic worsening resulting from the use of immediate cervical traction prior to obtaining an MRI.[29] Other centers have reported little risk if the reduction is performed with the patient awake.[82] However, in the obtunded patient an MRI should be obtained first. In all cases, an MRI is obtained after closed reduction to rule out spinal cord compression from disc herniation.[85]

SCI WITHOUT RADIOGRAPHIC ABNORMALITIES

The spinal cord can be damaged without any radiographic evidence of bony injury in all age groups,[11] but infants and children are particularly prone because of differences in anatomy and biomechanical properties that make the pediatric spine inherently unstable.[68] The heads of children are proportionately larger and heavier than adults', and the center of rotation is higher on the cervical spine, but descends as the spine matures. The zygopophyseal joints in the neck are aligned more horizontally, allowing for increased motion along the anteroposterior plane. The ligaments are also more elastic, and the neck musculature is not as well developed.[37] The uncinate processes on the superior border of the vertebral bodies are also underdeveloped and cannot help resist flexion and rotational forces.[83] These differences are much more prominent in the high cervical region, explaining why the upper cord is much more prone to injury after trauma.

The neonatal spinal column can elongate 2 inches before stability is compromised, but the spinal cord can tolerate only a ¼-inch increase in length before failure.[54] The high degree of flexibility of the cervical spine increases the risk of damage to the spinal cord in children. The cervical vertebrae may dislocate and spontaneously reduce without fracturing, damaging the cord.

SCI without radiographic abnormality, called SCIWORA by Pang and Wilberger, occurs commonly in children less than 16 years old before the pediatric spine fully develops adult characteristics, with children less than 8 years old especially vulnerable to upper cervical lesions.[69] Children who complain of neck pain or transient neurologic symptoms such as tingling, numbness, or weakness must be followed carefully because many of them develop delayed paralysis. SCI in the pediatric population is largely preventable. Kokoska et al. found that 80% of children with SCI from an MVA were improperly restrained.[52]

TIMING OF SURGERY

The timing of surgery following SCI remains controversial. Studies of spinal cord compression in animals have clearly shown the benefits of early decompression.[34,43] Guha et al. studied the relationship between force and duration of compression to neurologic recovery in a rat model. He concluded that the force of injury was the most important factor in predicting recovery, but when compressive forces were not high early decompression improved recovery.[43] Shorter periods of compression also correlated with return of evoked potentials.[23]

However, clinical studies have shown conflicting results. Several authors believe that early surgical intervention may lead to neurologic deterioration and an increase in complications. An early multicenter study found that 4.9% of spinal cord–injured patients did worse neurologically after surgery. All of the patients with cervical cord injury who deteriorated were operated on within the first 5 days.[61] More recently, Vaccaro et al., in a prospective study, did not find any significant difference between patients who had surgery less than 72 hours or more than 5 days after injury in terms of motor recovery or length of stay in the intensive care unit and inpatient rehabilitation unit.[86]

Other authors refute these findings. Croce et al. found that patients with thoracic fractures who had early spinal fixation, defined as less than 3 days, had fewer complications, less time on the ventilator, and lower hospitalization costs.[31] Mirza et al. compared outcomes in patients who had cervical stabilization within 72 hours to those who had surgery 10 to 14 days after injury. He concluded that the early stabilization group spent fewer days in the hospital and may have better neurologic recovery without a higher complication rate.[63]

Medical Interventions

Improvement in emergency medical procedures, critical care medicine, and the development of model centers for the treatment of acute SCI have improved survival in this population. With improved survival, strategies to maximize neurologic recovery are of paramount importance. Over the past 20 years, several pharmacologic agents have shown promise in improving neurologic recovery in SCI survivors.[14–18,39]

Following the publication of the results of the Second National Acute Spinal Cord Injury Study (NASCIS II),[15] methylprednisolone (MP) (bolus dose of 30 mg/kg followed by 5.4 mg/kg/hour maintenance dose for 23 hours) has been considered standard of care. However, the scientific integrity of these studies has recently been reevaluated based on the quality of evidence needed to change pattern of practice.[49] Hulbert expressed in this recent review that both NASCIS II and III were well-designed and well-executed trials; however, the data from NASCIS III were weak and noncompelling. The conclusions of three recent systematic reviews are that the use of 24 hours of MP remains experimental and the use of 48 hours of MP potentially harmful.[49,66,79] Because the evidence indicates that the use of MP is still experimental, clinicians should keep within strict inclusion and exclusion criteria described in NASCIS II and III.

Inclusion for steroids includes a traumatic SCI diagnosis within 8 hours of injury. Those who should not receive a steroid protocol include people aged less than 13 years, nerve root or cauda equina injury only, SCI secondary to gunshot wounds, life-threatening morbidity, pregnancy, and addiction to narcotics. Unfortunately, the use of MP has been extended to subgroups not included in NASCIS studies, such as those with penetrating SCI, ie, gunshot wounds. Two retrospective nonrandomized studies have shown that the use of MP in penetrating injuries is not supported.[45,55] Currently, many clinicians use this experimental protocol because of medicolegal concerns, which may not be in the best interest of the patient.[66]

References

1. American Spinal Injury Association/International Medical Society of Paraplegia International Standards for Neurological and Functional Classification of Spinal Cord Injury (revised). Chicago, American Spinal Injury Association, 1992.
2. American Spinal Injury Association/International Medical Society of Paraplegia International Standards for Neurological and Functional Classification of Spinal Cord Injury. Chicago, American Spinal Injury Association, 1996.
3. American Spinal Injury Association/International Medical Society of Paraplegia International Standards for Neurological and Functional Classification of Spinal Cord Injury. Chicago, American Spinal Injury Association, 2000.
4. An HS: Cervical spine trauma. Spine 23:2713–2729, 1998.
5. Atkinson PP, Atkinson JL: Spinal shock. Mayo Clin Proc 71:384–389, 1996.
6. Bauer RD, Errico TJ: Cervical spine injuries. In Errico TJ, Bauer RD, Waugh T (eds): Spinal Trauma. Philadelphia, JB Lippincott, 1991, pp 71–121.
7. Beatson TR: Fractures and dislocations of the cervical spine. J Bone Joint Surg Br 45:21–35, 1963.
8. Beattie MS, Farooqui AA, Bresnahan JC: Apoptosis and secondary damage after experimental spinal cord injury. Top Spinal Cord Injury Rehabil 6:14–26, 2000.
9. Beckner MA, Heggeness MH, Doherty BJ: Biomechanical study of Jefferson fractures. Spine 23:1832-1836, 1998.
10. Bedbrook GM: Spinal injuries with tetraplegia and paraplegia. J Bone Joint Surg Br 61:267-284, 1979.
11. Bhatoe HS: Cervical spinal cord injury without radiological abnormality in adults. Neurol India 48:243–248, 2000.
12. Bohlman HH: Acute fractures and dislocations of the cervical spine. An analysis of three hundred hospitalized patients and review of the literature. J Bone Joint Surg Am 61:1119–1142, 1979.

13. Bosch A, Stauffer ES, Nickel VL: Incomplete traumatic quadriplegia-a ten year review. JAMA 216:473–478, 1971.
14. Bracken MB, Collins WF, Freeman DF, et al: Efficacy of methylprednisolone in acute spinal cord injury. JAMA 251:45–52, 1984.
15. Bracken MB, Shepard MJ, Collins WF, et al: A randomized controlled trail of methylprednisolone or naloxone in the treatment of acute spinal-cord injury: results of the Second National Acute Spinal Cord Injury Study. N Engl J Med 322:405–411, 1990.
16. Bracken MB, Shepard MJ, Collins WF, et al: Methylprednisolone or naloxone in the treatment of acute spinal cord injury: 1-year follow-up data. Results of the second National Acute Spinal Cord Injury Study. J Neurosurg 76:23–31, 1992.
17. Bracken MB, Shepard MJ, Holford TR, et al: Administration of methylprednisolone for 24 or 48 hours or tirilazad mesylate for 48 hours in the treatment of acute spinal cord injury. Results of the Third National Acute Spinal Cord Injury Randomized Controlled Trial. National Acute Spinal Cord Injury Study. JAMA 277:1597–1604, 1997.
18. Bracken MB, Shepard MJ, Holford TR, et al: Methylprednisolone or tirilazad mesylate administration after acute spinal cord injury: 1-year follow up. Results of the third National Acute Spinal Cord Injury randomized controlled trial. J Neurosurg 89:699–706 1998.
19. Bresnahan NJ: An elecron-microscopic analysis of axonal alterations following blunt contusion of the spinal cord of the rhesus monkey (Macaca mulatta). J Neurol Sci 37:59–82, 1978.
20. Brown-Sequard CE: Lectures on the physiology and pathology of the central nervous system and the treatment of organic nervous affections. Lancet 2:593–595, 659–662, 755–757, 821–823, 1868.
21. Burney RE, Maio RF, Maynard F, Karunas R: Incidence, characteristics and outcome of spinal cord injury at trauma centers in North America. Arch Surg 128;596–599, 1993.
22. Burns SP, Golding DG, Rolle WA, et al: Recovery of ambulation in motor incomplete tetraplegia. Arch Phys Med Rehabil 78:1169–1172, 1997.
23. Carlson GD, Minato Y, Okada A, et al: Early time-dependent decompression for spinal cord injury: vascular mechanisms of recovery. J Neurotrauma 14: 951–962, 1997.
24. Castro-Moure F, Kupsky W, Goshgarian HG: Pathophysiological classification of human spinal cord ischemia. J Spinal Cord Med 20:74–87, 1997.
25. Cheshire WP, Santos CC, Massey EW, Howard JF: Spinal cord infarction: etiology and outcome. Neurology 47:321–330, 1996.
26. Clark CR, White AA III: Fractures of the dens. A multicenter study. J Bone J Surg Am 67:1340–1348, 1985.
27. Cohen M: Initial resuscitation of the patient with spinal cord injury. Trauma Q 9:38–43, 1993.
28. Corsolini TB, Brooks DW: Overview of motor vehicle accident statistics and insurance claims. Phys Med Rehabil State Art Rev 12(1):1–10, 1998.
29. Cotler JM, Herbison GJ, Nasuti JF, et al: Closed reduction of traumatic cervical spine dislocation using traction weights up to 140 pounds. Spine 18:386–390, 1993.
30. Crandall JR, Kuhlmann TP, Pilkey WD: Air and knee bolster restraint system. Laboratory sled tests with human cadavers and hybrid III dummy. J Trauma 28:517–520, 1995.
31. Croce MA, Bee TK, Pritchard E, et al: Does optimal timing for spine fracture fixation exist? Ann Surg 233:851–858, 2001.
32. Cushman LA, Good RG, States JD: Characteristics of motor vehicle accidents resulting in spinal cord injury. Accid Anal Prev 23:557–560, 1991.
33. Daniels L, Worthingham C: Muscle Testing Techniques Of Manual Examination, 5th ed. Philadelphia, WB Saunders, 1986.
34. Dimar JR II, Glassman SD, Raque GH, et al: Influence of spinal canal narrowing and timing of decompression on neurologic recovery after spinal cord contusion in a rat model. Spine 24:1623–1633, 1999.
35. Effendi B, Roy D, Cornish B, et al: Fractures of the ring of the axis. A classification based on the analysis of 131 cases. J Bone Joint Surg Br 63:319–327, 1981.
36. Eismont FJ, Arena MJ, Green BA: Extrusion of an intervertebral disc associated with traumatic subluxation or dislocation of cervical facets. Case report. J Bone Surg 73:1555–1560, 1997.
37. Farley FA, Hensinger RN, Herzenberg JE: Cervical spinal cord injury in children. J Spinal Disord 5:410–416, 1992.
38. Foerster O: Symptomatologie der erkrankungen des Ruclenmarks und seiner surzeln. Handbook Neurol 5:1–403, 1936.
39. Geisler FH, Dorsey FC, Coleman WP: Recovery of motor function after spinal cord injury-a randomized, placebo-controlled trial with GM-1 ganglioside. N Engl J Med 324:1829–1838, 1991.

40. Geisler FH: Acute management of cervical spinal cord injury. Md Med J 37:525–530, 1998.
41. Reference deleted.
42. Greene KA, Dickman CA, Marciano FF, et al: Acute axis fractures. Spine 22:1843–1852, 1997.
43. Guha A, Tator CH, Endrenyi L, Piper I: Decompression of the spinal cord improves recovery after acute experimental spinal cord compression injury. Paraplegia 25:324–339, 1987.
44. Harrington JF, Likavec MJ, Smith AS: Disc herniation in cervical fracture subluxation. Neurosurgery 29:374–379, 1991.
45. Heary RF, Vaccaro AR, Mesa JJ, et al: Steroids and gunshot wounds to the spine. Neurosurgery 41:576–583, 1997.
46. Heineman A, Goranson N, Ginsburg K, Schnoll S: Alcohol use and activity patterns following spinal cord injury. Rehabil Psychol 34:191–205, 1989.
47. Hopkins A, Rudge P: Hyperpathia in the central cervical cord syndrome. J Neurol Neurosurg Psychiatry 36:637–642, 1973.
48. Huelke DF, Moore JL, Ostrom M: Air bag injuries and occupant protection. J Trauma 33:894–898, 1992.
49. Hurlbert R: Methyprednisolone for acute spinal cord injury: an inappropriate standard of care. J Neurosurg 93:1–7, 2000.
50. Kearney PA, Ridella SA, Viano DC, Anderson TE: Interaction of constant velocity and cord compression in determining the severity of spinal cord injury. J Neurotrauma 5:187–208, 1988.
51. Koivikko MP, Myllynen P, Karjalainen M, et al: Conservative and operative treatment in cervical burst fractures. Arch Orthop Trauma Surg 120:448–451, 2000.
52. Kokoska ER, Keller MS, Rallo MC, Weber TR: Characteristics of pediatric cervical spine injuries. J Ped Surg 36:100–105, 2001.
53. Kraus JF, Franti CE, Riggins RS, et al: Incidence of traumatic spinal cord lesions. J Chronic Dis 28:471–492, 1975.
54. Leventhal HR: Birth injuries of the spinal cord. J Pediatr 56:447–453, 1960.
55. Levy ML, Gans W, Wijesinghe HS, et al: Use of methylprednisolone as an adjunct in the management of patients with penetrating spinal cord injury: outcome analysis. Neurosurgery 39:1141–1148, 1996.
56. Lintner DM, Knight RQ, Cullen JP: Neurologic sequelae of cervical spine facet injuries. Spine 18:725–729, 1993.
57. Little JW, Halar E: Temporal course of motor recovery after Brown-Sequard spinal cord injuries. Paraplegia 23:39–46, 1985.
58. Lyness SS, Simeone FA: Vascular complications of upper cervical spine injuries. Orthop Clin North Am 9:1029–1038, 1978.
59. Marar BC, Orth MC: Hyperextension injuries of the cervical spine. J Bone Joint Surg Am 56:1655–1662, 1974.
60. Marino RJ, Rider-Foster D, Maissel G, Ditunno JF: Superiority of motor level over single neurological level in categorizing patients. Paraplegia 33:510–513, 1995.
61. Marshall LF, Knowlton S, Garfin SR, et al: Deterioration following spinal cord injury. A multicenter study. J Neurosurg 66:400–404, 1987.
62. Merriam WF, Taylor TKF, Ruff SJ, McPhail MJ: A reappraisal of acute traumatic central cord syndrome. J Bone Joint Surg Br 68:708–713, 1986.
63. Mirza Sk, Krengel WF III, Chapman JR, et al: Early versus delayed surgery for acute cervical spinal cord injury. Clin Orthop 359:104–114, 1999.
64. Montane I, Eismont FJ, Green BA: Traumatic occipitoatlantal dislocation. Spine 16:112–116, 1991.
65. Nathan PW, Smith MC: Long descending tracts in man. Review of present knowledge. Brain 78:248–304, 1956.
66. Nesathurai S: Steroids and spinal cord injury: revisiting the NASCIS 2 and NASCIS 3 trials. J Trauma 45:1088–1093, 1998.
67. Neurological assessment: the motor examination. In Ditunno JF, Donovan WH, Maynard FM (eds): Reference Manual for the International Standards for Neurological and Functional Classification of Spinal Cord Injury. Chicago, American Spinal Injury Association, 1994.
68. Nobunga AI, Go BK, Karunas RB: Recent demographic and injury trends in people served by the Model Spinal Cord Injury Care Systems. Arch Phys Med Rehabil 80:1372–1382, 1999.
69. Pang D, Wilberger JE: Spinal cord injury without radiographic abnormalities in children. J Neurosurg 57:114–129, 1982.
70. Penrod LE, Hegde SK, Ditunno JF: Age effect on prognosis for functional recovery in acute, traumatic central cord syndrome. Arch Phys Med Rehabil 71:963–968, 1990.

71. Powers B, Miller MD, Kramer RS, et al: Traumatic anterior atlanto-occipital dislocation. Neurosurgery 4:12–17, 1979.
72. Quencer RM, Bunge RP, Egnor M, et al: Acute traumatic central cord syndrome: MRI pathological correlations. Neuroradiology 34:85–94, 1992.
73. Raynor RB, Koplik B: Cervical cord trauma. Spine 10:193–197, 1985.
74. Rizzolo SJ, Vaccaro, Cotler JM: Cervical spine trauma. Spine 19:2288–2298, 1994.
75. Roth EJ, Lawler MH, Yarkony GM: Traumatic central cord syndrome: clinical features and functional outcomes. Arch Phys Med Rehabil 71:18–23, 1990.
76. Sasso RC, Meyer PR, Heinemann AW, et al: Seat belt use and relation to neurologic injury in motor vehicle crashes. J Spinal Disord 10:325–328, 1997.
77. Schneider RC, Cherry GR, Patek H: Syndrome of acute central cervical spinal cord injury with special reference to mechanisms involved in hyper-extension injuries of cervical spine. J Neurosurg 11:546–577, 1954.
78. Senter HJ, Venes JL: Loss of autoregulation and posttraumatic ischemia following experimental spinal cord trauma. J Neurosurg 50:198–206, 1979.
79. Short DJ, El Masry WS, Jones PW: High dose methylprednisolone in the management of acute spinal cord injury—a systematic review from a clinical perspective. Spinal Cord 38:273–286, 2000.
80. Spence KF, Decker S, Sell KW: Bursting atlantal fracture associated with rupture of the transverse ligament. J Bone Joint Surg Am 52:543–549, 1970.
81. Spinal Cord Injury at a Glance. Facts and Figures. Birmingham, AL, National Spinal Cord Injury Statistical Center, 2001.
82. Star AM, Jones AA, Cotler JM, et al: Immediate closed reduction of cervical spine dislocations using traction. Spine 15:1068–1072, 1990.
83. Thurman DJ, Burnett CL, Beaudoin DE, et al: Risk factors and mechanisms of occurrence in motor vehicle-related spinal cord injuries: Utah. Accid Anal Prev 27:411–415, 1995.
84. Tondury G: The cervical spine: its development and changes during life. Acta Orthop Belg 25:602–607, 1959.
85. Vaccaro AR, An HS, Betz RR, et al: The management of acute spinal trauma: prehospital and in-hospital emergency care. Instr Course Lect 46:113–125, 1997.
86. Vaccaro AR, Daugherty RJ, Sheehan TP, et al: Neurologic outcome of early versus late surgery for cervical spinal cord injury. Spine 22:2609–2613, 1997.
87. Vale FL, Burns J, Jackson AB, et al: Combined medical and surgical treatment after acute spinal cord injury: results of a prospective pilot study to assess the merits of aggressive medical resuscitation and blood pressure management. J Neurosurg 87:239–246, 1997.
89. Viano DC: Causes and control of spinal cord injury in automotive crashes. World J Surg 16:410–419, 1992.
90. Waters RL, Adkins RH, Yakura JS: Definition of complete spinal cord injury. Paraplegia 29:573–581, 1991.
91. Waters RL, Adkins R, Yakura J, Vigil D: Motor and sensory recovery following complete tetraplegia. Arch Phys Med Rehabil 74:242–247, 1993.
92. West DH, Gough JP, Hsarper TK: Low speed collision testing using human subjects. Accid Reconstr J 5:22–26, 1993.
93. White AA III, Panjabi MM: Clinical Biomechanics of the Spine, 2nd ed. Philadelphia, JB Lippincott, 1990.
94. Wigglesworth EC: Motor vehicle crashes and spinal injury. Paraplegia 30;543–549, 1992.
95. Wolf A, Levi L, Mirvis S, et al: Operative management of bilateral facet dislocation. J Neursurg 75:883–890, 1991.
96. Yeo JD, Stabback S, McKenzie B: Central necrosis following contusion to the sheep's spinal cord. Paraplegia 14:276–285, 1977.
97. Ziai WC, Hulbert RJ. A six-year review of odontoid fractures: The emerging role of surgical intervention. Can J Neurol Sci 27(4):297–301, 2000.

13

Mild Traumatic Brain Injury and Postconcussion Syndrome

Benjamin N. Nguyen, M.D., and Stuart A. Yablon, M.D.

Traumatic brain injury (TBI) is a leading cause of neurologic disability. It is estimated that more than 3 million people are living with disability resulting from TBI in the United States.[27] The incidence of TBI is estimated to be more than 1 million new cases annually,[27] with 98 per 100,000 population requiring hospitalization yearly.[154] TBI also results in more than 50,000 deaths annually in the United States. These figures indicate that the incidence of TBI exceeds the combined annual incidence rates of the common neurologic diagnoses of multiple sclerosis,[12] Parkinson's disease,[107] and Alzheimer's disease.[23] Motor vehicle crashes cause 50% of TBIs in the United States, falls result in another 21%, and assaults and recreationally incurred injuries account for most of the remaining injuries.[27]

MILD TRAUMATIC BRAIN INJURY

TBI is commonly classified into categories based on injury severity. The three categories, severe, moderate, and mild, are usually classified according to the Glasgow Coma Scale (GCS) score of impaired consciousness.[151] Classification of injury severity facilitates appropriate medical treatment and assists in determination of prognosis for recovery. A GCS score of 3 to 8 indicates severe TBI, 9 to 12 indicates a moderate TBI, while a score of 13 to 15 indicates a mild TBI (MTBI). Because a GCS score of 15 does not differentiate MTBI from a person without injury, some have proposed adding measures of amnesia to the GCS scale, referred to as an extended Glasgow Coma Scale (GCS-E) to better identify MTBI.[116]

Many patients with MTBI sustain a brain "concussion," indicating a transient disturbance of neurologic function secondary to mechanical forces.[119] TBI can occur with or without evidence of external trauma following violent contact forces or rapid acceleration or deceleration movements of the head. Hallmarks of concussion are confusion and impaired memory, often without loss of consciousness. Early symptoms include headache, dizziness, nausea, vomiting, slurred speech, imbalance, and uncoordination. Signs of confusion include vacant stare, disorientation, delayed verbal or motor responses, and poor concentration or attention. Confusion and memory dysfunction may be immediate after trauma or may evolve gradually over several minutes.[171]

Epidemiology

While the incidence of MTBI has never been well defined, it is estimated that up to 80% of TBI cases meet the criteria for MTBI.[87] These figures likely represent an underestimation because millions of people who have "minor" head trauma every year either do not seek medical treatment or are discharged home from the emergency center without a diagnosis of MTBI. A recent population-based epidemiologic study estimates that more than 75% of individuals who sustain MTBI do not seek treatment.[19] A missed diagnosis can be significant because more than 50% of those with MTBI will manifest injury-related symptoms[5] and approximately 15% may develop persistent problems.[3] A recent study found that the rate of hospitalization for TBI-related injuries declined about 51% from 1995-1996 (199 to 98 per 100,000 per year), while the incidence of TBI-related emergency department visits for persons not subsequently hospitalized increased (392 per 100,000 in 1995-1996 vs 216 per 100,000 in 1991).[67] This indicates a rising incidence of MTBI but a reduced rate of hospitalization for people sustaining such injuries.

Definition of MTBI

Because MTBI can result in disabilities that can impact on social relationships, employment, and routine daily function, proper diagnosis and treatment are warranted to minimize morbidity and possible mortality. In response, the Brain Injury Special Interest Group (BI-SIG) of the American Congress of Rehabilitation Medicine published a set of guidelines establishing diagnostic criteria for MTBI.[82] BI-SIG defined MTBI as an event secondary to traumatically induced physiologic disruption of brain function and manifested by at least one of the following:
- Any loss of consciousness (LOC) 30 minutes or less
- Any loss of memory for the events immediately before or after the accident
- Any alteration in mental state at the time of the accident
- Focal neurologic deficit(s) that may or may not be transient
- After 30 minutes, an initial GCS of 13 to 15
- Posttraumatic amnesia not greater than 24 hours.

The American Psychiatric Association published a more stringent definition of MTBI in its Diagnostic and Statistical Manual of Mental Disorders, version 4 (DSM-IV).[8] Here, the diagnosis of MTBI requires at least two of the following criteria:
- Minimum of 5 minutes of LOC
- More than 12 hours of posttraumatic amnesia
- New onset of posttraumatic seizures.

Despite publication of these criteria, it is likely that some difficulties will persist with diagnosis of MTBI. Regarding the BI-SIG's criteria, transient subjective alteration of mental state is nonspecific and difficult to verify. The criteria for diagnosis according to the DSM-IV, on the other hand, are probably too stringent. The lack of consensus regarding an operational definition of MTBI complicates correct diagnosis and renders epidemiologic investigation more difficult.

Pathophysiology and Mechanism of Injury

Although postconcussive disorders have been described for several hundred years,[37] the underlying mechanisms of MTBI have yet to be fully elucidated. It was previously assumed that sudden deceleration or rotational acceleration generates shearing forces within the brain,[3] which disrupt small blood vessels and axons at the gray and white matter interface.[127] The resultant shear or tensile forces were assumed to physically disrupt the axons, leading to membrane retraction, extrusion of axoplasm, and formation of large reactive swelling.[55] The subsequent pattern of white matter change has been termed diffuse axonal injury (DAI). Pathologically, the classic triad of DAI presents as gross focal lesions in the corpus callosum and dorsolateral quadrants of the midbrain and pons.[100]

However, recent studies in animals and humans reveal that mechanical disruption per se is not the proximate cause for DAI.[129] Rather, trauma triggers focal changes in the permeability of the axolemma, allowing an influx of calcium. This, in turn, activates proteolytic enzymes in the subaxolemma. The resultant alteration of the intraaxonal cytoskeleton leads to impaired axoplasmic transport, contributing to axonal swelling and detachment. This is followed by Wallerian degeneration of the detached axonal segment and the synaptic terminals originating from the injured axon.[46,125]

Diagnosis and Neuroimaging

No definitive test exists for the diagnosis of MTBI other than postmortem microscopic changes of the injured brain tissue.[20] However, imaging studies are frequently indicated in the evaluation of MTBI. These include computed tomography (CT) and magnetic resonance imaging (MRI). Skull radiographs are no longer routinely ordered, because studies find no benefit from this procedure for evaluating MTBI.[51,105] Although neurologic complications of mild head injury are uncommon, a head CT is frequently obtained on patients with GCS below 15, abnormal mental status, or hemispheric deficits. Patients are often discharged from the emergency department with immediate treatment followed by observation at home after "negative" head CT results.[36] While most patients with MTBI lack significant neuroradiographic findings on CT scan, the early identification of epidural or subdural hematoma can be life saving.

MRI is more sensitive than CT in evaluating MTBI[98] and is able to detect parenchymal lesions in the frontal and temporal regions in 85% of patients in whom they are not detected by CT scan.[97] MRI is also superior in demonstrating brain contusions during subacute and chronic stages after TBI[76] and provides better estimates of the severity of DAI and possibility of delayed traumatic intracerebral hematoma.[173] Newer imaging modalities such as MR spectroscopy[147] and functional imaging modalities such as functional MRI,[108] single photon emission computed tomography,[158,178] and photon emission tomography[2,152] are being investigated as potential neurodiagnostic measures to assist with diagnosis of MTBI.

Neurophysiologic assessment of MTBI currently demonstrates limited utility in the clinical evaluation of MTBI. Reported neurophysiologic assessment techniques in MTBI include electroencephalography (EEG),[160] magnetic source imaging,[108] and brainstem auditory evoked responses (BAER).[52] While EEG findings are nonspecific among most patients with MTBI,[42,101] EEG studies may be helpful when a posttraumatic seizure disorder is suspected.[170] Similarly, routine use of EEG brain mapping is not recommended to evaluate cerebral cortical dysfunction following MTBI.[6] Although BAER abnormalities have been reported after MTBI,[115] no specific pattern of abnormality is noted. Furthermore, BAER abnormalities are found with the same prevalence in patients with and without postconcussion syndrome (PCS), limiting its utility in the evaluation of patients with these symptoms.[138]

In contrast, posturographic evaluation is useful in the characterization of impaired balance and planning treatment for related sensory integration deficits and visuovestibular disturbances.[142] Electronystagmography is useful in the evaluation of vestibular dysfunction as well as various eye movement disorders.[120] Polysomnography can document sleep architecture and posttraumatic sleep disturbances and may be particularly helpful with sleep disturbances intractable to sleep hygiene and or pharmacologic intervention.[178] No neurodiagnostic test, however, is diagnostic of MTBI and associated postconcussion syndrome. Rather, such tests serve as an adjunct to clinical history and examination in the evaluation of patients suspected of sustaining MTBI.

POSTCONCUSSION SYNDROME

PCS refers to a variable constellation of physical, behavioral, and cognitive symptoms among patients with a history of MTBI who experience persistence of symptoms months to years following injury.[30] PCS has been recognized in the medical literature for centuries,[146] with one of the first cases described involving a 26-year-old maid who complained of headaches, dizziness, tinnitus, and tiredness 6 months after she had been hit over the head with a stick in 1694.[37] Neurologic abnormalities are not associated with the syndrome and are not required for diagnosis. PCS is not synonymous with MTBI; patients with MTBI may not develop PCS.

PCS usually follows MTBI. The incidence of PCS among patients with MTBI varies, although some reports suggest that up to 55% of those with MTBI will develop PCS at 1 year after injury.[38] Symptoms of PCS are similar to those reported in MTBI and consist of headaches, dizziness, fatigue, irritability, anxiety, insomnia, loss of concentration and memory, and noise sensitivity.[104] Headaches are reported in more than half of patients with MTBI/PCS.[112] Other symptoms include tinnitus, hearing loss, blurred vision, diplopia, convergence insufficiency, light sensitivity, diminished taste and smell, depression, personality change, decreased libido, decreased appetite, slowing of reaction time, and slowing of information-processing speed.[16,47] These symptoms are not exclusive to PCS and may reflect injuries to the neck or back. Residual impairment may be present even after resolution of cognitive symptoms, and the sequelae of MTBI may be cumulative even in persons who have clinically recovered.[47]

Disagreements exist regarding diagnosis of PCS. Rigler raised the issue of compensation neurosis when he described the increased incidence of posttraumatic invalidism after a system for financial compensation was established for accidental injuries on the Prussian railways in 1871.[132] Other authors have characterized PCS as a compensation neurosis.[110] To assist with the diagnosis of PCS, the International Statistical Classification of Diseases and Related Health Problems, 10th edition (ICD-10),[169] published a set of guidelines based on epidemiologic studies in several countries and regions, including the United States, Great Britain, and Scandinavia. Here, PCS is defined as a ". . . history of head trauma with loss of consciousness [that] precedes symptom onset by maximum of 4 weeks with three or more symptoms of the following:

- Headache, dizziness, malaise, fatigue, noise intolerance
- Irritability, depression, anxiety, emotional lability
- Subjective concentration, memory, or intellectual difficulties without neuropsychological evidence of marked impairment
- Insomnia
- Reduced alcohol tolerance
- Preoccupation with above symptoms and fear of brain damage without hypochondriacal concern and adoption of sick role."

The DSM-IV also has published criteria for PCS.[8] This definition is more stringent than that of the ICD-10 in that, to meet criteria, the history of TBI should result in significant cerebral contusion with LOC, posttraumatic amnesia, or seizures and show neuropsychological evidence of difficulty in attention and memory. Additionally, the diagnosis of PCS by the DSM-IV requires three or more of the following symptoms for at least 3 months. Onset of symptoms must occur shortly after head trauma or represent substantial worsening of previous symptoms: fatigue; irritability; disordered sleep; anxiety, depression, or affective lability; headache; changes in personality; dizziness; and apathy or lack of spontaneity.

The primary difference between ICD-10 and DSM-IV criteria involves the cause of the symptoms in PCS. The ICD-10 recognizes that persistent cognitive complaints may have a psychological basis, while the DSM-IV requires objective evidence of cognitive impairment associated with ongoing neurologic abnormality. Those with significant cognitive or emotional difficulties and those who present later with persistent somatic complaints or worsening of symptoms are at risk for persistent PCS. Risk factors for persisting sequelae include age older than 40 years; lower educational, intellectual, and socioeconomic level; female gender; alcohol abuse; prior TBI; and multiple trauma.[47]

DIFFERENTIAL DIAGNOSIS OF MTBI/PCS

Diagnosis of PCS requires a history of TBI and the co-occurrence of several symptoms. There is a long-standing debate as to whether PCS results from neurologic or psychological etiologies.[114] It is felt that the acute MTBI/PCS syndrome likely has a neurologic basis while the chronic symptoms of PCS likely persist because of psychological factors. PCS shares features with anxiety and depressive disorders, such as anxiety, insomnia, irritability, and poor concentration. However, PCS is not associated with numbing of general responsiveness as observed with anxiety disorders. Similarly, it is not characteristically associated with changes in appetite, weight, psychomotor agitation or retardation, or suicidal ideation, as observed among patients with a history of depressive disorder.

Other considerations in the patient with suspected MTBI/PCS include the presence of preinjury cognitive difficulties, such as previous TBI, age-related dementia, advanced age, and repeat TBI, because they may diminish cerebral "reserves,"[135] making a causal relationship between subsequent MTBI and cognitive impairment more likely. The presence of posttraumatic stress disorder, somatoform disorder, conversion disorder, factitious disorder, as well as the possibility of substance abuse or dependency also should be considered.

Malingering is a condition considered in the differential diagnosis of MTBI and particularly in PCS. According to DSM-IV, malingering involves the intentional production of false or grossly exaggerated physical or psychological symptoms motivated by external incentives.[8] It has been reported in several studies following PCS,[17,156] and differentiating malingering from MTBI is especially difficult due to the nonspecific nature complaints associated with MTBI/PCS. Nonetheless, some authors suggest that malingering be identified and discriminated from patients with MTBI by their performance patterns on the Wechsler Intelligence and Memory Scales[111] and Halstead-Reitan Battery.[113] The Hiscock Forced Choice Test is considered to be a useful screening test for malingering and other nonorganic disorders and should be considered as part of a comprehensive postconcussion examination.[18] However, because no neuroimaging study currently excludes the possibility of MTBI, clinicians instead should rely upon a combination of subjective measures, radiographic findings, and clinical experience to evaluate potentially injured patients.[134]

ASSOCIATED SYMPTOMS OF MTBI/PCS

Headache

A number of symptoms are associated with MTBI (Table 1). Headache represents the most common neurologic symptom after MTBI.[5] Estimates of headache incidence following MTBI range from 30% to 90%. Posttraumatic headaches occur more often and with longer duration in patients with MTBI compared with patients with more severe degrees of trauma.[171,168] Little is known about the pathophysiology of posttraumatic headaches, making assessment and treatment challenging.[62]

Hines classified posttraumatic headaches into six subtypes[77]: (1) tension, (2) local tissue injury or scar pain without associated neuralgia, (3) migraine, (4) dysautonomic cephalgia, (5) cervicogenic associated with whiplash neck injuries, and (6) neuralgic.

According to the International Headache Society, tension-type headache should be nonpulsating in nature, bilateral, not severe, and not aggravated by routine physical activity, with the absence of nausea or vomiting.[74] Tension headaches associated with MTBI are usually related to pain of myofascial origin and may be worsened by physical activity. Examination reveals localized muscle tenderness, usually associated with trigger points. Likewise, local tissue injury without neurologic deficits can give rise to similar symptoms.

Migraine headaches, on the other hand, are felt to be secondary to vascular causes. By the International Headache Society criteria, migraine headaches are usually unilateral in location; of moderate or severe quality; associated with nausea, photophobia, and phonophobia; and usually aggravated by physical activities.[74] Specifically, the throbbing localized pain worsens with activities that increase abdominal or intracranial pressure, such as coughing, sneezing, and Valsalva maneuvers. Examples of posttraumatic migraine include basilar artery migraine, which is caused by vasomotor instability in the vertebrobasilar posterior cerebral circulation. This may occur with acceleration-deceleration injury affecting the cervical spine,[69] resulting in vasoconstriction followed by vasodilatation.[121]

The fourth subtype is dysautonomic cephalgia, which usually manifests prominent dysautonomic features. This subtype includes cluster headache, paroxysmal hemicrania, and short-lasting unilateral neuralgiform headache with conjunctival injection and tearing (SUNCT) syndrome.[61] These headaches are often accompanied by autonomic symptoms such as conjuntival injection, lacrimation, nasal congestion, rhinorrhea, forehead and facial sweating, miosis, ptosis, and eyelid edema.[74] Although pain usually occurs around the orbital and adjacent areas, it sometimes localizes over the face or the occipital-nuchal areas.[145]

Cervicogenic headache associated with whiplash neck injuries, the fifth subtype, is due to injury to the cervical muscles and other soft tissues. It can occur after a motor vehicle crash, resulting in neck hyperflexion followed by flexion,[53] and is likely myofascial in nature.[155] Not surprisingly, these headaches may be confused with tension headaches.

Lastly, headaches secondary to neuralgic cause are felt to be secondary to nerve injury due to focal nerve irritation, with resultant nerve compression, and entrapment, including cervical radiculopathies.[88] Injury to sympathetic nerve fibers following significant cervical hyperextension injury may result from anterior cervical sympathetic dysfunction (Bernard-Horner syndrome) or posttraumatic autonomic cephalalgia arising from posterior cervical sympathetic dysfunction (Barre-Lieou syndrome).[79]

Other causes for headache after MTBI not included among Hines' classification include inner ear disturbances, such as benign positional vertigo or perilymphatic fistulas with resultant leakage of fluid from the inner ear into the middle ear[65]; abuse of analgesic medications (also known as analgesic-rebound headaches)[163]; and trauma-induced alteration of cerebral blood flow patterns in patients with chronic posttraumatic headaches.[60] More importantly, headaches may herald the development of a serious delayed complication associated with a more severe injury. These include delayed manifestation of vascular injury, such as carotid, vertebral, or posterior inferior cerebellar artery dissection.[62,176]

Depression

Depression represents a frequent complaint among those with MTBI/PCS, with the incidence ranging from 14.6% to 35%.[25,72] Those with MTBI/PCS have been shown in multiple studies to be at increased risk for development of depression/posttraumatic stress disorders.[25,72,96,106,137] Accompanying symptoms include psychologic and somatic complaints as well as cognitive deficits (Table 1). Risk factors for development of acute stress disorder include scores consistent with depression on the Beck Depression Inventory as well as individuals exhibiting "avoidant coping mechanisms."[72] Although usually mild and self-limited, in susceptible individuals depression may persist and become a major obstacle to recovery.[62]

Table 1. Sequelae of Mild Traumatic Brain Injury/Postconcussion Syndrome

Psychologic and Somatic Complaints	Cranial Nerve Complaints
Headaches	Anosmia
• Muscle contraction (tension)	Blurred vision
• Secondary to local injury without	Diplopia
neuralgia (tempomandibular joint	Convergence insufficiency
syndrome, laceration)	Dizziness
• Migraine (classical, common, mixed,	Vertigo
vascular)	Tinnitus
• Dysautonomic cephalgia (cluster,	Hyperacousis
paroxysmal hemicrania, SUNCT	Light and noise sensitivity
syndrome)	**Cognitive Deficits**
• Cervicogenic associated with whiplash	Memory dysfunction
neck injuries	Impaired concentration and attention
• Neuralgic (occipital, supraorbital,	Impaired abstract thinking
infraorbital)	Increased distractibility
Anxiety	Decreased reaction time
Depression	Decreased information-processing speed
Fatigability	Apathy
Personality change	**Rare Sequelae**
Sleep disturbance	Seizures
Decreased libido	Subdural and epidural hematomas
Decreased appetite	Cold hypersensitivity
	Transient global amnesia
	Tremor
	Dystonia

Sleep Disturbances

Sleep disturbances and pain complaints are also common following MTBI. Among those with insomnia and pain, 65.5% complain of difficulty with sleep, while 70% complain of pain. Among those without pain, 55.3% complain of insomnia.[14] Poor sleep maintenance appears to be the most common problem among patients with insomnia and may represent a sleep-wake schedule disorder.[124] Other problems reported include alteration of sleep architecture[131] and excessive daytime sleepiness related to breathing difficulties.[68]

Other Sequelae of MTBI/PCS

MTBI may also cause other neurologic impairments. Dizziness is reported in 40% to 60% of individuals after MTBI,[4] usually due to traumatically induced benign positional vertigo or labyrinthine concussion.[179] Perilymphatic fistula, posttraumatic causes, or cervicogenic causes of dizziness are less common. Postural instability is also a frequent occurrence in one study among TBI patients. These patients, all without sensorimotor impairments by standard clinical neurologic examination, demonstrated an increase in anteroposterior and lateral sway and a decrease in weight-shifting speed as measured by dual-plate force platform.[58] Instability may also result from disruption of one or more components of the postural control system, where balance results from a complex interaction among the musculoskeletal and neural systems.[142] It may result from vestibular dysfunction, often with vertigo and dizziness.[54] Other factors contributing to postural instability include visual deficits arising from head trauma. These may result in a vitreous lesion, either prefoveal or foveal, or retinal injury, causing detachment or hemorrhage.[34] Signs and symptoms of visual dysfunction may include convergence insufficiency, diplopia, photophobia, eye movement disorders, or accommodative spasm.[11,86] Audiovestibular sequelae include sonophobia, tinnitus, sensorineural hearing loss, and vestibular dysfunction.[47,178]

Other sensory deficits include anosmia, or loss of smell following trauma.[93,150] Posttraumatic anosmia may result from injury to olfactory neurofibrils as they pass through the cribiform plate. Alternatively, it can result from compression of the olfactory bulbs, injury to the central pathways of olfaction, or injury to the nasal passages themselves.[153]

Seizures, a rare consequence of MTBI, occur at approximately the same rate as unprovoked seizures in the general population.[10,92] However, some studies suggest that a small number of patients with MTBI may experience partial seizures, many of which remit spontaneously with time.[66,159]

MTBI IN SPORTS

MTBI represents a significant percentage of all athletic injuries. Each year, about 300,000 sports-related brain concussions occur in the United States.[28] It is estimated that 62,816 cases of MTBI occur annually among high school varsity athletes participating in football, basketball, baseball, soccer, field hockey, field hockey, and volleyball.[130] In American football, more than 250,000 high school players (about 20%) experience a concussion in a given season,[57] and less than 12% experience two concussions in the same season.[166] At the college level, the incidence of concussion ranges from 5.3%[24] to 8.2% per 4-year career.[4] In rugby, concussions represent the most common injury among amateurs, with an incidence of 15%[141] and up to 17% among professionals if "mild concussion" not involving an LOC were counted.[59] MTBI also represents the most common injury in ice hockey, making up 12% to 14% of all injuries and affecting 10% of all participants.[56,180] In boxing, the "knockout" rate is estimated at 5% for amateurs and 6.3% for professionals.[167] Other arenas in which MTBI occurr include motor racing, equestrian sports, martial arts, wrestling, gymnastics, baseball, softball, soccer, volleyball, horse riding, cycling, downhill skiing, diving, and motorcycling. Symptoms and signs of MTBI/PCS in sports are listed in Table 2.

Table 2. Symptoms and Signs of MTBI/PCS in Sports

Symptoms	Signs
Confusion	Altered levels of consciousness, impaired memory and attention
Dizziness and light-headedness	Dazed appearance, impaired gait/balance
Memory loss	Amnesia
Blurry vision	Pupillary concordance
Photophobia/phonophobia	Increased symptoms with exertion
Headache	Facial expression, hypersensitivity to light and sounds
Fatigue	Poor concentration ability, slowed information-processing speed
Nausea	Apprehension

Diagnosis of MTBI/PCS in sports is complicated by the minimization of symptoms by players, parents, and coaches in deference to continued participation in the athletic contest. Therefore, a high index of suspicion and a greater awareness of the risks of denial can contribute to earlier and more accurate interventions among the people who are susceptible. The involved party should be evaluated for level of consciousness, gait, confusion, orientation, amnesia, pupillary size, and coexisting injuries following published protocols by the Colorado Medical Society Sports Medicine Committee[33] and the American Academy of Neurology.[7] Follow-up evaluations provide clues to the stability and severity of the insult; any athlete with LOC should be observed closely and transported to the emergency department should any clinical deterioration occur. Persistent symptoms may require inpatient observation, imaging, and neurosurgical or neuropsychological consultation. Regarding criteria for return to play, multiple guidelines exist based on injury classifications and recurrence, including those by the American Academy of Neurology,[7] Sturmi,[148] Kelly,[84] Cantu,[26] the Colorado Medical Society,[33] Nelson,[117] and Wilberger.[167] Despite some differences, all agree on the following:

- The concussed athlete should be removed from competition, examined, and observed.
- Serial assessment is important; those who show evidence of deterioration should be transferred to the hospital for imaging and neurosurgical consultation.
- Those with LOC or amnesia should be prevented from returning to play, and no athlete should be returned to play until he is completely asymptomatic.

A recent study found that concussed athletes were much more likely to fail recent memory questions pertaining to simple game facts than a nonconcussed control group.[103] Additionally, a history of learning disability or multiple concussions can result in poor outcome, and the combination of these factors may be "detrimentally synergistic."[32] Because the effects of recurrent concussions may be cumulative,[103] those who return to play before their symptoms have resolved are completely at risk for a second impact syndrome if they sustain another concussion.[84,109,136] This phenomenon is termed "second impact syndrome" and is felt to result from acute autoregulatory dysfunction in the reinjured brain, leading to a rapid rise in transcranial pressure and brainstem failure. Fortunately, it is relatively rare compared with the total number of concussions per year and can be prevented with insistence on total resolution of all symptoms in every case of MTBI. Careful evaluations, adhering to conservative return-to-play criteria, selective imaging, and consultation will decrease the incidence of potential sequelae associated with MTBI/PCS in sports.

MTBI/PCS AMONG CHILDREN, ADOLESCENTS, AND THE ELDERLY

The challenges of defining what constitutes MTBI/PCS also exist among other patient populations, making proper diagnosis, treatment guidelines, and epidemiologic collection difficult. A recent attempt to establish a clinical practice guideline for the American Academy of Pediatrics concluded that the existing scientific literature on MTBI in children was insufficient to provide a scientific basis for evidence-based recommendations about most of the key issues in clinical management.[78] MTBI occurs more commonly in the young. Boys are twice as likely to experience these injuries, with the most common cause being low-velocity injury due to falls, recreational, or sporting activities.[140] The incidence of long-term sequelae of MTBI/PCS appears lower in children than in adults. In most studies, difficulties in attention, memory, and cognition appear to resolve between 3 to 12 months after injury in most injured children.[50,95] Nonetheless, persisting and troublesome difficulties exist in a number of children following MTBI.[13] These include difficulties with social, emotional, and behavioral deficits, which may have negative implications with regard to academic and educational performance, including issues relating to school reentry.[143,173] Given that the number of potential future years of significant disability are obviously greater in children, early diagnosis and management is important.[71]

With increasing survival and growth of the elderly population, an increase in the number of elderly trauma patients can be expected.[129] Epidemiologic studies indicate that the incidence of brain injury for older adults begins to increase gradually around 60 years of age, with a more dramatic increase after age 70.[63] Among the elderly, most MTBI occurs as a result of falls, followed by motor vehicle crashes and automobile-pedestrian accidents.[44] Among those younger than 80 years of age, there is a male preponderance, whereas among those older than 80 years old, there is a female preponderance. The greater number of females with MTBI/PCS among those older than 80 years, however, may be a reflection of the longer life expectancies of females in most studied populations.

The mortality rate after a mild head injury is significantly higher in the elderly—up to 20% in one study.[85] The increased mortality rate is generally ascribed to the existence of higher comorbidity among the elderly. Another study, composed of 411 hospitalized patients with TBI followed for 1 year, found that older adults experienced less complete recovery after TBI "either because they have reduced reserves with which to tolerate brain injury or because their physiologic status creates a more destructive injury." The authors cautioned against generalizing expectations of recovery in the elderly based on data obtained among younger individuals.[133]

TREATMENT CONSIDERATIONS

Because most patients have genuine complaints, treatment is warranted and should be individualized based on the specifics complaints. Simple reassurance is often a major treatment for MTBI and PCS because most patients will improve after 3 months.

For headache, response to optimal treatment reflects the accuracy of diagnosis. Different types of headache respond to different forms of treatment. Amitriptyline may help posttraumatic muscle contraction–type headaches as well as associated symptoms of irritability, dizziness, depression, fatigue, and insomnia.[155] Other antidepressants, such as maprotiline[89] and fluoxetine,[122] have been shown to be effective in treating posttraumatic muscle contraction-type headache. Headaches secondary to local injury respond well to acetaminophen or nonsteroidal anti-inflammatory medications. First-line abortive agents in the treatment of migraine headaches include a combination of isometheptene mucate-dichloralphenazone-acetaminophen (Midrin) or butalbital-aspirin-caffeine (Fiorinal).[161] Prophylaxis or preventative agents in the treatment of migraine consist of beta blockers,[81] calcium channel blockers,[90] selective serotonin antagonists,[126] and ergot alkaloids.[15] Similarly, posttraumatic migraine responds well to amiltriptyline or propanolol, with a 70% response rate.[164] Paroxysmal hemicrania almost uniformly responds to indomethicin but not to other anti-inflammatory drugs.[118] Greater occipital neuralgia can be treated with greater occipital nerve block with a local anesthetic.[144] Other treatments include transcutaneous electrical nerve stimulation, muscle relaxants, physical therapy, manipulation, biofeedback, acupuncture, psychotherapy, and counseling.

Depression following MTBI/PCS, though often mild in relative severity and self-limited in duration, may persist for many years. Moreover, symptoms of depressed mood may ultimately manifest as major depression among individuals who are "vulnerable."[25] As such, patients with MTBI/PCS with symptoms of depressed mood should be treated to help prevent further progression of illness. Treatment of contributing conditions, such as pain, sleep disruption,[14] removal of environmental or behavioral stressors, and cognitive retraining,[161] can be attempted. If the symptoms persist, pharmacologic treatment may be attempted. No evidence-based guideline for specific pharmacologic treatment exists, but selective serotonergic reuptake inhibitors are often preferred because of their favorable efficacy and adverse effect profile,[49] with little retardation on psychomotor performance.[70]

An initial step in the treatment of sleep disturbance involves identifying the underlying etiology. If pain contributes to the sleep disturbance, aggressive treatment of pain is warranted.[14] If the problem lies with sleep initiation or maintenance, pharmacologic treatment with low-dose trazodone or nortriptyline may be helpful.[178] Importantly, daytime administration of sedating medications should be withdrawn when possible, and behavioral treatment to improve sleep hygiene should also be considered.[73]

Treatments for postural instability include adaptation and motor learning,[142] exercises for vestibular hypofunction,[75] or benign paroxysmal positional benign paroxysmal vertigo.[22,45] If visual symptoms contribute to postural instability, a thorough ophthalmologic examination including a visual field test and electronystagmography is warranted.[34]

Although MTBI generally presents with less potential for disabling injury than moderate or severe TBI, clinicians must be cognizant of the potential for severe sequelae. Specifically, rare intracranial complications such as hematomas may occur and are usually seen in conjunction with skull fractures and late neurologic deterioration.[176,179] Detection of other potentially operative conditions is important, such as depressed skull fractures, elevated intracranial pressure, cerebrospinal fluid leaks, and injury to cranial adnexal structures. Controversy exists regarding whether hospital admission for MTBI results in better or worse outcomes.[43,102] Nevertheless, recommendations for hospitalization presently include a GCS score of 13 or 14, focal neurologic deficit, skull fracture, abnormal findings on CT scan, suspicion of abuse, confounded clinical evaluation due to alcohol or drug intoxication, and the absence of a caregiver at home to monitor for progression of symptoms.[35,36]

CONCLUSION

Most sequelae of MTBI will resolve or leave limited deficits among individuals without prior compromising conditions such substance abuse or a psychiatric disorder.[39,40,97] While not all MTBIs can be prevented, accurate and consistent medical management of injuries will minimize the potential for reinjury and subsequently reduce the potential for the long-term disability. Diagnosis and treatment remain challenging, in part because the symptoms of MTBI are nonspecific, the symptom severity may be magnified, the associated cognitive deficits may be apparent only in particularly stressful situations,[41,48] and current neuroimaging techniques fail to yield a definitive diagnosis. If not identified and treated appropriately, up to 15% of patients may develop lingering problems impairing daily functioning. Other appropriate diagnoses must also be considered before a diagnosis of MTBI is made, because treatment options will differ reflecting the specific type and severity of the complicating conditions.

Treatment of MTBI/PCS centers upon the identification of factors responsible for ongoing symptoms. Among those who present early after injury, intervention should be directed at evaluation and treatment of somatic complaints. Among those with MTBI sustained in sports events, subsequent morbidity can be decreased by careful evaluation, cautious return-to-play criteria, selective imaging, and consultation.[148] Importantly, the incidence of MTBI can also be reduced with simple prevention strategies through which interventions are aimed at controlling the participating environment, including modification of player skills, teaching techniques, playing rules, and protective equipment.[130]

To optimize outcome from MTBI/PCS, patients and family members should be educated regarding the rationale for specific interventions and expectations for treatment outcome, with incorporation of close family members into the long-term treatment plan. Those with persistent postconcussive symptoms may benefit from referral to a specialized pragmatic cognitive therapy program consisting of psychotherapy, occupational/vocational interventions, and an adaptive strategy training.[31,123] Diagnosis, recognition, and management of MTBI/PCS are facilitated by keeping abreast of current advances in neurodiagnosis and familiarity with the current literature on the neurologic, rehabilitative, psychological, and neuropharmacologic approaches relevant to this patient population.

References

1. Akpunonu BE, Ahrens J: Sexual headaches: case report, review, and treatment with calcium channel blocker. Headache 31:141–145, 1991.
2. Alavi A, Hirsch LJ: Studies of central nervous system disorders with single photon emission computed tomography and positron emission tomography: evolution over the past two decades. Semin Nucl Med 21:58–81, 1991.
3. Alexander MP: Mild traumatic brain injury: pathophysiology, natural history, and clinical management. Neurology 45:1253–1260, 1995.
4. Alves WM: Football-induced mild head injury. In Torg JS (ed): Athletic Injuries to the Head, Neck, and Face, 2nd ed. St. Louis, Mosby-Yearbook, 1991.
5. Alves W, Macciocchi SN, Barth JT: Postconcussive symptoms after uncomplicated mild head injury. J Head Trauma Rehabil 8(3):48–59, 1993.
6. American Academy of Neurology: EEG brain mapping. Neurology 39:1100–1101, 1989.
7. American Academy of Neurology Report of the Quality Standards Subcommittee: Practice parameter: the management of concussion in sports [summary statement]. Neurology 48:581–585, 1997.

8. American Psychiatric Association: Diagnostic and Statistical Manual of Mental Disorders, version 4. Washington, DC, American Psychiatric Association, 1994.
9. Anderson DW, McLaurin RL: Report on the National Head and Spinal Cord Injury Survey. J Neurosurg 53(suppl):S19–S31, 1980.
10. Annegers JF, Grabow JD, Groovr RV, et al: Seizures after head trauma: a population study. Neurology 30:683–689, 1980.
11. Baker RS, Epstein AD: Ocular motor abnormalities from head trauma. Surv Ophthalmol 35:245–267, 1991.
12. Baun HM, Rothschild BB: The incidence and prevalence of reported multiple sclerosis. Ann Neurol 10:420–428, 1981.
13. Beers SR: Cognitive effects of mild head injury in children and adolescents. Neuropsychol Rev 3:282–320, 1992.
14. Beetar JT, Thomas JG, Sparadeo FR: Sleep and pain complaints in symptomatic traumatic brain injury and neurologic populations. Arch Phys Med Rehabil 77:1298–1302, 1996.
15. Bell KR, Kraus EE, Zasler ND: Medical management of post-traumatic headaches. Pharmacological and physical treatments. J Head Trauma Rehabil 14:34–48, 1999.
16. Binder LM: Persisting symptoms after mild head injury. A review of the postconcussive syndrome. J Clin Exp Neuropsychol 8:323–346, 1986.
17. Binder LM: Malingering following mild head trauma. Clin Neuropsychol 4:25–36, 1990.
18. Binder LM: Forced choice testing provides evidence of malingering. Arch Phys Med Rehabil 72:377–380, 1992.
19. Binder LM, Rohling ML: Money matters: a meta-analytic review of the effects of financial incentives on recovery after closed-head injury. Am J Psychiatry 153:7–10, 1996.
20. Blumbergs PC, Scott G, Manavis J, et al: Staining of amyloid precursor protein to study axonal damage in mild brain injury. Lancet 344:1055–1056, 1994.
21. Bohenen N, Jolles J, Twijnstra A: Neuropsychological deficits in patients with persistent symptoms six months after mild head injury. Neurosurgery 30:692–696, 1992.
22. Brandt T, Daroff RB: Physical therapy for benign paroxysmal positional vertigo. Arch Otolaryngol 106:485–485, 1980.
23. Brookmeyer R, Gray S, Kawas C: Projections of Alzheimer's disease in the United States and the public health impact of delaying disease onset. Am J Public Health 88:1337–1342, 1998.
24. Buckley WE: Concussions in college football. Am J Sports Med 16:51–56, 1988.
25. Busch CR, Alpern HP: Depression after mild traumatic brain injury: a review of current research. Neuropsychol Rev 8:95–108, 1998.
26. Cantu RC: Cerebral concussion in sport: management and prevention. Sports Med 14:64–74, 1992.
27. Centers for Disease Controls and Prevention, National Center for Injury Prevention and Control: Traumatic Brain Injury in the United States. A Report to Congress. Atlanta, CDC, 1999.
28. Centers for Disease Controls and Prevention: Sports-related recurrent brain injuries-United States. MMWR Morb Mortal Wkly Rep 48:224–227, 1997.
29. Centers for Disease Control and Prevention: Traumatic brain injury-Colorado, Missouri, Oklahoma, and Utah, 1990-1993. Morb Mortal Wkly Rep 46(1):8–11, 1997.
30. Cicerone KD, Kalmar K: Persistent postconcussion syndrome: the structure of subjective complaints after mild traumatic brain injury. J Head Trauma Rehabil 10(3):1–17, 1995.
31. Cicerone KD, Smith CL, Ellmo W, et al: Neuropsychological rehabilitation of mild traumatic brain injury. Brain Inj 10:277–286, 1996.
32. Collins MW, Grindel SH, Lovell MR, et al: Relationship between concussion and neuropsychological performance in college football players. JAMA 282:964–970, 1999.
33. Colorado Medical Society Sports Medicine Committee: Guidelines for the Management of Concussion in Sports, rev. ed. Denver, Colorado Medical Society, 1990.
34. Cytowic R, Stump DA, Larned DC: Closed head trauma: somatic, ophthalmic and cognitive impairments in non-hospitalized patients. In Whitake HA (ed): Neuropsychological Studies of Non-Focal Brain Damage. New York, Springer-Verlag, 1988, pp 226–264.
35. Dacey RG: Complications after apparently mild head injury and strategies of neurosurgical management. In Levin HS, Eisenber HM, Benton AL (eds): Mild Head Injury. Oxford, Oxford University Press, 1989, pp 83–101.
36. Dacey RG, Alves WM, Rimel RW, et al: Neurosurgical complications after apparent minor head injury. Assessment of risk in a series of 610 patients. J Neurosurg 65:203–210, 1986.
37. de Morsier G: Les encephalopathies traumatiques. Etude neurologique. Schweiz Arch Neurol Neurochir Psychiat 50:161, 1943.

38. Deb S, Lyons I, Koutzoukis C: Neuropsychiatric sequelae one year after a minor head injury. J Neurol Neurosurg Psychiatry 65:899–902, 1998.
39. Dikmen SS, Machamer JE, Winn HR, Temkin NR: Neuropsychological outcome at 1-year post head injury. Neuropsychology 9:80–90, 1995.
40. Dikmen S, McLean A, Temkin N: Neuropsychological and psychosocial consequences of minor head injury. J Neurol Neurosurg Psychiatry 49:1227–1232, 1986.
41. Dixon CE, Hamm RJ, Taft WC, Hayes RL: Increased anticholinergic sensitivity following closed skull impact and controlled cortical impact traumatic brain injury in the rat. J Neurotrauma 11:275–287, 1994.
42. Dow RS, Ulett G, Raaf J: Electroencephalographic studies immediately following head injury. Am J Psychiatry 101:174–183, 1944.
43. Edna T-H, Cappelen J: Late postconcussional symptoms in traumatic brain injury. An analysis of frequency and risk factors. Acta Neurochir 86:12–17, 1987.
44. Englander J, Cifu DX: The older adult with traumatic brain injury. In Rosenthal M, Griffith ER, Kreutzer JS, Pentland B (eds): Rehabilitation of the Adult and Child with Traumatic Brain Injury, 3rd ed. Philadelphia, FA Davis, 1999, pp 453–470.
45. Epley J: The canalith repositioning procedure for treatment of benign postional vertigo. Otolaryngol Head Neck Surg 107:399–404, 1992.
46. Erb DE, Povlishock JT: Neuroplasticity following traumatic brain injury: a study of GABAergic terminal loss and recovery in the cat dorsal lateral vestibular nucleus. Exp Brain Res 83:253–267, 1991.
47. Evans RW: The postconcussion syndrome and the sequelae of mild head injury. Neurol Trauma 10:815–847, 1992.
48. Ewing R, McCarthy C, Gronwall D, Wrightson P: Persisting effects of minor head injury observable during hypoxic stress. J Clin Neuropsychol 2:147–155, 1980.
49. Fann JR, Uomoto JM, Katon WJ: Sertraline in the treatment of major depression following mild traumatic brain injury. J Neuropsychiatry Clin Neurosci 12:226–232, 2000.
50. Fay GC, Jaffe KM, Polissar NL, et al: Outcome of pediatric traumatic brain injury at three years. A cohort study. Arch Phys Med Rehabil 75:733–741, 1994
51. Feuerman T, Wackym PA, Gade GF, Becker DP: Value of skull radiography, head computed tomographic scanning, and admission for observation in cases of minor head injury. Neurosurgery 22:449–453, 1988.
52. Ford MR, Khalil M: Evoked potential findings in mild traumatic brain injury. 1: Middle latency component augmentation and cognitive component attenuation. J Head Trauma Rehabil 11:1–15, 1996.
53. Foreman S, Croft A: Whiplash Injuries: The Cervical Acceleration/Deceleration Syndrome, 2nd ed. Baltimore, Williams & Wilkins, 1995.
54. Furman JM, Cass SP: Benign paroxysmal positional vertigo. N Engl J Med 341:1590–1596, 1999.
55. Gennarelli TA, Segawa H Wald U, et al: Physiological responses to angular acceleration of the head. In Grossman RG, Gildenberg PL (eds): Head Injury: Basic and Clinical Aspects. New York, Raven, 1982, pp 129–140.
56. Gerberich SG, Finke R, Madden M, et al: An epidemiological study of high school ice hockey injuries. Child Nerv Syst 3:59–64, 1987.
57. Gerberich SG, Priest JD, Boen JR, Straub CP, Maxwell RE: Concussion incidences and severity in secondary school varsity football players. Am J Public Health 73:1370–1375, 1983.
58. Geursts ACH, Ribbers GM, Knoop JA, Limbeek JV: Identification of static and dynamic postural instability following traumatic brain injury. Arch Phys Med Rehabil 77:639–644, 1996.
59. Gibbs N: Injuries in professional rugby league. Am J Sports Med 21:696–700, 1993.
60. Gilkey SJ, Ramadan NM, Aurora TK, Welch KM: Cerebral blood flow in chronic posttraumatic headache. Headache 37:583–587, 1997.
61. Goadsby PJ, Lipton RB: A review of paroxysmal hemicranias, SUNCT syndrome and other short-lasting headaches with autonomic features, including new cases. Brain 120:193–209, 1997.
62. Goldberg G: Mild traumatic brain injury and concussion. Phys Med Rehabil State Art Rev 15(2):363–398, 2001.
63. Goldstein FC, Levin HS: Neurobehavioral outcome of traumatic brain injury on older adults: initial findings. J Head Trauma Rehabil 10:57–73, 1995.
64. Greiffenstein MF, Gola T, Baker WJ: MMPI-2 validity scales versus domain specific measures in detection of factitious traumatic brain injury. Clin Neuropsychol 9:230–240, 1995.
65. Grimm RJ, Hemenway WG, Lebay PR, Black FO: The perilymph fistula syndrome defined in mild head trauma. Acta Otolaryngol Suppl (Stockh) 464:1–40, 1989.

66. Gualtieri T: Neuropsychiatry and Behavioral Pharmacology. New York, Springer-Verlag, 1991.
67. Guerrero JL, Thurman DJ, Sniezek JE: Emergency department visits associated with traumatic brain injury: United States, 1995–1996. Brain Inj 14:181–186, 2000.
68. Guilleminault C, Faull KF, Mile L, van den Hoed J: Posttraumatic excessive daytime sleepiness: a review of 20 patients. Neurology 33:1584–1589, 1983.
69. Haas DC, Lourie H: Trauma triggered migraine: an explanation for common neurological attacks after mild head injury: review of the literature. J Neurosurg 68:181–188, 1988.
70. Hale MS: New antidepressants: use in high-risk patients. J Clin Psychiatry 54(suppl):61–70, 1993.
71. Harrington DE, Malec J, Cicerone K, Katz HT: Current perceptions of rehabilitation professionals towards mild traumatic brain injury. Arch Phys Med Rehabil 74:579–586, 1993.
72. Harvey AG, Bryant RA: Predictors of acute stress following mild traumatic brain injury. Brain Inj 12:147–154, 1998.
73. Hauri PJ: Sleep hygiene, relaxation therapy, and cognitive interventions. In Hauri PJ (ed): Case Studies in Insomnia. New York, Plenum Medical Book Company, 1991.
74. Headache Classification Committee of the International Headache Society: Classification and diagnostic criteria for headache disorders, cranial neuralgias, and facial pain. Cephalalgia 8(suppl 7):1–96, 1988.
75. Herdman SJ: Treatment of vestibular disorders in traumatically brain-injured patients. J Head Trauma Rehabil 5(4):63–76, 1990.
76. Hesselink JR, Dowd CF, Healy ME, et al: MR imaging of brain contusions: a comparative study with CT. AJR 150:1133–1142, 1988.
77. Hines ME: Posttraumatic headaches: In Varney NR, Robert RJ (eds): The Evaluation and Treatment of Mild Traumatic Brain Injury. Mahwah, NJ, Lawrence Erlbaum Associates, 1999, pp 375–410.
78. Homer CJ, Kleinman L: Technical report: minor head injury in children. Pediatrics 104:E78, 1999.
79. Horn LJ, Zasler ND (eds): Rehabilitation of Post-Concussive Disorders. Philadelphia, Hanley & Belfus, 1992.
80. Jorgensen U, Schmidt-Olsen S: The epidemiology of ice hockey injuries. Br J Sports Med 20:7–9, 1986.
81. Kaniecki RG: A comparison of divalproex with propanolol and placebo for the prophylaxis of migraine without aura. Arch Neurol 54:1141–1145, 1997.
82. Kay T, Harrington DE, Adams R, et al: Definition of mild traumatic brain injury. J Head Trauma Rehabil 8(3):86–87, 1993.
83. Kelly JP: Concussion in sports and recreation. Semin Neurol 20:176–171, 2000.
84. Kelly JP, Nichols JS, Filley CM, et al: Concussion in sports: guidelines for the prevention of catastrophic outcome. JAMA 266:2867–2869, 1991.
85. Kotwica Z, Jakubowski JK: Acute head injuries in the elderly: an analysis of 136 consecutive patients. Acta Neurochir 118:98–102, 1992.
86. Kowal L: Ophthalmic manifestations of head injury. Aust N Z J Ophthalmol 20:35–40, 1992.
87. Krauss JF, Nourjah P: The epidemiology of mild un-complicated brain injury. J Trauma 28:1637–1643, 1988.
88. Kushner D: Mild traumatic brain injury. Toward understanding manifestations and treatment. Arch Intern Med 158:1617–1624, 1998.
89. Label LS: Treatment of post-traumatic headaches: maprotilline or amiltriptyline? Neurology 41(suppl 1):247, 1991.
90. Lamsudin R, Sadjimin T: Comparison of the efficacy between flunarizine and nifedipine in the prophylaxis of migraine. Headache 33:335–338, 1993.
91. Larrabee GJ: Somatic malingering on the MMPI and MMPI-2 in personal injury litigants. Clin Neuropsychol 12:179–188, 1998.
92. Lee ST, Lui TN: Early seizures after mild closed head injury. J Neurosurg 76:435–439, 1992.
93. Leigh AD: Defects of smell after head injury. Lancet 1:38–40, 1943.
94. Levin HS, Amparo E, Eisenberg HM, et al: Magnetic resonance imaging and computerized tomography in relation to the neurobehavioral sequelae of mild and moderate head injuries. J Neurosurg 66:706–713, 1987.
95. Levin HS, Ewing-Cobbs L, Eisenberg HM: Neurobehavioral outcome of pediatric closed head injury. In Broman SH, Michel ME (eds): Traumatic Head Injury in Children. New York, Oxford University Press, 1995, pp 70–116.
96. Levin HS, Goldstein FC, MacKenzie EJ: Depression as a secondary condition following mild and moderate traumatic brain injury. Semin Clin Neuropsychiatry 2:207–215, 1997.

97. Levin HS, Mattis S, Ruff RM, et al: Neurobehavioral outcome following minor head injury: a three-center study. J Neurosurg 66:234–243, 1987.
98. Levin HS, Williams DH, Eisenberg HM, et al: Serial MRI and neurobehavioral findings after mild to moderate closed head injury. J Neurol Neurosurg Psychiatry 55:255–262, 1992.
99. Lewine JD, Davis JT, Sloan JH, et al: Neuromagnetic assessment of pathophysiologic brain activity induced by minor head trauma. Am J Neuroradiol 20:857–866, 1999.
100. Liau LM, Bergsneider M, Becker DP: Pathology and pathophysiology of head injury. In Youmans JR (ed): Neurological Surgery, 4th ed. Philadelphia, WB Saunders, 1996, pp 1549–1594.
101. Lorenzoni E: Electroencephalographic studies before and after head injuries. Electroencephalogr Clin Neurophysiol 28:216, 1970.
102. Lowden IMR, Briggs M, Cockin J: Post-concussional symptoms following minor head injury. Injury 20:193–194, 1989.
103. Maddocks DL, Dicker GD, Saling MM: The assessment of orientation following concussion in athletes. Clin J Sport Med 5:32–35, 1995.
104. Mandel S: Minor head injury may not be "minor." Postgrad Med 85:213–225, 1989.
105. Masters SJ, McClean PM, Arcarese JS, et al: Skull x-ray examinations after head trauma: recommendations by a multi-disciplinary panel and validation study. N Engl J Med 316:84–91, 1987.
106. Mathias JL, Coats JL: Emotional and cognitive sequelae to mild traumatic brain injury. J Clin Exp Neuropsychol 21:200–215, 1999.
107. Mayeux R, Marder K, Cote LJ, et al: The frequency of idiopathic Parkinson's disease by age, ethnic group, and sex in northern Manhattan. Am J Epidemiol 142:820–827, 1995.
108. McAllister TW, Saykin AJ, Flashman LA, et al: Brain activation during working memory 1 month after mild traumatic brain injury: a functional MRI study. Neurology 53:1300–1308, 1999.
109. McCrory PR, Berkovic SF: Second impact syndrome. Neurology 50:677–683, 1998.
110. Miller H: Accident neurosis. Br Med J 1:919, 1961.
111. Mittenberg W, Azrin R, Millsaps C, Heilbronner R: Identification of malingered head injury on the Wechsler Memory Scale-Revised. Psychol Assess 5:34–40, 1993.
112. Mittenberg W, Burton DB: A survey of treatment of post-concussion syndrome. Brain Inj 8:429–437, 1994.
113. Mittenberg W, Rotholc A, Russell E, et al: Identification of malingered head injury on the Halstead-Reitan Battery. Arch Clin Neuropsychol 11:271–282, 1996.
114. Mittenberg W, Tremont G, Zielinski RE, et al: Cognitive-behavioral prevention of postconcussion syndrome. Arch Clin Neuropsychol 11:139–145, 1996.
115. Montgomery A, Fenton GW, McClelland RJ: Delayed brainstem conduction time in post-concussional syndrome. Lancet 1(8384):1011, 1984.
116. Nell V, Yates DW, Kruger J: An extended Glasgow Coma Scale (GCS-E) with enhanced sensitivity to mild brain injury. Arch Phys Med Rehabil 81:614–617, 2000.
117. Nelson WE, Jane JA, Gieck JH: Minor head injury in sports: management and prevention. Sports Med 14:64–74, 1984.
118. Newman LC, Gordon ML, Lipton RB, et al: Episodic paroxysmal hemicrania: two new cases and a literature review. Neurology 42:964–966, 1992.
119. Ommaya AK, Gennarelli TA: Cerebral concussion and traumatic unconsciousness. Brain 97:633–654, 1974.
120. Oosterveld WJ, Kortschot HW, Kingma GG, et al: Electronystamographic findings following cervical whiplash injuries. Acta Otolanryngol (Stockh) 111:201–205, 1991.
121. Packard RC, Ham LP: Pathogenesis of posttraumatic headache and migraine: a common headache pathway? Headache 37:142–152, 1997.
122. Packard RC, Ham LP: Posttraumatic headache. J Neuropsychiatry Clin Neurosci 6:229–235, 1994.
123. Parker RS: The spectrum of emotional distress and personality changes after minor head injury incurred in a motor vehicle accident. Brain Inj 10:287–302, 1996.
124. Patten SB, Lauderdale WM: Delayed sleep phase disorder after traumatic brain injury. J Am Acad Child Adolesc Psychiatry 1:100–102, 1992.
125. Pettus EH, Povlishock JT: Characterization of a distinct set of intra-axonal ultrastructural changes associated with traumatically induced alteration in axolemmal permeability. Brain Res 722:1–11, 1996.
126. Plosker GL, McTavish D: Sumatriptan. A reappraisal of its pharmacology and therapeutic efficacy in the acute treatment of migraine and cluster headache. Drugs 47:622–651, 1994.

127. Povlishock JT: Pathobiology of traumatically induced axonal injury in animals and man. Ann Emerg Med 22:980–986, 1993.
128. Povlishock JT, Erb DE, Astruc J: Axonal response to traumatic brain injury: reactive axonal change, deafferentation, and neuroplasticity. J Neurotrauma 9(suppl 1):189–200, 1992.
129. Povlishock JT, Jenkins LW: Are the pathological changes evoked by traumatic brain injury immediate and irreversible? Brain Pathol 5:415–426, 1995.
130. Powell JW, Barber-Foss KD: Traumatic brain injury in high school athletes. JAMA 282:958–963, 1999.
131. Prigatano GP, Stahl ML, Orr WC, Zeiner HK: Sleep and dreaming disturbances in closed head injury patients. J Neurol Neurosurg Psychiatry 45:78–80, 1982.
132. Rigler J: Ueber die Verletzungen auf Eisenbahnen Insbesondere der Verletzungen des Rueckenmarks. Berlin, Reimer, 1879.
133. Rothweiler B, Temkin NR, Dikmen SS: Aging effect on psychosocial outcome in traumatic brain injury. Arch Phys Med Rehabil 79:881–887, 1998.
134. Ruff RM, Wylie T, Tennant W: Malingering and malingering-like aspects of mild closed head injury. J Head Trauma Rehabil 8(3):60–73, 1993.
135. Satz P: Brain reserve capacity on symptom onset after brain injury. A formulation and review of evidence for threshold theory. Neuropsychology 7:273–295, 1993.
136. Saunders RL, Harbaugh RE: The second impact in catastrophic contact-sports head trauma. JAMA 252:538–539, 1984.
137. Schoenhuber R, Gentilini M: Anxiety and depression after mild head injury: a case control study. J Neurol Neurosurg Psychiatry 51:722–724, 1988.
138. Schoenhuber R, Gentilini M, Orlando A: Prognostic value of auditory brainstem responses for late postconcussion symptoms following minor head injury. J Neurosurg 68:742–744, 1988.
139. Schwab CW, Kauder DR: Trauma in the geriatric patient. Arch Surg 127:727–739, 1992.
140. Segalowitz SJ, Brown D: Mild head injury as a source of developmental disabilities. J Learn Disabil 24:551–559, 1991.
141. Shawdon A, Brukner P: Injury profile of amateur Australian rules footballers. Aust J Sci Med Sport 26:59–61, 1994.
142. Shumway-Cook A, Horak FB: Rehabilitation strategies for patients with vestibular deficits. Diagn Neurol 8:441–457, 1990.
143. Shurtleff HA, Massagli TL, Hays RM, et al: Screening children and adolescents with mild to moderate traumatic brain injury to assist school reentry. J Head Trauma Rehabil 10:64–79, 1995.
144. Sjaastad O: The headache of challenge in our time: cervicogenic headache. Funct Neurol 5:155–158, 1990.
145. Solomon S, Lipton RB, Newman LC: Nuchal features of cluster headaches. Headache 30:347–349, 1990.
146. Strauss I, Savitsky N: Head injury: neurologic and psychiatric aspects. Arch Neurol Psych 31:893–955, 1934.
147. Stringer W, Balseiro J, Fidler R: Advances in traumatic brain injury neuroimaging techniques. NeuroRehabilitation 1:11–30, 1991.
148. Sturmi JE, Smith C, Lombardo JA: Mild brain trauma in sports, diagnosis and treatment guidelines. Sports Med 25:351–358, 1998.
149. Stuss DT: A sensible approach to mild traumatic brain injury. Neurology 45:1251–1252, 1995.
150. Sumner D: Post-traumatic anosmia. Brain 87:107–120, 1964.
151. Teasdale G, Jennett B: Assessment of coma and impaired consciousness. A practical scale. Lancet 2(7872):81–84, 1974.
152. Tenjin H, Ueda S, Mizukawa N, et al: Positron emission tomographic studies on cerebral hemodynamics in patients with cerebral contusion. Neurosurgery 26:971–979, 1990.
153. Thomas MD, Zasler ND: Sensory-perceptual disorders after traumatic brain injury. In Horn LJ, Zasler ND (eds): Medical Rehabilitation of Traumatic Brain Injury. Philadelphia, Hanley & Belfus, 1996, pp 499–513.
154. Thurman D, Guerrero J: Trends in hospitalization associated with traumatic brain injury. JAMA 282:954–957, 1999.
155. Treleaven J, Jull G, Atkinson L: Cervical musculoskeletal dysfunction in postconcussional headache. Cephalgia 14:273–279, 1994.
156. Troncoso B: The malingering of neuropsychological deficits following mild closed head trauma. Dissert Abst Int 48:1524, 1987.
157. Tyler GS, McNeely HE, Dick ML: Treatment of post-traumatic headache with amitriptyline. Headache 20:213–216, 1980.

158. Varney NR, Bushnell D, Nathan M, et al: NeuroSPECT correlates of disabling "mild" head injury: Preliminary findings. J Head Trauma Rehabil 10:18–28, 1995.
159. Verduyn WH, Hilt J, Roberts MA, Roberts RJ: Multiple partial seizure-like symptoms following "minor" closed head injury. Brain Inj 6:245–260, 1992.
160. Voller B, Benke T, Benedetto K, et al: Neuropsychological MRI and EEG findings after very mild traumatic brain injury. Brain Inj 13:821–827, 1999.
161. Volpe BT, McDowell FH: The efficacy of cognitive rehabilitation in patients with traumatic brain injury. Arch Neurol 47:220–222, 1990.
162. Von Seggern RL, Adelman JU: Cost considerations in headache management, part 2: acute migraine treatment. Headache 36:493–502, 1996.
163. Warner JS, Fenichel GM: Chronic posttraumatic headache often a myth? Neurology 46:915–916, 1996.
164. Weiss H, Stern B, Goldberg J: Posttraumatic migraine: chronic migraine precipitated by minor head or neck trauma. Headache 31:451–456, 1991.
165. White K, Simpson G: The combined use of MAOIs and tricyclics. J Clin Psychiatry 45(7 Pt 2): 67–69, 1984.
166. Wilberger JE: Minor head injuries in American football. Sports Med 15:338–343, 1993.
167. Wilberger JE, Maroon JC: Head injuries in athletes: emergency management of the injured athlete. Clin Sports Med 8:1–9, 1989.
168. Wilkinson M, Gilchrist I: Posttraumatic headache. Ups J Med Sci 31:48–51, 1992.
169. World Health Organization: International Statistical Classification of Diseases and Related Health Problems, 10th ed. Geneva, Switzerland, World Health Organization, 1992.
170. Yablon SA, Dostrow VG: Post-traumatic seizures and epilepsy. Phys Med Rehabil State Art Rev 15(2):301–326, 2001.
171. Yamaguchi M: Incidence of headache and severity of head injury. Headache 32:427–431, 1992.
172. Yarnell PR, Lynch R: Retrograde memory immediately after concussion. Lancet 1(7652):863–864, 1970.
173. Ylvisaker M, Feeney T, Mullins K: School reentry following mild traumatic brain injury. A proposed hospital to school protocol. J Head Trauma Rehabil 10:42–49, 1995.
174. Yokota H, Kurokawa A, Otsuka T, et al: Significance of magnetic resonance imaging in acute head injury. J Trauma 31:351–357, 1991.
175. Young HA, Gleave RW, Schmidek HH, Gregory S: Delayed traumatic intracerebral hematoma: report of 15 cases operatively treated. Neurosurgery 14:22–25, 1984.
176. Zafonte RD, Horn LJ: Clinical assessment of posttraumatic headaches. J Head Trauma Rehabil 14:22–33, 1999.
177. Zasler ND: Mild traumatic brain injury: medical assessment and intervention. J Head Trauma Rehabil 8:13–29, 1993.
178. Zasler ND: Neuromedical diagnosis and treatment of postconcussive disorders. In Horn LJ, Zasler ND (eds): Rehabilitation of Post-Concussive Disorders. Philadelphia, Hanley & Belfus, 1992.
179. Zasler ND, Billings K: Single photon emission computerized tomogaphy in mild traumatic brain injury. Arch Phys Med Rehabil 73:975, 1992.

14

Myofascial Pain After Whiplash Injury

Scott F. Nadler, D.O.

Whiplash injury, which can result in injury to the soft tissue structures of the neck, including muscle, tendon, and ligament, occurs immediately after impact and may persist for a prolonged period.[22,28,51] Squires et al[59] followed 40 patients 10 to 15 years after whiplash and found that 70% continued to report neck pain. Many factors, including older age, preexisting osteoarthritic changes, loss or reversal of lordosis, restricted motion, congenital abnormalities, and psychological disturbance may contribute to this delayed recovery.[18,27,28,43,50,59,72] The accident mechanism may also play a role in the ultimate failure to improve. Both rear-end collision while stationary[50,62] or with concomitant front-end impact have previously been described.[43] The head position at the time of accident may also be important. Sturzenegger[62] demonstrated a rotated or inclined head position to be the primary feature related to symptom persistence. Uhlig et al[70] showed in 1995 that soft tissue injuries of the neck can elicit muscular changes that are interpreted as muscle fiber transformations. They biopsied neck muscles from 64 patients with cervical dysfunction, including whiplash, and found signs of muscle fiber transformation as evidenced by an increased relative amount of type IIC fibers. Neck pain, which was the primary symptom in all the patients, must be integrally related to this pattern of muscular reaction. Therefore, myofascial pain is most likely a key player in whiplash-associated soft tissue injury to the neck and needs to be thoroughly evaluated and treated.

PATHOPHYSIOLOGY
Whiplash injury of the cervical spine commonly causes a painful condition. Various structures may be involved in producing pain and are considered pain generators (Table 1). This discussion focuses on the pathophysiology of whiplash injury related to the development of myofascial pain; a detailed review of the overall pathophysiology of whiplash is provided in Chapter 4.

Acceleration, deceleration, and rotational forces place great stress on the anatomic structures of the neck.[44] Instead of thinking of the pain as referred from only one of these pain generators, it should be considered more of a symptom complex. Hyperextension-hyperflexion injury in which physiologic motion is exceeded causes the deformity of the intervertebral disc and damage of the posteriorly situated ligaments and the facet joint capsule (Fig. 1). Disc deformity may be the precipitating injury in cases of whiplash, setting up the symptom complex. Narrowing of the disc decreases the amount of compressive

Table 1. Pain Generators in the Cervical Spine Implicated in Whiplash Injury

Anterior longitudinal ligament	Outer layers of the intervertebral disc anulus
Posterior longitudinal ligament	Nerve root dura
Intervertebral ligaments	Anterior/posterior musculature
Zygapophyseal joints	

load it can absorb, eventually leading to increased compression in the posteriorly situated zygapophyseal joints (Fig. 2). Loss of disc height may also lead to segmental instability of the vertebral motion segment, necessitating greater dynamic control from the surrounding musculature. The increased demand upon muscular control results in tissue overload and muscule fatigue. This fatigue is secondary to numerous factors, but decreased blood flow, ischemia, and the buildup of metabolic by-products are considered the likely causes.[38] The trigger point is the classic sign of focal muscle fatigue and, when active, causes significant pain both local and distant from the involved site.[69] Continued muscle spasm or irritability eventually leads to an inflammatory response, causing myofascial shortening or scarring.[73] This leads to further restrictions of facet motion, leading to or exacerbating the facet syndrome (Fig. 3).

Barnsley et al[6] in 1995 demonstrated chronic zygapophyseal pain in 54% of whiplash victims 5 to 272 months after injury. An understanding of the intimate relationship of both the posterior (splenius, semispinalis, multifidi) and anterior (scalenes) musculature to zygapophyseal function facilitates the explanation of concomitant involvement of the facet syndrome with cervical myofascial pain. Hilton's law states that the nerve supplying a joint also supplies the muscles, which move the joint and the skin covering the articular insertion of

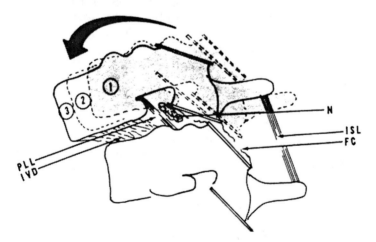

Figure 1. Hyperextension-hyperflexion injury. Normal physiologic flexion (see 1 to 2) is possible with no soft tissue damage. When motion is exceeded (see 3) the intervertebral disc (IVD) is pathologically deformed, the posterior longitudinal ligament (PLL) is strained or torn, the nerve (N) is acutely entrapped, the facet capsule (FC) is torn or stretched, and the interspinous ligament (ISL) is damaged. (From Caillet R: Neck and Arm Pain, 3rd ed. Philadelphia, FA Davis Co., 1991, pp 81–123; with permission.)

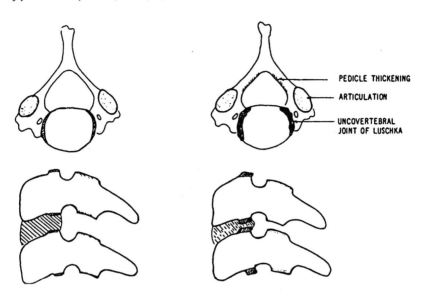

Figure 2. Disc degeneration with formation of spondylosis. *Left*, normal relationship of the vertebral bodies separated by an intact disc, normal uncovertebral joints of Luschka, and normal posterior articulations (facets). *Right*, changes resulting from disc degeneration. (From Caillet R: Neck and Arm Pain, 3rd ed. Philadelphia, FA Davis Co., 1991, pp 81–123; with permission.)

those muscles.[60] Cavanaugh et al[13] performed microdissection and electrophysiologic and neuroanatomic studies of the dorsal ramus in the lumbar spine of the rat. They found that reflex neural activity recorded from the dorsal ramus innervating the facet joint may be part of a cycle leading to paraspinal muscle spasm. Thus, it may be postulated that myofascial irritation in the form of trigger points seen in whiplash injury may be secondary to the zygapophyseal joint pain itself.

It becomes apparent that any condition that places greater stress or endurance requirements on the cervical musculature can precipitate myofascial pain. Treating clinicians must be aware of the coexistence of the various conditions, including cervical disc or facet pathology and/or spondylolisthesis in conjunction with cervical myofascial pain. Jonsson et al[33] demonstrated loss of disc signal intensity on magnetic resonance imaging 6 weeks after injury in 34% of discs. Via postmortem evaluation, Taylor and Twomey[64] compared the cervical spines of patients with major trauma to control cadavers of people who died from natural causes. Fifteen of 16 patients dying of trauma had clefts in the cartilaginous endplates of the intervertebral discs, as compared with none of 16 controls.

MYOFASCIAL SYNDROME

Myofascial pain is described as a regional rather than focal disorder characterized by muscle tenderness and pain. A trigger point is the pathognomonic sign demonstrated on physical examination of individuals with myofascial pain. The trigger point has several characteristics that define its presence, including

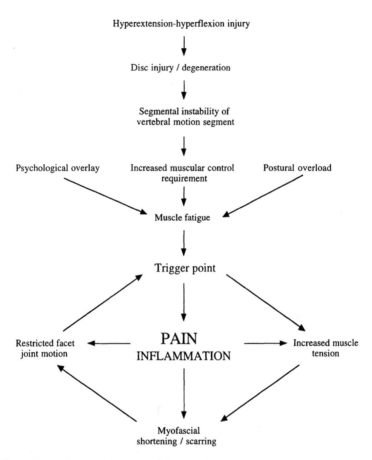

Figure 3.   The cyclic involvement of the myofascial component of the tissue overload complex seen in whiplash-associated injury.

a taut bandlike consistency, pain radiation far from the site of palpation, a twitchlike response when rolled between the fingers, reproducibility of the pain referral pattern, and autonomic phenomena.[65,69] Trigger points can be further described as latent or active. A latent trigger point is not clinically painful but may cause restriction of motion and weakness of involved muscles and may persist for years after whiplash injury.[68] Sola et al[57] demonstrated latent trigger points in 54% of asymptomatic women and 45% of asymptomatic men. Active trigger points, on the other hand, cause the previously described painful syndrome.

The exact nature of what causes myofascial pain after whiplash is still unclear. Numerous theories abound, but it appears to have a multifaceted etiology consisting of biochemical, biomechanical, and electrophysiologic components.

Biochemically, post-whiplash muscle has been characterized by lymphatic infiltration, myofibrillar degeneration, increased acid mucopolysaccharide and glycogen deposition, and abnormal mitochondria.[80] Alterations in adenosine triphosphate, tissue oxygenation, lactose dehydrogenase, and aldolase have also been observed.[8,30,41] In individuals with symptoms of neck pain persisting for 6 to 16 months, a significant increase in transitional type IIC muscle fibers in the sternocleidomastoid and omohyoid muscles was noted. This may indicate some ongoing muscular adaptation or transformations in patients with cervical spine pain.[73] McPartland et al[45] demonstrated atrophy of the suboccipital muscles along with fatty infiltration in those with chronic neck pain as compared with normal controls. Force platform assessment of balance demonstrated a decrease in standing balance, indicating a deficit in proprioception.

The impact of injury to the disc, as previously discussed, may play a large role in the biomechanical etiology of this syndrome. In addition, posture, in the form of the forward-head position, may play a role secondary to the increased load on the posteriorly situated zygapophyseal joints and narrowing of the neural foramina.[12] Travell[69] implicated various postural abnormalities in relation to overload of the various neck muscles. The "bird-watching position" stresses the splenius cervicis, as sustained upward gaze aggravates the suboccipital muscles, and sustained neck flexion irritates the semispinalis and multifidi. Griegel-Morris et al[24] demonstrated that individuals with a forward-head posture had an increased incidence of cervical and interscapular pain and headache. Naragasawa et al[49] also showed that a straightened cervical spine and low-set shoulders played a role in development of tension-type headaches.

Increased muscle activity related to improper posture has been demonstrated electromyographically as noted in the trapezius.[26,54] The cause of this increased tension is debatable, but it appears to be a reflection of local muscle fatigue. Larsson et al[38] demonstrated a significant fall in the mean frequency determined electromyographically. This decrease is thought to be caused by a lowered pH due to accumulation of lactate. Sjogaard[56] demonstrated a loss of potassium ions from the intracellular to extracellular space causing a reduction in resting membrane potential. Larsson also demonstrated a reduced ability to increase blood flow to the fatiguing trapezius by laser Doppler flowmetry.[38] These changes in resting membrane potentials and blood flow may account for fatigue-related pain after whiplash. Needle electromyography of the trigger point has shown no increased resting activity, although increased polyphasic potentials have been reported in uncontrolled studies.[4,5,36] Overall, electromyography, especially the use of the power spectral analysis, may be a valuable tool to improve the understanding of the muscular adaptations in myofascial pain associated with whiplash. The etiology of cervical myofascial pain remains a mystery, although it is most likely a combination of postural and mechanical abnormalities along with underlying biochemical and electrophysiologic influences. More research is required to better understand this multifactorial relationship.

HISTORY AND PHYSICAL EXAMINATION

History

In the evaluation of the individual suffering from post-whiplash neck discomfort, the history is of key importance. At the outset, the date and specific details of the accident should be determined. The accident mechanism, as previously described, may play a role in continuation of symptomatology.[43,50,62] The exact nature of the pain, including intensity, duration, frequency, and radiation pattern, should be elucidated. Factors that exacerbate or alleviate the symptoms and response to previous treatments need to be determined. One must not forget to identify the relative impact on the individual's normal daily functioning as well as underlying occupational and recreational risk factors. A thorough evaluation of the amount of standing, sitting, lifting, typing, and telephone responsibilities and the occurrence of discomfort is needed. When considering myofascial pain, the clinician must have a high index of suspicion that this entity exists. Too often, any radiation of pain is considered to be related to a herniated disc or nerve root compression. In our experience, myofascial pain can occur not only as an isolated phenomenon but, more commonly, concurrently with disc, facet, or nerve root injury.

Physical Examination

The physical examination in the post-whiplash patient should be performed in a comprehensive manner (Table 2). Inspection should begin by noting the position of head in relation to the line of gravity, which passes through the external auditory meatus; odontoid process; cervical, thoracic, thoracolumbar, and lumbosacral spine; and the sacral promontory. One should carefully assess not only the upper cervical region but also the relative curvature of the thoracolumbar and lumbosacral spines, because the relative positioning of the cervical spine may be influenced by the curvature below. The forward-head position can also be the direct cause of the loss of cervical motion. Caillet[12] reports a 25% to 50% loss of head rotation with a forwardly protruded head (Fig. 4) and a significant increase in the gravity-induced weight of the head brought on by this postural abnormality. The forward-head posture thus increases the work requirements of the capital and cervical musculature (Fig. 5).

Range of motion should ideally be assessed actively using a goniometer placed at the external auditory meatus for flexion or extension, at the top of the head for rotation, and at the nares for side-bending (Fig. 6). More commonly, range of motion is assessed based on the percentage of normal cervical motion or on the presence of any side-to-side asymmetry (Fig. 7). A segmental evaluation can be incorporated for those skilled in manual treatment, realizing that at C1-C2 almost pure rotation is present while coupled side-bending and rotation is the general rule for C2-C7 region. This may be performed by translating segments from right to left and left to right in flexed, extended, and neutral positions of the neck to identify segments with limited mobility.

Table 2. Components of the Physical Examination in Assessment of Myofascial Pain after Whiplash Injury

Inspection	Palpation
Postural assessment	Provocative testing
Range of motion	Spurling maneuver
	Scalene cramp test
Neurologic screen (strength, sensation reflexes)	Scalene relief test

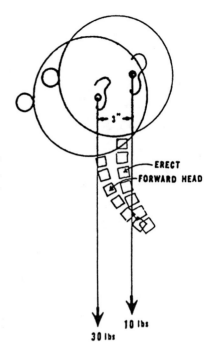

Figure 4. Weight of the head in forward-head posture. (From Caillet R: Neck and Arm Pain, 3rd ed. Philadelphia, FA Davis Co., 1991, pp 81–123; with permission.)

The neurologic screen should be performed on any individual being evaluated for whiplash-related pain, along with the Spurling maneuver (Fig. 8). Palpation is a key component of the evaluation for cervical myofascial pain. For the purpose of this section, palpation discussion is limited to the trapezius,

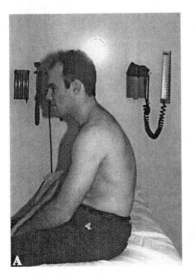 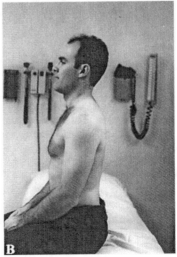

Figure 5. Demonstration of forward-head posture with **A**, rounded shoulders and **B**, correct upright posture.

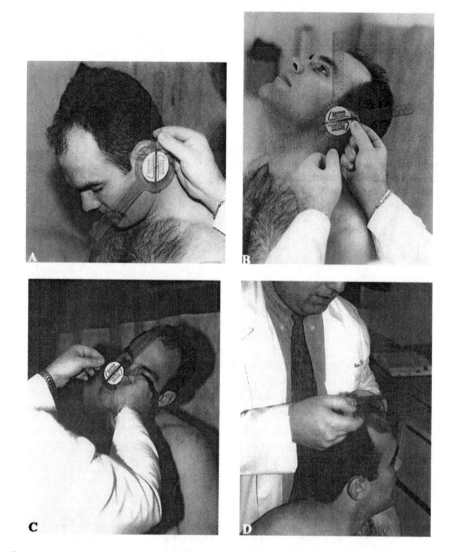

Figure 6.   Assessment of active cervical range of motion using a goniometer, for **A**, flexion, **B**, extension, **C**, side bending, and **D**, rotation.

sternocleidomastoid, scalenes, and the posterior cervical/capital musculature (Fig. 9). Other muscles, including the masseter and digastric, may be involved but are not the focus of this section. The clinician evaluating these various structures must have a thorough understanding of both structural and functional anatomy. Upon encountering a taut band in any of these muscles, various steps should be undertaken.

The first step is to assess whether the trigger point is active or latent. Activity is determined by a reproduction of pain often radiating far distal from its initial focus. Latent trigger points cause only restriction in motion without pain.

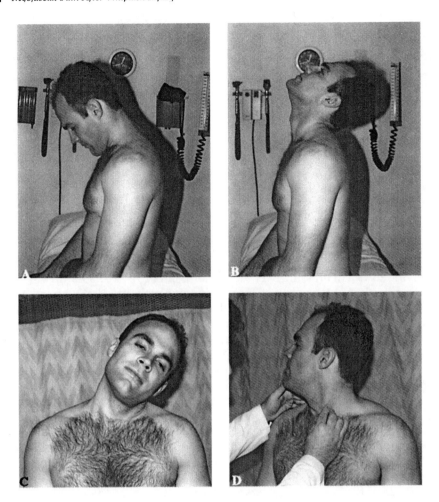

Figure 7. Cervical active range of motion is more commonly evaluated visually by comparison to the expected normal range in **A**, flexion, **B**, extension, **C**, side bending, and **D**, rotation.

Figure 8. The Spurling maneuver should be part of a comprehensive neurologic screen.

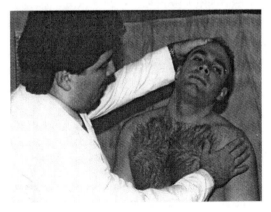

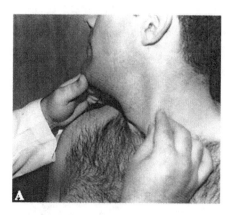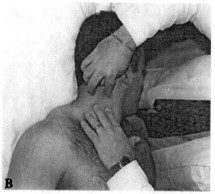

Figure 9.   Palpation of the **A**, sternocleidomastoid muscle and **B**, scalenes.

Applying sufficient pressure over the trigger point occasionally induces a "jump sign" on the part of the patient. This may involve withdrawal of the head, wrinkling of the face or forehead, or a verbal response that the pain has been located. More commonly, a twitch response and various autonomic disturbances are noted. These autonomic features include pallor, sweating, piloerection, and dermatographism.[65] Also noted is an increase in electromyographic activity within the pain reference zone.[68] Trigger points within the sternocleidomastoid are reported to cause eye symptoms, including excessive lacrimation, conjunctival reddening, spasm of the orbicularis oculi, and dizziness.[67,74] Headache can also result from palpation of trigger points in the posterior cervical muscles, including the suboccipital muscles along with the scalenes and sternocleidomastoid.[34,40] This should be distinguished from third occipital nerve headache described by Bogduk.[10] This entity is considered to be secondary to dysfunction at the C2-C3 zygapophyseal joint, which is innervated by the third occipital nerve. Segmental evaluation of the various facet joints determining translatory motion of the individual segments can be helpful in diagnosing headache related to the C2-C3 facet joint. Sandmark and Nisell[53] reported in 1995 that palpation over the facet joints was the most appropriate screening to corroborate replies of self-reported neck dysfunction. Range of motion assessment had poor overall sensitivity.

The trapezius is a large muscle group with upper, middle, and lower fibers. The large area of this muscle makes it susceptible to the effects of whiplash injury. Trigger points may be encountered in any of the portions and invariably cause radiating pain into the interscapular region and up into the head, causing muscle tension-type headaches (Figs. 10–12). The upper trapezius is greatly affected by postural insufficiency and has been noted in dentists, secretaries, and sewing machine operators.[2,42,47] The sternocleidomastoid, as previously mentioned, is associated with many facial symptoms as well as dizziness and headaches.[67,74] The clinician should palpate along both sternal and clavicular heads when evaluating the trigger point activity (Fig. 13).

Evaluation of the posterior musculature, including the splenius, semispinalis, multifidi, and suboccipital muscles, should be included. All of these muscle groups can cause radiation of pain in or about the head (Fig. 14).

Figure 10. Referred pain pattern and location (Xs) of trigger point 1 in the upper trapezius muscle. Solid areas show the essential referred pain zone; stippling maps the spillover zone. (From Travell JG, Simons DG: Myofascial Pain and Dysfunction: The Trigger Point Manual. Vol. 1: The Upper Extremities. Baltimore, Williams & Wilkins, 1983; with permission.)

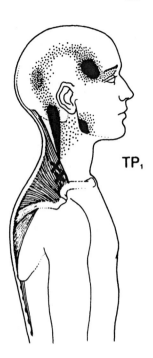

TP₁

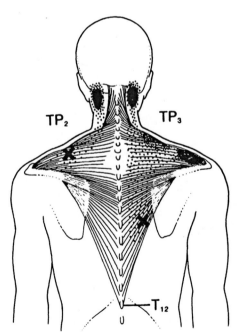

Figure 11. Referred pain patterns and locations (Xs) of trigger point 2 in the left upper trapezius, and of trigger point 3 in the right lower trapezius. Conventions are as in Fig. 10. (From Travell JG, Simons DG: Myofascial Pain and Dysfunction: The Trigger Point Manual. Vol. 1: The Upper Extremities. Baltimore, Williams & Wilkins, 1983; with permission.)

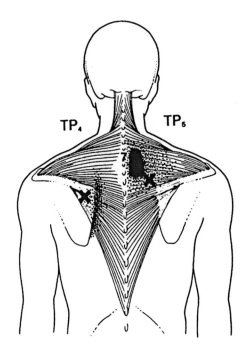

Figure 12. Referred pain patterns and locations (Xs) of trigger point 4 in the left lower trapezius, and of trigger point 5 in the right middle trapezius. Conventions are as in Fig. 10. (From Travell JG, Simons DG: Myofascial Pain and Dysfunction: The Trigger Point Manual. Vol 1: The Upper Extremities. Baltimore, Williams & Wilkins, 1983; with permission.)

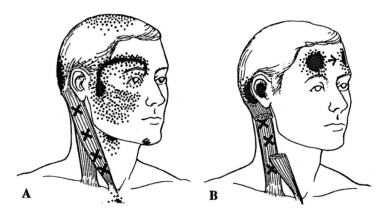

Figure 13. Referred pain patterns (solid black shows essential zones and stippling shows the spillover areas) with location of corresponding trigger points (Xs) in the right sternocleidomastoid muscle. **A**, the sternal (superficial) division. **B**, the clavicular (deep) division. (From Travell JG, Simons DG: Myofascial Pain and Dysfunction: The Trigger Point Manual. Vol 1: The Upper Extremities. Baltimore, Williams & Wilkins, 1983; with permission.)

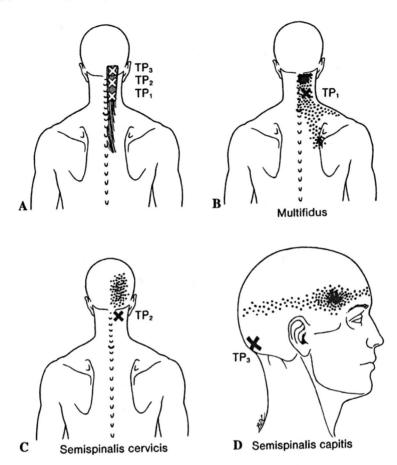

Figure 14. Referred pain patterns and their trigger points (Xs) in the medial posterior cervical muscles. **A,** Three major trigger point locations. **B,** TP$_1$ lies deep at the C4 or C5 level in the multifidi or rotatores; it is the posterior cervical trigger point most commonly found and often leads to entrapment of the greater occipital nerve. **C,** TP$_2$ in the third-layer semispinalis cervicis. **D,** The uppermost TP$_3$ in the semispinalis capitis. (From Travell JG, Simons DG: Myofascial Pain and Dysfunction: The Trigger Point Manual. Vol 1: The Upper Extremities. Baltimore, Williams & Wilkins, 1983; with permission.)

Trigger points within the scalenes can cause variable symptoms of radiating pain into the distal upper extremity (Fig. 15). For example, the scalenes have long been implicated as a cause of the thoracic outlet syndrome.[15,71] Muscular hypertrophy, adaptive shortening, and postural abnormalities such as the forward-head position have been implicated.[1,71,77] The scalenes can be evaluated during physical examination by the "scalene cramp test" (Fig. 16), which is performed by having the patient turn the head toward the painful side and pulling the chin down into supraclavicular fossa. This position causes contraction of the scalenes and should reproduce distal radiation of pain. The individual scalene muscles can be evaluated by stretching the head to the opposite side, looking

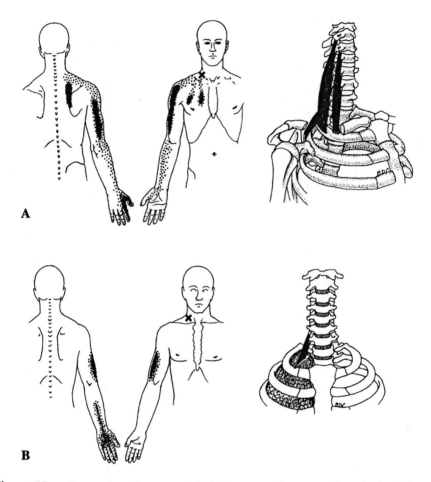

Figure 15. Composite pain patterns (solid areas are the essential, and stippled areas are the spillover pain reference zones) with location of trigger points (Xs) in the right scalene muscles. **A,** Scalenus anterior, medius, and posterior. Some trigger points may have only one essential reference zone. **B,** Scalenus minimus. (From Travell JG, Simons DG: Myofascial Pain and Dysfunction: The Trigger Point Manual. Vol 1: The Upper Extremities. Baltimore, Williams & Wilkins, 1983; with permission.)

straightforward (middle scalene), looking away (anterior scalene), and looking toward the elbow (posterior scalene) (Fig. 17). Stretching of the various portions of the scalenes may also reproduce symptoms. The "scalene relief test" (Fig. 18) attempts to relax the scalenes by increasing the space between the clavicle and the scalenes.

In making the diagnosis of cervical myofascial pain, the clinician must rule out other more serious problems prior to initiating treatment. The appropriate use of diagnostic testing, including x-ray, computed tomography, magnetic resonance imaging, and electromyography should be incorporated into the evaluation. Finally, a thorough understanding of any coexisting conditions is needed prior to giving an isolated diagnosis of cervical myofascial pain.

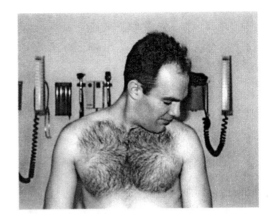

Figure 16. The scalene cramp test.

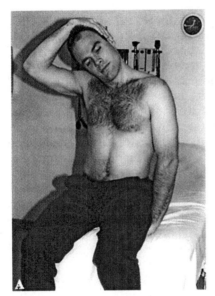

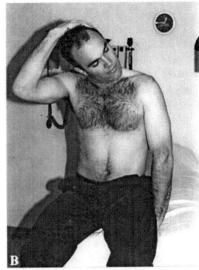

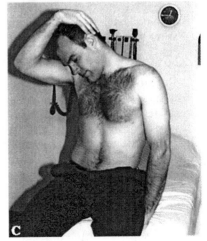

Figure 17. Scalene stretching exercises performed by the patient, for **A**, the middle scalene, **B**, anterior scalene, and **C** posterior scalene muscles.

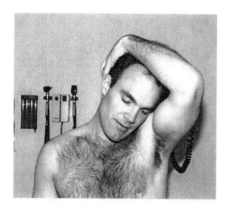

Figure 18.   The scalene relief test.

TREATMENT OF MYOFASCIAL PAIN IN WHIPLASH INJURY

Myofascial pain is a difficult process to treat because it may be initiated by both peripheral and central mechanisms. Central sensitization refers to the central mechanism whereby an increased excitability of spinal and supraspinal regions results from injury or inflammation-induced activation of peripheral nociceptors.[9] Central sensitization leads to nociceptive nerve impulses being perceived as being painful (hyperalgesia) and nonnociceptive nerve impulses being perceived as painful (allodynia). The phenomenon of nonnociceptive pain may correlate very strongly with myofasical pain with many similar characteristics: The description of pain seems inappropriate in comparison with tissue pathology or lack of discernible tissue pathology; noxious stimuli result in a pain experience greater than normally expected; normally nonnoxious stimuli result in pain; and the extent of the pain boundary is greater than would be normally expected based on the site of the original tissue injury.[9] If one thinks of the trigger point and the characteristics of pain and pain referral, it becomes clear how the phenomena of central sensitization and nonnociceptive pain may be related.

In addressing the central sensitization phenomenon, various pharmacologic and nonpharmacologic strategies can be employed. In regard to pharmacologic intervention, the tricyclic antidepressants have been used with some success in treating this phenomenon through an impact on noradrenergic and serotonergic reuptake inhibition. Muscle relaxants may offer some assistance with improving sleep, but no significant effect on true muscle relaxation has been demonstrated. Newer antispasticity medications such as baclofen and tizanidine have some promise, but increased weakness associated with baclofen limits its beneficial effects.[29] Tizanidine, an alpha-2 adrenergic agonist, exerts effects in both the brain and spinal cord, having effects at the second-order dorsal horn neurons and wide dynamic-range neurons, the same location implicated in the central sensitization process.[16] Tizanidine decreases spasticity by reinforcing presynaptic inhibition and reinforcing Ia reciprocal and Ib nonreciprocal postsynaptic inhibition.[79] The exact mechanism by which the alpha-2 adrenergic agonists reduce pain is unknown; however, it is theorized to occur via modulation of excitatory amino acids glutamate and aspartate along with substance P.[35,48] This medication therefore demonstrates promise in the treatment of myofascial pain by reducing both pain and associated tone. Opiate analgesics may be considered for a limited course to treat severe whiplash-associated myofascial pain for the purpose of returning the patient to his usual activities as quickly as possible. There is evidence to suggest that an endogenous opioid system is a mediator of decreased pain and improved physical findings following trigger point injection (TPI) with local anesthetic.[19]

In regard to the peripheral component of myofasical pain, many strategies have been employed. Modalities such as ice, moist heat, ultrasound, and massage were recommended by the Quebec Task Force in 1995 as optional adjuncts during the first 3 weeks of treatment.[58] In addition, transcutaneous electrical nerve stimulation has also been proposed for treatment of acute whiplash pain[52] but has not been proven to be effective in a scientifically controlled study. A major complication of modality usage in the treatment of whiplash is the potential effects on outcome. Jette and Jette[32] demonstrated a significantly poorer outcome in subjects with neck pain treated with heat and cold modalities as compared with active exercise-based treatment. The reason for this phenomenon may be linked to the need for immobilization during modality usage without active exercise-based treatment. Continuous low-level heat therapy is a newer concept in modality usage that allows for the benefit of a therapeutic modality without the need for the subject to remain immobile. The therapeutic effect, derived from a wearable heat wrap generating temperatures to 40° C, lasts more than 8 hours. Steiner et al[61] demonstrated improved pain relief, decreased muscle tension, and disability in individuals with trapezius myalgia treated with the continuous low-level heat wrap (Thermacare, by Proctor & Gamble, Cincinnati, OH) as compared with subjects treated with nonprescription dosages of acetaminophen or ibuprofen.[61] The continuous low-level heat wrap may therefore replace the need for passive use of modalities with their inherent negative impact on outcome.

Another strategy in addressing the peripheral aspect of myofasical pain involves treatment of the biomechanical components. Mealy et al[46] demonstrated that patients receiving mobilizing physical therapy showed significant improvements in cervical movement and pain 8 weeks after the accident compared with a group receiving the standard treatment of rest and a cervical collar. Manual mobilization is useful for a short-term benefit in the acute injury process. In addition, a limited course of manipulation performed by qualified personnel was a consensus-based recommendation of the Quebec Task Force.[58] Postural training (see Fig. 5) is another key biomechanical component of treatment in preventing acute myofascial pain symptoms from becoming chronic. Stretching exercises for cervical musculature, particularly the scalenes and posterior muscle group, are important to maintain cervical range of motion (see Fig. 17).[70] These should ideally be done several times per day and are often an essential component of the home exercise program for cervical myofascial pain syndrome. Hanten et al[26] demonstrated sustained stretching to be superior to active range of motion when used as part of a home exercise program. Overall, education in and review of the home exercise program is paramount to the success any clinician treating myofascial pain.

TPIs have been shown to increase range of motion, exercise tolerance, and circulation in muscle and to reduce pain.[31] It is thought that the mechanical disruption of the trigger point by the needle is critical to its inactivation and ultimately interrupts nociceptive transmission to the central nervous system.[39] Another new TPI technique involves the use of botulinum toxin, which inhibits muscle contraction by blocking the release of acetylcholine from peripheral nerves. In addition to addressing the peripheral component of myofascial pain, botulinum toxin may also have effects centrally, mediated through afferent pathways coming from the injected site, possibly originating within the muscle spindles.[23] In regard to research into the use of botulinum toxin, In 1994 Cheshire et al[14] studied six patients—who were followed for 12 weeks—with chronic cervical myofascial pain syndrome in a randomized, double-blind, placebo-controlled study. Results showed a statistically significant reduction in pain following botulinum toxin injection but not with placebo. The response was transient, with the benefit lasting 5 to 6 weeks. Newer research into the use of botulinum toxin has offered increasing promise. In 1998 Wheeler et al[76] demonstrated a high percentage of subjects to be asymptomatic after a second injection of botulinum toxin for treatment of myofascial pain. In 2000 Freund et al[20] reported a significant improvement in pain and range of motion in subjects with whiplash-associated muscle spasm treated with botulinum toxin as compared with placebo. This is an interesting area of further research that could have a significant impact on future treatment of chronic myofascial pain syndrome. However, it should be noted that performing TPIs in isolation treats an effect of the condition without addressing the underlying causes. TPIs should be reserved for when they are specifically needed to break the vicious cycle of tissue overload that has been described (see Fig. 3). They have not been shown to be of any benefit in the acute phase and may contribute to an increase in tissue injury and psychological overlay during that stage. Finally, acupuncture may be effective in treating myofascial pain, but this has not been clearly demonstrated in the literature.

In addition to the peripheral and central components of myofascial pain, one must not forget the impact of the behavioral milieu. The psychological, behavioral, or social issues associated with myofascial pain can certainly impact upon the subject's response to treatment. A study of 40 patients 15 years after whiplash injury revealed that 52% of patients with persistent symptoms showed evidence of an abnormal psychological profile. This was mostly in the form of diagnoses of anxiety or depression.[59] An interdisciplinary team approach may be useful in these cases, with the team consisting of the treating physician, a physical or occupational therapist, psychologist, the patient, and his family member or friend. In this situation, each team member approaches the common goals of reducing the symptoms and restoring function. The use of aerobic exercise may be especially helpful in individuals with strong behavioral components to their pain. Aerobic activity has been demonstrated to be effective in improving mood, decreasing depression, and increasing the pain threshold.[3,63] It has also been shown electromyographically that aerobic exercise has a greater relaxing effect on musculature than a sedative medication such as meprobamate.[17] The clinician treating myofascial pain should be aware of the impact of psychosocial issues and be positive and supportive in regard to the education of the involved subject. The Quebec Task Force[58] emphasized that clinicians should reassure patients about the good prognosis in whiplash—that it is essentially a benign, self-limited condition from which most patients recover.

These patients should be encouraged to return to their usual activities as soon as possible.

In conclusion, cervical myofascial pain after whiplash injury is a poorly understood phenomenon with broad clinical implication. The clinician managing this condition must be aware of the entire complex and be able to address its various components. Unfortunately, most clinicians treat only the pain without considering the underlying condition. We hope that a better understanding of this complex entity is achieved through this and other resources to provide for better management of whiplash-associated myofascial pain.

References

1. Adson A, Coffey JR: Cervical rib: a method of anterior approach for relief of symptoms by divisions of the scalenes anticus. Ann Surg 85:839–857, 1927.
2. Anderson JH, Gaardbol O: Musculoskeletal disorders of the neck and upper limb in serving machine operators: a clinical investigation. Am J Ind Med 24:689–700, 1993.
3. Anshel MH, Russell KG: Effect of aerobic and strength training on pain tolerance, pain appraisal and mood of unfit males as a function of pain location. J Sports Sci 12:535–547, 1994
4. Arroyo P Jr: Electromyography in the evaluation of reflex muscle spasm. Simplified method for direct evaluation of muscle-relaxant drugs. J Fla Med Assoc 53:29–31, 1966.
5. Awad EA: Interstitial myofibrositis: hypothesis of the mechanism. Arch Phys Med Rehabil 54:440–453, 1973.
6. Barnsley L, Lord S, Bogduk N: Clinical review: whiplash injury. Pain 58:283–307, 1994.
7. Barnsley L, Lord SM, Wallis BJ, Bogduk N: The prevalence of chronic cervical zygopoplyseal joint pain after whiplash. Spine 20:20–26, 1995.
8. Bengtsson A, Henriksson KJ, Larsson J: Reduced high energy phosphate levels in the painful muscles of patients with primary fibromyalgia. Arthritis Rheum 29:817–821, 1986.
9. Bennett RM: Emerging concepts in the neurobiology of chronic pain: evidence of abnormal sensory processing in fibromyalgia. Mayo Clin Proc 74:385–398, 1999.
10. Bogduk N, Musland A: On the concept of third occipital headache. J Neurol Neurosurg Psychiatry 49:775–780, 1986.
11. Bovim G, Schrader H, Sand T: Neck pain in the general population. Spine 19:1307–1309, 1994.
12. Caillet R: Neck and Arm Pain. Philadelphia, FA Davis, 1991.
13. Cavanaugh JM, El-Bohy A, Hardy W, et al: Sensory innervation of soft tissues of the lumbar spine in the rat. J Orthop Res 7:378–388, 1989.
14. Cheshire WP, Abashian SW, Mann JD: Botulinum toxin in the treatment of myofascial pain syndrome. Pain 59:65–69, 1994.
15. Cuetter AC, Bartoszak DM: The thoracic outlet syndrome: controversies, overdiagnosis, overtreatment, and recommendations for management. Muscle Nerve 12:410–419, 1989.
16. Davies J, Johnston SE, Hill DR, Quinlan JE: Tiazanidine (DS 103-282), a centrally acting muscle relaxant, selectively depresses excitation of feline dorsal horn neurons to noxious stimuli by an action at alpha 2 adrenoreceptors. Neurosci Lett 48:197–202, 1984.
17. De Vries HA, Adams GM: Electromyographic comparison of single doses of exercise and meprobamate as to effects on muscular relaxation. Am J Phys Med Rehabil 51:130–141, 1972.
18. Evans RW: Some observations of whiplash injuries. Neurol Clin 10:975–977, 1992.
19. Fine PG, Milano R, Hare BD: The effects of myofascial trigger point injections are naloxone reversible. Pain 32:15–20, 1988.
20. Freund BJ, Schwartz M: Treatment of whiplash associated with neck pain with botulinum toxin-A: a pilot study. J Rheumatol 27:481–484, 2000.
21. Fricton J, Kroening R, Haley D: Myofascial pain syndrome of the head and neck: a review of clinical characteristics of 164 patients. Oral Surg Oral Med Oral Pathol 60:615–623, 1985.
22. Gargan MF, Bannister GC: Long-term prognosis of soft tissue injuries of the neck. J Bone Joint Surg Br 72:901–903, 1990.
23. Giladi N: The mechanism of action of botulinum toxin A in focal dystonia is most probably through its dual effect on efferent (motor) and afferent pathways at the injected site. J Neurol Sci 152:132–135, 1997.
24. Griegel-Morris P, Larson K, Mueller-Klaus K, Catis CA: Incidence of common postural abnormalities in the cervical, shoulder, and thoracic region and their association with pain in two age groups of healthy subjects. Phys Ther 72:425–431, 1992.

25. Hanten WP, Olson SL, Butts NL, Nowicki AL: Effectiveness of a home program of ischemic pressure followed by sustained stretch for treatment of myofascial trigger points. Phys Ther 80:997–1003, 2000.
26. Herberts P, Kadefors R, Broman H: Arm positioning in manual tasks: an electromyographic study of localized muscle fatigue. Ergonomics 23:655–665, 1980.
27. Hirsch SA, Hirsh PF, Hiramoto H, Weiss A: Whiplash syndrome: fact or fiction? Orthop Clin North Am 19:791–795, 1988.
28. Hohl M: Soft tissue injuries of the neck in automobile accidents. J Bone Joint Surg Am 56:1675–1682, 1974.
29. Hoogstraten MC, van der Ploeg RJ, vd Burg W, et al: Tizanidine versus baclofen in the treatment of spasticity in multiple sclerosis patients. Acta Neurol Scand 77:224–230, 1988.
30. Ibraluim GA, Awad EA, Katke FJ: Interstitial myofibrositis: serum and muscle enzymes and lactate dehydrogenase isoenzymes. Arch Phys Med Rehabil 35:23–28, 1974.
31. Jaeger B, Skootsky SA: Double-blind controlled study of different myofascial trigger point injection techniques. Pain 4(suppl):560, 1987.
32. Jette DU, Jette AM: Physical therapy and health outcomes in patients with spinal impairments. Phys Ther 76: 930–944, 1996.
33. Jonsson H, Cesarini K, Sahestedt B, Rauschning W: Findings and outcome in whiplash-type neck distortions. Spine 19:2733–2743, 1994.
34. Kellgren JH: Observations on referred pain arising from muscle. Clin Sci 3:175–190, 1938.
35. Koyuncuoglu H, Kara I, Gunel MA, et al: N-methyl-D-aspartate antagonists, glutamate release inhibitors, 4 aminopyridine at neuromuscular transmission. Pharmacol Res 37:485–491, 1998.
36. Kraft GH, Johnson EW, LaBan MM: The fibrositis syndrome. Arch Phys Med Rehabil 48:155–162, 1968.
37. Kurtzke JF: The current neurological burden of illness and injury in the United States. Neurology 32:1207–1214, 1982.
38. Larsson SE, Alund M, Cai H, Oberg PA: Chronic pain after soft tissue injury of the cervical spine: trapezius muscle blood flow and electromyography at static load and fatigue. Pain 57:173–180, 1994.
39. Lewit K: The needle effect in relief of myofascial pain. Pain 6:83–90, 1979.
40. Long C: Myofascial pain syndromes: Part 2: Syndromes of the head, neck and shoulder girdle. Henry Ford Hosp Bull 4:22–28, 1956.
41. Lund N, Bengtsson A, Thorborg P: Muscle tissue oxygen pressure in primary fibromyalgia. Scand J Rheumatol 15:165–173, 1986.
42. Lundervold AL: Electromyographic investigation during sedentary work, especially typewriting. Br J Phys Med 14:32–36, 1951.
43. Macnab I: The "whiplash" syndrome. Orthop Clin North Am 2:389–403, 1971.
44. Maimaris C, Barnes MR, Allen MJ: Whiplash injuries of the neck: a retrospective study. Injury 19:393–396, 1988.
45. McPartland JM, Brodeur RR, Hallgren RC: Chronic neck pain, standing balance and suboccipital muscle atrophy: a pilot study. J Manipulative Physiol Ther 20:24–29, 1997.
46. Mealy K, Brennan H, Fenelon GC: Early mobilization of acute whiplash injuries. BMJ 292:656–657, 1986.
47. Milerad E, Ericson MO, Nisell R, Kilbom A: An electromyographic study of dental work. Ergonomics 34:953–962, 1991.
48. Moon DE, Lee DH, Han HC, et al: Adrenergic sensitiviy of the sensory receptors modulating mechanical allodynia in a rat neuropathic pain model. Pain 80:589–595, 1999.
49. Naragasawa A, Sakakibara T, Takahashi A: Roentgenographic findings of the cervical spine in tension-type headaches. Headache 33:90–95, 1993.
50. Norris SH, Watt I: The prognosis of neck injuries resulting from rear-end vehicle collisions. J Bone Joint Surg Br 65:608–611, 1983.
51. Parmar HV, Raymalcers R: Neck injuries from rear-impact road traffic accidents: prognosis in persons seeking compensation. Injury 24:75–78, 1993.
52. Richardson RR, Siqueira EB: Transcutaneous electrical neurostimulation in acute cervical hyperextension-hyperflexion injuries. Ill Med J 159:227–230, 1981.
53. Sandmark H, Nisell R: Validity of five common manual neck pain provoking tests. Scand J Rehabil Med 27:131–136, 1995.
54. Sigholm G, Herberts P, Almstrom C, Kadeforo R: Electromyographic analysis of shoulder muscle load. J Orthop Research 1:379–386, 1984.
55. Simons DG: Myofascial trigger points: a need for understanding. Arch Phys Med Rehabil 62:97–99, 1981.

56. Sjogaard G: Water and electrolyte fluxes during exercise and their relation to muscle fatigue. Acta Physiol Scand 556:129–136, 1986.
57. Sola AE, Rodenberger ML, Getlys BB: Incidence of hypersensitive areas in posterior shoulder muscles. Am J Phys Med Rehabil 34:585–590, 1955.
58. Spitzer WO, Skovron ML, Salmi LR, et al: Scientific monograph of the Quebec Task Force on whiplash-associated disorders: redefining "whiplash" and its management. Spine 20(8 suppl):S1–S73, 1995.
59. Squires B, Gargan MF, Bannister GC: Soft tissue injuries of the cervical spine. J Bone Joint Surg Br 78:955–957, 1996.
60. Stedman's Medical Dictionary, 26th ed. Baltimore, Williams & Wilkins, 1995.
61. Steiner, D, Erasala G, Hengehold, D, et al: Continuous low level topical heat therapy for trapezius myalgia. Proc Am Pain Society 19th annual meeting, 2000, p 171.
62. Sturzenegger M, Radanov BP, Di Stefano G: The effect of accident mechanisms and initial findings on the long-term course of whiplash injury. J Neurol 242:443–449, 1995.
63. Szymanski LM, Pate RR: Effects of exerciser intensity, duration, and time of day on fibrinolytic activity in physically active men. Med Sci Sports Exerc 26:1102–1108, 1994.
64. Taylor JR, Twomey LT: Acute injuries to cervical joints: an autopsy study of neck sprain. Spine 18:1115–1122, 1993.
65. Travell J: Pain mechanisms in connective tissue. In Ragan C (ed): Transactions of the Second Conference of Josiah Macy Jr. Foundation. New York, 1952, pp 96–111.
66. Travell J: Referred pain from skeletal muscle: the pectoralis major syndrome of breast pain and soreness and the sternocleidomastoid syndrome of headache and dizziness. N Y State J Med 55:331–339, 1953.
67. Travell J: Referred pain from skeletal muscle: sternocleidomastoid syndrome of pectoralis major syndrome of breast pain and soreness of headaches and dizziness. N Y State J Med 55:331–339, 1955.
68. Travell J, Berry C, Bigelow N: Effects of referred somatic pain on structures in the reference zone. Fed Proc 3:49, 1944.
69. Travell J, Simons DG: Myofascial Pain and Dysfunction: The Trigger Point Manual. Baltimore, Williams & Wilkins, 1983.
70. Uhlig Y, Weber BR, Grob D, Muntener M: Fiber composition and fiber transformation in neck muscles of patients with dysfunction of the cervical spine. J Orthop Res 13:240–249, 1995.
71. Walsh MT: Therapist management of thoracic outlet syndrome. J Hand Ther 7:131–144, 1994.
72. Watkinson A, Gargan MF, Bannister GC: Prognostic factors in soft tissue injuries of the cervical spine. Injury 22:307–309, 1991.
73. Weber Br, Uhlig Y, Grob D, et al: Duration of pain and muscular adaptations in patients with dysfunction of the cervical spine. J Orthop Res 11:805–810, 1993.
74. Weeks VD, Travell J: Postural vertigo due to trigger areas in the sternocleidomastoid muscle. J Pediatr 47:315–327, 1995.
75. Westerling D, Jonsson BG: Pain from the neck shoulder region and sick leave. Scand J Soc Med 8:131–136, 1980.
76. Wheeler AH, Goolkasian P, Gretz SS: A randomized, double-blind, prospective pilot study of botulinum toxin injection for refractory, unilateral, cervicothoracic, paraspinal, myofascial pain syndrome. Spine 23:1662–1666, 1998.
77. Willshire WH: Supernumerary first rib: clinical records. Lancet 2:633, 1860.
78. Wolfe F, Simons DG, Fricton J, et al: The fibromyalgia and myofascial pain syndromes: a preliminary study of tender point and trigger points in persons with fibromyalgia: myofascial pain and no disease. J Rheumatol 19:944–951, 1992.
79. Yanagisawa N, Tanaka R, Ito Z: Reciprocal Ia inhibition in spastic hemiplegia of man. Brain 99:555–574, 1976.
80. Yunus MB, Kalyan-Raman U, Kalyan-Raman K, Masi AT: Pathologic changes in muscle in primary fibromyalgia syndrome. Am J Med 81:34–43, 1987.

15

Psychological Factors in the Treatment of Chronic Pain Associated with Whiplash

J. Bradley Williams, Ph.D.

Psychological factors that contribute to the experience of pain and suffering in chronic benign neck pain are common concomitants of whiplash.[8,11] The treatment of chronic nonmalignant pain, including neck pain, is often complicated by clinicians' failure to consider its multifactorial nature. In the case of chronic benign pain such as that which often follows whiplash injuries, the severity of pain and level of disability are poorly predicted by physical pathology.[12] Therefore, treating the symptom (the sensory component of the experience of pain) independent of other components of the broader pain problem often results in prolonged suffering for the patient and frustration for the clinician.

The internationally accepted definition of pain is, "An unpleasant sensory and emotional experience associated with actual or potential tissue damage, or described in terms of such damage."[9] This definition acknowledges the role of emotional factors in the pain experience and the necessity to treat all aspects of the pain problem rather than focusing only on the symptom. To treat the pain problem, clinicians must understand the context in which the pain is experienced, identify factors from multiple domains that contribute to suffering, and develop a multidisciplinary treatment plan that addresses those factors in a coordinated manner. This chapter identifies psychological factors that often contribute to the suffering experienced by patients with chronic nonmalignant neck pain, elucidates concepts that account for those factors, and describes strategies that clinicians of any specialty can use to address those factors. The strategies should not be construed to constitute psychological treatment or replace the necessity of employing the services of a qualified clinical psychologist in the multidisciplinary treatment of whiplash injuries.

To treat chronic nonmalignant pain effectively, clinicians must understand the goal of pain management in a rehabilitation model. An understanding of basic definitions and concepts that facilitate the rehabilitation goal of development and independent implementation of multiple strategies for making the quality of life independent of the experience of pain and suffering is important. Some of the definitions provided in this chapter are purposely simplified to maximize their usefulness in a clinical setting. A more thorough discussion of physiologic and medical distinctions is beyond the scope of this chapter and may be in some cases confusing and possibly distressing to some patients.

A brief overview of two of the three major psychological theories that are typically used to explain psychological factors in the experience of chronic benign pain is presented. These theories were chosen because they explain psychological factors in a parsimonious manner, they can be understood without specialized training in psychology, and it is from these theories that the recommendations for addressing psychological factors are derived. The second section of the chapter describes these recommendations in a concise and useable manner. The major category of theories (psychodynamic) that is not described is perhaps the most interesting to psychologists, but it does not contribute to the recommendations that are the focus of this chapter. Additionally, interventions based on psychodynamic theories are quite specialized and should be left to qualified psychologists.

DEFINITIONS

There are two definitions that are fundamental to addressing psychological factors in chronic neck pain and that are derived directly from the theories that are described. These are the definitions of acute and chronic pain and the distinction between pain and suffering.

To treat chronic nonmalignant pain effectively, clinicians must understand the distinction between acute and chronic pain and, most importantly, be able to effectively communicate this distinction to patients. A simple and useful way to differentiate these two types of pain is to identify acute pain as pain that is expected to resolve when the injury is healed and chronic pain as pain that lasts longer than expected and that serves no useful purpose. Acute pain serves a useful purpose of protecting an injured area and often results in recommendations that include rest, assistance, guarding, and other strategies that facilitate healing, recovery, and recuperation. Chronic pain persists beyond the resolution of an acute injury and lacks the biological value of acute pain.[7] It represents a threat to quality of life but does not represent a threat to survival as does acute pain.

It is necessary to differentiate the sensory experience of pain from the emotional experience. As will be seen in the discussion of behavioral and cognitive factors in the experience of chronic benign pain, the emission of pain behaviors exacerbates emotional distress, ie, suffering. Although this aspect of the pain experience can be independent of the sensory component, one must realize that the suffering experience is real. It is experienced exactly the same as the sensation of pain. Suffering and the behaviors that represent it are multidetermined.[10] While everyone is aware that pain and suffering are often correlated, we rarely think of them as independent factors. In fact, our language betrays this fact in that we use the word "feeling" to describe both sensation and emotion. However, the psychologically savvy pain practitioner is aware of the independence of these factors and not only treats them independently but emphasizes their independence to patients. An example of the independence of pain and suffering can be seen in athletes who ascribe a positive meaning to the pain experience (eg, "no pain, no gain"). To individualize treatment for every patient suffering chronic neck pain, it is necessary to understand that each patient differs in the relative contributions of the physical and psychological factors in the experience of pain and suffering. It is obvious then that close collaboration among the physician, therapists, and psychologist is necessary for coordinated assessment and treatment.

PSYCHOLOGICAL THEORIES THAT ADDRESS CHRONIC NECK PAIN

Factors that contribute to the experience of suffering can be broken down into two categories: intrinsic and extrinsic. Intrinsic factors include intrapsychic experiences including cognition, affect, and behavior. Extrinsic factors refer to the effects of outside forces (the responses of others to expressions of suffering) and include associative learning, operant conditioning, and learning by observation. Practitioners' understanding of extrinsic factors provides us with techniques that can facilitate the patient's modulation of intrinsic factors. Provided here is an overview of psychological theories that explain these intrinsic and extrinsic factors. Because the purpose of this chapter is to identify specific strategies in the treatment of chronic benign neck pain that facilitate coping with pain and minimizing suffering, thereby avoiding treatment strategies that exacerbate suffering, the elucidation of these theoretical perspectives are limited. The theoretical models discussed, and from which the treatment recommendations are drawn, are the behavioral and the cognitive behavioral models.

The Behavioral Model: Extrinsic Factors

The actions of caregivers in response to patients' expressions of pain and suffering can promote either coping or suffering. This principle is elucidated by understanding behavioral principles. The behavioral theoretical perspective of chronic benign neck pain is based on the principles of learning. Specifically, focus is on associative learning and operant conditioning. In **associative learning**, the patient learns that seemingly good things can come from expressions of suffering. Fordyce identified the importance of the natural human response to pain as expressed in behaviors that signify suffering.[5] Some of these "pain behaviors" include verbal expressions of injury ("It's killing me.") or emotion ("It's excruciating."); nonverbal expressions of injury or disability (antalgic gait, facial expressions such as grimacing); functional evidence of injury or disability (maladaptive rest and diminished activity); and maladaptive prescription drug use (maladaptive reliance on external sources for coping, eg, pills and pill-taking behavior). As a result of the naturally occurring behaviors that accompany the experience of acute pain, we learn as children that under most circumstances caring behavior is elicited from others around us. Some forms of caring behavior that typically occur include sympathy, nurturance, medical treatment, financial compensation, and relief.

Relief is most notable in that it often includes relief from pain, relief from responsibilities, and relief from relationship problems, ie, relief from stressors. A primitive example of this principle is demonstrated by the young child who awakens with a scratchy throat and emits suffering behavior in the form of hoarseness and entreaties for Mommy's help, which often comes in the form of nurturant behavior (soothing voice, hugging) and the pleasant taste of a cherry-flavored lozenge. Additionally, if the young child had a history test planned for that day for which he did not prepare, he has learned that his expressions of pain and suffering have resulted not only in the addition of something desirable (nurturance and tasty treats) but also relief from his anxiety over the impending test. Thus, under normal circumstances we learn at an early age that expressions of suffering result in the acquisition of desirable things and relief from some undesirable things.

The second form of learning that is pertinent to chronic neck pain is **operant conditioning.** In operant conditioning, the patient produces pain behavior, ie, expressions of pain and suffering, to elicit the acquisition of desirable things and/or relief from something undesirable. Operant conditioning has been described as the effects of consequences and context on overt behavioral responses. The application of operant conditioning to chronic benign pain can be attributed to Fordyce.[4] In operant conditioning a fundamental principle of learning is the concept of reinforcement. Reinforcement is defined as anything that increases the likelihood that a behavior will be repeated. It comes in two forms: positive and negative. Positive reinforcement is the addition of something desirable, and negative reinforcement is the subtraction of something undesirable. In other words, positive reinforcement can be described as reward, while negative reinforcement can be described as relief.

The implications of both reward and relief are significant. For clinicians treating chronic pain, relief (often the primary goal of intervention) becomes a most salient factor that if not recognized and accounted for can inadvertently facilitate the suffering experience (see page 246). Whenever a caregiver provides reward or relief, he is reinforcing some set of behaviors. If these behaviors include expressions of pain and suffering, these expressions will be likely to recur, ie, suffering will be facilitated. This paradoxical response to treatment frustrates clinicians and sets up a cycle in which the patient experiences repeated treatment disappointments with subsequent despair. Negative reinforcement is one of the most powerful forms of reinforcement and often includes relief from responsibilities, such as work, school, domestic, and interpersonal responsibilities.[10]

Notable to physicians is that relief from pain is a significant example of a negative reinforcer. While relief from pain is highly desirable, the prescriber needs to realize that in providing such relief he is reinforcing the set of behaviors that precedes the relief. In acute pain settings, it is normal and often adaptive to express pain to get relief. Postsurgical patients may be well advised to make their pain experience known in order to acquire adequate analgesia that is the standard of care in such settings.[1] In the case of chronic benign pain, however, by definition treatment will be ongoing and management of the pain should not require the expressions of pain that would normally occur in an acute pain situation.

If caregivers require expressions of suffering in order to provide caring, those expressions of suffering are by definition reinforced and will be likely to recur. Fordyce[6] has identified these behaviors as a target of treatment. As seen in the issue of caring responses to acute pain, normal caring responses are appropriate and adaptive. In the case of chronic benign pain, however, the same caring behaviors become maladaptive and promote suffering. It is of primary importance to realize that these processes happen to normal people. While the practitioner in the field of chronic pain often encounters people with psychopathology, the learning principles described above are normal. Therefore, pain practitioners should avoid concluding that recognition of and intervention for these principles implies the presence of psychopathology.

The Cognitive Behavioral Model: Intrinsic Factors

Patients' thoughts and actions can promote either coping or suffering. This principle is elucidated by understanding cognitive behavioral principles. The cognitive behavioral theoretical position on the experience of chronic benign neck pain incorporates and is an extension of the behavioral theory previously described. In addition to learning principles that are a function of extrinsic factors (ie, the response of others to the patient's expressions of pain and suffering), the intrinsic factors of affect, cognition, and behavior are incorporated. In 1957, Festinger[3] established the theory of cognitive dissonance, which states that humans are motivated to maintain consistency in their behavior, thoughts, and emotions. Inconsistency in these factors results in a psychological dissonance that is difficult to tolerate. If either of these factors is in dissonance, one or more of the factors will change to resolve the dissonance. In the case of chronic benign pain, the sensory experience and concomitant physiologic arousal results in emotional distress. Subsequently, cognitive and behavioral factors will be consistent with this distress. Cognitive factors include appraisal of the situation as an emergency, and behavioral factors include exhibition of behaviors that would be consistent with an acute emergency, including cessation of normal activity and pleas for assistance. In this way, it can be seen that affect determines cognition and behavior. The unpleasant emotional experience spawns thought processes and behaviors that are consistent with the natural response to pain. Such thoughts include appraising the situation as signifying danger to life and limb. In the case of chronic benign pain, the normal response is actually maladaptive.

Again, this can be seen as a natural response to the experience of pain that is appropriate in the case of acute pain but becomes maladaptive in the case of chronic benign pain. Therefore, in the normal response pattern to the sensation of pain, the affect determines the cognition and behavior. While these cognitions and behaviors are adaptive in the case of acute pain, they are maladaptive in the case of chronic pain. Therefore, in the case of chronic pain the goal is to alter this psychological process so that adaptive behavior and cognitions moderate the distressed affect that accompanies the sensory experience of pain. Specifically, the presence of a sensation of pain results in an undesirable affect that is moderated by cognitive appraisal of a benign situation and behaviors that signify to self and others that the sensation is inconsequential. In other words, the goal of a cognitive behavioral approach to coping with chronic benign pain is a deemphasis on the importance of the pain sensation. Therefore, the cognitive process of accurate appraisal of the meaning of pain becomes a fundamental psychological factor in coping with chronic benign neck pain. Again, the distinction between acute and chronic benign pain is crucial.

Another important cognitive behavioral factor of is self-efficacy. In the instance of acute pain, it is appropriate to stop and get help. With chronic benign pain, the opposite is true; the goal is to be active in managing and coping with the pain problem. It has been well established by Bandura[2] and others that self-efficacy is an important element of the experience of depression. One of the most common phrases heard among patients suffering chronic benign pain is, "The pain is controlling my life." This is one significant contributor to the depression that so often accompanies the experience of chronic neck pain. Self-efficacy can be defined as a conviction that one can act in a manner that provides a desired outcome in any given situation.[12] By its very nature, the presence of persistent pain undermines this important conviction, and the subsequent pleading for assistance further undermines the sense of self-efficacy.

With regard to cognitive appraisal, learning is not limited to didactic instruction. Patients also learn by observation. Thus, if clinicians respond to chronic pain as if it were an acute emergency, patients will do so as well and their behaviors will reflect the perceived catastrophe. In contrast, if all members of the treatment team consistently respond to patients' expressions of suffering with a calm measured demeanor that encourages independent implementation of coping skills, the likelihood that patients will learn and accept this crucial distinction with subsequent diminution of suffering is enhanced.

CONSIDERING PSYCHOLOGICAL FACTORS IN THE TREATMENT OF CHRONIC NECK AND BACK PAIN

Four simple concepts exist that, when integrated into the multidisciplinary treatment plan, can help patients to use adaptive thoughts and actions to decrease emotional suffering associated with the experience of chronic nonmalignant pain. Behavioral and cognitive behavioral principles are implemented in a format that treats chronic nonmalignant pain in the context of a rehabilitation perspective that focuses on the goal of making the quality of life independent of the pain problem.

To treat chronic nonmalignant pain effectively, clinicians must understand the distinction between acute and chronic pain and, most importantly, be able to effectively communicate this distinction to patients. The difference between acute and chronic pain should be emphasized. The importance of this distinction is that the *emotional* response that is appropriate (adaptive) in an emergency is not appropriate (maladaptive) if maintained beyond the duration of the crisis. If maintained for a prolonged period, the psychophysiologic arousal associated with the emergency response reinforces suffering and often results in the development and maintenance of psychological symptoms, including anxiety and depression. The clinician must remember that from the patient's perspective chronic and acute pain feel the same. Although they feel the same, they have very different meanings. Acute pain means, "Stop! Get help." Ideally the patient learns that chronic pain means, "Do something to manage your pain problem." Because these sensory experiences are essentially the same, patients are reliant upon clinicians to help them learn the difference and to develop emotional responses that are more appropriate for chronic pain. Learning is not limited to didactic instruction. Patients also learn by observation. Thus, if clinicians respond to chronic pain as if it were an acute emergency, patients will do so as well. In contrast, if all members of the treatment team consistently respond to patients' expressions of suffering with a calm measured demeanor that encourages independent implementation of coping skills, the likelihood that patients will learn and accept this crucial distinction is enhanced. In summary, when treating chronic benign pain, it is therapeutic to remind the patient that "this is not an emergency."

The relationship of pain and suffering is another important concept that can facilitate the development of effective skills for coping with chronic pain. While it is easy to understand that pain causes suffering, it is important to assist patients in interrupting this effect. If this is accomplished, a person with intractable pain has the opportunity to learn that even if he cannot reduce his pain sensation he can reduce emotional suffering and thus improve his quality of life. To accomplish this, it is helpful to define pain as the sensory component of the pain problem and suffering as the emotional component of the pain problem, ie, "Pain is a sensation; suffering is an emotion." Note the relationship of this concept to the distinction of acute and chronic pain: The emotional response (emergency) that is appropriate for acute pain typically results in an experience of distress (suffering) that is relieved when the acute pain resolves. Because, by definition, the chronic pain is expected to continue indefinitely, if distress can be modulated the suffering can be addressed *independently* of the pain sensation.

We have seen that appropriate appraisal of the chronic pain experience as chronic and not an emergency diminishes suffering by promoting appropriate emotional reactions. In a similar manner behavior also contributes to emotional experience. The presentation of behaviors appropriate for acute pain in the presence of chronic pain is known as "pain behavior." Pain behaviors not only express suffering to others but also reinforce the patient's perception that he is suffering. One effect of pain behaviors is that the patient's expression of emergency exacerbates his distress and inhibits his ability to moderate his emotional response. An effective way of expressing this is, "What you say about your pain not only reflects how you feel, it *affects* how you feel." Additionally, pain behaviors typically elicit responses from others. Fordyce[6] has shown that operant conditioning in the form of benefits (caring behavior of others) that result from pain behaviors actually increases the likelihood that suffering will be maintained or even increased. Essentially, normal people experiencing chronic pain and expressing pain as if it were acute come to expect caring behavior appropriate for acute pain. While such special treatment is appropriate for emergencies, it typically ends when the emergency is resolved. When pain and the perception of emergency persist, the normal expectation is that special treatment will continue. Patients quickly learn that the caring from others to which they have become accustomed is contingent upon expressions of pain and suffering. Thus, if the rehabilitation goal of independence and maximized functioning is pursued, the behavior that elicits special treatment that is appropriate for acute pain is contraindicated for chronic pain. Here, too, it can be seen that the differentiation between acute and chronic pain is fundamental.

The final concept in this treatment model is the emphasis on independence in managing the pain problem. Patients frequently report that pain controls their lives. This sense of decreased self-efficacy has been shown to contribute to depression and diminished coping abilities. To this end, emphasizing the difference in management of pain as opposed to curing pain promotes the perception that one is not helpless in the presence of the pain sensation. Even if he cannot eliminate (cure) the pain, the patient can learn to manage the effects of the pain problem. In other words, he can "take charge of his pain problem." Emphasizing that strategies the patient implements to manage the effects of pain and minimize pain sensations are the core elements of treatment allows him to begin to combat the sense of helplessness and dependency that often robs him of his self-worth and self-esteem.

CONCLUSION

In summary, understanding and implementation of psychological principles is an important component in the treatment of chronic benign neck pain. From a rehabilitation perspective, the goal of treatment is to make the quality of life independent of the pain problem. To attain this goal, four concepts are employed: the difference between acute and chronic pain ("This is not an emergency."); the difference between pain and suffering ("Pain is a sensation; suffering is an emotion."); behavioral affects on suffering ("What you say about your pain not only *reflects* how you feel, it *affects* how you feel."); and independence in managing chronic pain ("Take charge of your pain problem."). Treating the pain symptom without considering the broader aspects of the pain problem often results in increased suffering for the patient and frustration for the clinician. Incorporating these concepts into a multidisciplinary approach to managing chronic benign neck pain allows the patient to maximize functioning and independence, thus enhancing quality of life despite the pain sensation.[13]

References

1. American Pain Society: Perioperative Analgesia: Approaching the 21st Century. Study Guide. Fair Lawn, NJ, MPE Communications, 1997.
2. Bandura A: Self-efficacy: toward a unifying theory of behavioral change. Psychol Rev 84:191–215, 1977.
3. Festinger L: A Theory of Cognitive Dissonance. Evanston, IL, Rowe, Peterson, 1957.
4. Fordyce WE: Behavioral Methods for Chronic Pain and Illness. St. Louis, Mosby, 1976.
5. Fordyce WE: Learned pain: pain as behavior. In Bonica JJ (ed): The Management of Pain, Vol 1. Philadelphia, Lea and Febiger, 1990, pp 291–299.
6. Fordyce W (ed): Back Pain in the Workplace: Management of Disability in Nonspecific Conditions. Taskforce on Pain in the Workplace. Seattle, IASP Press, 1995.
7. Galer BS, Dworkin RH: Neuropathic Pain. New York, McGraw Hill, 2000.
8. Mayou R, Bryant B: Outcome of whiplash neck injury. Injury 27:617–623, 1996.
9. Merskey H, Bogduk N: Classification of Chronic Pain: Descriptions of Chronic Pain Syndromes and Definition of Pain Terms, 2nd ed. Seattle, IASP Press, 1994.
10. Sanders HS: Operant conditioning with chronic pain. In Gatchel RJ, Turk DC (eds): Psychological Approaches to Pain Management: A Practitioner's Guide. New York, Guilford Press, 1996, pp 112–130.
11. Schwartz DP: Cognitive Deficits. In Lynch NY, Vasudevan SV (eds): Persistent Pain: Psychosocial Assessment and Intervention. Boston, Kluwer Academic Publishers, 1988, pp 23–40.
12. Turk DC: Biopsychosocial perspective on chronic pain. In Gatchel RJ, Turk DC (eds): Psychological Approaches to Pain Management: A Practitioner's Guide. New York, Guilford Press, 1996, pp 3–32.
13. Williams JB: Psychological concepts and strategies in the treatment of chronic nonmalignant pain. Pain Clin 2(4):44–46, 2000.

16

Imaging of Whiplash Injuries

Joseph D. Fortin, D.O., and Edward C. Weber, D.O.

This chapter is reprinted from **Spine: State of the Art Reviews** *12(2):419–436, 1998, published by Hanley & Belfus, Inc.*

Acceleration-hyperextension injuries were originally described in 1867 associated with railroad accidents. Since the time of railroad injuries to the present, with frequent high-speed rear-end motor vehicle collisions, our ability to image the resultant pathology has grown from nonexistent (since x-rays were discovered in 1895) to the startling multiplanar and three-dimensional near "real-time" CT and MRI acquisitions.

Modern imaging technology is, nonetheless, "put to the test" in evaluating whiplash injuries since the tremendous deceleration forces result in a spectrum of lesions. Violent acceleration of the brain within the closed confines of the osseous skull, movement of the head on the shoulders, and bending of the torso on the pelvis, all occur within approximately 0.2 seconds.[29] Consequently, it is not surprising that a host of pathology has been reported, which includes traumatic brain injury,[10] cardiac contusion,[13] vertebral artery traction,[17] occipital neuralgia,[16] carotid artery dissection,[14] as well as sternoclavicular, cervical, and lumbar fracture-dislocation injuries. Imaging findings are also diverse and may be as subtle as prevertebral muscle and fascial strain or as gross as fracture-dislocation of the cervical spine with neurologic sequelae.

Determining the imaging needs of a whiplash victim may be confounded by a myriad of symptoms that span many organ systems (e.g., vertigo, tinnitus, hoarseness, facial dysesthesia, bizarre visual disturbances, memory difficulties, temporomandibular joint, neck, shoulder, chest, or low back pain, and paralysis). Imaging is indicated not by the occurrence of "whiplash" (a mechanism of injury) but rather by specific clinical signs and symptoms resulting from a whiplash injury. Since imaging needs are complex, it is imperative to have a systematic approach to the various imaging modalities that can be applied.

Our work will focus on the cervical spine, since it is the primary region of interest in the investigation of whiplash injuries. The scope of this chapter is admittedly limited and does not obviate the need to apply imaging modalities to other organ systems as indicated by the clinical presentation.

PHYSICAL AND TECHNICAL PRINCIPLES

An image of an object is a graphical representation of the spatial distribution of one or more of its properties. An image is a reflection of not only of the structure being observed, but also of the physical principles of the imaging modality.

Radiography

Plain films or x-rays are often the screening modality of choice for patients presenting to the emergency department (ED) who have sustained whiplash injuries.[1,8] They may disclose frank fracture-dislocation, retropharyngeal edema, tracheal displacement, or instability. Several authors have demonstrated a high incidence of cervical spine pathology despite normal radiographs.[8,24]

The process of acquiring plain films or radiographs involves positioning an x-ray tube opposite the interposed body part and film cassette. Within the x-ray tube, electrons are "boiled off" a heated cathode filament. Subsequently, the electrons are rapidly accelerated across high voltage, striking an anode target, which results in the production of electromagnetic energy (i.e., x-rays) and heat. The emerging beam is constricted by collimators to the area being imaged. X-rays which have not been absorbed or scattered (by structures in the patient) then strike the film cassette. Within the cassette, rare earth phosphorus atoms efficiently capture the x-ray photons and emit visible light which exposes photographic film. A physicochemical reaction in the film ensues, according to the radiographic density and volume of the interposed body part, resulting in an image. The fundamental radiographic densities are water density (i.e., muscle), fat density, air density, and calcium density (bone).

An x-ray beam is diverging, therefore objects closer to the x-ray tube may be magnified. The ratio of the distances between the tube, patient structures, and film cassette affect the geometry of the image. The quality of plain radiographs depends upon tube, cassette, and patient positioning, exposure settings, film and cassette technology, and processing factors. Parenthetically, some large sites are testing filmless digital systems for radiography.

Even with many other imaging technologies available, radiographs still fulfill a basic role within our diagnostic armamentarium for screening trauma victims, ruling out instability or segmental motion aberration, ascertaining segmentation, and providing exquisite bone detail. The spatial resolution of transmission radiography provides a unique perspective on bone morphology and texture which remains unsurpassed.

Computed Tomography (CT) Scanning

In the 1970s, CT provided the first direct view of discs, nerve roots, and spinal canals. Employing an array of electronic detectors directly opposite a rapidly rotating x-ray tube, CT produces cross-sectional images, opening the window for three-dimensional conceptualization of the spine.

The patient lies on a moveable bed placed within the imaging device or "gantry." Within the gantry, an x-ray tube rotates around the patient during the exposure (typically one second for a 360° rotation), while an x-ray detector rotates on the side of the patient opposite the tube. A xenon or solid state detector captures the x-ray photons which pass through the patient.

Tissues which absorb or deflect a large number of x-ray photons are said to have high attenuation. In classic axial (nonhelical) scanning, the pattern of attenuation detected during a single rotation (i.e., each exposure or slice) is computer-processed into a cross-sectional image. The thickness of that slice depends upon the collimation of the x-ray beam. The number of slices needed depends upon the area to be covered, the thickness of each slice, and the relationship of adjacent slices, whether contiguous (most common), overlapped, or with some interslice gap.

Shades of gray for each point on the displayed image are chosen to represent the attenuation of the tissue at that point. Window and level controls on the CT computer allow for choices in gray scale (contrast) and brightness, which enhance the viewer's perception of various tissues. For example, a broad gray scale (wide window setting) provides greater bone detail, while a narrow window setting enhances soft tissue.

In classic axial CT scanning, each section viewed is the result of a single exposure as described above, followed by movement of the patient bed to the next slice location. In helical (also called "spiral") CT the entire anatomic area under study is scanned in a single long exposure while the tube and detector array make many rotations around the patient. Thus a cylindrical volume is scanned, and the data from that volume can be used to produce cross-sectional images. For mathematical reasons beyond the scope of this text, the effective width of each slice produced is slightly greater than the width—collimation— of the x-ray beam. Compared to axial scanning, some resolution is lost, especially along the axis of patient movement.

While the slice thickness in helical scanning is limited by the physical size of the x-ray beam, the number of slices computed from the data acquisition has virtually no limitation beyond storage capacity and patience of the viewer. The scanner could produce, for example, slices with an effective width of 5.5 mm, each slice beginning just 1 mm from the beginning of the previous slice, resulting in many greatly overlapped CT images. Most commonly, either contiguous sections or 50% overlapped sections are produced.

Because a CT image represents a "slice" of tissue of a given thickness, each point on the image represents a volume which could contain more than one tissue type.[16a] For example, a calcified pulmonary granuloma (very high attenuation) could "share" a location with aerated lung (very low attenuation). The measured attenuation for that point would be an average of the two tissues. The attenuation value or shade of gray at that position would thus represent neither tissue accurately. This artifact is known a "partial volume averaging." Understanding this limitation of CT is important for those who are responsible for determining CT protocols, as well as for all those who interpret CT images.

The measurement of attenuation by a tissue on a CT image is given in Houndsfield units (HU). Tissues measuring above 100 Houndsfield units usually contain calcium. Structures measuring near 0 HU are water density, near −100 HU are fatty, and near −1000 are air-containing.

The images presented in axial scanning are usually just those cross-sections created in-plane with the scanner, possibly oblique to the patient's anatomy, e.g., if they have a scoliosis. In helical scanning, the volume acquisition allows more freedom to produce a variety of multiplanar displays, including curved

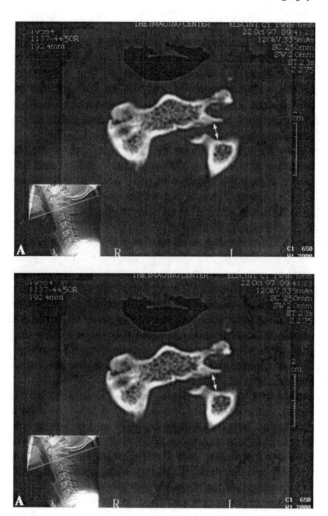

Figure 1. CT scan of a 25-year-old male (in halo brace) two months after injury. **A,** axial CT section ("fused" 2 mm section from pair of dual axial 1 mm slices) shows fracture separating left lateral mass from body of C2 (double arrow within fracture); **B,** sagittal reconstruction from helical CT acquisition (dual spiral 2.5 mm collimation; slice reconstruction interval 1.3 mm). *(Figure continued on facing page.)*

planes following a deformity or parallel to a normal spinal curvature, as well as three-dimensional shaded surface displays (Fig. 1).[3]

Despite the latest fast MR imaging techniques, newer pulse sequences, improved receiver coils, and computer postprocessing enhancement of MR images, CT still has higher spatial resolution for better definition of fractures and other bone morphology. CT provides excellent visualization of osseous detail,[16a] including post-traumatic changes, facet arthropathy, spondylolysis, spondylolisthesis, osseous stenosis, and structural alignment. Spatial and contour changes from disc pathology are adequately evaluated by CT, yet beam

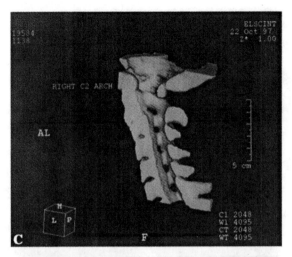

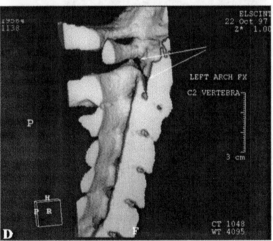

Figure 1 *(Cont).* C and D, shaded surface displays three-dimensional reconstructions from the same helical CT acquisition.

attenuation may occur at the cervicothoracic junction. The main limitations of CT include radiation exposure, slightly restricted field of view, and poor delineation of intrathecal pathology. The overwhelming majority of soft tissue processes are best imaged by MRI[16a]; however, post-discography CT is more sensitive in detecting sometimes painful annular fissures (Fig. 2), and post-myelography CT may still be more sensitive than MRI in detecting nerve root avulsion.[26]

Routine post-traumatic cervical spine CT with multiplanar reconstructions should include contiguous thin transaxial sections from the craniocervical junction to the mid-pedicle of T1. High-resolution helical CT (collimation down to 1 mm) is crucial[25] in order to define complex or subtle fractures and to prevent misregistration artifact. Overlapping slice reconstruction is necessary for high

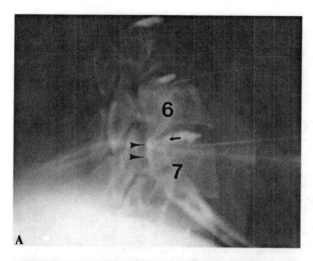

A

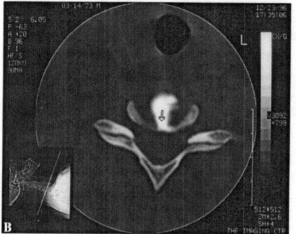

B

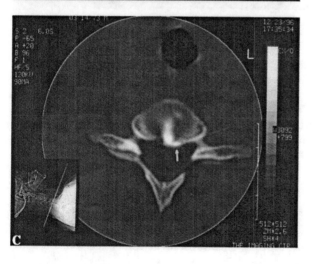

C

Figure 2. A 23-year-old male with right triceps weakness who had prior MR scan which was interpreted as showing C4–5 disc protrusion. CT revealed that this was a punctate bone spur unrelated to his symptoms. Other levels were thought to be normal on the MR scan. **A,** lateral projection nucleography disclosed complete posterior annular rent (*arrow*) of the C6–7 disc allowing contrast material to extravasate into the epidural space (*arrowheads*); **B** and **C,** axial CT images immediately after discography show annular rent (*open arrow*) and posterior disc protrusion (*closed arrow*).

quality multiplanar reconstruction images. The speed of helical scanning usually overcomes the traditional difficulty of trying to get an acutely injured patient to hold still for imaging. The inferior margin of the foramen magnum must be included in order to exclude fracture of an occipital condyle.[27]

Functional craniocervical CT (Fig. 3) involves scanning during axial rotation of the head in order to demonstrate dynamic C0-1 and C1-2 instability.[7] CT data can be acquired in 20–25 minutes with conventional CT but this takes only seconds with helical scanners.

Modern rapid scanning techniques significantly reduce radiation exposure, yet the risk must be considered when ordering a CT examination. Plain film evaluations are, unfortunately, limited by their lack of sensitivity and specificity and changes noted on plain films (including post-traumatic deformation) may not manifest themselves until they are subacute or chronic.

Magnetic Resonance Imaging (MRI)

In the 1980s, MRI allowed us to view soft tissue with stunning resolution. For the first time, we could visualize changes in hydration in the nuclear matrix, tiny fissures in the annulus, and detailed intrathecal anatomy.

MRI images are based on the interaction of nuclei (usually the single proton in hydrogen) with a magnetic field.[28] A spinning nucleus will tend to align its axis with an external magnetic field. An applied radiofrequency (RF) pulse will force that spin out of alignment, causing the nucleus to "wobble"—the axis of spin will precess around the axis of the external field. When the radiofrequency pulse is discontinued, protons realign with the external field, and while doing so emit a radiofrequency pulse which is detected by the receiver coils. The frequency of this emitted RF pulse is related to the strength of the magnetic field.

Superimposed upon the main magnetic field are "gradient" fields, so that there is a slight rise in magnetic field strength from one end of the scanner to the other, as well as from side to side. These gradients which vary the field strength result in slight frequency variations in the RF signals emitted by protons in the intervals when the external or applied pulses are turned off. These frequency differences provide spatial information along two axes. In order to obtain spatial information along a third axis, the applied pulses are "phase-encoded" and the phase differences provide information for that third axis.

The very complicated radio signal emitted by the patient's protons (the radiofrequency "echoes") are detected by receiver coils which are very sensitive antennae. This signal is computer-processed into a cross-sectional image using mathematical formulas similar to those used in CT scanning.

The MR signal of a given tissue is related to two independent **time constants** (T1 or longitudinal relaxation time and T2 or transverse relaxation time). These constants vary with the intrinsic physical properties of a given tissue and produce varied signal intensities or contrast within the images. **T1** is the time required for the excited protons to return to their equilibrium state and **T2** is the loss of coherence or harmonic convergence of the precessing nuclei following discontinuation of the radiofrequency signal. T1 "weighted" images emphasize the T1 properties of a tissue and are generated with a short TR (repetition time between radiofrequency signals) of 400–600 ms and a short TE

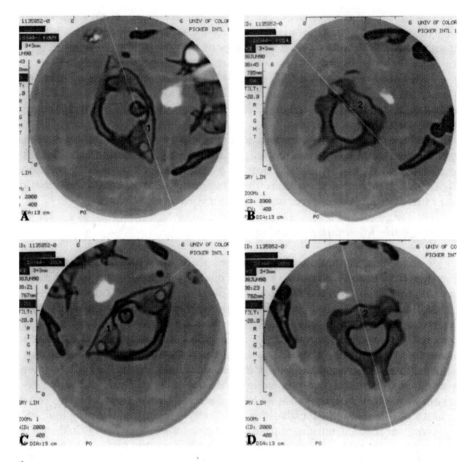

Figure 3. CT scans of a 19-year-old female following neck injury that occurred while her head was turned. *A–D*, images from craniocervical functional CT. White lines were drawn for consistent anatomic relationships necessary for accuracy. **A**, C1 rotation left; **B**, C2 rotation left; **C**, C1 rotation right; **D**, C2 rotation right.   *(Figure continued on facing page)*

or echo time of 15–30 ms. Fat, subacute, and chronic hemorrhage, as well as proteinaceous fluid all yield high signal on T1. T1-weighted images are known for their excellent delineation of anatomic structures and are sometimes thought of as "fat images." T2-weighted images relate to the state of hydration of the tissue and are produced with a long TR of 1500-3000 ms and a long TE of 60–120 ms. Tissues that are rich in free or extracellular water generate high signal on T2 (e.g., cerebrospinal fluid,[16a] necrotic or inflammatory tissue, cystic structures, nucleus pulposus, and tumors).

Proton density or spin density images have long TR-like T2-weighted images, and short TE-like T1-weighted images. Hence, they retain a significant amount of anatomic detail (like T1), yet structures that are rich in water yield high signal (like T2). Proton density images reflect the absolute number of mobile hydrogen protons in a tissue. Mineral-rich tissues such as cortical bone contain few mobile protons and generate very little signal in all pulse sequences.

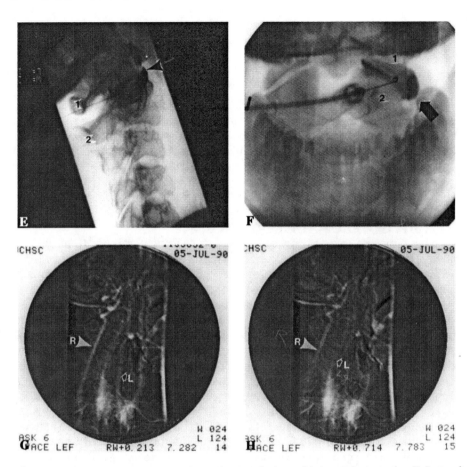

Figure 3 (Cont.)   E–F, images from C1–2 right lateral joint arthrography. E, Lateral view (arrowhead indicates extravasation of contrast material from an anterolateral joint capsule tear); F, PA projection (arrow points to irregular margin of lateral joint recess). G–H, images from dynamic vertebral angiography with patient's head turned to the left. G, Early image showing both vertebral arteries (open and closed arrows); H, Later image showing normal washout of contrast material from normal left vertebral artery, but retained contrast in abnormal right vertebral artery because of extrinsic compression.

Gas, which contains no mobile hydrogen protons, generates no MRI signal. T2-weighted images are prone to degradation from motion artifact because of the long acquisition time. The above discussion refers to "conventional spin echo" sequence of RF pulses.

A large variety of newer pulse sequences have been developed to mitigate motion artifacts and other MR imaging limitations. Unfortunately, there is no "free lunch" with MRI. For instance, fast spin echo T2-weighted images have less signal to noise, generate less magnetic susceptibility (which may obscure some hematomas), and generate high signal from fat (obscuring some tumors). Gradient echo images are prone to excess magnetic susceptibility causing some pathology to appear larger than it actually is while obscuring others. On another

MRI technical "battle front," higher field strength magnets have mitigated the never ending struggle to limit signal-to-noise constraints, yet are subject to obscuring from chemical shift artifact and eddy currents. Newer receiver coil designs continue to improve detection of the MR signal, leading to further improvements in image quality.

Dynamic MR studies acquire sagittal images with the patient in flexion and extension. These may demonstrate atlantoaxial and other intersegment instabilities. In a patient with otherwise unexplained neurologic signs or symptoms, a functional study may reveal cord impingement or nerve root entrapment in only one position (Fig. 4). Routine cervical spine MR scans should involve acquisition of T1- and T2-weighted images in multiple planes.

AN ALGORITHMIC APPROACH TO INTERPRETING THE POST-TRAUMATIC CERVICAL SPINE

The choice of imaging procedure(s) after cervical spine trauma has not always been universally agreed upon. Imaging algorithms have been evolving with newer technology and recent studies which shed light on the relationship between patient symptoms and the mechanism of injury.

A systematic approach to post-traumatic imaging must include an understanding of the structures vulnerable to injury within each phase of the injury mechanics. During the extension phase of whiplash, the anterior column will be strained, while the posterior elements are compressed. At the craniocervical junction, the head resists forward acceleration transmitted by the neck. During the flexion phase, the posterior structures (including the PLL, interspinous ligaments, ligamentum nuchae, muscles, and zygapophyseal joint capsule are subjected to strain while the intervertebral discs and bodies undergo compression.[15,16,20]

The American College of Radiology (ACR) has published Appropriateness Guidelines[1] for imaging in a variety of clinical situations, including cervical spine trauma. An expert multidisciplinary panel reviewed available literature (studies which reported on 15,000 cervical spine trauma cases) and reached a consensus on imaging choices. This consensus addressed two stages of imaging after acute cervical spine trauma. First, an initial radiographic evaluation is indicated in the acutely symptomatic patient, with or without neurologic deficit. If there is clinical suspicion of ligamentous injury, flexion and extension films are indicated unless there is obvious instability, such as with flexion teardrop vertebral fracture. Even patients with unstable spinal injuries may not present with immediate neurologic symptoms. Cross-sectional imaging, either MR or CT, is appropriate for patients with neuromuscular changes or radiographic abnormalities suggesting an unstable injury. In particular, for injuries at the craniovertebral junction, the ACR panel recommended CT scanning with multiplanar reconstruction. They were unable to reach a consensus on the use of MR scanning for injuries to the craniovertebral junction.

The ACR criteria mentioned above do not address the patient with delayed onset of symptoms or persistent symptoms after an initial negative screening evaluation. For this group of patients the authors recognize the need to include a third stage of imaging.

General guidelines for imaging do not always address the needs of individual patients. For example, it is well known that claustrophobic patients may

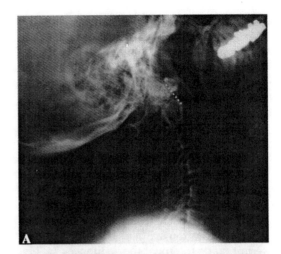

Figure 4. A 54-year-old female who sustained a whiplash injury at the age of 18 which resulted in a nonunited odontoid fracture with pseudarthrosis. **A,** Lateral film in extension showing normal alignment (dotted line along anterior margin of C2 and odontoid); **B,** Lateral film in flexion showing anterior displacement of odontoid fragment in relation to body of C2; **C,** Sagittal T1 weighted spin echo MR sequence (TR 482, TE 25) performed with as much flexion as allowed by the neck coil. Pannus at posterior margin of pseudarthrosis mildly impinges on cervicomedullary junction.

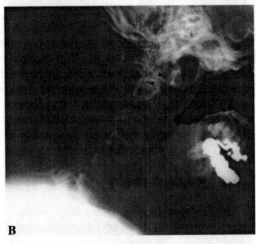

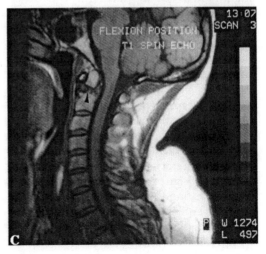

become agitated with resultant motion degrading the quality of the MR scan. Pain, hyperactive gag or swallow reflex, erratic respiration, or decreased sensorium may all degrade image quality through patient motion artifact; therefore, it is imperative to use clinical judgment in selecting the appropriate examination for each patient. Imaging of the cervical spine should include the basic principles discussed below.

General Observations

When initially evaluating any images, one should inspect the overall quality of the study. Was the area in question adequately surveyed? For example, is there a sufficient number of images, images in multiple planes, osseous and soft tissue window/level settings for CT, and multiple pulse sequences for MRI? Is there poor resolution or degradation of MR images by physiologic or aperiodic motion artifact? If a scan was degraded by patient motion, was an attempt made to repeat the sequences involved, or use alternative sequences less subject to such artifact?

There are a number of important technical factors that affect the quality of MR images. What type of scanner was employed and what type of pre- and postprocessing factors could affect the quality of the study? If the study was an MRI, was the magnet low-, mid-, or high-field strength? Were appropriate section thicknesses used? What was the field of view, matrix size, and number of excitations? Were appropriate and sufficient pulse sequences obtained in multiple planes? In addition to technical factors, interpersonal factors (patient handling) may greatly influence the quality of an imaging study. Was the patient made comfortable for the exam both physically and psychologically?

Gross Morphometry

Alterations in alignment may be the "footprints" of trauma and lead to asymmetrical loading and degeneration. Segmentation anomalies should be identified. Major supporting ligaments (such as the anterior longitudinal ligament, annulus, posterior longitudinal ligament, and osseous structures, including the odontoid, C1 arch, vertebral bodies, and zygapophyseal joints) are all vulnerable during different phases of the whiplash mechanism. Hence, it is imperative to exclude changes in alignment which may be the "telltale" signs of ligamentous or osseous disruption and unstable spine.[6]

Soft Tissue Structures

Myofascial elements should be symmetrical. Prevertebral edema or hematoma may be the warning sign of cervical instability, although many cervical spine fractures are not associated with thickened prevertebral tissues.[5] The esophagus, pharynx, longus capitus, longus coli, and sternocleidomastoid muscles are vulnerable during the extension phase and the nuchal ligament and posterior neck muscles subjected to strain during the extension phase. The vertebral artery undergoes dynamic elongation, most notably while the spine assumes an S-type compressed configuration immediately, before the skull undergoes extension.[12]

Muscle strains or tears cause characteristic MRI signal changes resulting from edema and/or hemorrhage within the muscle or between the muscles and adjacent structures.[16] Likewise, dissection of the vertebral artery may be visible on MR scanning because of the signal hyperintensity of subacute hematoma in a false lumen.

Osseous Detail

Fat suppression (i.e., STIR) MRI pulse sequences can be helpful in evaluating some bone tumors and fractures. MRI is the most sensitive modality for detecting marrow space abnormalities, and consequently might show bone marrow edema as a precursor to a stress fracture. However, plain radiographs are fundamental in furnishing a comprehensive view of anatomic relationships. A single radiograph may lead to an understanding of a three-dimensional structure which can facilitate the comprehension of cross-sectional images. An AP radiograph of the cervical spine may display the presence of cervical ribs which clarifies the appearance of an otherwise confusing axial image.

Plain radiographs, sometimes combined with CT scanning, may yield the best appreciation of bone texture and associated features such as periosteal reaction. While MR scanning is more sensitive for detecting bone marrow changes, radiographic and CT findings have higher specificity for identifying bone lesions and in a recent study was found to be more sensitive in detecting cervical spine fracture.[18]

Anterior Column

The anterior column undergoes distraction followed by compression during whiplash. Extension mechanics may lead to an attenuated or avulsed anterior longitudinal ligament, avulsion of the involved vertebrae from the adjacent discs, frank nuclear extrusion (Figs. 5 and 6), or horizontal rupture of the

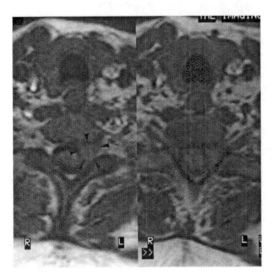

Figure 5. A 50-year-old female suffered cervical hyperextension injury resulting in acute disc rupture. Axial T1-weighted spin echo MR sequence (TR 575, TE 20) shows large sequestered disc fragment (*arrowheads*) in left lateral recess at the level of the C6–7 neuroforamen.

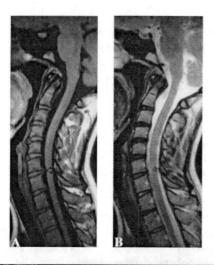

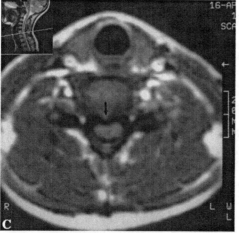

Figure 6. A 27-year-old female with no prior history of cervical spine problems suffered a whiplash injury to her neck during an amusement park ride and immediately experienced neck pain and paresthesias in all four extremities. **A,** Sagittal T1-weighted spin echo sequence (TR 450, TE 20) shows moderately sized posterocentral C6/7 disc extrusion indenting the ventral margin of the cord (*open arrow*). A smaller disc protrusion is visible at C7/T1. **B,** Sagittal T2-weighted fast spin echo sequence (TR 2390, TE 110) shows the hyperintense extruded disc material (*open arrow*), which is isointense with CSF and therefore less conspicuous than on the comparable T1-weighted sequence. **C,** Axial T1-weighted image (TR 435, TE 15) at the level of the C6/7 disc demonstrates the midline position of the extruded disc material (*arrow*) and its relationship to the cord. **D,** Axial T2* gradient echo sequence (flip angle 30°) at the level of the C6/7 disc demonstrates hyperintense extruded disc material (*solid arrow*) within the disrupted annulus (*open arrow*).

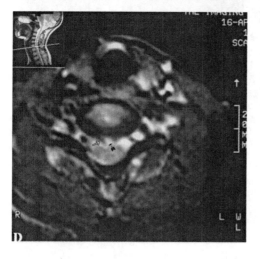

disc. (Fig. 1B illustrates mechanism of injury for horizontal disc rupture.) Annular fissures may result from strain on the annulus. Vertebral body compression, wedge-type ventral compression deformity, and radiographically occult anterior vertebral end-plate fractures result from the flexion phase.[4]

Posterior Elements

The posterior elements include the components of the neural arch. Embryologically, the transverse processes are not associated with the neural arch, but for this discussion will be included. The zygapophyseal joints share the load with the anterior column in hyperextension injuries. While the anterior column is undergoing distraction, the posterior elements are subject to compression during the extension phase and vice versa for the flexion phase. Compression may lead to cortical defects, fractures, capsular tears, hemorrhage, or rupture of the articular pillars. In one study, zygapophyseal joint pain was demonstrated to be the most common cause of chronic neck pain after whiplash injury.[2] During the flexion phase, the tips of the spinous processes can be avulsed and interspinous ligaments strained or ruptured.

Neuraxial Canals

Spinal cord injury manifesting as characteristic signal changes of edema and hemorrhage within the spinal cord on MRI can result from compression of the spinal cord between the ligamentum flavum and retrodisplaced vertebrae above a disrupted disc. Degenerative spondylosis and congenital spinal stenosis may result in spinal cord entrapment, anteriorly by osteophytes or vertebral bodies and posteriorly by thickened or buckled ligamentum flavum. A narrow spinal canal has been shown to correlate with persistent symptoms after whiplash.[21]

MRI allows excellent visualization of the morphology and position of the cord,[8,11] nerve roots, thecal sac, cord, or nerve root edema, hemorrhage, myelomalacia, and syrinx (Fig. 7). MRI also provides superior categorization of predisposing pathology, such as Arnold Chiari malformation.

There remains a role for high-resolution thin-section CT in evaluating osseous stenosis, especially in the cervical spine due to the following pitfalls of MRI: variable signal intensity in degenerative osseous ridges, magnetic susceptibility, and thicker slices (resulting in partial volume averaging).

Craniocervical Junction

The craniocervical junction is the link between the forces acting on the head and the neck. Moreover, the forward acceleration of the trunk must be transmitted to the head through the craniocervical junction. As the neck moves forward, the odontoid process impacts the ventral arch of the atlas which in turn transmits the forces through the atlanto-occipital joint and longus capitus muscles. Any torsion forces imparted in the axial plane at the time of the accident will subject the atlantoaxial joint capsules and alar ligaments, as well as vertebral arch to additional strain.

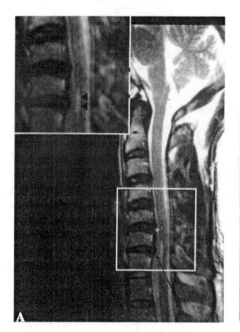

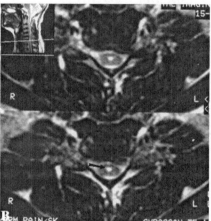

Figure 7. A 42-year-old male with posttraumatic syrinx at C6–7. **A**, Sagittal T2-weighted fast spin echo MR sequence (TR 2200, TE 110) with zoomed inset image (*arrowheads* indicate syrinx in cord, and low arrow points to mold disc prolapse abutting cord); **B**, Axial T2-weighted fast spin echo sequence (TR 1800, TE 130) shows hyperintensity (fluid signal) in cord syrinx (*arrow*).

Associated Extraspinal Injuries

During whiplash injury, the head undergoes rapid acceleration and deceleration movements which may cause impaction of the brain on the inner table of the calvarium and contra-coup injury. A recent report has shown a link between whiplash injury and movement disorders.[9] Neuropsychiatric evaluations after whiplash injury have not been consistent in providing objective evidence of brain injury in whiplash patients.[10,23] However, with quantitative SPECT scanning, Otte et al.[19] have recently demonstrated parieto-occipital hypoperfusion in patients with late whiplash syndrome. This finding may provide some insight into the protean delayed onset or chronic CNS symptoms of some whiplash patients.

Indirect forces acting upon the temporomandibular joint during motor vehicle injuries are a major cause of TMJ dysfunction.[22] During whiplash, hyperextension of the head results in excessive mouth opening and potential tearing of the posterior attachments of the TMJ meniscus or forceful anterior movement of the meniscus. MR scanning of the TMJ may reveal anterior displacement of the meniscus (Fig. 8).

Experimental studies have shown elongation of the vertebral artery during whiplash simulation.[17] This mechanism may explain, in addition to direct trauma, the reported cases of vertebral artery dissection or thrombosis after

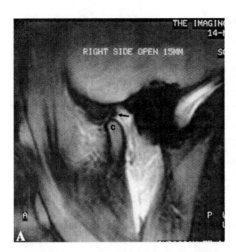 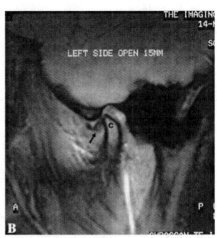

Figure 8. A 21-year-old female whose symptoms of left TM joint clicking and pain began after whiplash injury. Oblique sagittal T2* gradient echo (TR 264, TE 25, flip angle 30°) MR sequences obtained with mouth opened to an interincisural distance of 15 mm. **A,** Normal right side showing position of posterior band of TM joint meniscus (*arrow*) at 2:00 position of mandibular condyle (c); **B,** Abnormal left side showing displacement of the meniscus (*arrow*) anterior to condyle (c).

whiplash injury. Carotid artery dissection without direct trauma has been reported and the mechanism of vessel injury attributed to whiplash.[14] In addition, shoulder injuries, thoracic outlet syndrome, and carpal tunnel syndrome have been associated with whiplash injury.[16] These should be further evaluated based on history and clinical examination.

CONCLUSION

It is important to have an understanding of the indications and limitations of imaging techniques of the spine in the evaluation of cervical whiplash injuries. It is imperative that clinicians follow a systematic approach based on clinical history and examination and then choose the appropriate imaging study to assist in a more accurate diagnosis and proper treatment.

References

1. American College of Radiology Task Force on Appropriateness Criteria: Appropriateness Criteria for Imaging and Treatment Decisions. American College of Radiology, 1996.
2. Barnsley L, Lord SM, Wallis BJ, Bogduk N: The prevalence of chronic zygapophyseal joint pain after whiplash. Spine 20:20–25, 26 [discussion], 1995.
3. Brink JA: Technical aspects of helical (spiral) CT. Radiol Clin North Am 33:825–841, 1995.
4. Davis SJ, Teresi LM, Bradley WG, et al: Cervical spine hyperextension injuries: MR findings. Radiology 180:245–251, 1991.
5. DeBehnke DJ, Havel CJ: Utility of prevertebral soft tissue measurements in identifying patients with cervical spine fractures. Ann Emerg Med 24:1119, 1994.
6. Dvorak J: Functional roentgen diagnosis of the upper cervical spine. Orthopade 20:121–126, 1991.
7. Dvorak H, Hayek J, Vehnder R: CT functional diagnostics of the rotary instability of upper cervical spine. Part II: An evaluation of healthy adults with suspected instability. Spine 12:726–731, 1987.

8. El-Koury GY, Kathol MH, Daniel WW: Imaging of acute injuries of the cervical spine: Value of plain radiography, CT, and MR imaging. Am J Roentgenol 164:43–50, 1995.
9. Ellis SJ: Tremor and other movement disorders after whiplash type injuries. J Neurol Neurosurg Psychiatry 63:110–112, 1997.
10. Ettlin TM, Kischka U, Reichmann S, et al: Cerebral symptoms after whiplash injury of the neck: A prospective clinical and neuropsychological study of whiplash injury. J Neurol Neurosurg Psychiatry 55:943–948, 1992.
11. Flanders AE, Schaefer DM, Doan JT, et al: Acute cervical spine trauma: Correlation of MR imaging findings with degree of neurologic deficit. Radiology 177:25–33, 1990.
12. Grauer JN, Panjabi MM, Cholewicki J, et al: Whiplash produces an S-shaped curvature of the neck with hyperextension at lower levels. Spine 22:2489–2494, 1997.
13. Hamilton JR, Dearden C, Rutherford WHH: Myocardial contusion associated with fracture of the sternum: Important features of the seat belt syndrome. Injury 16:155–156, 1984.
14. Janjua KJ, Goswami V, Sagar G: Whiplash injury associated with acute bilateral internal carotid arterial dissection. J Trauma 40:456–458, 1996.
15. Johnson G: Hyperextension soft tissue injuries of the cervical spine: A review. J Accid Emerg Med 13:3–8, 1996.
16. LaBan MM: Whiplash: Its evaluation and treatment. Phys Med Rehabil State Art Rev 4:293–307, 1990.
16a. Murphy RB, Humphreys SC, Fisher DL, et al: Imaging of the cervical spine and its role in clinical decision making. J South Orthop Assoc 9(1):24–35, 2000.
17. Nibu K, Cholewicki J, Panjabi MM, et al: Dynamic elongation of the vertebral artery during an in vitro whiplash simulation. Eur Spine J 6:286–289, 1997.
18. Orrison WW, Benzel EC, Willis BK, et al: Magnetic resonance imaging evaluation of acute spine trauma. Emerg Radiol 2:120–128, 1995.
19. Otte A, Ettlin T, Fierz L, Mueller-Brand J: Parieto-occipital hypoperfusion in late whiplash syndrome: First quantitative SPET study using technetium 99m bicisate (ECD). Eur J Nucl Med 23:72–74, 1996.
20. Panjabi MM, Cholewicki J, Nibu K, et al: Simulation of whiplash trauma using whole cervical spine specimens. Spine 23:17–24, 1998.
21. Pettersson K, Karrholm J, Toolanen G, Hildingsson C: Decreased width of the spinal canal in patients with chronic symptoms after whiplash. Spine 20:1664–1667, 1995.
22. Pressman, BD, Frank GS, Schames J, Schames M: MR imaging of temporomandibular joint abnormalities associated with cervical hyperextension/hyperflexion (whiplash) injuries. J Magn Reson Imaging 2:569–574, 1992.
23. Radanov BP, Dvorak J: Spine update: Impaired cognitive functioning after whiplash injury of the cervical spine. Spine 21:392–397, 1996.
24. Reid DC, Henderson R, Saboe L, Miller JDR: Etiology and clinical course of missed spine fractures. J Trauma 27:980–986, 1987.
25. Rubinstein D, Escott EJ, Mestek MF: Computed tomographic scans of minimally displaced type II odontoid fractures. J Trauma 40:204–210, 1996.
26. Volle E, Assheuer J, Hedde JP, Gustorf-Aeckerle R: Radicular avulsion resulting from spinal injury: Assessment of diagnostic modalities. Neuroradiology 34:235–240, 1992.
27. Wasserber J, Bartlett RJV: Occipital condyle fractures diagnosed by high-definition CT and coronal reconstructions. Neuroradiology 37:370, 1995.
28. Wehrli FW, Shaw D, Kneeland BJ: Biomedical Magnetic Resonance Imaging. New York, VCH Publishers, Inc., 1988.
29. Wolf RA: Four facets of automotive crash injury research. N Y State J Med 66:1798-1813, 1966.

17

The Electrodiagnostic Evaluation of Whiplash Injuries: A Practical Approach

Gregory J. Mulford, M.D.

It is well established that numerous structures may be damaged as a result of whiplash mechanism injuries. The significant challenge for clinicians is to determine the etiology of the patient's symptoms by identifying the symptom generators as precisely and accurately as possible. Only after a specific diagnosis is made can a focused, specific, and appropriate treatment plan be implemented. Electrodiagnostic testing can be an important component of the diagnostic assessment of the individual who has sustained a whiplash mechanism injury. Electrodiagnostic studies provide useful information on the physiologic and functional status of the nervous system. This information complements imaging studies such as x-rays, computed tomography, and magnetic resonance imaging, which give information on the status and integrity of anatomic structures.[1] Importantly, neither electrodiagnostic nor imaging studies are able to definitively determine the presence or absence of pain. In fact, pain is a complex subjective and multifactorial phenomenon for which there is no "gold standard" diagnostic test. Electrodiagnostic studies may be useful as one component of a thorough, rational, and objective assessment when an individual presents with complaints of numbness, sensory disturbance, weakness, pain, cramping, or loss of function.

There is no substitute for a thorough history and physical examination in the evaluation of individuals who present with pain or other undesirable symptoms following trauma. The relevant findings on the history and physical examination should form the basis for establishing a differential diagnosis.[2] Only after establishing a differential diagnosis, as supported by relevant findings on the history and/or physical examination, should additional diagnostic studies be considered.[3] The routine performance of any test or battery of tests is inappropriate and should be discouraged. If the clinician suspects that mechanical structures have been injured and if the test results will affect the course of treatment, imaging studies may be indicated. If, on the other hand, the injured individual has complaints or physical findings that suggest abnormalities of nervous system function, electrodiagnostic consultation may be more appropriate. It is important to emphasize the complementary nature of imaging tests and electrodiagnostic studies. For example, magnetic resonance imaging that demonstrates a disc herniation provides little information on the presence or absence of radiculopathy (nerve root injury). Conversely, electrodiagnostic studies that identify the presence of radiculopathy, plexopathy, or peripheral neuropathy are not able to determine whether a structural abnormality is causing or contributing to the electrophysiologic abnormalities. Therefore, it is not uncommon for both imaging and electrodiagnostic studies to be performed, when warranted based on the clinical scenario, to develop a clearer understanding of the pathophysiologic processes that may be present. The relative frequency of false positives with both imaging and electrodiagnostic studies further validates the importance of identifying significant relevant findings in the history along with objective findings on the physical examination.

Symptoms of numbness, weakness, sensory disturbance, or pain may be the result of injury to neural structures. Physical signs of atrophy, weakness not due to painful inhibition of muscle contraction, disordered sensation, or abnormal reflexes may also indicate neuropathic abnormalities and justify the performance of electrodiagnostic studies.[4] Not all individuals with such complaints or findings require electrodiagnostic testing, which should be performed when the test results will help guide further diagnostic work-up, establish a definitive diagnosis, determine optimal treatment, or aid in prognostication.

Appropriate performance of electrodiagnostic testing should always begin with a history and physical examination by the treating clinician that corroborates subjective complaints and identified objective abnormalities on physical examination such as weakness, atrophy, reflex loss, or sensory deficit. Upon receiving the referral, the electrodiagnostic consultant should also repeat the history and physical examination because this is essential in determining which specific electrodiagnostic tests will be most appropriate and useful in the particular clinical situation.[5] The failure of the electrodiagnostic consultant to adequately examine the patient only leads to the performance of unnecessary or inappropriate tests and diminishes the value of the electrodiagnostic consultation. For this reason, the physician who is responsible for the electrodiagnostic testing should always personally examine the patient and either perform the testing directly or directly oversee the technician who performs the studies. Additionally, the practice of routinely performing a standard battery of tests regardless of the clinical situation is inappropriate and should be avoided.

Electrodiagnostic medicine consultations should be performed by physicians who, by virtue of their education, training, credentialing, and experience, are qualified to practice electrodiagnostic medicine.[6] To arrive at an accurate diagnosis, the electrodiagnostic medicine consultant must be intimately involved in obtaining and reviewing the relevant history and physical examination, performing the studies, and interpreting the data. Performing and, most importantly, interpreting electrodiagnostic studies constitutes the practice of medicine because establishing a diagnosis and making recommendations on diagnosis, treatment, and prognosis are all components of a quality electrodiagnostic consultation and report. Performing tests and reporting data without interpreting the electrophysiologic findings in the context of the clinical picture is of limited value and is discouraged.

Electrodiagnostic studies assist in assessing the function of central and peripheral nervous system structures. Studies such as electroencephalography, visual evoked potentials, and brainstem auditory evoked responses offer useful information regarding the functional status of the brain, brainstem, and spinal cord and are not addressed in this text. Electrodiagnostic studies commonly used to evaluate function of peripheral nervous system elements such as nerve roots, cervical and lumbosacral plexuses, and peripheral nerves include nerve conduction studies (NCSs), late responses (F waves and H reflexes), needle electromyography examination (NEE), spinal nerve root stimulation, and somatosensory evoked potentials (SSEPs). Quantitative sensory testing (QST) and surface electromyography (sEMG), which are less valuable and infrequently used electrophysiologic techniques, are discussed briefly.

NERVE CONDUCTION STUDIES

NCSs are a valuable means of assessing the functional status of peripheral motor and sensory nerves.[7] NCSs evaluate the ability of a peripheral nerve to transmit an electric signal. Motor NCSs are performed by stimulating a peripheral motor nerve with an electrical stimulus and recording a compound motor action potential (CMAP) response with either surface or needle electrodes from a distal muscle supplied by that particular motor nerve. In a similar fashion, sensory NCSs are performed by electrically stimulating a peripheral sensory nerve and recording a sensory nerve action potential (SNAP) directly from the peripheral sensory nerve branch.

Electrophysiologic parameters that are commonly measured include the size of the CMAP or SNAP, distal motor or sensory latency, peak sensory latency, and nerve conduction velocity (Figs. 1–4). These parameters are used to evaluate the functional status of peripheral nerve axon and myelin structures. In general, decreases in CMAP or SNAP amplitude suggest the presence of axonal damage or conduction block, and prolongation of latency or slowing of conduction velocity implies some element of demyelination.[8]

NCSs may have limited value in the assessment of radiculopathies, but they are useful for assessing peripheral nerve and plexus function and can assist in determining whether a more diffuse or distal neuropathic process is present.[9] NCSs also offer the ability to assist in categorizing the type and severity of peripheral nerve injuries[10,11] (Table 1). A mild nerve injury may result in a neuropraxia, which is defined as a mild and temporary failure of

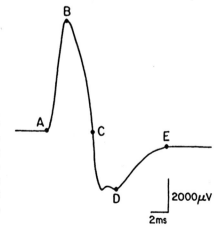

Figure 1. Thenar muscle CMAP. Example of a typical CMAP recorded from the thenar eminence following median nerve excitation at the wrist. The time represented by the segment A-B is referred to as the rise time, whereas A-C is the duration of the negative spike. Segment A-E represents the duration of the total potential. The amplitude of A-B is the baseline-to-peak magnitude of the potential, while B-D is the peak-to-peak amplitude. That portion of the CMAP between A-C and C-E each constitutes one phase of this biphasic potential. The latency of point A is the onset latency, while point B represents the peak latency. (From Dumitru D: Electrodiagnostic Medicine. Philadelphia, Hanley & Belfus, 1995; with permission.)

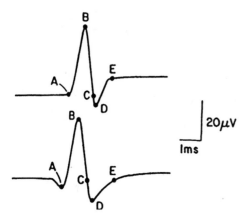

Figure 2. Antidromic median SNAP recorded from the third digit. The same descriptions noted in Fig. 1 for the potential's various segments apply here. In the upper trace, a bipolar recording montage (both recording electrodes on the third digit) is shown. The lower trace depicts the result of relocating the reference (E-2) electrode to the fifth digit, resulting in a referential recording montage and an initially positive triphasic SNAP. (From Dumitru D: Electrodiagnostic Medicine. Philadelphia, Hanley & Belfus, 1995; with permission.)

nerve conduction without disruption of the nerve axons or architecture. A neuropraxia is usually identified by a normal amplitude response when stimulating distal to the site of injury and a reduced or absent response when stimulating proximally. Slowing of conduction velocity across the injured nerve segment may also be present. A more significant focal nerve injury that results

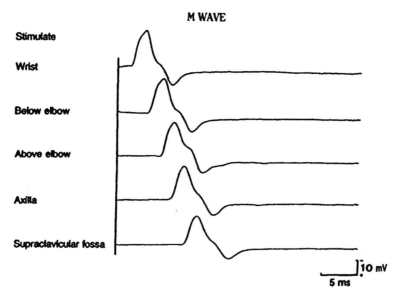

Figure 3. The M wave, or motor wave, recorded with surface electrodes over the abductor digiti quinti elicited by electric stimulation of the ulnar nerve at several levels. The M wave is a compound action potential evoked from a muscle by a single electric stimulus to its motor nerve. The latency, commonly called the motor latency or distal latency, is the latency (ms) to the onset of the first phase of the M wave. The amplitude (mV) is the baseline-to-peak amplitude of the first phase. (From the AAEM Glossary of Terms in Neurodiagnostic Medicine. Muscle Nerve, Supplement no. 10, 2001; with permission.)

COMPOUND SENSORY NERVE ACTION POTENTIALS

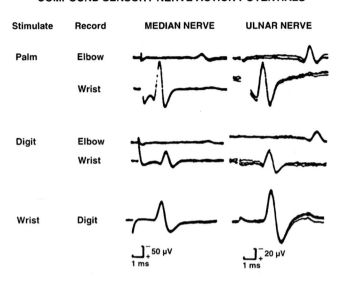

Figure 4. Compound SNAP recorded with surface electrodes in a normal subject. A compound nerve action potential is considered to have been evoked from afferent fibers if the recording electrodes detect activity in only a sensory nerve or in a sensory branch of a mixed nerve. The compound SNAP has been referred to as the sensory response or sensory potential. (From the AAEM Glossary of Terms in Neurodiagnostic Medicine. Muscle Nerve, Supplement no. 10, 2001; with permission.)

in axonal damage is called an axonotmesis, and NCSs classically demonstrate decreased amplitudes when stimulating both proximal and distal to the site of nerve injury. In a neurotmesis, the most severe degree of nerve injury, motor

Table 1. Sunderland and Seddon Classification and Degrees of Peripheral Nerve Injury

	First Degree	Second Degree	Third Degree	Fourth Degree	Fifth Degree
	Neurapraxia	Axonotmesis		Neurotmesis	
Electrophysiology	Conduction block		Axonal loss		
Pathology	Segmental demyelination	Loss of axons, with intact supporting structures	Loss of axons, with disrupted endoneurium	Loss of axons, with disrupted endoneurium and perineurium	Loss of axons, with distion of all supporting structures (discontinuous)
Prognosis	Excellent, recovery is usually complete in 2 to 3 mo	Slow recovery; dependent on sprouting and reinnervation	Protracted and recovery may fail because of misdirected axonal sprouts	Unlikely without surgical repair	Impossible without surgical repair

and sensory conduction responses, are usually completely unobtainable. With neuropraxic nerve injuries, there is little structural damage to the axons or myelin sheaths of the affected nerves and there is only a partial and temporary decrease in the ability of the nerve to conduct electric signals across the affected segment. Axonal damage and axon death occurs with axonotmesis injuries, and the prognosis as well as the rate of recovery is significantly worse for axonotmesis injuries than for neuropraxic injuries. In injuries resulting in neurotmesis, damage occurs to the endoneurium, perineurium, and epineurium in addition to the nerve axons and myelin sheaths. Prognosis for nerve recovery is much less favorable for neurotmesis injuries because of the presence of such severe damage to the ultrastructural and architectural elements of the peripheral nerve. It may be difficult to differentiate between these various degrees of nerve injury with NCSs alone, and needle electromyography is helpful in further differentiating among neuropraxia, axonotmesis, and neurotmesis.

LATE RESPONSES

H reflexes, F waves, and A waves are typically referred to as late responses. They are secondary, or late, responses that are observed several milliseconds following the direct CMAP response when stimulating a peripheral motor nerve.[12] F waves are recorded by stimulating a peripheral motor nerve with a supramaximal stimulus and recording the action potential that travels along the alpha motor neuron. F waves have much smaller, more variable amplitudes and longer latencies than the CMAP and generally occur between 25 to 35 msec when stimulating the upper extremity at the wrists and between 50 and 60 msec when stimulating the lower extremity at the ankles.[13] F waves are felt to represent a "backfiring" of the anterior horn cell, and the latency, amplitude, and shape vary in size from one stimulation to the next. The shortest reproducible response, or minimal latency, is the most widely measured component and represents conduction time along the largest-diameter motor fibers in the stimulated nerve. Other parameters that are sometimes measured include F-wave amplitude, mean latency, extent of latency scatter (or "chronodispersion"), and persistence of the F-wave response.[14–16] F waves provide a means of indirectly evaluating motor nerve conduction proximally at the root level and have been used for more than two decades in the evaluation of radiculopathies. Initially thought to be valuable in detecting proximal peripheral nervous system lesions such as radiculopathies, their usefulness is somewhat limited because they can be normal in patients with unequivocal radiculopathies, they do not detect sensory lesions, and abnormalities are often redundant with needle EMG abnormalities.[17,18] For these reasons, routine performance of F-wave responses on all peripheral motor nerves in the electrodiagnostic evaluation of radiculopathies is difficult to justify.

A waves, sometimes referred to as axon reflexes, are nonreflex, monosynaptic responses that may occur between the CMAP and F wave when performing F-wave studies. Unlike the variable latency of the F wave, which is obtained with a supramaximum stimulus, the A wave has a constant latency and is usually elicited with a submaximal stimulus. It represents a "backfiring" response from collateral sprouting of a proximal portion of the motor nerve and is believed to be a pathological response that may be seen in radiculopathies, plexopathies, peripheral neuropathies, and motor neuron disease.[19]

The H reflex, first described by Hoffman, is a CMAP that arises through the electrical activation of a monosynaptic reflex arc involving sensory afferent and motor efferent pathways.[20] It is most commonly used in assessing S1 fibers in the lower extremities and is elicited by stimulating the tibial nerve in the popliteal fossa with a long-duration, low-intensity stimulus and recording over the gastrocnemius-soleus muscles. H reflexes are sometimes used in the evaluation of C6-C7 nerve roots by stimulating the median nerve at the elbow and recording from the flexor carpi radialis muscle.[21] Parameters that are frequently measured include side-to-side comparisons of latencies or amplitudes.[22-24] Side-to-side latency differences[25] and side-to-side amplitude differences[26,27] have been used to diagnose radiculopathies. Importantly, an abnormal H reflex alone is not synonymous with a radiculopathy, because the reflex is mediated over a long pathway and abnormalities may be due to pathology of the peripheral nerve, plexus, or nerve roots.[28]

NEEDLE ELECTROMYOGRAPHY EXAMINATION

NEE involves the insertion of a sterile monopolar or concentric needle electrode directly into skeletal muscle and allows the examiner to evaluate the muscle electrical activity. It is a diagnostic procedure that directly evaluates the electrical properties of skeletal muscle membranes. It is the oldest electrophysiologic method used to evaluate patients with suspected radiculopathies and is still the single most useful electrodiagnostic procedure, having a higher diagnostic yield than other techniques.[29-31] The steps of the NEE generally include examination of muscle electrical activity during needle insertion with the muscles at rest and with minimal to moderate muscle contraction. The electromyographer must continuously synthesize the information and be formulating an impression while performing the examination because the dynamic nature of the NEE often requires the physician to modify the study based on findings seen during the NEE itself. Unlike an x-ray or electrocardiogram, the NEE is an interactive test. The value and validity of the NEE is determined by the real-time feedback, interaction, and decision making that occur during the actual performance of the study itself.

Needle insertion into normal muscle gives rise to brief bursts of electrical activity that usually last less than 300 msec following needle movement.[32] These discharges originate from muscle fibers that are mechanically stimulated or injured by the penetrating needle.[33-35] Insertional activity is decreased in fibrotic muscle and increased in the presence of motor axonal damage, denervation, and myopathy. In normal muscles, no electrical activity is seen at rest except when the needle is near the end-plate region at the neuromuscular junction. Low-amplitude (10–50 µV) miniature end-plate potentials, with a characteristic sound like a seashell held to the ear, and end-plate spikes of 100 to 200 µV that fire irregularly at 5 to 50 pulses per second, constitute normal end-plate activity.[36] They are believed to be due to the spontaneous release of acetylcholine from the presynaptic nerve terminal.[37-39]

These normal findings, which are often accompanied by an increase in patient discomfort, can be incorrectly mistaken for abnormal spontaneous activity by the inexperienced electromyographer. Fibrillation potentials, positive sharp waves, and complex repetitive discharges are forms of abnormal spontaneous activity arising from abnormal muscle generators. Fasciculation potentials and myokymic discharges are abnormal spontaneous potentials that arise from neural generators.[40]

Positive sharp waves and fibrillation potentials are the most common forms of abnormal spontaneous activity seen on NEE, and both are generally believed to represent muscle membrane instability and the spontaneous depolarization of single muscle fibers.[41] **Positive sharp waves**, which usually fire at regular rates between 2 to 50 times per second, demonstrate a classic "popping" sound or "dull thud" and have a characteristic morphology of an initial positive (downward) deflection followed by a slower return to baseline (Fig 5). **Fibrillation potentials** also have an initial positive deflection, sharp return to baseline with biphasic or triphasic morphology, amplitude of 20 to 1000 µV, firing rates of up to 20 per second, and a high-pitched sound described as "rain on a tin roof" (Fig. 6). The initial positive deflection, slower rate of firing, and more regular rhythm generally help to differentiate abnormal fibrillation potentials from normal end-plate spikes (Fig. 7). Positive sharp waves and fibrillation potentials may be recorded in both neurogenic and myopathic diseases. They typically develop within 1 to 3 weeks following nerve injury and take longer to appear in muscles more distal to the site of nerve injury. In radiculopathies, such membrane instability may be seen in the paraspinal muscles

POSITIVE SHARP WAVE

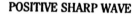

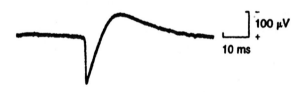

TRAIN OF POSITIVE SHARP WAVES

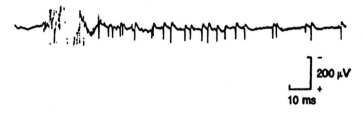

Figure 5. A positive sharp wave is a biphasic action potential initiated by needle movement and recurring in a uniform, regular pattern. A "train" of such waves can be recorded from a damaged area of fibrillating muscle fibers. This is one of the hallmarks of axonal degeneration. (From the AAEM Glossary of Terms in Neurodiagnostic Medicine. Muscle Nerve, Supplement no. 10, 2001; with permission.)

FIBRILLATION POTENTIAL

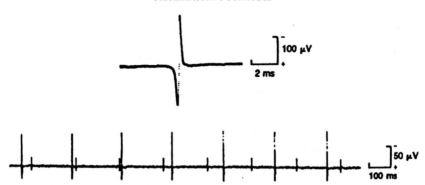

Figure 6. Fibrillation potential. A fibrillation potential is the electric activity associated with a spontaneously contracting (fibrillating) muscle fiber. This is one of the hallmarks of axonal degeneration. (From the AAEM Glossary of Terms in Neurodiagnostic Medicine. Muscle Nerve, Supplement no. 10, 2001; with permission.)

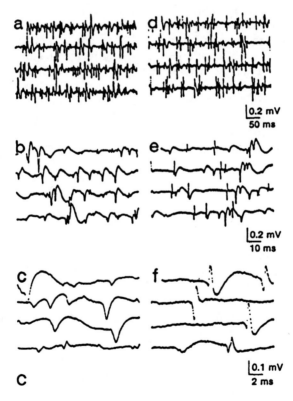

Figure 7. Spontaneous single-fiber activity of the paraspinal muscle in a 40-year-old man with radiculopathy, consisting of positive sharp waves (a-c) and fibrillation potentials (d–f). (From Kimura J: Electrodiagnosis in Diseases of Nerve and Muscle: Principles and Practices, 2nd ed. Philadelphia, FA Davis, 1989; with permission.)

within 7 to 10 days and in the corresponding myotomal limb muscles in approximately 21 days.[42-45]

Complex repetitive discharges, sometimes called bizarre, high-frequency, or pseudomyotonic discharges, are spontaneously firing groups of action potentials. They fire regularly at frequencies up to 150 times per second, start and stop abruptly, and often sound like heavy machinery or an idling motorcycle. They have been associated with chronic radiculopathies and neuropathies as well as motor neuron disease and myopathies.[46]

Myotonic discharges may also be seen in chronic radiculopathy or peripheral neuropathy and have a characteristic sound much like a dive-bomber. Myotonic discharges demonstrate a waxing and waning of the amplitude and firing rate of the spontaneously discharging single muscle fibers generating the potentials.[47] **Fasciculations** are the spontaneous intermittent contraction of a portion of a muscle, and fasciculation potentials are the electrically summated voltage of multiple spontaneously depolarizing muscle fibers belonging to one motor unit.[48] Their amplitude, duration, and phases are similar to those of normal motor units and discharge irregularly and spontaneously from one to several times per second.[49]

Myokymic discharges, usually seen in association with visible rippling movements of the skin, or myokymia, represent bursts of normal-appearing motor units with interburst intervals of silence in a semirhythmic pattern.[50] Myokymic discharges often sound like the sputtering of a low-powered motorboat engine. Myokymic discharges, representing groups of motor units, may be distinguished from complex repetitive discharges, which represent groups of single muscle fibers.[51] They do not typically start and stop abruptly, and the motor unit action potentials (MUAPs) of each burst of motor units are variable, unlike complex repetitive discharges, which usually start and stop abruptly and have consistent morphologies of each burst. Myokymic discharges may be seen in segmental patterns in chronic radiculopathies.[52]

The MUAP recruitment pattern and morphology can be evaluated during minimal to moderate muscle contraction. Single motor units usually fire at a rate of 5 to 10 times per second.[53,54] Small, type I muscle fibers are activated first, and larger, type II units are recruited later during stronger voluntary contractions.[55] Abnormalities of motor unit firing rates may occur at the onset of nerve injury—long before abnormal spontaneous activity develops[56,57]—but considerable experience is needed to be able to recognize more subtle changes in MUAP firing patterns.[58] At just-perceptible levels of muscle contraction, when motor unit firing begins, the needle electrode will record from one to three single motor units. MUAP morphology as well as onset and recruitment firing rates can be assessed best at this low level of muscle activation.[59]

A decrease in the number of MUAPs contracting due to nerve injury will result in a decreased recruitment pattern and incomplete interference. Objective analysis of interference and recruitment patterns can be difficult because of a lack of patient effort or because of pain during the attempted muscle contraction. Single motor units firing at rates of greater than 20 Hz are abnormal.[60] Normally, by the time a motor unit is firing at a rate of 10 Hz, a second motor unit begins firing, and when the first unit reaches a firing rate of approximately 15 Hz, a third motor unit becomes activated. Under these normal conditions, the recruitment ratio, defined as the firing rate of the fastest motor unit divided by the total number of motor units firing, is 3. In pathological states with reduced numbers of normally contracting motor units, single motor units often fire at rates greater than 20 Hz, and recruitment ratios are greater than 5.[61]

For example, if a motor unit is firing at 20 Hz when the second motor unit begins firing, the recruitment ratio is 20:2, or 10, which is abnormal. In situations with mild abnormalities and minimal weakness, recruitment may be normal at minimal to moderate levels of contraction. The electromyographer should gradually increase the force of muscle contraction to allow recruitment of high-threshold motor units that may be firing at abnormally high rates.[62]

MUAP amplitudes normally range from several hundred microvolts to a few millivolts with a concentric needle and are often substantially greater when using a monopolar needle electrode. MUAP duration normally varies from 5 to 15 msec.[63] The number of phases of a MUAP equals the number of baseline crossings plus 1, and normal motor unit potentials usually have four or fewer phases. MUAPs with more than four phases are designated polyphasic.[64] Because up to 20% of MUAPs may be polyphasic in any normal muscle, the electromyographer should be cautious about determining that a study is abnormal based solely on the presence of polyphasic MUAPs. Furthermore, the presence of polyphasic potentials seen in the paraspinal muscles alone has little if any value in determining the presence of a radiculopathy.

NEE is useful in the evaluation of patients with suspected radiculopathies, plexopathies, or peripheral neuropathies but is most useful in determining the presence of motor axon loss. "Identification of cervical radiculopathies: optimizing the electromyographic screen" demonstrated that, when cervical paraspinal muscles were included, screening seven muscles on NEE identified 96% to 100% of cervical radiculopathies.[65] Furthermore, evaluating eight distal limb muscles recognized 92% to 95% of radiculopathies when paraspinal muscles were not examined. The exact muscles evaluated on NEE will be dependent upon the differential diagnosis and the innervation of the various muscles sampled. Careful muscle selection can assist in determining whether the location of a nerve injury lies at the level of the nerve root, plexus, or peripheral nerve. In radiculopathies, NEE abnormalities are seen in a myotomal distribution, and paraspinal muscles are often involved. NEE of the paraspinal muscles is necessary for proper assessment of radiculopathy. Normal paraspinal NEE findings do not rule out the presence of a radiculopathy because reinnervation to the paraspinal muscles may have already occurred or the pathology may involve only anterior ramus fibers. Precise localization of a specific nerve root involved in a radiculopathy is difficult to determine based on the presence of paraspinal abnormalities alone due to the overlapping innervation of most paraspinal muscles. Therefore, identifying the specific abnormal nerve root is most accurately accomplished by finding abnormalities in limb muscles in a myotomal distribution, and it is important to sample limb muscles supplied by the nerve root(s) in question as well as muscles supplied by nerve roots above and below. A study is said to be positive if abnormalities are present in two or more muscles receiving innervation from the same nerve root, preferably from different peripheral nerves.[66] While the primary innervation of

Table 2.   Minimal Screen Needle Electromyographic Examination

Upper Extremity		Lower Extremity	
Muscle	*Root Level*	*Muscle*	*Root Level*
Cervical paraspinal muscles	C4–T2	Lumbosacral paraspinal muscles	L1–S1
Deltoid	C5, C6	Quadriceps femoris	L2, L3, L4
Biceps brachii	C6, C6	Gluteus medius	L4, L5, S1
Triceps	C6, C7, C8	Tibialis anterior	L4, L5, S1
Extensor carpi radialis	C6, C7, C8	Peroneus longus	L5, S1
Flexor carpi radialis	C6, C7, C8	Medial gastrocnemius	S1, S2
Pronator teres	C6, C7	Lateral Gastrocnemius	L5, S1, S2
Thenar muscles	C8, T1	Extensor hallucis longus	L5, S1
Dorsal interossei	C8, T1		
Hypothenar muscles	C8, T1		

If the diagnosis is unclear, additional muscles should be investigated. In the paraspinal regions, the root level designations refer to the bony level that should be examined, ie, the multifidi muscle layer.

many muscles remains debatable, myotomal maps are helpful as approximate guides (Table 2).

SPINAL NERVE ROOT STIMULATION

It is possible to directly stimulate the spinal nerve roots using an EMG needle as the stimulating cathode.[67,68] Recording from the biceps brachii allows evaluation of the C5-C6 nerve roots, upper trunk, lateral cord, and musculocutaneous nerve.[69] A normal side-to-side latency difference is less than 0.6 msec.[70] Nerve roots from C6-C8 are evaluated by recording from the biceps, and it is difficult to exactly localize specific nerve roots involving these levels. The posterior divisions and posterior cord of the brachial plexus can also be evaluated with this technique.[71] Stimulation of the C8-T1 nerve roots is one of the more commonly performed nerve root stimulation procedures. It is helpful in evaluating the C8-T1 nerve roots, lower trunk, and medial cord of the brachial plexus and is often useful in the evaluation of a patient suspected of having thoracic outlet syndrome because it provides objective electrophysiologic means of evaluating the involved neurologic structures.[72] Normal values for side-to-side latency and amplitude differences are conservatively less than 1.0 msec and 20%, respectively.[73,74] Limitations to this method include its relatively invasive and uncomfortable nature, risk of injury to spinal or neurovascular structures, difficulty in determining the exact site of neural stimulation, and potential for technical factors to result in abnormal side-to-side results and thereby produce false positive findings.

SOMATOSENSORY EVOKED POTENTIALS

SSEPs have been used increasingly in recent years to evaluate the function of peripheral and central sensory pathways.[75] They are elicited by electrical stimulation of an accessible mixed or cutaneous nerve or of the skin in the territory of a particular nerve or nerve root and are conceptualized as NCSs over a

SHORT-LATENCY SSEPs

MEDIAN NERVE

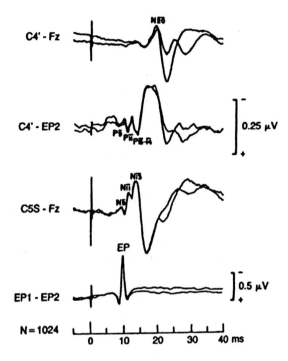

Figure 8. Evoked potential tracings from the median nerve. The different peaks of the evoked potentials are assessed and compared side to side and against normal values. (From the AAEM Glossary of Terms in Neurodiagnostic Medicine. Muscle Nerve, Supplement no. 10, 2001; with permission.)

relatively long portion of both the peripheral and central nervous systems[76] (Fig. 8). They are helpful in evaluating patients with suspected sensory root lesions because they provide a means of studying sensory function in proximal portions of the peripheral nervous system. Limitations to their use include the potential masking of any focal slowing of conduction by the long distance between the site of peripheral stimulation and the site at which the response is recorded. Focal conduction block in some fibers may be undetected because conduction in the unaffected fibers generates a normal response. Additionally, precise localization of a lesion is very limited. SSEP abnormalities provide little clue to the nature or age of a lesion involving the sensory pathways. Normal individuals may have up to 70% variation of amplitude between one trial and another for the same nerve or from one side to the other.[77,78] With proper technique and preparation, SSEPs are no more difficult to obtain than routine peripheral sensory NCSs. Waveforms can be recorded from the peripheral nerve, spinal cord, or sensory cortex following peripheral stimulation of a sensory nerve, mixed nerve, or dermatomal location. Standard locations for electrode placement have been recommended by the American Electroencephalographic Society. Short-latency responses are defined as waveforms occurring within approximately 25 msec of upper extremity stimulus in normal people and within approximately 50 msec following lower extremity stimulation.[79,80]

Table 3. Upper Extremity Dermatomal/Segmental SSEPs

Nerve	Cord	Trunk	Segment	Latency (N$\overline{2}$0)
Musculocutaneous (forearm)	Lateral	Upper	C6	17.4 ± 1.2
Median (digit 1)	Lateral	Upper	C6	22.5 ± 1.1
Median (digits 2 and 3)	Lateral	Middle	C7	21.2 ± 1.2
Superficial radial (digit 1)	Posterior	Upper	C6	22.5 ± 1.1
Ulnar (digit 5)	Medial	Lower	C8	22.5 ± 1.1

Modified from Eisen A, Hoirch M: Electrodiagnostic evaluation of radiculopathies and plexopathies using somatosensory evoked potentials. Electroencephalogr Clin Neurophysiol 1982;36(Suppl): 349–357. Eisen A: The use of somatosensory evoked potentials for the evaluation of the peripheral nervous system. Neurol Clin 1988;6:825–838.

Dermatomal/segmental SSEPs (Table 3) are relatively easy to perform but remain controversial in the diagnosis of nerve root injury, and there are questions regarding the sensitivity and specificity of these studies.[81–89] In Dumitru's opinion, cervical root lesions are not particularly amenable to diagnostic SSEPs and frankly positive needle EMG findings have been accompanied by completely symmetric cortical SSEPs in the face of obvious clinical motor and sensory findings.[90] The diagnostic yield of SSEPs appears to be somewhat higher in the lumbosacral region,[91–93] but controversies on the usefulness of these studies in the diagnosis of radiculopathy still exist.[94,95] A detailed review of the literature failed to identify any studies evaluating the sensitivity, specificity, or efficacy of SSEPs in whiplash injuries. In general, patients with pain and paresthesias who lack abnormal neurologic signs have normal median, ulnar, or radial SSEPs, and only rarely among patients with objective evidence of root compression is the mixed nerve SSEP abnormal when the NEE is normal.[96] Therefore, routine performance of mixed nerve SSEPs in particular as part of the standard evaluation of the individual with whiplash injury has not been established and cannot be recommended.

QUANTITATIVE SENSORY TESTING

Lesions that involve small, unmyelinated sensory fibers or that occur proximal to the dorsal root ganglion may go undetected by NCS, EMG, and SSEP techniques, which evaluate only the large-diameter, myelinated motor and sensory fibers.[97] Various QST methods theoretically offer means by which different sensory nerve populations can be evaluated.[98,99] Controlled, prospective studies using QST in the evaluation of acute neuromusculoskeletal injuries are lacking, and there is still controversy regarding the usefulness of QST,[100] but QST appears to hold promise in the evaluation of individuals who present with sensory complaints and pain. A recent article by Mironer et al[101] demonstrated 80% positive QST results but there was a lack of correlation between changes in pain scores and sensory test results in a group of patients with clinical radiculopathy following treatment with epidural steroid injections. BenEliyahu at al[102] identified a statistically significant correlation between magnetic resonance imaging findings and QST in a group of patients with signs and symptoms of cervical and lumbosacral intervertebral disc disease. Other studies[103-105] identified changes in QST findings following spinal anesthesia. While this literature raises intriguing possibilities regarding the potential use of this technology in the clinical setting and the Texas Workers Compensation Commission recently incorporated QST measures into its spinal treatment guidelines,[106] it is the author's opinion that there appears to be insufficient clinical research to support its routine use in the standard evaluation of patients with whiplash mechanism injuries. Additional, well-designed, prospective clinical studies evaluating the usefulness and efficacy of QST are necessary before it is incorporated into the routine electrodiagnostic evaluation of acute neuromusculoskeletal injuries.

SURFACE ELECTROMYOGRAPHY
Surface EMG refers to recording of electrophysiologic signals from skeletal muscles using surface recording electrodes. Summated muscle electrical activity is observed when muscles are activated or contracting. A technology review approved by the American Association of Electrodiagnostic Medicine and endorsed by the American Academy of Physical Medicine and Rehabilitation in 1995 concluded that there are no clinical indications for the use of sEMG in the diagnosis and treatment of disorders of nerve or muscle.[107] Surface EMG studies are more routinely used as components of gait and motion analysis and have considerable potential in the evaluation of movement, ergonomics, and kinesiology. At this time, there appears to be little evidence to support their use in the routine diagnostic evaluation of acute radiculopathy, plexopathy, peripheral nerve injury, or other acute neuromusculoskeletal injury.[108]

CONCLUSIONS
Electrodiagnostic studies assist in identifying and quantifying injuries to nerve roots, plexuses, and peripheral nerves using techniques as identified and described above. Cervical radiculopathies, brachial plexopathies, and peripheral nerve injuries are certainly of primary concern when evaluating the individual with neck and upper extremity complaints following a whiplash mechanism injury. Cervical radiculopathies are most commonly identified by finding needle EMG abnormalities in the cervical paraspinal muscles or in limb muscles in a myotomal distribution.[109] Sensory NCSs are typically normal in cervical radiculopathies. Table 4 summarizes neurophysiologic changes in radicular lesions.

Any abnormalities of sensory nerve function should raise the possibility of a lesion distal to the dorsal root ganglion and should lead the electrodiagnostic consultant to search diligently for the possibility of a brachial plexopathy or peripheral nerve pathology.[110] Reduced motor amplitudes may be seen in severe radiculopathies, but focal conduction block or segmental slowing of motor conduction velocities should also suggest the possibility of a lesion or lesions distal to the nerve root. Brachial plexus or peripheral nerve injuries should be suspected when motor or sensory amplitudes are abnormal and/or when needle EMG abnormalities are present in the distribution of a peripheral nerve or portion of the brachial plexus and not in a myotomal distribution. Therefore, intimate knowledge of brachial plexus anatomy and physiology (Figs. 9, 10 and Table 5) and the various electrodiagnostic techniques available to evaluate the various portions of the brachial plexus is essential when performing

Table 4. Neurophysiologic Changes in Radicular Lesions

	< 1 Week	1–6 Weeks	6 Weeks to 3 Months	> 3 Months
SNAP	Normal	Normal	Normal	Normal
CMAP	Normal	Reduced	Reduced	Reduced
M. NCV	Normal	Minor reduction	Minor reduction	Minor reduction
H-reflex	Prolonged or absent	Prolonged or absent	Prolonged or absent	Prolonged or absent
F-wave	Prolonged or absent	Prolonged or absent	Prolonged or absent	Prolonged or absent
SEPs	Prolonged or absent, decreased amplitude	Prolonged or absent, decreased amplitude	Prolonged or absent, decreased amplitude	Prolonged or absent, decreased amplitude
Fibs/PSW	Absent	Present in proximal muscles first (7 d in paraspinal muscles) and then in distal muscles (3–5 wk; > 300 µV)	Present	Decreased numbers and small amplitude (< 100–200 µV)
Fascics	Rare	Rare	Rare	Rare
CRD	Absent	Absent	Absent	Present but rare
MUAPs*	Reduced recruitment	Reduced recruitment; may see increased numbers of poly-phasic potentials	Reduced re-recruitment; with increased duration, ampli-tude, and poly-phasics	Essentially the same as 6 wk to 3 mo

M. NCV indicates motor nerve conduction velocity; Fibs/PSW, fibrillation potentials and positive sharp waves; fascics, fasciculation potentials; CRD, complex repetitive discharges. This table is only a rough approximation and may vary with individual patients.
* Data obtained with quantitative motor unit analysis only.
Modified from Albers JW: Common EMG problems. In AAEM Course A: Fundamentals of EMG (Fifth Annual Continuing Education Course). Rochester, Minnesota, 1982, pp 59–67.

electrodiagnostic studies. NCSs, particularly sensory conduction studies, are generally abnormal with all but the mildest axon loss brachial plexopathies.[111] Table 6 summarizes electrophysiologic changes seen in plexopathies.

A detailed review of the literature identified a paucity of information on electrodiagnosis and whiplash injuries and failed to identify any studies that support the routine performance of bilateral needle EMG or NCSs in the standard evaluation of the individual with whiplash mechanism injuries. Only when bilateral symptoms or signs are present, or when multilevel abnormalities are documented on the symptomatic side, is there a good chance that bilateral disease is present. Therefore, there seems to be little justification for the routine performance of bilateral studies in patients presenting with unilateral complaints when electrophysiologic findings are normal in the symptomatic extremity. A thorough and thoughtful electrodiagnostic study, as an extension of a detailed history and physical examination, can be an important and useful component of the proper evaluation of the individual with a whiplash mechanism injury.

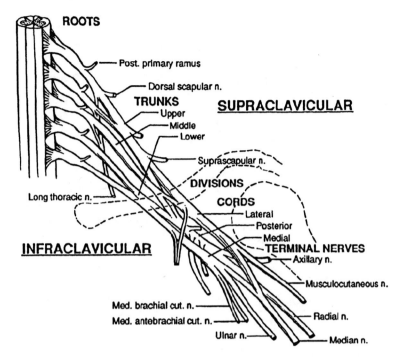

Figure 9. The brachial plexus and its relation to the clavicle and humeral head. (From Wilbourn AJ: Brachial plexus disorders. In Dyck PJ, Thomas PK (eds): Peripheral Neuropathy, 3rd ed. Philadelphia, WB Saunders, 1993; with permission.)

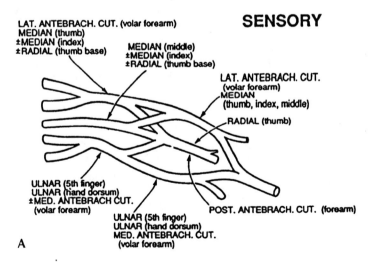

Figure 10. Components of the brachial plexus assessed by the various **A,** sensory and **B,** motor nerve conduction studies. "Unusual" conduction studies must be performed to assess some portions, especially the upper trunk. (From Wilbourn AJ: Brachial plexus disorders. In Dyck PJ, Thomas PK (eds): Peripheral Neuropathy, 3rd ed. Philadelphia, WB Saunders, 1993; with permission.) *(B shown on next page.)*

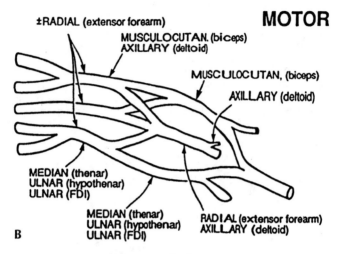

MOTOR

Figure 10B (Cont.).

Table 5.   Nerve Conduction Studies

| | Brachial Plexus | | |
	Trunk	Cord	Peripheral Nerves
Sensory studies	Upper	Lateral	Lateral antebrachial cutaneous
	Upper	Lateral	Median to first/second digit
	Upper	Posterior	Radial to base of first digit
	Middle	Posterior	Posterior antebrachial cutaneous
	Middle	Lateral	Median to second digit
	Middle	Lateral	Median to third digit
	Lower	Medial	Ulnar to fifth digit
	Lower	Medial	Ulnar: dorsal ulnar cutaneous
	Lower	Medial	Medial antebrachial cutaneous
Motor studies	Upper	Lateral	Musculocutaneous
	Upper	Posterior	Axillary
	Upper		Suprascapular
	Middle	Posterior	Radial
	Lower	Medial	Median
	Lower	Medial	Ulnar

Modified from Wilbourn AJ: Electrodiagnosis of plexopathies. Neurol Clin 1985;3:511–529.

Table 6.   Sequence of Electrophysiologic Changes

	Abnormality	Onset	Peak
Nerve conduction studies			
SNAP	Decreased amplitude	5–6 d	9–10 d
CMAP	Decreased amplitude	2–4 d	6–7 d
Needle electromyography			
Rest activity	Increased insertional activity	≥ 7–8 d	—
	PSW and fibrillation potentials	10–30 d	21–30 d
Voluntary activity	Decreased recruitment	Immediately	—

PSW indicates positive sharp wave.
Modified from Wilbourn AJ: Electrodiagnosis of plexopathies. Neurol Clin 1985;3:511–529.

References

1. Cole A, Herring S (eds): The Low Back Pain Handbook: A Practical Guide For The Primary Care Clinician. Philadelphia, Hanley & Belfus, 1997.
2. DeLisa J (ed): Rehabilitation Medicine: Principles and Practice. Philadelphia, JB Lippincott, 1988.
3. Dumitru D: Electrodiagnostic Medicine. Philadelphia, Hanley & Belfus, 1995.
4. Malanga G (ed): Cervical flexion-extension/whiplash injuries. Spine State Art Rev 12(2), 1998.
5. Reference deleted.
6. American Association of Electrodiagnostic Medicine: Guidelines in electrodiagnostic medicine. Muscle Nerve (suppl 8), 1999.
7. Lambert EH: Neurophysiological techniques useful in the study of neuromuscular disorders. In Adams, RD, Eaton, LM, Shy G (eds): Neuromuscular Disorders. Baltimore, Williams & Wilkins, 1960, pp 247–273.
8. Martinez AC, Perez Conde M, DelCampo F, et al: Ratio between the amplitude of sensory evoked potentials at the wrist in both hands of left-handed subjects. J Neurol Neurosurg Psychiatry 43:182–184, 1980.
9. Reference deleted.
10. Kimura J: Electrodiagnosis in Diseases of Nerve and Muscle: Principles and Practice, 2nd ed. Philadelphia, FA Davis, 1989.
11. Reference deleted.
12. Reference deleted.
13. Kimura J: F-wave determination in nerve conduction studies. In Desmedt JE (ed): Motor Control Mechanisms in Health and Disease. New York, Raven Press, 1983, pp 961–975.
14. Fisher MA: F response latency determination. Muscle Nerve 5:730–734, 1982.
15. Reference deleted.
16. Panayiotopoulos CP, Scarpalezos S, Nastas PE: F-wave studies on the deep peroneal nerve. J Neurol Sci 31:319–329, 1977.
17. Aminoff MJ, Goodin DS, Parry GJ: Electrophysiologic evaluation of lumbosacral radiculopathies: electromyography, late responses, and somatosensory evoked potentials. Neurology 34:1514–1518, 1985.
18. Young RR, Shahani BT: Clinical value and limitations of F-wave determination. Muscle Nerve 1:248–249, 1978.
19. Reference deleted.
20. Eisen A: Electrodiagnosis of radiculopathies. Neurol Clin 3:495–510, 1985.
21. Jabre JF: Surface recording of the H-reflex of the flexor carpi ulnaris. Muscle Nerve 4:435–438, 1981.
22. Jankus WR, Robinson LR, Little JW: Normal limits of side-to-side H-reflex amplitude variability. Arch Phys Med Rehabil 75:3–7, 1994.
23. Nishida T, Kompoliti A, Janssen I, Levin KF: H reflex I S-1 radiculopathy: latency versus amplitude controversy revisited. Muscle Nerve 19:915–917, 1996.
24. Schuchmann J: H-reflex latency in radiculopathy. Arch Phys Med Rehabil 59:185–187, 1978.
25. Falco FJE, Hennessey WJ, Goldbert G, et al: H reflex latency in the healthy elderly. Muscle Nerve 17:161-167, 1994.
26. Reference deleted.
27. Scarberry S, AlHakim M, Jatirji B: H-reflex amplitude in the healthy elderly. Muscle Nerve 17:1350–1351, 1994.
28. Wilbourn AJ: The value and limitations of electromyographic examination in the diagnosis of lumbosacral radiculopathy. In Hardy RW (ed): Lumbar Disc Disease. New York, Raven Press, 1982, pp 65–109.
29. Aminoff MJ: Electromyography in Clinical Practice, 3rd ed. New York, Churchill Livingstone, 1998.
30. Reference deleted.
31. Kuruoglu R, Oh SJ, Thompson B: Clinical and electromyographic correlations of lumbosacral radiculopathy. Muscle Nerve 17:250–251, 1994.
32. Goodgold J, Eberstein A: Electrodiagnosis of Neuromuscular Diseases, 3rd ed. Baltimore, Williams & Wilkins, 1983.
33. Reference deleted.
34. Wiechers DO: Mechanically provoked insertional activity before and after nerve section in rats. Arch Phys Med Rehabil 58:402–405, 1977.
35. Wiechers DO, Stow R, Johnson EW: Electromyographic insertional activity mechanically provoked in the biceps brachii. Arch Phys Med Rehabil 58:573–578, 1977.

36. Reference deleted.
37. Elmqvist D, Johns TR, Thesleff S: A study of some electrophysiological properties of human intercostal muscle. J Physiol 154:602–607, 1960.
38. Elmqvist D, Hofmann WW, Kugelberg J, Quastel DMJ: An electrophysiological investigation of neuromuscular transmission in myasthenia gravis. J Physiol 174:417–434, 1964.
39. Elmqvist D, Quastel DMJ: A quantitative study of endplate potentials in isolated human muscle. J Physiol 1965;178:505–529.
40. Reference deleted.
41. Reference deleted.
42. Reference deleted.
43. Buchthal F, Rosenfalck P: Spontaneous electrical activity of human muscle. Electroencephalogr Clin Neurophysiol 20:321–336, 1966.
44. Buchthal F: Fibrillations: clinical electrophysiology. In Culp WJ, Ochoa J (eds): Abnormal Nerves and Muscle Generators. New York, Oxford University Press, 1982, pp 632–662.
45. Thesleff S: Physiological effects of denervation of muscle. Ann N Y Acad Sci 228:89–103, 1974.
46. Emeryk B, Hausmanowa-Petrusewicz I, Nowak T: Spontaneous volleys of bizarre high frequency potentials in neuromuscular diseases. Electromyogr Clin Neurophysiol 14:339–354, 1974.
47. Brumlik J, Dreschler B, Vannin TM: The myotonic discharge in various neurological syndromes: neurophysiologic analysis. Electromyography 10:369–383, 1970.
48. Brown WF: The Physiological and Technical Basis of Electromyography. Boston, Butterworth, 1984.
49. Litchy WJ: A practical demonstration of EMG activity. In AAEM Course C: Standard Needle Electromyography of Muscles. Rochester, MN, American Association of Electrodiagnostic Medicine, 1988, pp 23–33.
50. Daube JA, Kelly JJ, Martin RA: Facial myokymia with polyradiculoneuropathy. Neurology 29:662–669, 1979.
51. Stalberg EV, Trontelj JV: Abnormal discharges generated within the motor unit as observed with single-fiber electromyography. In Culp WJ, Ochoa J (eds): Abnormal Nerves and Muscles as Impulse Generators. New York, Oxford University Press, 1982, pp 445–474.
52. Albers JW, Allen AA, Bastron JD, et al: Limb myokymia. Muscle Nerve 4:494–504, 1981.
53. Clamann HP: Activity of single motor units during isometric tension. Neurology 20:254–260, 1970.
54. Petajan JH: Clinical electromyographic studies of diseases of the motor unit. Electroencephalogr Clin Neurophysiol 36:395–401, 1974.
55. Warmolts JR, Engel WK: Open-biopsy electromyography. I. Correction of motor unit behavior with histochemical muscle fiber type in human limb muscle. Arch Neurol 27:512–517, 1972.
56. Clairmont AC, Johnson EW: Evaluation of the patient with possible radiculopathy. In Johnson EW, Pease WS (eds): Practical Electromyography, 3rd ed. Baltimore, William & Wilkins 1997, pp 115–130.
57. Eisen A: Electrodiagnosis of radiculopathies. Neurol Clin 3:495–510, 1985.
58. Wilbourn A, Aminoff M: AAEM Minimonograph No. 32: The Electrodiagnostic Examination in Patients with Radiculopathies. Rochester, MN, American Association of Electrodiagnostic Medicine, 1998.
59. Petajan J: AAEM Minimonograph No. 3: Motor Unit Recruitment. Rochester, MN, American Association of Electrodiagnostic Medicine, 1991.
60. Reference deleted.
61. Reference deleted.
62. Reference deleted.
63. Reference deleted.
64. Reference deleted.
65. Dillingham TR, Lauder TD, Andary M, et al: Identification of cervical radiculopathies: optimizing the electromyographic screen. Am J Phys Med Rehabil 80:84–91, 2001.
66. Reference delted.
67. Cherington M: Long thoracic nerve. Conduction studies. Dis Nerv Syst 33:49–51, 1972.
68. Davis FA: Impairment of repetitive impulse conduction in experimentally demyelinated and pressure injured nerves. J Neurol Neurosurg Psychiatry 35:537–544, 1972.
69. Hollinshead WH: Anatomy for Surgeons: The Back and Limbs, 3rd ed. Philadelphia, Harper & Row, 1982.
70. MacLean IC: Spinal nerve stimulation. In AAEM Course B: Nerve Conduction Studies–A Review. Rochester, MN, American Association of Electrodiagnostic Medicine, 1988.
71. Reference deleted.

72. Reference deleted.
73. Reference delted.
74. Dawson GD, Merton PA: "Recurrent" discharges from motoneurons [abstract of communications]. Brussels, Twentieth International Congress of Physiology, 1956, pp 221–222.
75. Reference deleted.
76. Reference delted.
77. Aminoff MJ, Goodin DS, Barbaro NM, et al: Dermatomal somatosensory evoked potentials in unilateral lumbosacral radiculopathy. Ann Neurol 17:171–176, 1985.
78. Aminoff MJ: Use of somatosensory evoked potentials to evaluate the peripheral nervous system. J Clin Neurophysiol 4:135–144, 1987.
79. American Electroencephalographic Society: Recommended standards for short-latency somatosensory evoked potentials. J Clin Neurophysiol 1:41–53, 1984.
80. American Electroencephalographic Society: Recommended standards for the clinical practice of evoked potentials. J Clin Neurophysiol 1:6–14, 1984.
81. Reference deleted.
82. Reference deleted.
83. Aminoff MJ, Goodin DS: Dermatomal somatosensory evoked potentials in lumbosacral root compression [letter]. J Neurol Neurosurg Psychiatry 51:740–741, 1988.
84. Aminoff MF: Evoked potential studies in neurological diagnosis and management. Ann Neurol 28:706–710, 1990.
85. Eisen A, Elleker G: Sensory nerve stimulation and evoked cerebral potentials. Neurology 30:1097–1105, 1980.
86. Eisen A, Hoirch M, Moll A: Evaluation of radiculopathies by segmental stimulation and somatosensory evoked potentials. Can J Neurol Sci 10:178–182, 1983.
87. Eisen A: Electrodiagnosis of radiculopathies. Neurol Clin 3:495–510, 1985.
88. Perlik S. Fisher MA, Patel DV, Slack C: On the usefulness of somatosensory evoked responses for the evaluation of lower back pain. Arch Neurol 43:907–913, 1986.
89. Rodriquez AA, Kanis L, Rodriquez AA, et al: Somatosensory evoked potentials from dermatomal stimulation as an indicator of L5 and S1 radiculopathy. Arch Phys Med Rehabil 68:366–368, 1987.
90. Reference deleted.
91. Reference deleted.
92. Scarff TB, Dallman DE, Toleikis JR, Bunch WH: Dermatomal somatosensory evoked potentials in the diagnosis of lumbar root entrapment. Surg Forum 32:488–491, 1981.
93. Walk D, Fisher MA, Doundoulakis SH, Hemmati M: Somatosensory evoked responses in the evaluation of lumbosacral radiculopathy. Neurology 43:1197–1202, 1991.
94. Dumitru D, Dreyfuss P: Dermatomal/segmental somatosensory evoked potential evaluation of L5/S1 unilateral/unilevel radiculopathies. Muscle Nerve 19:442–449, 1996.
95. Seyal M, Sandhu LS, Mack YP: Spinal segmental somatosensory evoked potentials in lumbosacral radiculopathies. Neurology 39:801–805, 1989.
96. Reference deleted.
97. Reference deleted.
98. Zhu PY, Starr A: Neuroselective CPT evaluation in syringomyelia. Presented at NA Spine Society, Washington, DC, 1995.
99. Lius, Kopacz DJ: Quantitative assessment of differential sensory nerve block after lidocaine spinal anesthesia. Anesthesia 83:60–63, 1995.
100. Technology review: the Neurometer Current Perception Threshold (CPT). AAEM Equipment and Computer Committee. American Association of Electrodiagnostic Medicine. Muscle Nerve 22:523–531, 1991.
101. Mironer YE, Somerville JJ: The current perception threshold evaluation in radiculopathy: efficacy in diagnosis and assessment of the treatment results. Pain Digest 8:37–38, 1998.
102. BenEliyahu DH, Tartaglia SV, Spinelle R: Assessment: current perception threshold/quantitative sensory testing and MRI findings in patients with signs and symptoms of cervical or lumbar disc herniation: a correlative study of the neurosensory diagnosis of discogenic pain. Am J Pain Manage 10:2, 2000
103. Tay B, Wallace M, Irving G: Quantitative assessment of differential sensory blockade after lumbar epidural lidocaine. J Anesth Analg 84:10751–10755, 1997.
104. Liu S, Kopacz D, Carpenter R: Quantitative assessment of differential sensory nerve block after lidocaine spinal anesthesia. Anesthesiology 82:60–63, 1995.
105. Sakura S, Sumi M, Yamada Y, et al: Quantitative and selective assessment of sensory block during lumbar epidural anesthesia with 1% or 2% lidocaine. Br J Anaesth 81:718–722, 1998.

106. Adopted amendments to §134.1001 (Spine Treatment Guideline). Adopted at the 12/2/99 public meting and scheduled to be published12/17/99 in the Texas Register. Effective date: 2/1/00.
107. Reference deleted.
108. Pullman SL, Goodin DS, Marquinez AI: Clinical utility of surface EMG: report of the therapeutics and technology assessment subcommittee of the American Academy of Neurology. Neurology 55:171–177, 2000.
109. Reference deleted.
110. Reference deleted.
111. Wilbourn AJ: Brachial plexus disorders. In Dyck PJ, Thomas PK (eds): Peripheral Neuropathy, 3rd ed. Philadelphia, WB Saunders, 1993.

18
Rehabilitation of Whiplash Injuries

Todd A. Edelson, M.A., P.T., Dip. MDT

The term *whiplash* was first introduced in 1928 by the American orthopedist H. E. Crowe.[10] It was defined as the effects of sudden acceleration-deceleration forces on the neck and upper trunk due to external forces exerting a "lash-like effect." In 1995, The Quebec Task Force on Whiplash-Associated Disorders (WADs) redefined whiplash as follows: "Whiplash is an acceleration-deceleration mechanism of energy transfer to the neck which may result from rear-end or side impact, predominantly in motor vehicle collisions, but also from diving accidents, and from other mishaps." The energy transfer may result in bony or soft tissue injuries (whiplash injury), which in turn may lead to a wide variety of clinical manifestations (whiplash-associated disorders),[52] most commonly neck pain (88–100%) and headache (54–66%). Other symptoms include neck stiffness, shoulder pain, arm pain and numbness, paresthesia, weakness, dysphagia, visual and auditory symptoms, and dizziness.[26,39,47]

The Quebec Task Force on Whiplash-Associated Disorders reported that more than 10,000 studies focusing on whiplash and neck sprain injuries have been published.[52] Borchgrevink et al[5] reported that the studies cited by the Quebec Task Force recommended various types of treatment for acute-onset injuries, including analgesics, sedatives, antihistamines, nonsteroidal anti-inflammatory medications, antidepressives, codeine, muscle relaxants, and local anesthetic injections. The efficacy of other conservative treatments is still under debate, including local heat and ice treatment, neck collar immobilization, ultrasound, traction, (active) mobilization, exercises, pulsed electromagnetic therapy, and multimodal rehabilitation. In a recent systematic review of clinical trials, Peeters et al[45] reported that despite the many treatments available for patients with whiplash injury, there continues to be no evidence for their accepted use. The investigators cautiously concluded that active interventions have a tendency to be more effective for patients with whiplash injuries. The reason for the caution was the overall poor methodology of the available studies. To date, the literature does not support the use of passive modalities for the treatment of whiplash disorders.[45,65] Because these modalities appear to have limited or palliative value, this chapter focuses on the rationale for the use of active interventions, their application, and the safe progression of treatment programs.

A number of physical therapy modalities are employed in managing pain of musculoskeletal origin. These can be broadly categorized as electrotherapeutic (eg, transcutaneous electrical nerve stimulation [TENS], interferential therapy), thermal (eg, moist heat, ultrasound, ice), manual therapies (eg, manipulation or massage), and exercise. There are many specific therapies or specific dosage regimens that have not been subjected to scientific investigation. In adopting an evidence-based approach to patient management, the physical therapist must select those therapeutic modalities for which there is scientific evidence indicating effectiveness.[65]

PHYSICAL THERAPY MODALITIES

Electrotherapy Modalities

Electrical stimulation is used to produce sensory effects or to facilitate motor function. By varying the parameters of frequency, waveform, pulse duration electrode placement or configuration, and duration of stimulation, it is possible to produce a range of therapeutic effects. **TENS** and **interferential therapy** are two forms of electrical stimulation commonly used for pain control. With regard to treatment of musculoskeletal pain, clinical studies show mixed results and few studies compare the effects to placebo treatment.

Many studies do not standardize the stimulus parameters of TENS, making interpretation between groups and studies difficult.[65] Deyo et al[11] compared the effects of TENS with those of placebo TENS (with and without exercise) in patients with chronic low back pain. The effects were the same in the TENS group and placebo TENS group. However, the parameters were not standardized, and other modalities such as hot packs were used. In contrast, animal models of inflammation have shown that TENS partially reduces hyperalgesia at the site of injury.[20]

Interferential therapy is thought to have a similar mechanism of action to that of TENS, through activating the descending pain-inhibitory systems. In addition, it is thought to have a positive influence on blood flow, which may contribute to tissue healing.[40] The evidence base for determining clinical effectiveness of interferential therapy is less compelling than that for TENS. In a study by van der Heijden et al, there was no additional benefit for interferential therapy and exercise beyond that produced by exercise therapy alone in the management of patients with musculoskeletal pain in the shoulder region at 12-month follow-up.[57] Although interferential therapy has the potential for providing stimulation of deep musculoskeletal structures, the evidence base to determine the effectiveness of the intervention is not adequate. The studies that have been reported do not suggest significant therapeutic benefit.[65]

Thermal Modalities

The use of thermal modalities to relieve musculoskeletal pain is common. The most common method of delivering superficial heat is **moist heat** pack application. The physiologic effects of heat have been studied thoroughly; heat increases skin and joint temperature and blood flow and decreases joint stiffness.[43,53] The use of superficial heat has been studied by several different groups, with little support for its use in the treatment of painful conditions.[65] Toomey et al studied patients with Colles fractures and compared warm whirlpool baths with exercise to exercise alone and found no difference between groups, although each group had increased range of motion and decreased pain.[53] No difference between groups was observed when superficial heat was compared with cold treatment. Thus, there is little evidence to support the use of superficial heat in the treatment of musculoskeletal pain. However, outcome measures have been limited, and the quality of trials needs to be improved.[65]

Therapeutic **ultrasound**, as a modality for pain relief, is applied through the skin overlying the painful area. Ultrasound preferentially heats deeper tissues, and the effects are not normally perceived by the patient, making placebo-controlled studies relatively easy. Heating occurs predominantly at tissue interfaces.[65] Several studies have examined the effects of ultrasound for a variety of musculoskeletal conditions.[13,42,59] In a double-blind, randomized trial, Downing and Weinstein found no difference in pain relief, range of motion, or functional activities between sham ultrasound and ultrasound in patients with shoulder pain.[13] In two nonrandomized studies with blind evaluators, ultrasound was compared with other noninvasive physical modalities, such as ice, TENS, superficial heat, and massage. There was no difference between groups, although significant pain relief occurred with all treatments.[39,42] There is more evidence to support the use of ultrasound, although all heating modalities showed similar short-term effects with little long-term carry-over.[66]

Manual Therapy

Massage techniques encompass a wide range of procedures designed to mobilize soft tissues, specifically skin and underlying muscle tissue. Massage is considered to have a number of beneficial physiologic effects that may contribute to tissue repair, pain modulation, and relaxation.[20] At this stage, there is no evidence to suggest that massage produces effects superior to those of other physical modalities. Although massage may have a number of beneficial physiologic effects, the available research does not clearly demonstrate that these effects translate into beneficial clinical outcomes.[66]

PHYSIOLOGY OF TISSUE HEALING

An understanding of the mechanism of healing is essential if we are to have a positive influence on the repair of damaged tissue following injury. Hardy[23] states that "a knowledge of wound healing and repair enables the clinician to design and implement treatment regimens based on scar biology. Understanding the sequence of repair permits flexibility in management as the wound changes." Because mechanical therapy uses the principles of repeated movement and graded force based on clinical presentation, it fits the criteria of flexibility necessary for the management of an injured structure that is undergoing repair.

A basic understanding of the biology of the healing process is necessary prior to a discussion of treatment modalities and the effects they may have on healing tissues. The three stages of tissue healing are well defined in the literature and include the following: (1) the inflammatory phase, (2) the fibroplastic phase, and (3) the remodeling phase.[8,15,23]

Phase 1—The inflammatory phase is characterized by a period of inflammation that prepares the area for healing by increasing blood flow through the release of chemicals such as prostaglandins and histamines. In addition, peripheral neutrophils and then monocytes migrate into the wound.[8] These cells destroy

bacteria and maintain a clean environment for healing to continue. Mast cells release proteoglycans that help bind the wound. The final stage of the inflammatory process is neovascularization, which brings increased oxygen to the damaged area. For healing to commence, two prerequisite events must occur:
- The wound must be decontaminated (phagocytosis).
- A new blood supply (neovascularization) must then be available.[23]

Phase II—The fibroplastic phase is characterized by the laying down of collagen by fibroblasts and the formation of scar tissue. The purpose of this phase is to impart strength to the wound. The fibroblasts synthesize collagen simultaneously with epithelialization and wound contraction. Wound contraction is carried out by a specialized cell called a myofibroblast and serves to close the damaged tissue. If the wound is not closed by 14 to 21 days postinjury, contraction stops because of the restraint of the surrounding stretched tissue. In addition to collagen production, the fibroblasts also synthesize glycosaminoglycans (GAGs), which fill in the space in and around collagen fibers. This GAG ground substance, combined with water, provides lubrication and acts as a spacer between moving collagen fibers.[23] Akeson et al[1] have demonstrated that immobilization causes a loss of ground substance. Therefore, mobilization of the wound during this phase is essential. Hardy[23] states: "When this important buffer interface [GAG] is diminished, new cross-links are formed, rendering mobile tissue immobile." It is believed that the composition of this nonfibrous substance is also related to the amount and location of cross-links formed; therefore, a relationship between GAG ground substance and collagen dictates scar architecture. The classification of connective tissue is determined by the ratio of collagen (tensile strength) to proteoglycans (compressive strength) in the extracellular matrix, which is determined in part by the mechanical environment of the tissue.[25,30] The mechanical environment is especially important during the final two stages of healing, when the architectural make-up of the tissue is being formed.[23] The forming tissues adapt their structure and composition, and therefore their length and extensibility, in response to the forces and movements they experience.[25,29]

Phase III—The remodeling phase provides the final form to the scar. The process of scar remodeling continues for up to 12 months or more, as collagen turnover allows the randomly deposited scar tissues to be rearranged in linear and lateral orientation.[15,23,62] It is during the fibroplastic and remodeling phases that mechanical therapy can have the greatest benefit on healing tissue. The amount of scar to be remodeled is inversely related to the return of function.[15,23] There are two theories to explain the repair of damaged tissue by collagen synthesis. The induction theory proposes that scar formation attempts to mimic the characteristics of the tissue it is healing. Many authors have demonstrated experimentally that a weak, fibrous, dense scar is formed in the absence of controlled stress.[1,2,6,43,51,57,65] These studies refute the notion that collagen inherently "knows" the type of tissue it is repairing and, as a result, adopts specific characteristics of that tissue. The tension theory states that internal and external stresses placed on the wound during the remodeling phase will influence the characteristics of the collagen repair. Arem and Madden showed that the application of stress during the appropriate phase of healing could change scar length. Their work lends support to the tension theory of wound healing.[2]

The use of controlled force to remodel scar tissue has been clearly demonstrated in experimental models.[2,28,43,51] How much force should be applied during the healing process, and when? A major consideration in treatment of WADs is whether the application of early mobilization to traumatic neck injuries is beneficial. Pennie[47] published a prospective (but not randomized) treatment study consisting of two treatment groups with a 2-year follow-up. One group received early neck traction and physiotherapy, while the other group was told to rest in a neck collar and was given instructions for mobilization. Immobilization in a collar molded in slight flexion provided the best outcome. Contrary results were reported in randomized studies by Mealy et al[37] and McKinney et al.[36] In the study by Mealey et al, one group of patients received daily training in neck movements, while a second group of patients was given a soft collar and instructed to rest before mobilization. The McKinney study evaluated the outcome of 3 treatment groups. One group received instruction in self-mobilization, another group received supervised physiotherapy, and a third group received general instruction to rest for 10 to 14 days before mobilization. Each patient was fitted with a soft collar and given an analgesic. The groups that performed self-training with early mobilization improved significantly faster than the groups receiving immobilization and advice to rest, as measured by the number of recovered patients at monthly follow-up.

Controlled mobilization should begin as soon as the stage of collagen repair allows and with long-duration loading.[2] In practical terms, this relies upon regular, controlled application of tension on several occasions throughout the day over a period of weeks to months.[62] The concept of repeated movements, as outlined by McKenzie,[32] provides safety guidelines for the commencement of controlled movement following injury: Any exercise that becomes progressively more painful or peripheralizes with repetition should be abandoned because continuation will either produce recurrence of injury or disrupt the repair process. Additionally, an exercise that causes pain at end range, does not get progressively worse, or becomes less painful with repetition is safe to continue.

Brickley-Parsons and Glimcher,[6] studying the chemistry of collagen in the intervertebral disc, demonstrated that active cellular activity and tissue remodeling occur in the anulus fibrosus. They suggest that specific changes in cellular activity are initiated in response to overall increases in compressive loading on the concave side and tensile loading on the convex side of the spine (Wolff's law). The apparent biological response of the anulus fibrosus to the application of mechanical force suggests a correlation to Wolff's law. The researchers also give two opposing scenarios for active molecular remodeling of the anulus:

1. The remodeling is viewed as a *favorable* and *desirable* response, an adaptive change to better meet the new and altered external and internal forces.

2. The molecular reorganization of the tissue and organ in response to altered mechanical forces is considered *undesirable:* The changes in collagen content, collagen type, and posttranslational cross-link chemistry *decrease* the biological and or mechanical properties of the discs.[6]

In both instances, the application of mechanical therapy would fit the model of Brickley-Parsons and Glimcher[6]; graded stress, based on response of the tissue to the mechanical force applied, guides the quality and direction of the force. By following this guideline, mechanical therapy provides an inherent safety factor. If too much force is applied, or the direction of force being applied is inappropriate, the tissue will be damaged. If the quality and direction of force is appropriate, tissue strength will be enhanced. Osti et al,[45] studying anular tears and intervertebral disc degeneration in an animal model, found that surgically induced cuts in the outermost layer of the anulus led initially to deformation and bulging of the collagen bundles and eventually to inner extension of the tear and complete failure of the disc despite the ability of the outer anulus to heal. The researchers intimate that peripheral tears of the anulus fibrosus may play an important role in the degeneration of the intervertebral disc. Similar findings were shown by Hampton et al,[22] who state that a stab wound of the anulus has a limited healing potential and the persisting defect could provide a pathway for nuclear fluid to escape onto the perineural tissue, possibly resulting in persistent pain. If these scenarios are seen in vivo, mechanical therapy would have little, if any, effect on a disc lesion.

The question must then be asked: Is this type of puncture injury the sequela to physiologic loading, or is there a more circumferential stress placed on the anulus as a result of the biomechanical stresses of translation and shear? Twomey and Taylor[57] reported that rim lesions of the anulus fibrosus are the most common pathology observed in the intervertebral disc as a result of traumatic whiplash injuries. They also reported, in a separate study, a higher incidence of rim lesions in the upper cervical discs, possibly due to the greater translational movement that accompanies sagittal plane motion in the upper segmental levels, where the plane of the facet joints is close to horizontal.[45] The outer layers of the anulus fibrosus are well innervated,[4] and the rim lesions described usually involve this area of the disc. The delayed healing and early degeneration following experimental rim lesions in animals suggests that similar lesions in humans may contribute, in part, toward the chronic pain so often associated with acute soft tissue damage to the neck.[57] In addition to the intervertebral disc, there are other known generators of pain arising from the spine. These include muscles, the zygapophyseal joints, ligaments, nerve roots, and the dura.[4,24,50,52]

The application of movement and force (either patient-generated or externally applied) in a controlled and graded manner, based on clinical presentation, is the hallmark of mechanical therapy. Early mobilization and controlled stress has been shown to be beneficial for remodeling of injured tissue,[2,19,28,35,37,51,65] while immobilization has been shown to have a deleterious effect that is often long-lasting or permanent.[1,18,60] Evans[16] reported that with repeated intermittent stress (10 to 20 times per each waking hour), there was only one report of a ruptured extensor tendon and no reports of tenolysis in a 10-year study of patients with complex extensor tendon injury. Hunter[29] supports early and regular mobilization for the extensibility of scar tissue and states that "patients need to be aware that wound contraction will continue long after treatment has ceased, and they must continue to stretch the area on a regular basis."

The methods of mechanical therapy, specifically those described by McKenzie,[32,33] highlight the principles of controlled, graded stress for the treatment of spinal disorders by encouraging repeated movements during the course of the day. In addition, the concept of controlled, intermittent stress was shown by Evans to be safe and effective in the treatment of tendon injury. The treatment of spinal pain has been littered by trial and error approaches. As Deyo[12] reports, "Much of the history of back pain therapy appears to be a succession of fads." The use of a system that is supported by the scientific principles of tissue healing deserves close scrutiny and adequate consideration.

TREATMENT

The treatment of a patient with cervical trauma must be preceded by a thorough subjective history and appropriate objective testing to rule out serious pathology. A full radiographic evaluation should be obtained in patients with significant trauma to rule out fracture, instability, or other pathology that would be a contraindication for active therapy. Physical tests should also be employed to rule out rupture of the transverse ligament, vertebrobasilar artery insufficiency, and central cord signs; then assessment should proceed with caution. Frequently, the patient's report of pain prevents adequate assessment so that in the early stages following injury the extent of soft tissue damage remains obscure.[33] As soon as the patient's condition permits, assessment by repetitive motion should be performed so the patient can be classified in a diagnostic category and treated accordingly. As previously discussed, a short period of rest is essential during the initial inflammatory phase of injury. Care must also be taken to avoid excessive motion during this phase because disruption of the healing process can delay recovery. The goals of treatment should be to correct the patient's posture, reduce internal derangement (if present), remodel adaptively shortened tissue (dysfunction), educate the patient in prophylaxis, and restore functional mobility. During the course of treatment it is imperative to encourage return to normal activity as soon as possible.

Posture Correction

Correction of Sitting Posture: Posture correction is accomplished by demonstrating cause and effect to the patient. It is imperative that the patient be educated about the effects of static, end-range loading on his symptoms. If prolonged, end-range positions (eg, slouched sitting with the head in a protruded position) produce the patient's symptoms, the patient must be instructed in proper posture. To correct the patient's sitting posture, McKenzie uses a technique called "slouch-overcorrect" (Fig. 1). The patient is instructed to slump into the extreme of the bad sitting posture and then to come to the extreme of good sitting posture by going into full extension and restoring lordosis. The patient is then instructed to "let off the strain" (approximately 10%) to find his correct sitting position. The procedure should be repeated several times throughout the course of the day, especially during periods of prolonged sitting.

Correction of Lying Posture: The therapist must be careful to avoid the temptation of correcting what needs no correction. If the patient reports in the subjective history that his sleep is undisturbed and that he is not worse in the morning after a night's sleep, there is no reason to change his sleeping posture. If the patient's sleep is interrupted during the night, the patient awakes with symptoms that are worse in the morning, or the patient has symptoms that were not present the night before, the patient may be using an inappropriate

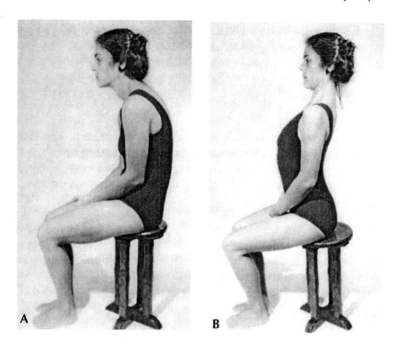

Figure 1.   McKenzie's "slouch-overcorrect" technique. **A,** Extreme of the bad sitting posture. **B,** Extreme of the good sitting posture. (From McKenzie RA: Treat Your Own Neck. Waikanai, New Zealand, Spinal Publications, 1997, with permission.)

pillow or adopting poor lying postures. If the former is suspected, "Under no circumstances should patients with neck pain use molded form or rubber pillows,"[33] because they do not accommodate for the normal lordotic cervical curve. If an excessively high pillow or more than one pillow is used, excessive flexion will result from supine lying, and excessive lateral flexion will be the result of side-lying. Patients who sleep in a prone position are subjected to extremes of cervical rotation. Although position of the head and neck is difficult to control during sleep, the patient with altered sleep, as a result of whiplash symptoms, should be encouraged to use a supportive pillow that keeps the head in a neutral position and to avoid prone-lying and end-range positions. The patient should also be encouraged to resume his normal sleeping position as soon as symptoms permit.

Treatment of Internal Derangement

As soon as the symptoms permit, repeated movement testing should be performed to identify the presence of derangement syndrome. Because protracted symptoms are common with whiplash disorders, identification of an internal derangement is imperative. The derangement syndrome is characterized by a rapid change in mechanical and/or symptomatic response to repeated movements or loading strategies. The syndrome is treated by first identifying a direction of preference—a movement or position that centralizes,

Table 1. Derangements and Their Classification

Derangement No. Quebec Task Force (QTF) Classification	Location of Symptoms	Deformity	Principle of Treatment	Rapidly Reversible
1; QTF = 1	Central/symmetrical; not beyond the elbow	None	Extension	Yes
2; QTF = 1 or 2	Central/symmetrical; not beyond the elbow	Kyphosis	Extension (allow time)	Yes
3; QTF = 1 or 2	Unilateral/asymmetrical; not beyond the elbow	None	Extension (may or may not need lateral compartment procedures)	Yes
4; QTF = 1 or 2	Unilateral/asymmetrical; not beyond the elbow	Torticollis	Correction of torticollis, extension principle	Yes
5; QTF = 3	Unilateral/asymmetrical; beyond the elbow	None	Extension (may or may not need lateral compartment procedures)	Yes, although failure may be more common
6; QTF = 3 or 4	Unilateral/asymmetrical; beyond the elbow	Torticollis	Attempt correction of torticollis, extension principle	No
7; QTF = 1 or 2	Central/symmetrical; unilateral/asymmetrical; often includes H/A; never beyond the elbow	Lordosis (may not be obvious)	Flexion (may or may not need lateral compartment procedures)	Yes

From McKenzie RA: The Cervical Spine: Mechanical Diagnosis and Therapy. Waikani, New Zealand, Spinal Publications, 1981; with permission..

decreases, or abolishes the presenting symptoms, which then remain better (Table 1) (Fig. 2).

The patient is then instructed in the performance of these movements (with posture correction), to be carried out every 1 to 2 hours during the course of the day. McKenzie states that 70% of patients are able to self-treat, while 30% will require therapist assistance (externally applied force or mobilization).[32,33] The application of force is graded, and based on the patient's response to repeated movement:

Patient generated force → patient overpressure → therapist overpressure(mobilization → manipulation.

Treatment should begin in the sitting position because the loaded position is more functional. The lying position should only be used if the patient is unable to

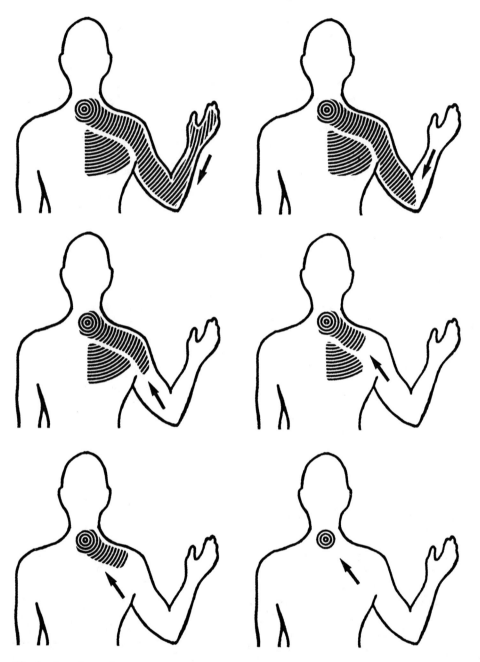

Figure 2. Centralization phenomenon. To determine the appropriateness of exercise, pay close attention to any change in location of the patient's symptoms. A change from a position distal to the spine (e.g., hand or arm) to a position closer to the spine (e.g., neck) indicates the correct direction of movement or exercise (directional preference). (From McKenzie RA: The Cervical Spine: Mechanical Diagnosis and Therapy. Waikanai, New Zealand, Spinal Publications, 1990, with permission).

tolerate a sitting position. If the patient requires treatment in the lying position, we must return him to a sitting position as quickly as the symptomatic response to treatment allows. Sitting is much more functional than lying, and the patient is more likely to perform their exercises with the required frequency.

Treatment of the internal derangement should begin in the sagittal plane, progressing to the frontal or coronal planes only after the initial treatment plane has been exhausted (the patient has been taken through the aforementioned progression of force). When we move out of the sagittal plane, the same progression of force should be followed and return to the sagittal plane accomplished as soon as the symptoms have centralized. Allow the patient ample opportunity to explore self-treatment, thus avoiding dependency. Where possible, avoid mobilization techniques on day 1 of treatment. If the patient requires mobilization, perform the technique with the purpose of enhancing the patient's self-treatment. When treating the patient with an internal derangement, it is important to not give too many interventions at one time. The reasons for this are: (1) Most patients are unlikely to perform a cadre of exercises, requiring significant amounts of time, during the day. They simply will not perform the exercises. (2) If patients are given many exercises (they perform them properly and with the prescribed frequency) and they report on follow-up that their symptoms are worse, it is difficult to know which exercises made them worse. Too many variables have been introduced, and it is difficult to ascertain the mechanical effect of the intervention. If patients are given only one or two exercises (moving in one direction), they will be more inclined to perform them and the therapist will be able to determine the effect of the treatment. Understanding the mechanics of an intervention allows the therapist to develop an appropriate treatment program based on sound rationale and the principles of tissue healing.

Treatment of Dysfunction

Dysfunction is a common sequela of WADs and the derangement syndrome. If the patient has been immobile during the stages of healing, adaptive shortening of soft tissues and collagenous tissues occurs and the repair itself can become symptomatic. It is not uncommon to see limitation of range in all motions. The very nature of adaptive shortening of soft tissues adjacent to articular structures prohibits the rapid recovery of function, and progress must be measured in terms of weeks and months rather than days.[32,33] It is important to reiterate that collagen formation and remodeling occur in response to regularly applied stress.[16,29,38] The stretching must be intermittent in nature and performed frequently and at regular intervals throughout the day. Intermittent stress, applied at regular intervals, strengthens collagenous structures, remodels, and increases the extensibility of scar tissue. If the time between stretching procedures is too long, the rest period will negate the effects of the stretch. Sustained stress, if applied regularly, may damage ligamentous, capsular, and scar tissue.[26,57,65]

The same principles of treatment apply for patients presenting with symptoms arising from dysfunction (adaptively shortened tissue) as for patients presenting with internal derangement. The therapist should follow the progression of force previously described; the exercises must be performed frequently throughout the course of the day, and the patient must be instructed in proper posture. Unlike the treatment for derangement (where the patient is instructed to perform the exercises that decrease, centralize, or abolish the symptoms), the patient with dysfunction is instructed to stretch in the direction that produces the symptoms. McKenzie outlines the following instructions for patients with dysfunction:

- Because posterior derangement is so common, patients with dysfunction in the cervical region must maintain correct posture at all times and will at the end of each session of exercise perform retraction and extension;
- If the exercises do not produce some minor pain, the movement has not been performed far enough into the end range;
- The type of discomfort sought is not unlike the pain felt when bending the finger backward beyond the normal position;
- The pain should have subsided within 10 to 20 minutes after completion of the exercises;
- When pain produced by the stretching procedures lasts continuously and is still evident the next day, overstretching has taken place; in this case the number of exercises in each sequence or the frequency of sequences must be reduced;
- When stretching results in rapidly increasing and peripheralizing pain, the procedures should be stopped immediately because derangement is likely to develop.

In addition, the patient must be advised that pain cannot be used as a barometer for progress. As the patient's range of motion increases, each new end-range position will be productive of symptoms. In the presence of dysfunction, an increase in range of motion and improved functional mobility should be used as a gauge for improvement. For the recovery of extension in the lower cervical spine, patient-generated force is usually sufficient. The exercises should be performed every 2 hours for 10 repetitions (Fig. 3).

If patient-generated forces are not adequate to restore full motion, common extension mobilization techniques may be required. These techniques are indicated *only* when the patient alone is unable to fully restore cervical extension. The patient must be instructed to continue with his exercises in addition to the mobilization techniques.

For the treatment of rotation dysfunction, the patient must again be educated regarding the importance of frequent repetition throughout the day and the production of discomfort when performing the exercises. Discomfort will usually be felt unilaterally (to the side of the dysfunction). The exercises should be performed every 2 hours for 10 to 15 repetitions (Fig. 4).

To apply full passive stretch, the patient is instructed to perform rotation with overpressure. If patient-generated forces are not adequate to restore full motion, common rotation mobilization techniques may be required. Again, these techniques are indicated *only* when the patient alone is unable to fully restore cervical rotation.

Patients rarely present with a complaint of loss of lateral flexion. Because lateral flexion and rotation are biomechanically the same motion, limitation of lateral flexion frequently coexists with limitation of rotation. The instructions are the same as previously described (Fig. 5). Lateral flexion mobilization techniques

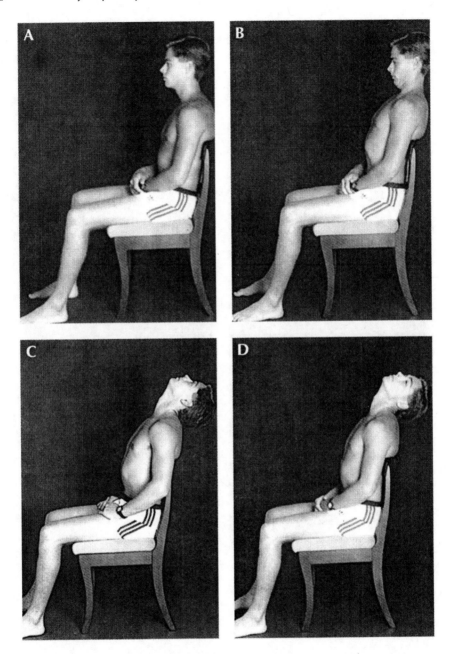

Figure 3. For recovery of extension range of motion, the patient is instructed to sit in a straight-backed (supportive) chair (*A*) and tuck the chin as far back as possible while keeping it parallel to the ground (*B*). When full retraction is achieved, the patient rolls the head backward until end range extension is reached (*C*). At this point, the patient rotates the head 1–2 inches to the left and right (*D*) and then returns to the starting position (*A*). (From McKenzie RA: The Cervical Spine: Mechanical Diagnosis and Therapy. Waikanai, New Zealand, Spinal Publications, 1990, with permission).

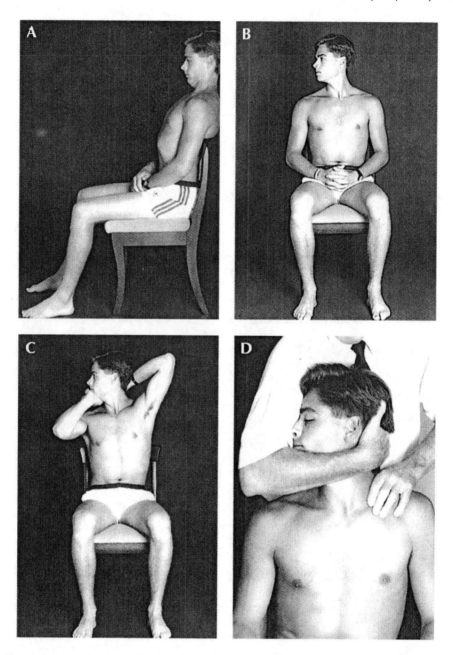

Figure 4. For recovery of rotation range of motion, the patient sits in a straight-backed (supportive) chair, tucks the chin (*A*), and rotates to the end of the available range (*B*). Overpressure may be added by the patient placing one hand on the chin (right hand for right rotation and left hand for left rotation) and one hand on the occiput to apply a self-mobilizing force (*C*). The therapist can also provide overpressure to achieve rotation (*D*). (From McKenzie RA: The Cervical Spine: Mechanical Diagnosis and Therapy. Waikanai, New Zealand, Spinal Publications, 1990, with permission).

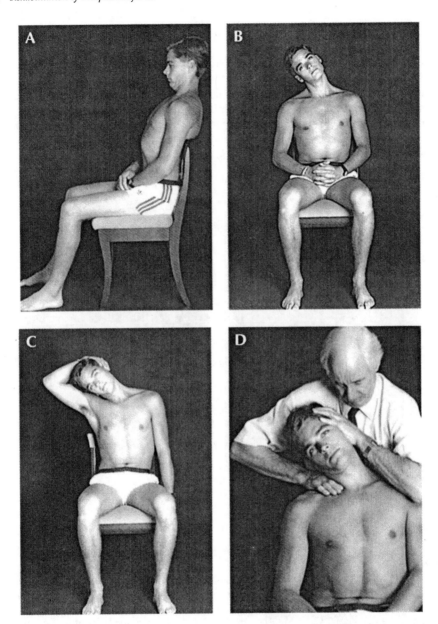

Figure 5. For recovery of lateral flexion range of motion, the patient sits in a straight-backed (supportive) chair, tucks the chin (*A*), and brings the ear to the shoulder (laterally flex) to the end of the available range (*B*). Overpressure may be added by the patient placing one hand on the head just above the opposite ear (right hand for right lateral flexion and left hand for left lateral flexion); the opposite arm is used to grab the seat of the chair to apply a stabilizing component (*C*). The therapist also can apply overpressure to achieve lateral flexion (*D*). (From McKenzie RA: The Cervical Spine: Mechanical Diagnosis and Therapy. Waikanai, New Zealand, Spinal Publications, 1990, with permission).

can be employed with the same guidelines as extension and rotation mobilization techniques.

Treatment of flexion dysfunction should begin in the sitting position, and full recovery can usually be achieved without moving to the lying position. For the recovery of flexion in the cervical spine, patient-generated force is usually sufficient. Flexion stresses should initially be applied without overpressure and performed two to three times per day for 5 to 10 repetitions. At the end of one week, the patient may increase the frequency to 10 repetitions every 2 hours. When active flexion becomes painless, the patient may be instructed to apply overpressure (Fig. 6).

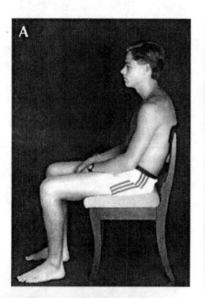
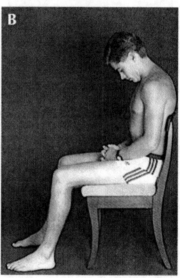
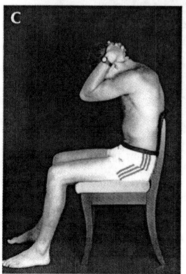

Figure 6. For recovery of flexion range of motion, the patient slouches in a chair (*A*) and bends the chin to the chest (*B*). If active flexion is pain-free after 1 week of repetitive performance of this exercise, the patient is instructed to grasp the back of the head at the level of the occiput and apply force until a stretch is felt, then return to the neutral sitting position (*C*). (From McKenzie RA: The Cervical Spine: Mechanical Diagnosis and Therapy. Waikanai, New Zealand, Spinal Publications, 1990, with permission).

If patient-generated forces are not adequate to restore full motion, common flexion mobilization techniques may be required. Again, these techniques are indicated *only* when the patient is unable to fully restore cervical flexion. Because flexion stresses have the potential to cause a posterior derangement, care must be taken when applying flexion techniques. At the end of each set of flexion stretches, the patient is instructed to retract and extend the cervical spine prophylactically to decrease the likelihood of any untoward effects.

Adverse Neural Tension

Treatment for adverse neural tension or adherent nerve root is approached in the same manner as for cervical dysfunction, because the symptoms arise from adaptively shortened structures. The symptoms from adverse neural tension disorders can often persist for months or years. Treating the pathomechanics of this disorder inevitably involves some discomfort.[7] Because adherent neural structures are strictly dysfunctions, they are treated with the same frequency and progression as previously described. Upper limb tension positions that specifically target the injured neural structures have been described in detail by Butler[7] and Elvey.[13] Two common procedures used for upper extremity symptoms are seen in Figures 7 and 8.

Care must be taken not to overstretch the healing tissue. As in the treatment of connective tissue dysfunction, if symptoms are produced, increased, or peripheralized in response to treatment (and they remain worse as a result), the stretch is too vigorous. The patient must then be instructed to decrease the frequency and intensity of the exercise. In addition, if a symptom that is initially intermittent has become constant, overstretching has occurred. In the presence of an adherent neural structure, the symptoms must be continually monitored. This requires constant feedback from the patient. The techniques of neural mobilization should begin slowly, starting at a point distal to the injury (eg, elbow or wrist). As the patient progresses, more tension can be applied to the nervous system, the number of repetitions may be altered, the amplitude of the technique may be varied, or techniques to address the more proximally situated symptoms (from provoking structures such as the shoulder or neck) should be initiated.

FUNCTIONAL RESTORATION AND PREVENTION

Functional restoration does not occur in isolation. The muscles of the cervical and cervicothoracic spine must be exercised in a manner that supports the patient's normal activities of daily living. For example, if the patient works in a sedentary occupation, it would not suit the patient's needs to merely strengthen the cervical extensor muscles. The extensor muscles of the cervical spine are postural muscles-thus, built for endurance, not strength. A simple analogy would be training for a marathon by exclusively running sprints. Sufficient training of the fast-twitch (type II) muscle fibers required for explosive strength, ignoring the slow-twitch fibers required to complete the ultimate goal of finishing the race, leads to an undesirable result. If the patient is not instructed in proper posture and maintenance of that posture, the muscles will be ill-trained to perform the tasks required without putting undo stress on the articular and noncontractile structures of the cervical spine.

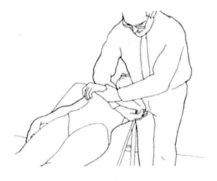

ULTT2 (median nerve bias) stage 1

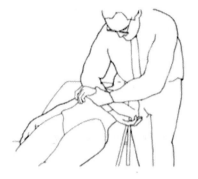

ULTT2 (median nerve bias) stage 2

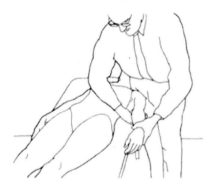

ULTT2 (median nerve bias) stage 3

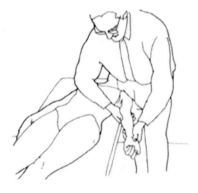

ULTT2 (median nerve bias) stage 4

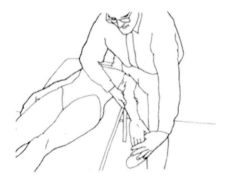

ULTT2 (median nerve bias) stage 5

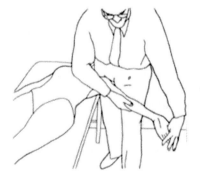

ULTT2 (median nerve bias) stage 6

Figure 7. The upper limb tension test (ULTT) shown here is designed for the assessment and treatment of injuries resulting in adverse neural tension of the median nerve. (From Butler D: Mobilization of the Nervous System. Melbourne, Churchill Livingstone, 1991, with permission.)

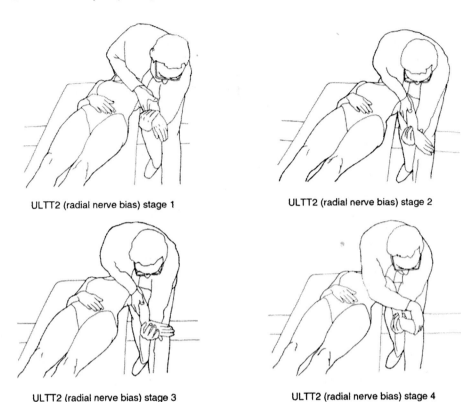

ULTT2 (radial nerve bias) stage 1   ULTT2 (radial nerve bias) stage 2

ULTT2 (radial nerve bias) stage 3   ULTT2 (radial nerve bias) stage 4

Figure 8.   The upper limb tension test (ULTT) shown here is designed for the assessment and treatment of injuries resulting in adverse neural tension of the radial nerve nerve. (From Butler D: Mobilization of the Nervous System. Melbourne, Churchill Livingstone, 1991, with permission.)

Stabilization exercises use muscular control and proprioceptive input from joint receptors to allow for normal, functional range of movement during static and dynamic activities. There are many different stabilization exercises (limited only by the creativity of the clinician) that are appropriate for rehabilitation of cervical spine injuries. The exercises must be well understood by the patient, performed frequently throughout the day, and should not require expensive or large amounts of equipment. Maintenance of posture is a form of stabilization exercise that fits the aforementioned criteria. The patient can easily perform posture correction while working; it does not require expensive equipment, and it requires approximately 1 minute to perform a set of 10 repetitions of slouch-overcorrect exercises, allowing for frequent performance throughout the day.

There are four key factors of particular importance when returning the patient to activity following injury[63]:

1. **Fitness for the task.** Most people spend a considerable amount of time in one position-either sitting or standing at work, driving, reading, or watching television. Prolonged periods of limited activity lead to adaptive

shortening of connective tissue and ultimately to a loss of flexibility. A program of regular exercise and stretching will enable the patient to maintain a level of flexibility necessary to safely perform more strenuous tasks.

2. **Warming up and cooling down.** A warm-up period before beginning repetitive or strenuous work prepares the body (specifically the injured tissue) for the activity by increasing blood flow, elevating the body temperature, and increasing the extensibility of soft tissues. Stretching subsequent to activity will maintain the extensibility of soft tissue.

3. **Maintaining flexibility.** As previously discussed, scar tissue formed following injury has a tendency to contract and shorten. Regular, frequent stretching postinjury is vital for maintaining the flexibility required for normal function.

4. **Appropriate environment, technique, and equipment.** Ensuring that the patient performs the activities in the appropriate environment, with good technique, minimizes the risk of injury. Instruct the patient in proper work positions, and make sure the patient has the proper supports and equipment to maintain those positions. Good technique also includes frequent interruption of sustained work positions, thus minimizing stress on the healing tissues.

CONCLUSION

Physical therapy following acute damage to the discs, joints, and soft tissues of the neck should be approached with a clear understanding of the physiology of tissue healing and how healing can be facilitated. Passive modality treatment such as heat, electrical stimulation, and massage has not been scientifically validated and does not promote tissue healing. The current literature supports an early, active intervention for treatment of WADs rather than immobilization in a soft collar, rest, or passive treatment.[5,35,36,37,47,49,53,57] Active treatment is seen as more effective in reducing pain and restoring function than treatment with initial rest, recommendation of a soft collar, and gradual introduction of home exercises. An initial period of active, small-amplitude movements of the neck (dictated by the patient's symptomatic and mechanical response to loading) performed at regular, frequent intervals throughout the day is essential for tissue healing, because collagen in healing tissues occurs along the lines of stress. Movement encourages fluid transport and aids nutrition to the collagenous and largely avascular joint structures, facilitates the removal of exudates, and allows healing to occur.[57] The force should be gradually increased over a period of weeks, progressing to resisted motion designed to restore functional mobility and a return to the premorbid activity level. A major recommendation of the Quebec Task Force on Whiplash-Associated Disorders is that "early return to usual activities for WAD patients should be vigorously encouraged by clinicians."

A word of caution: Manipulation is ill advised during the initial stages of healing, because considerable strain is placed on the anulus fibrosus during a high-velocity, end-range thrust. The anulus is an avascular structure (thus slow to heal), and cervical manipulation is likely to increase the size of any rim lesion rather than assist in the healing process. Manipulation should be considered only in the later stages of whiplash syndrome, when it is clear that healing has occurred.[57] By following the principles of mechanical diagnosis and therapy (the application of graded force), we are provided with an inherent safety mechanism that allows both patient and therapist a guideline for progression to restoration of motion and function.

One final note: The Rosenfeld study points out that an average of four sessions of physical therapy was needed for the patients who underwent active treatment (early, frequent submaximal movements to be performed 10 times per hour, combined with mechanical diagnosis and therapy as described by McKenzie[32,33]) for WADs. Only 10% of properly managed patients continued to have clinically relevant symptoms at 6 months, compared with more than 50% of patients who received standard care (delayed onset of exercise commencing 2 weeks postinjury, to be performed only a few times every day).[49]

References

1. Akeson WH, Amiel D, Abel MF, et al: Effects of immobilization on joints. Clin Orthop 219:28–36, 1987.
2. Arem A, Madden JW: Effects of stress on healing wounds: I. Intermittent noncyclical tension. J Surg Res 20:93–102, 1976.
3. Bogduk N: Cervical causes of headache and dizziness. In Grieve GP (ed): Modern Manual Therapy of the Vertebral Column. Edinburgh, Churchill Livingstone, 1986.
4. Bogduk N: The clinical anatomy of the cervical dorsal roots. Spine 7:319–329, 1982.
5. Borchgrevink GE, Kaasa A, McDonagh D, et al: Acute treatment of whiplash neck sprain injuries. Spine 23:25–31, 1998.
6. Brickley-Parsons D, Glimcher M: Is the chemistry of collagen in intervertebral discs an expression of Wolff's Law? A study of the human lumbar spine. Spine 9:148–163, 1984.
7. Butler D: Mobilization of the Nervous System. Melbourne, Churchill Livingstone, 1991.
8. Carrico T, Merhoff A, Cohen K: Biology of wound healing. Surg Clin North Am 64:721–732, 1984.
9. Cassidy JD, Carroll LJ, Cote P, et al: Effect of eliminating compensation for pain and suffering on the outcome of insurance claims for whiplash injury. N Engl J Med 342:1179–1186, 2000.
10. Crowe H: Injuries to the cervical spine. Presented at the Annual Meeting of the Western Orthopaedic Association, San Francisco, 1928.
11. Deyo RA, Walsh NE, Martin DC, et al: A controlled trial of transcutaneous electrical nerve stimulation (TENS) and exercise for chronic low back pain. N Engl J Med 322:1627–1634, 1990.
12. Deyo R: Practice variations, treatment fads, rising disability. Do we need a new clinical research paradigm? Spine 18:2153–2162, 1993.
13. Downing DS, Weinstein A: Ultrasound of subacromial bursitis. A double blind trial. Phys Ther 66:194–199, 1986.
14. Elvey R: Brachial plexus tension tests and the pathoanatomical origin of arm pain. In Idczak RM (ed): Aspects of Manipulative Therapy. Carlton, Australia, Lincoln Institute of Health Sciences, 1981.
15. Evans P: The healing process at the cellular level: a review. Physiotherapy 66:256–259, 1980.
16. Evans R: Clinical applications of controlled stress to the healing extensor tendon: a review of 112 cases. Phys Ther 69:1041–1049, 1989.
17. Falconer MA, McGeorge M, Begg AC: Observations on the cause and mechanism of symptom production in sciatica and low back pain. J Neurol Neurosurg Psychiatry 11:2–26, 1948.
18. Finsterbush A, Friedman B: Reversibility of joint changes produced by immobilization in rabbits. Clin Orthop 111:290–298, 1975.
19. Gelberman R, Botte M, Spiegelman JJ, Akeson W: The excursion and deformation of repaired flexor tendons treated with protected early motion. J Hand Surg [Am] 11:106–110, 1986.
20. Goats GC. Massage—the scientific basis of an ancient art: part 2. Physiologic and therapeutic effects. Br J Sports Med 28:153–156,1994.
21. Gopalkrishnan P, Sluka KA: Effect of varying frequency, intensity, and pulse duration of transcutaneous electrical nerve stimulation on primary hyperalgesia in inflamed rats. Arch Phys Med Rehabil 81:984–990, 2000.
22. Hampton D, Laros G, McCarron R, Franks D: Healing potential of the anulus fibrosus. Spine 14:398–401, 1989.

23. Hardy M: The biology of scar formation. Phys Ther 69:1014–1024, 1989.
24. Hasue M: Pain and the nerve root; an interdisciplinary approach. Spine 18:2053–2058, 1993.
25. Herbert R: Preventing stiff joints. In Crosbie J, McConnell J (eds): Key Issues in Musculoskeletal Physiotherapy. Oxford, Butterworth-Heinenmann, 1993.
26. Hickey DS, Hukins DW: Relationship between the structure and function of the annulus fibrosus and the function and failure of the intervertebral disc. Spine 5:106–112, 1980.
27. Hildingsson C, Toolanen G: Outcome after soft-tissue injury of the cervical spine: a prospective study of 93 car-accident victims. Acta Orthop Scand 61:357–359, 1990.
28. Houlbrooke K, Vause K, Merrilees M J: Effects of movement and weight bearing on the glycosaminoglycan content of sheep articular cartilage. Aust Physiother 36:88–89, 1990.
29. Hunter G: Specific soft tissue mobilization in the treatment of soft tissue lesions. Physiotherapy 80:15–21, 1994.
30. Jayson MIV: Fibrosis, chronic inflammation and vascular damage in back pain syndromes. In Weinstein JN, Weisel S (eds): The Lumbar Spine. Philadelphia, WB Saunders, 1990.
31. King EW, Sluka KA: The effect of varying frequency and intensity of transcutaneous electrical nerve stimulation on the treatment of secondary mechanical hyperalgesia in an animal model of inflammation. J Pain. In press.
32. McKenzie RA: The Lumbar Spine: Mechanical Diagnosis and Therapy. Waikanai, New Zealand, Spinal Publications, 1981.
33. McKenzie RA: The Cervical Spine: Mechanical Diagnosis and Therapy. Waikanai, New Zealand, Spinal Publications, 1990.
34. McKenzie RA: Treat Your Own Neck. Waikanai, New Zealand, Spinal Publications, 1997.
35. McKinney LA: Early mobilization and outcome in acute sprains of the neck. BMJ 299:1006–1008, 1989.
36. McKinney LA, Dornan JO, Ryan M: The role of physiotherapy in the management of acute neck sprains following road-traffic accidents. Arch Emerg Med 6:27–33, 1989.
37. Mealy K, Brennan H, Fenelon GCC: Early mobilization of acute whiplash injuries. BMJ 292:656–657, 1986.
38. Merrilees MJ, Flint MH: Ultrastructural study of tension and pressure zones in a rabbit flexor tendon. Am J Anat 157:87–106, 1980.
39. Munting E: Ultrasonic therapy for painful shoulders. Physiotherapy 64:180–181, 1978.
40. Norris SH, Watt I: The prognosis of neck injuries resulting from rear-end vehicle collisions. J Bone Joint Surg Br 65:608–611, 1983.
41. Noble JG, Henderson G, Cramp AF, et al: The effect of interferential therapy upon cutaneous blood flow in humans. Clin Physiol 20:2–7, 2000.
42. Nwuga VC: Ultrasound in treatment of back pain resulting from prolapsed intervertebral disc. Arch Phys Med Rehabil 64:88–89, 1983.
43. O'Driscoll SW, Keeley FW, Salter RB: Durability of regenerated articular cartilage produced by free autogenous periosteal grafts in major full-thickness defects in joint surfaces under the influence of continuous passive motion. J Bone Joint Surg Am 70:595–606, 1988.
44. Oosterveld FGJ, Rasker JJ, Jacobs JWG, et al: The effect of local heat and cold therapy on the intraartiular and skin surface temperature of the knee. Arthritis Rheum 35:146–151, 1992.
45. Osti OL, Vernon-Roberts B, Fraser RD: Annulus tears and intervertebral disc degeneration; an experimental study using an animal model. Spine 15:762–767, 1990.
46. Peeters GM, Verhagen AP, de Bie RA, Oostendorp AB: The efficacy of conservative treatment in patients with whiplash injury. Spine 26:E64–E73, 2001.
47. Pennie BH, Agambar LJ: Whiplash injuries: a trial of early management. J Bone Joint Surg Br 72:277–279, 1990.
48. Radanov BP, Di Stefano G, Schnidrig A, et al: Role of psychosocial stress in recovery from common whiplash. Lancet 338:712–715, 1991.
49. Rosenfeld M, Gunnarsson R, Borenstein P: Early intervention in whiplash-associated disorders. Spine 25:1782–1787, 2000.
50. Rydevik B, Brown MO, Lundborg G: Pathoanatomy and pathophysiology of nerve root compression. Spine 9:7–15, 1984.
51. Salter RB: The biological concept of continuous passive motion. The first 18 years of basic research and its clinical application. Clin Orthop 242:12–25, 1989.
52. Spencer OL, Miller JAA, Bertolini JE: The effect of intervertebral disc space narrowing on the contact force between the nerve root and a simulated disc protrusion. Spine 9:422–426, 1984.
53. Spitzer WO, Skovron ML, Salmi LR, et al: Scientific monograph of the Quebec Task Force on Whiplash-Associated Disorders: redefining "whiplash" and its management. Spine 20(8 suppl): 21S–73S, 1995.

54. Toomey R, Greif-Schwartz R, Piper MC: Clinical evaluation of the effects of whirlpool on patients with Colles' fractures. Physiother Can 38:280–284, 1986.
55. Twomey LT, Taylor JR: Physical Therapy of the Low Back. New York, Churchill Livingstone, 1987.
56. Twomey LT, Taylor JR: Flexion creep deformation and hysteresis in the lumbar vertebral column. Spine 7:116–122, 1982.
57. Twomey LT, Taylor JR: The whiplash syndrome: pathology and physical treatment. J Manipulative Manual Ther 1:26–29, 1993.
58. van der Heijden GJ, Leffers P,Wolters PJ, et al: No effect of bipolar interferential electrotherapy and pulsed ultrasound for soft tissue shoulder disorders: a randomized controlled trial. Ann Rheum Dis 58:530–540, 1999.
59. van der Windt DA, van der Heijden GJ, van der Berg SG, et al: Ultrasound therapy for musculoskeletal disorders. Pain 81:257–271, 1999.
60. Videman T: Connective tissue and immobilization. Key factors in musculoskeletal degeneration? Clin Orthop 221:26–32, 1987.
61. Wainner RS, Gill H: Diagnosis and nonoperative management of cervical radiculopathy. J Orthop Sports Phys Ther 30:728–741, 2000.
62. Watson G, Lindsay R: The treatment of soft tissue injuries: A review. N Z J Sports Med 4:66–68, 1993.
63. Watson G, Lindsay R, Hickmott D, et al: Treat Your Own Strains, Sprains and Bruises. Waikanai, New Zealand, Spinal Publications, 1994.
64. Wilder DG, Pope MH, Frymoyer JW: The biomechanics of lumbar disc herniation and the effect of overload and instability: J Spinal Disord 1:16–32, 1988.
65. Woo SL, Gelberman RH, Cobb NG, et al: The importance of controlled passive mobilization on flexor tendon healing. A biomechanical study. Acta Orthop Scand 52:615–622, 1981.
66. Wright A, Sluka KA: Nonpharmacologic treatments for musculoskeletal pain. Clin J Pain 17:33–46, 2001.

19

The Role of Chiropractic Treatment in Whiplash Injury

Craig Liebenson, D.C., and Clayton D. Skaggs, D.C.

Whiplash or whiplash-associated disorders (WADs) commonly involve the cervical spine. The natural history of neck pain is poorly understood, and little research about its causes or treatments has been performed.[6] The severity of symptoms and the severity of trauma are not always directly related. Few objective findings are correlated with the symptoms reported in the head, neck, or upper quarter. The duration of symptoms and signs associated with whiplash are reported by numerous authors to be between 2 to 6 months.[13,27,35] However, the magnitude of this problem cannot be overestimated. In a survey of more than 10,000 cases of WAD pain, it persisted in 25% of the cases for 5 years after the accident.[11]

Neck pain is not only common following an automobile accident but is common independently of traumatic origin as well. The incidence of neck and shoulder pain is quite high in the general population. The point prevalence (number of individuals suffering at a given point in time) of neck and shoulder pain is between 10% to 22%.[7,29,33] The 1-year prevalence is 16% to 40% (number of individuals who will have discomfort during a 1-year period).[33,44,49] The lifetime prevalence falls between 50% and 70%.[10,33]

The Quebec WAD guideline recommended early, active intervention (including manipulation) as a basic approach to managing symptoms (Table 1).[43] Treatment following these guidelines has recently been shown to be much more effective than traditional passive-based care.[38] Clinically important symptoms at 6 months postaccident were present in only 10% of properly managed patients (early active intervention with submaximal movements identified by McKenzie evaluation) as compared with more than 50% of those given standard care (soft collar, initial rest, gradual mobilization).

Similar positive results for early activation were found in two other studies. Encouragement to continue with activities of daily living (ADLs) had a superior outcome over prescription of sick leave and immobilization.[5] Physical therapy or exact instruction in self-mobilization were both better than 2 weeks of rest with a soft collar at 1-month, 2-month, and 2-year follow-ups.[31]

A recent meta-analysis of manual therapy (mobilization, manipulation, massage) concluded that, when used alone, there was insufficient data to recommend it.[14] But, when manual therapy was used in combination with other active treatments, there is moderate evidence of benefit. In a systematic review of the literature, Hurwitz reported that there is evidence, although limited, on the short-term effectiveness of spinal manipulation.[16] In a prospective study of

Table 1.   Treatment Guidelines for Whiplash-Associated Disorders (WADs)

- Clinical diagnosis
- Reassurance
- Immobilization (< 4 days for WADs II & III)
- Activation
- Manipulation, mobilization/traction, exercise, postural advise, passive modalities (first 3 weeks only)
- Multidisciplinary team management (WAD I, 6 weeks; II or III, 12 weeks).

1000 clinical patients, Jette determined that manipulation and mobilization were associated with better outcomes for neck disorders.[18] One of the most recent reviews also supports manipulation and mobilization for disorders of the head and neck.[30]

A recent study found that chronic neck pain patients receive more benefit from a combination of low-technology exercise and manipulation than with high-technology exercise or manipulation alone.[8] Most outcomes were similar for the two exercise groups except that patient satisfaction was higher for the combined exercise and manipulation group. In another study comparing exercise, manipulation, and physical therapy for chronic neck pain, no significant differences in outcome were seen at 2, 6, and 12 months after treatment.[19]

It is apparent that the evidence suggests that reactivation approaches are central to any strategy attempting to improve the health status of patients with WAD. The role of reactivation advice versus specific exercises is not so clear. It also is not certain what role manual therapy or manipulation plays. More qualitative research is clearly needed in this area.

CLINICAL ASSESSMENT

In the patient suffering from acute or chronic WAD, diagnostic triage should be carried out to determine the complexity of the condition and thus the appropriate strategy for management (Table 2). Unfortunately, there is a dearth of objective findings that are correlated with the more common grades I and II. A

Table 2.   Quebec Whiplash-Associated Disorders Guidelines*

Grade	WAD Classification Clinical Presentation
0	No complaint or physical sign†
I	Neck complaint of pain, stiffness, or tenderness
	No physical signs
II	Neck complaint and musculoskeletal signs†
III	Neck complaint and neurologic signs
IV	Neck complaint and fracture or dislocation

* Classification system based on signs and symptoms
† Physical or musculoskeletal signs—range of motion loss or tenderness.
Data from Spitzer WO, Skovron ML, Salmi LIR, et al: Scientific monograph of the Quebec Task Force on Whiplash-Associated Disorders: redefining "whiplash" and its management. Spine 20(suppl):S1–S73, 1995.

Table 3. Goals of Functional Examination

History
    Identify the clinical symptom complex.

Examination
    Identify the tissue injury complex (or pain generators).
    Identify the source of biomechanical overload.
    Identify the dysfunctional kinetic chain.
    Identify the functional adaptations.

Data from Kibler WB, Herring SA, Press JM: Functional Rehabilitation of Sports and Musculo-skeletal Injuries. Gaithersburg, MD, Aspen Publishers, 1998.

new objective sign of musculoskeletal dysfunction associated with whiplash grade II patients was recently reported.[34] Nederhand et al demonstrated that a decreased ability to relax the upper trapezius muscles during static tasks and following exercise distinguised chronic WAD II patients from healthy control subjects. In a restropective cohort, Hartling et al demonstrated a high prognostic value for the Quebec classification system and recommended it as a tool for emergency department settings.[15]

Because the overall goal of care is to reduce pain and restore function, the history and examination are focused on determining the primary pain generator or injured tissue, the source of biomechanical overload, related disturbance of function in the kinetic chain and, finally, adaptive mechanisms. These overarching goals are shown in Table 3.

Using this approach helps to identify likely suspects in the patient's presentation and creates a treatment pathway that can be easily fine-tuned to determine if the goals of pain relief and functional restoration are being achieved. For instance, a neck pain patient (clinical symptom complex) who has pain with cervical extension (source of biomechanical overload) may be found to have an increased thoracic kyphosis (dysfunctional kinetic chain) and trigger points in the upper trapezius (functional adaptation). The treatment path would include palliative measures directed at the cervical spine, but if it is determined that cervical extension is less pain-provoking following thoracic mobilization, treatment should be focused on this "key link" in the kinetic chain rather than the site of symptoms. Further empirical evidence that the fixed kyphosis is a central determinant of the patient's persistent symptoms is present if restoration of thoracic mobility not only decreases neck pain with cervical extension but also eliminates the upper trapezius trigger points. The hypothesis that there is a causal relationship linking decreased thoracic extension mobility to sensitivity of the injured cervical spine tissues is thus strengthened.

Essential to the success of the functional approach is appropriate reactivation of the patient and an appreciation of the biopsychosocial model of care. An overemphasis on the biomedical model can be disabling. Radanov et al found that 2 years after a neck sprain injury there were no significant differences in the reporting of symptoms between the symptomatic patients who were able to work and the symptomatic patients who were disabled.[37] In the neck, the false-positive rate for imaging has been reported to be as high as 75% with an asymptomatic population.[4,45] Thus, imaging tests have high sensitivity (few false negatives) but low specificity (high false-positive rate) for identifying disc problems. Such poor specificity marks imaging as an inappropriate screening method. Bush found that most cervical disc herniations regress with time without the need to resort to surgery.[9] Additionally, he found that the larger the disc herniation the more likely it is to spontaneously reabsorb. Therefore, it is important to avoid "labeling" patients as being damaged because this may have disabling effects in terms of promoting the "sick role" and interfering with functional reactivation.[28]

Functional Instability

Functional instability has been defined by Anderson as "the loss of the ability of the spine under physiologic loads to maintain relationships between vertebrae in such a way that there is neither initial nor subsequent damage to the spinal cord or nerve roots, and in addition, there is neither development of incapacitating deformity or severe pain."[1] This type of poor stability establishes faulty movement patterns (kinetic chain dysfunction), which are sources of biomechanical overload. These patterns lead to perpetuation of muscle imbalance, abnormal joint loads, and are the most likely perpetuating factor of pain.

Panjabi theorized that most WAD patients experience mild soft tissue injury that does not cause tissue failure and thus goes undetected by static imaging procedures.[36] In these sub-failure injuries the soft tissues are not torn, but are stretched beyond their elastic limit, resulting in instability and poor healing.

Instability will render the osteoligamentous structures vulnerable to repeated strain with normal ADLs and be compensated for in the muscle system. Lauren et al discuss the associations between motor skills and coordination as they relate to neck pain. They describe appropriate timing and amplitude of muscle reactions and how poor motor control of arm motion was correlated with neck pain.[23]

Edgerton et al studied altered muscle activation ratios of synergist spinal muscles during a variety of motor tasks in whiplash patients.[12] They discovered that underactivity of agonists and overactivity of synergists was able to discriminate chronic neck pain patients from those who had recovered with 88% accuracy. They concluded: "The nervous system apparently can detect a reduced capacity to generate force from a specific muscle or group of muscles and compensate by recruiting more motoneurons. This compensation can be made by recruiting motor units from an uninjured area of the muscle or from other muscles capable of performing the same task."

Lauren et al demostrated strong support for this element of compensation with their functional study of neck and shoulder pain incidence.[23] Their study showed a higher incidence of neck and shoulder pain in individuals who performed tasks either extremely fast or extremely slow. Those performing them in a medium range had a low incidence of neck and shoulder pain. Nederhand's study showing a decreased ability to relax the upper trapezius muscles during static tasks as well as following exercise in WAD grade II patients also correlates well with these motor control studies.[34]

Watson and Trott found that two examination findings could differentiate headache from nonheadache patients[48]:

• Forward head posture
• Decreased isometric strength and endurance of neck flexors.

Treleaven et al found that the following three factors could distinguish post-concussional headache patients from asymptomatics[46]:

• Upper cervical joint dysfunction
• Weak neck flexors
• Tight suboccipitals.

Reduced endurance of the deep neck flexors is also found in a number of other published studies.[3,20,21,40]

Functional Tests

Posture is an important starting point for functional assessment. Poor posture takes joints out of their aligned "centrated" positions and alters muscle balance between antagonist muscles (Figs. 1 and 2). A typical example is a person working on a computer with a head forward position. This overstresses both the upper and lower cervical spine.

Movement patterns are important to assess because classic muscle tests evaluate strength but not the quality of movement.[17,24–26] A number of muscles participate in any movement pattern. There is a great difference in the strain in the cervical spine if, for instance, neck flexion is performed with or without hyperextension of C0-C1. The deep neck flexors keep the chin tucked in while the sternocleidomastoid (SCM) can raise the head with C0-C1 extended.[20,46] In either case, the neck flexors could test as strong.

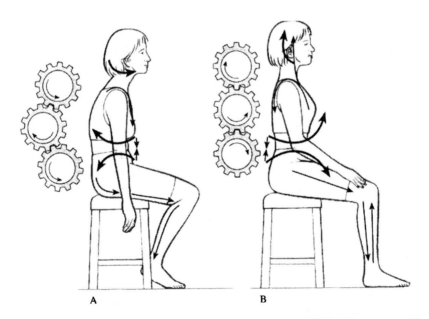

Figure 1. Cogwheels from Brügger. (*A*) Slumped posture. (*B*) Upright posture. (From Liebenson C: Self-treatment of mid-thoracic dysfunction: a key link in the body axis. Part 1: overview and assessment. J Body Move Ther 5:91, 2001; with permission.)

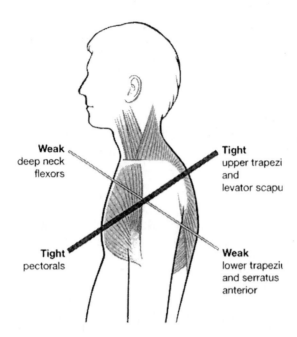

Figure 2. Upper crossed syndrome after Janda. (From Liebenson C: Manual resistance techniques. In Chaitow L (ed): Rehabilitation in Muscle Energy Procedures. Edinburgh, Churchill Livingstone, 2001; with permission.)

Poor posture and faulty movement patterns are typical kinetic chain dysfunctions that cause biomechanical overload. Such repetitive strain irritates pain-sensitive structures and can be a key perpetuating factor of pain due to WADs. Common clinical relationships are shown in Table 4.

These same faulty movement patterns or postures are associated with typical patterns of trigger points in overloaded muscles and accompanying muscle imbalances (short and inhibited muscle antagonists) (Table 5).

Pain referred from the SCM muscle(s) or upper cervical joints is related to muscle imbalance involving shortened suboccipitals combined with overactivity of the SCM and inhibition of the deep neck flexors (DNFs) (Figs. 3 and 4). A simple screen is to perform the head/neck flexion test (Fig. 5).

Upper cervical flexion is important for maintainance of good spinal statics. The results of the head/neck flexion test can often be predicted on the basis of postural analysis of the head and neck. In standing analysis, a head-forward

Table 4. Relationship Between Key Sources of Biomechanical Overload and Painful Joints

Painful Joint	Faulty Posture	Faulty Movement Pattern
Cervicocranial	Head forward	Neck flexion
Glenohumeral	Rounded shoulder	Scapulohumeral rhythm
Upper ribs	Slumped posture	Respiration
TMJ	Chin poke	Mouth opening

Table 5.   Key Myofascial or Osteoligamentous Pain Syndromes and Muscle
Imbalances Associated with Head and Neck Dysfunction

Painful Joint	Trigger Points	Shortened Muscle	Inhibited Muscle
Cervico-cranial	SCM	Suboccipitals	DNFs
Gleno-humeral	Upper trapezius	Levator scapulae or subscapularis	Lower trapezius
Upper ribs	Scalenes	Pectorals	Diaphragm
TMJ	Lateral pterygoids	Masseter	Digastricus

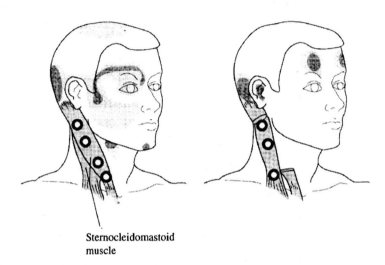

Sternocleidomastoid
muscle

Figure 3.   SCM-referred pain. (From Liebenson C: Self-treatment of mid-thoracic dysfunction: a key link in the body axis. Part 1: overview and assessment. J Body Move Ther 5:92, 2001; with permission).

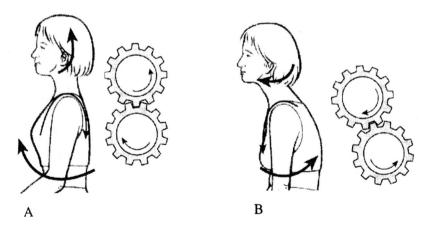

A   B

Figure 4.   Head-forward posture. (From Liebenson C: Self-treatment of mid-thoracic dysfunction: a key link in the body axis. Part 1: overview and assessment. J Body Move Ther 5:93, 2001; with permission.

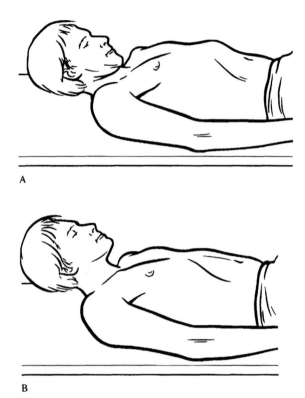

A

B

Figure 5. Deep neck flexor (head/neck flexion) test after Janda. (A) Correct. (B) Incorrect. (From Liebenson C: Self-treatment of mid-thoracic dysfunction: a key link in the body axis. Part 1: overview and assessment. J Body Move Ther 5:94, 2001; with permission.)

posture with a chin poke indicates agonist/antagonist/synergist muscle imbalance. In particular, the cervical extensors (the upper trapezius and suboccipitals) are not balanced by the coactivation of the DNFs: longus colli and capitis. As a result, SCM substitution occurs.

The clinical relevance of this imbalance is that treatment of the myofascial or articular pain generators without subsequent neuromuscular reeducation will likely not correct the underlying problem. The key is to look for chin poking during head/neck flexion, which signifies abnormal synergist substitution of the SCM for the DNFs. Possible suboccipital shortening exists. Head and neck syndromes can result from the cervicocranial hyperextension repetitive strain. Certainly WAD pain can be perpetuated by this disturbed function.

Pain referred from the upper trapezius or pectoral muscles or glenohumeral joint is related to muscle imbalance involving shortened pectorals combined with overactivity of the upper trapezius and inhibition of the lower trapezius and dorsal erector spinae (Figs. 6–8). A simple screen is to perform the arm abduction test (Fig. 9).

Poor scapulohumeral rhythm coordination is related to head/neck (ie, headache, whiplash) and shoulder disorders (ie, impingement).[2] This stereotypical movement pattern screens for functional pathology during tasks involved with prehension.[2,12,34] Inadequate fixation of the scapulae from below will overstress both the cervical spine and shoulder joint complex. This is eval-

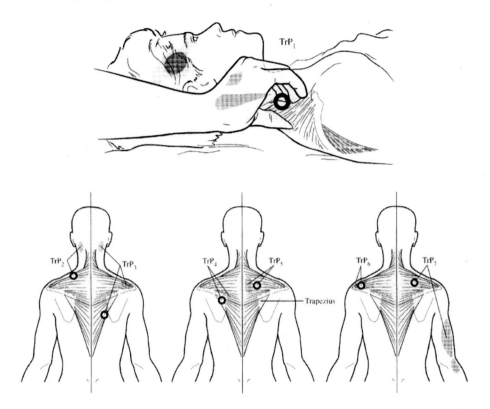

Figure 6. Upper trapezius–referred pain. (From Liebenson C: Self-treatment of mid-thoracic dysfunction: a key link in the body axis. Part 1: overview and assessment. J Body Move Ther 5:94, 2001; with permission.)

Figure 7. Shrugged (gothic) shoulder posture. (From Tunnell P: Self-treatment of mid-thoracic dysfunction: a key link in the body axis. Part 1: overview and assessment J Body Move Ther 1:24, 1996; with permission.)

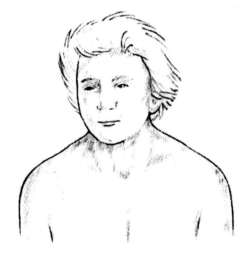

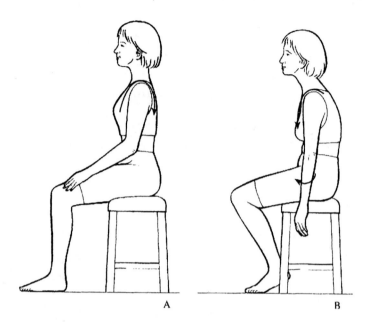

Figure 8. Round shouldered posture. (*A*) Internally rotated arms. (*B*) Secondary to kyphosis. (From Liebenson C: Self-treatment of mid-thoracic dysfunction: a key link in the body axis. Part 1: overview and assessment J Body Move Ther 5:91, 2001.)

uated during reaching and carrying tasks. Coactivation of the upper and lower scapular fixators maintains a "neutral" position of the scapulae during arm movements.

Pain referred from the scalenes or upper trapezius muscles or upper ribs is related to muscle imbalance involving overactivity of the scalenes and upper trapezius combined with inhibition of the diaphragm (Fig. 10). A simple screen is to perform an evaluation of respiration during inhalation (Fig. 11).

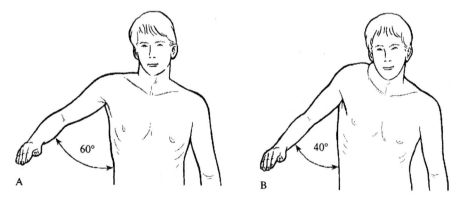

Figure 9. Arm abduction test after Janda. (*A*) Correct. (*B*) Incorrect. (From Liebenson C: Self-treatment of mid-thoracic dysfunction: a key link in the body axis. Part 1: overview and assessment J Body Move Ther 5:95, 2001; with permission.)

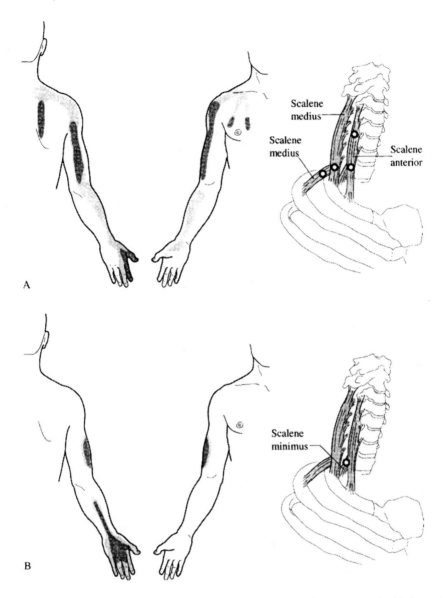

Figure 10. Scalene-referred pain. ((From Liebenson C: Self-treatment of mid-thoracic dysfunction: a key link in the body axis. Part 1: overview and assessment J Body Move Ther 5:95, 2001; with permission.)

Dysfunctional respiration can be related to lumbopelvic, head/neck, orofacial, and cervicothoracic disorders. Respiration is perhaps the most important of all movement patterns. In the thoracic spine, widening of the thorax posteriorly during inhalation should be visible as a respiratory wave observed in a prone patient. Exhalation has a mobilizing effect on thoracic spine extension and is particularly important in those suffering from a forward drawn posture and

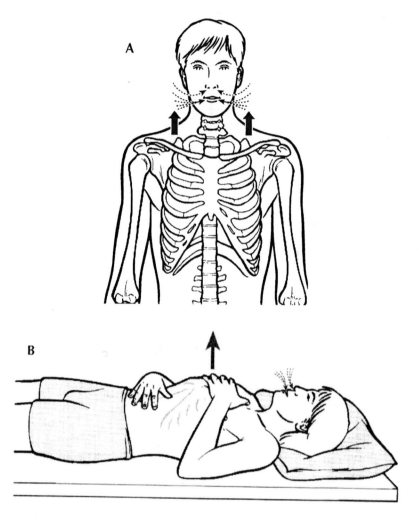

Figure 11. Faulty respiration. (A) Seated. (B) Supine. (From Liebenson C: Re-education of faulty respiration. (From J Body Move Ther 3:225, 1999; with permission.)

kyphosis. The most important fault during breathing is lifting the thorax with the scalenes instead of widening it in the horizontal plane. This can lead to overstrain of the cervical spine.

Pain referred from the masseter or lateral pterygoid muscles and/or the temporomandibular joint (TMJ) is related to shortened masseters and lateral pterygoids combined with inhibition of the digastricus (Figs. 12 and 13). A simple screen is to perform the mouth-opening test (Fig. 14).[41,42]

Dysfunctional mouth opening signifies muscle imbalance with overactive mouth closers (masseters, medial pterygoids) and inhibited mouth openers (digastricus). The lateral pterygoid will also become overactive and often shortened as it begins to dominate mouth opening. Due to the high utilization of the muscles of mastication, improper mouth opening and poor mandibular

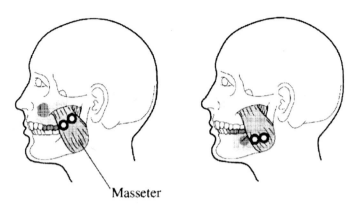

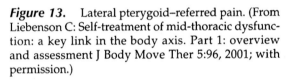

Figure 12. Masseter-referred pain. (From Liebenson C: Self-treatment of mid-thoracic dysfunction: a key link in the body axis. Part 1: overview and assessment J Body Move Ther 5:96, 2001; with permission.)

Figure 13. Lateral pterygoid–referred pain. (From Liebenson C: Self-treatment of mid-thoracic dysfunction: a key link in the body axis. Part 1: overview and assessment J Body Move Ther 5:96, 2001; with permission.)

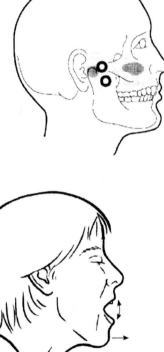

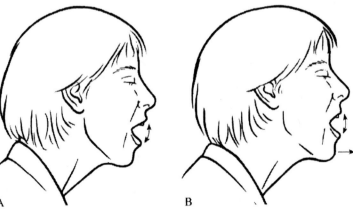

Figure 14. Faulty mouth opening test. (*A*) Correct (*B*) Incorrect. (From Liebenson C: Self-treatment of mid-thoracic dysfunction: a key link in the body axis. Part 1: overview and assessment J Body Move Ther 5:96, 2001; with permission.)

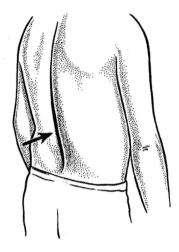

Figure 15. Thoracolumbar erector spinae dysfunction. (From Liebenson C: Self-treatment of mid-thoracic dysfunction: a key link in the body axis. Part 1: overview and assessment J Body Move Ther 5:93, 2001; with permission.)

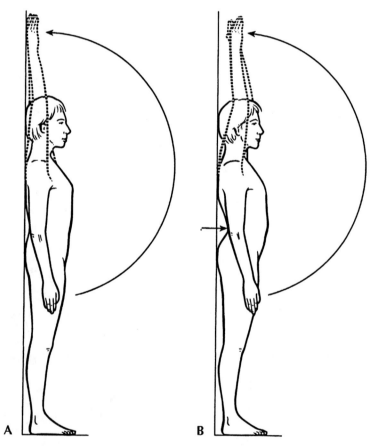

Figure 16. Faulty arm elevation test after Norris. (*A*) Correct. (*B*) Incorrect. (From Liebenson C: Self-treatment of mid-thoracic dysfunction: a key link in the body axis. Part 1: overview and assessment J Body Move Ther 5:96, 2001; with permission.)

locomotion can frequently sabatoge the healing and functional restoration of the WAD patient. This can result in TMJ and cervicocranial overstrain.

Pain referred from the thoracolumbar erector spinae muscle(s) or T10-L5 joints is related to overactivity of the thoracolumbar erector spinae combined with inhibition of the dorsal erector spinae (Fig. 15). A simple screen is to perform the standing arm elevation test (Fig. 16).

Fixed kyphosis of the mid-thoracic region is important because of its potential to cause the head-forward or round shouldered postures. It is a key perpetuating factor of any pain in the upper body.

TREATMENT OF WHIPLASH PATIENTS IN THE SUBACUTE PHASE

According to Turner[47] patients have two goals: first, to receive information about how to manage their pain, and second, to receive advice on how to resume normal activities. The modern approach focuses on function, not just relief of symptoms. In the report of findings it is important to establish the following goals of care: to reduce pain, restore function, and keep the patient independent.

Most WAD patients require a relatively straightforward evaluation and treatment approach because the prognosis is reasonably good for most. Unless there are **"red flags"** of serious disease, the patient should be reassured and reactivated. If needed, one can provide pain-relief treatments. Avoidance of unnecessary surgery, overmedication, and overexamination, especially with diagnostic imaging, is important to prevent "medicalizing" the problem. In contrast, patients who are not satisfactorily recovering by the subacute phase require more aggressive management because it is easier to prevent than to treat chronic pain. The key time frame in which aggressive management should be considered is between 4 and 12 weeks. Those with **"yellow flag"** (psychosocial or medical) risk factors of chronicity should be more aggressively managed even earlier. This still does not indicate magnetic resonance imaging on every patient, but it does mean a rehabilitation specialist should be involved and, in particular, one with training in cognitive-behavorial approaches. The most important point is that when a full diagnostic work-up is recommended it should not be limited to magnetic resonance imaging or other structural evaluations but also include functional/physiologic testing such as a functional capacity evaluation and a psychosocial evaluation. Table 6 presents an overview of the key steps to recovery.

Table 6.   Keys to Recovery: The 5 R's

1. Reassurance that no serious disease is present and that improvement is likely to begin rapidly

2. Relief of pain with medication or manipulation

3. Reactivation advice that normal activities can be resumed (walking, swimming, biking) and education about simple activity modifications to reduce biomechanical strain (ie, Brügger relief position, chin tucks)

4. Reevaluation of those entering the subacute phase for structural, functional, or psychosocial factors

5. Rehabilitation/reconditioning/reeducation of muscles with McKenzie, stabilization, progressive strengthening, or cognitive-behavorial (indicated if high "yellow flags" score) approaches.

The chiropractic or musculoskeletal medicine approach to whiplash has reached a new standard of care. It embraces the current evidence for advice, manipulation, and exercise. Most importantly it recognizes the importance of reassurance and reactivation for promoting a quick recovery and minimizing the risk of chronicity.

Advice

Advice for patients with WADs is designed to reassure them about the positive prognosis for their condition and the safety of gradually resuming normal activities. It includes activity modification advice to improve postural habits, such as when working at a computer and performing movement stereotypes such as carrying a briefcase and reaching overhead. Advice should teach the difference between hurt and harm, focusing on the need to avoid activities that cause symptoms to peripheralize, while being less anxious about mild, local symptoms that accompany typical activities or light exercises.

While improved biomechanics during sustained static tasks or repetitive dynamic tasks is important, patients should not be overly vigilant about posture in all activities. Full range of motion will be lost if one is educated to stay in a "neutral range" all of the time. Full-range activities that involve light load will beneficially stretch and mobilize tissues. Traditional back school education emphasizing "proper form" all of the time is to be avoided in favor of a modern cognitve-behavorial approach emphasizing that hurt does not necessarily equal harm.

Patients with WADs do have injured tissues. They should be informed that these tissues will heal better with light activity than with rest. Pain flare-ups are normal and to be expected and are not a sign of further injury. Stress and emotional tension will tend to reduce an individual's pain threshold and intensify the symptoms associated with such "flare-ups". Patients should be educated that stress plays a role but that it does not cause injury and that the pain will run a course. Advice about physiologic coping strategies, such as breathing techniques, light exercise, and meditation is also important.

Manipulation

Manual therapy and manipulation are important for facilitating recovery from WADs. Normalization of afferent information from joints, muscles, skin, and fascia is important for the promotion of healing and rehabilitation of function. Joints that are stiff, such as in the mid-thoracic region, should be mobilized to improve load-sharing and thus take pressure off sensitive cervical joints. Any joint that is painful or stiff can be mobilized gently with postisometric relaxation, muscle energy, or other nonthrust techniques. However, only joints that are carefully examined and found not to be hypermobile should be considered as candidates for high-velocity, short-amplitude thrust manipulation. (Figs. 17 and 18).

Muscles that are typically shortened should be relaxed to improve the quality of movement patterns. The latissmus dorsi, pectorals, and hip flexors are prime examples. Soft tissue manipulation including fascial release is an important method in the manual therapy field. Such techniques are usually very gentle and can be used early in the care of WAD patients. Subacute or chronic

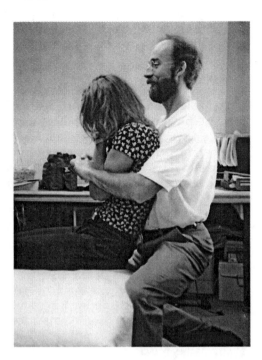

Figure 17. Long-axis mobilization of mid-thoracic spine.

WAD patients may require more advanced forms of connective tissue manipulation, including an active release technique to resolve areas of shortening.

Adjunctive therapy to manual therapy can include physical agents such as heat and ice, electrical muscle stimulation, and traction. Many of these methods are well-suited for early care in the acute phase, but they become progressively less valuable as more time has elapsed since the trauma. These passive

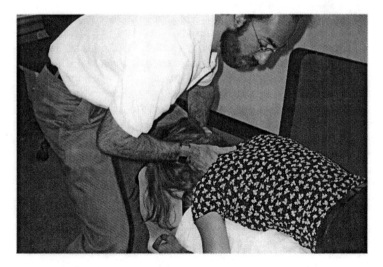

Figure 18. High-velocity thrust to cervicothoracic junction.

modalities should be seen as means to facilitate active rehabilitation and not as ends in themselves.

Exercise

Rehabilitation focuses on the identification of key functional pathologies related to spinal instability and their management by reactivation and reconditioning. Exercise is thus important alongside the advice and manipulation to improve the patient's functional performance in their daily activities.

Patients learn to appreciate that the quality of the movement is more important than the number of repetitions. This is very different from how most people view exercise, and patients thusly are reeducated about "therapeutic" exercise. The first goal is for the patient to learn how to produce and control the movement in his functional training range. This is the painless range within which movements are performed in a coordinated way. Such training for coordination during arm abduction tasks has been demonstrated to be successful.[2]

Because the results of exercise training are highly specific to the movement, velocity, and range trained, the goal is to include ADLs and demands of employment into the training program. Exercises initially require conscious control, but the goal is to automatize coordination to lessen the consequences of poor motivation and compliance. Patients should first become consciously aware of the muscle or part of the body that is to be activated. Exercises and coordinated activities are prescribed that train the patient how to gain this volitional control. Finally, the motor program becomes a subcortical engram, and the patient achieves the desired affect without having to concentrate on the function (Table 7). Thus, the patient is able to protect the vulnerable region during ADLs and when exposed to unexpected perturbations.

The **cognitive-kinesthetic** stage involves learning the *kinesthetic awareness* of the "functional range." First, the clinician must find the patient's **functional range**—the position or movement that centralizes or decreases pain without unwanted superficial muscle activity (ie, upper trapezius). The patient should demonstrate that he has the **kinesthetic awareness** to produce isolated movements of different joints and that he can find and maintain a "neutral position" of certain key joints such as the cervicocranial or scapulothoracic. This will show that he has learned to coordinate and coactivate antagonist muscles.

An example is teaching the patients to disassociate related movements such as scapulothoracic from scapulohumeral or cervicocranial from cervicothoracic. The patient should be able to move his arm in abduction or flexion while fixing the scapulae inferior against the thorax. Excessive shrugging of the shoulder signifies poor scapulothoracic kinesthetic awareness. Another example is that the patient should be able to perform a chin tuck and use this skill dynamically so that when he rises from a chair or a bed he can avoid poking his chin.

Table 7.   Stages of Motor Learning

• Cognitive-kinesthetic
• Associative
• Autonomous

The **associative stage** involves training endurance of the "deep" stabilizers repetitively. The key is to find two or three faulty or pain-producing movements and focus on improving their function. One should train "inner-range" endurance of the deep stabilizers, such as the DNFs, digastricus, and lower scapular stabilizers. The exercises should train endurance, not strength. This involves gentle loading (less than 50% of maximum voluntary contraction ability), frequent repetitions (8-10), and sustained hold times (5-6 sec). These exercises should be performed approximately twice a day with durations as long as 3 months possibly being necessary.

The **autonomous stage** involves integration of improved motor control into ADLs on an automatic basis. The goal is to incorporate control of the functionalrange into ADLs so that a low degree of attention is required on an automatic basis.

Training hints for teaching patients the exercises:
- Remind patients that they can do as many repetitions as necessary to feel the burn of the targeted muscle being exercises, but they must stop if the quality of the movement is altered in any way.
- Always have patients demonstrate the exercise on the next office visit to correct any errors that they may have adopted.
- Whenever possible, have patients work toward mimicking activities that they do in real life as part of their exercise.

Self-Treatments
Postural management: see Figure 19
Lower and middle trapezius: see Figure 20
Neck flexion: supine and seated chin tucks (see Figure 5)
Training track for an inhibited diaphragm: see Figure 21
T4–T8 dorsal extension: see Figures 22–27
TMJ: see Figure 28

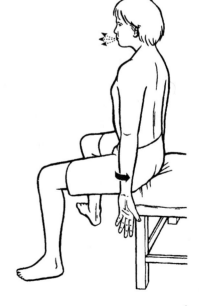

Figure 19. Brügger relief position. (From Liebenson C: Self-treatment of the slump posture. J Body Move Ther 5:100, 2001; with permission.)

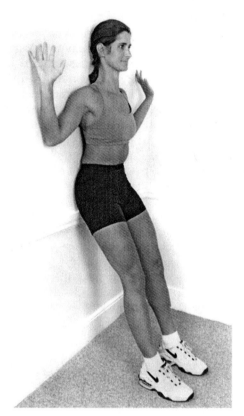

Figure 20. Wall angel: sliding arms down and back up along the wall without shrugging the shoulders. (From DeFranca C, Liebenson C: The Upper Body Book. San Diego, The Gym Ball Store, 2001; with permission.)

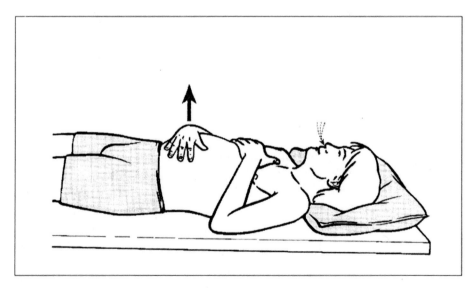

Figure 21. Lower abdomen belly breathing. (From Liebenson C: Re-education of faulty respiration. J Body Move Ther 3:227, 1999; with permission.)

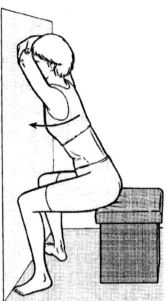

Figure 22. Lewit wall mobilization with postisometric relaxation. (From Liebenson C: Self-treatment of the slump posture. J Body Move Ther 5:100, 2001; with permission.)

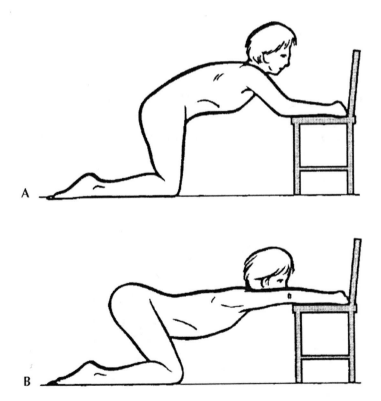

Figure 23. Upper back cat. (*A*) Beginning phase. (*B*) Final phase. (From Liebenson C: Self-treatment of the slump poisture. J Body Move Ther 5:100, 2001; with permission.)

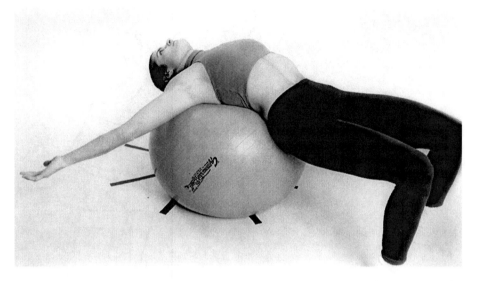

Figure 24. Ball stretches. (From DeFranca C, Liebenson C: The Upper Body Book. San Diego, The Gym Ball Store, 2001; with permission.)

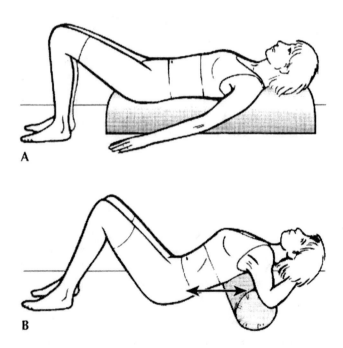

Figure 25. Foam roll stretches. (*A*) Vertical; easier. (*B*) Horizontal; more advanced. (From Liebenson C: Self-treatment of mid-thoracic dysfunction: a key link in the body axis. Part 2: treatment. J Body Move Ther 5:193, 2001; with permission.)

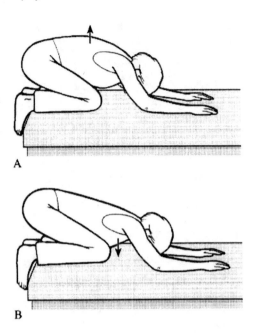

Figure 26. Active prayer stretch after Kolár (*A*) Inhalation phase. (*B*) Active exhalation phase. (From Liebenson C: Self-treatment of mid-thoracic dysfunction: a key link in the body axis. Part 2: treatment. J Body Move Ther 5:194, 2001; with permission.)

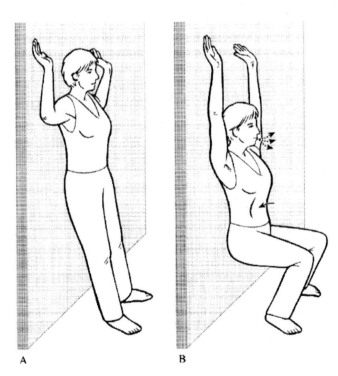

Figure 27. Wall slide with arm elevation after Kolár. (*A*) Inhalation phase. (*B*) Active exhalation phase. (From Liebenson C: Self-treatment of mid-thoracic dysfunction: a key link in the body axis. Part 2: treatment. J Body Move Ther 5:194, 2001; with permission.)

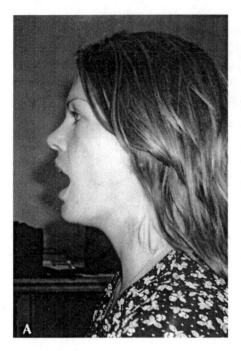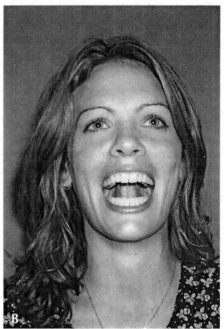

Figure 28. Mandibular rotation exercises. (*A*) Side view. (*B*) Frontal view.

CONCLUSION

Appropriate management of WADs depends on focusing on functional reactivation. A biopsychosocial approach is needed not a biomedical one. Because structural diagnosis is limited, functional/physiologic and psychosocial factors must become the paramount concern in WAD grades I through III. Functional assessment is the most important step and establishes the ability for immediate reexamination to validate the treatment prescription. To reactivate patients requires a careful approach that is not too aggressive in the acute phase or too passive in the subacute phase. In fact, the subacute phase is the ideal time for aggressive treatment to prevent the onset of a chronic pain syndrome.

Reassurance, activity modification advice, and pain-relieving treatments are the mainstay of acute care. Manipulation and exercise are also needed for patients still suffering significant symptoms in the subacute phase. A cognitive-behavioral and perhaps multidisciplinary approach is needed for chronic patients. When appropriate decision points are used to guide the type and intensity of assessment and treatment approaches, patient comfort and recovery can be enhanced without the iatrogenic effect of encouraging the patient to take on the "sick role."

References

1. Anderson GBJ, Ortengren R: Lumbar disc pressure and myoeelctric activity during sittin III: studies on an office chair. Scand J Rehabil Med 13:122–177, 1974.
2. Babyar SR: Excessive scapular motion in individuals recovering from painful and stiff shoulders: causes and treatment strategies. Phys Ther 76:226–238, 1996.

3. Barton PM, Hayes KC. Neck flexor muscle strength and relaxation times in normal subjects and subjects with unilateral neck pain and headache. Arch Phys Med Rehabil 77:680–687, 1996.
4. Boden SD. McCowin PR, Davis Do, Dina TS, et al: Abnormal magnetic-resonance scans of the cervical spine in asymptomatic subjects. J Bone Joint Surg Am 72:1178–1184, 1990.
5. Borchgrevink GE, Kaasa A, McDonoagh D, et al: Acute treatment of whiplash neck sprain injuries. Spine 23:25–31, 1998.
6. Borghouts JAJ, Koes BW, Bouter LM: The clinical course and prognostic factors of nonspecific neck pain: a systematic review. Pain 77:1–13, 1998.
7. Bovim G, Schrader H, Sand T: Neck pain in the general population. Spine 19:1307–1309, 1994.
8. Bronfort G, Evans R, Nelson B, et al: A randomized clinical trial of exercise and spinal manipulation for patients with chronic neck pain. Spine 26:788–799, 2001.
9. Bush K, Chaudhuri R, Hillier S, Penny J: The pathomorphologic changes that accompany the resolution of cervical radiculopathy. Spine 22:183–187, 1997.
10. Cote P, Cassidy JD, Carroll L: The factors associated with neck pain and its related disability in the Saskatchewan population. Spine 25(9):1109–1117, 2000.
11. Dvorak J, Valach L, Schmidt S: Cervical spine injuries in Switzerland. J Man Med 4:7–16, 1989.
12. Edgerton VR, Wolf SL, Levendowski DJ, Roy RR: Theoretical basis for patterning EMG amplitudes to assess muscle dysfunction. Med Sci Sports Exerc 28:744–751, 1996.
13. Gargan MR, Bannister GC: Long-term prognosis of soft-tissue injuries of the neck. J Bone Joint Surg Br 72:901–903, 1990.
14. Harms-Ringdahl K, Nachemson A: Acute and subacute neck pain: nonsurgical treatment. In Nachemson A, Jonsson E (eds): Swedish SBU report. Evidence-Based Treatment for Back Pain. Philadelphia, Swedish Council on Technology Assessment in Health Care (SBU)/Lippincott, 2000, pp 327–338.
15. Hartling L, Brison R, Ardern C, Pickett W: Prognostic value of the Quebec classifiction of whiplash-associated disorders. Spine 26:36–41, 2001.
16. Hurwitz EL, Aker PD, Adams AH, et al: Manipulation and mobilization of the cervical spine: a systematic review of the literature. Spine 21:1746–1760, 1996.
17. Janda V: Evaluation of muscle imbalance. In Liebenson C (ed): Rehabilitation of the Spine: A Practitioner's Manual. Baltimore, Williams & Wilkins, 1996.
18. Jette A: Physical therapy and health outcomes in patients with spinal impairments. Phys Ther 76:930–941, 1996
19. Jordan A, Bendix T, Nielsen H, et al: Intensive training, physiotherapy, or manipulation for patients with chronic neck pain: a prospective single-blinded randomized clinical trial. Spine 23:311–319, 1998.
20. Jull G, Barret C, Magee R, Ho P: Further clincial clarification of the muscle dysfunction in cervical headache. Cephalgia 19:179–185,1999.
21. Jull GA: Deep cervical flexor muscle dysfunction in whiplash. J Musculoskel Pain 8:143–154, 2000.
22. Kibler WB, Herring SA, Press JM: Functional Rehabilitation of Sports and Musculoskeletal Injuries. Gaithersburg, MD, Aspen Publishers, 1998.
23. Lauren H, Luoto S, Alaranta H, et al: Arm motion speed and risk of neck pain. Spine 22:2094–2099, 1997.
24. Lewit K: Manipulative Therapy in Rehabilitation of the Motor System, 3rd ed. London, Butterworths, 1999.
25. Liebenson C, DeFranca C, Lefebvre R: Rehabilitation of the spine: functional evaluation of the cervical spine [videotape]. Baltimore, Lippincott Williams & Wilkins, 1998.
26. Liebenson C: Rehabilitation of the Spine: A Practitioner's Manual. Baltimore, Lippincott Williams & Wilkins, 1996.
27. Maimaris C, Barnes MR, Allen MJ: 'Whiplash injuries' of the neck: a retrospective study. Injury 19:393–396, 1988.
28. Main CJ, Watson PJ: Psychological aspects of pain. Man Ther 4:203–215, 1999.
29. Makela M, Heliovaara M, Sievers K, et al: Prevalence, determinants and consequences of chronic neck pain in Finland. Am J Epidemiol 134:1356–1367, 1991.
30. McCrory D, Penzien D, Hasselblad V, Gray R: Evidence Report: Behavioral and Physical Treatments for Tension-Type and Cervicogenic Headache. Durham, NC, Duke University/Foundation for Chiropractic Education and Research, 2001.
31. McKinney LA: Early mobilisation and outcome in acute sprains of the neck. BMJ 299:1006–1008, 1989.
32. Murphy D: Conservative Care of Cervical Spine Disorders. McGraw Hill, New York, 1999.

33. Nachemson A, Vingard E: Assessment of neck and back pain syndromes. In Nachemson A, Jonsson E (eds): Swedish SBU report. Evidence-based Treatment for Back Pain. Philadelphia, Swedish Council on Technology Assessment in Health Care (SBU)/Lippincott, 2000, pp 189–236.
34. Nederhand MJ, Ijzerman MJ, Hermens HK, et al: Cervical muscle dysfunction in the chronic whiplash associated disorder grade II (WAD-II). Spine 15:1938–1943, 2000.
35. Olsson I, Bunketorp O, Carlsson G, et al: An in-depth study of neck injuries in rear end collisions. IRCOBI 269–280, 1990.
36. Panjabi MM, Nibu K, Cholewicki J: Whiplash injuries and the potential for mechanical instability. Eur Spine J 7:484–492, 1998.
37. Radonov BP, Sturzanegger M, Di Stefano G: Long term outcome after whiplash injury: a 2 year follow-up considering features of injury mechanism and somatic, radiological and psychosocial findings. Medicine 74:281–297, 1995.
38. Rosenfeld M, Gunnarsson R, Borenstein P: Early intervention in whiplash-associated disorders: a comparison of two treatment protocols. Spine 25:1782–1787, 2000.
39. Shumway-Cook A, Woollacott M: Motor Control—Theory and Practical Applications. Baltimore, Lippincott Williams & Wilkins, 1995.
40. Silverman JL, Rodriguez AA, Agre JC: Quantitative cervical flexor strength in healthy subjects and in subjects with mechanical neck pain. Arch Phys Med Rehabil 72:679–681, 1991.
41. Skaggs C, Liebenson CS: Orofacial pain. Top Clin Chiropract 7:43–50, 2000.
42. Skaggs C: Diagnosis and treatment of temporomandibular disorders. In Murphy D (ed): Conservative Care of Cervical Spine Disorders. New York, McGraw Hill, 1999.
43. Spitzer WO, Skovron ML, Salmi LIR, et al: Scientific monograph of the Quebec Task Force on Whiplash-Associated Disorders: redefining "whiplash" and its management. Spine 20(suppl): S1–S73, 1995.
44. Takala J, Sievers K, Klaukka T: Rheumatic symptoms in the middle aged population in southwestern Finland. Scand J Rheumatol 47(suppl):15–29, 1982.
45. Teresi LM, Lufkin RB, Reicher MA, et al: Asymptomatic degenerative disk disease and spondylosis of the cervical spine: MR Imaging. Radiology 164:83–88, 1987.
46. Treleavan J, Jull G, Atkinson L: Cervical musculoskeletal dysfunction in post-concussion headache. Cephalalgia 14:273–279, 1994.
47. Turner JA: Educational and behavorial interventions for back pain in primary care. Spine 21:2851–2859, 1996.
48. Watson DH, Trott PH: Cervical headache: an investigation of natural head posture and cervical flexor muscle performance. Cephalgia 13:272–284, 1993.
49. Westerling D, Jonsson BG: Pain from the neck-shoulder region and sick leave. Scand J Soc Med 8:131–136, 1980.

20

Medications in the Treatment of Whiplash-Associated Disorders

Gerard A. Malanga, M.D., Steven Roman, M.D., and Scott F. Nadler, D.O.

Although whiplash is a common disorder, there is little scientific evidence on the topic of pharmacologic management. Unlike low back pain, where evidence is plentiful, there is a paucity of evidence focusing on the pharmacologic management of whiplash or acute neck pain. Various classes of pharmacologic agents are frequently prescribed for the symptoms of whiplash injury, but there is very little evidence to support their use. This chapter attempts to provide a logical approach to the use of pharmacologic agents in the treatment of whiplash injury.

The Quebec Task Force, a board of international experts commissioned by the Quebec Automobile Insurance Society, analyzed the clinical, public health, social, and financial determinants of whiplash.[85] The goal of the recommendations of the Quebec Task Force was to assure fairness and compassion, medical care of the highest scientific standards, realistic strategies of primary prevention, and judicious management of society's resources to individuals who have suffered whiplash injuries following a motor vehicle collision. Evidence used by the task force showed that analgesics and nonsteroidal anti-inflammatory drugs (NSAIDs) combined with other treatment modalities were associated with short-term benefit for whiplash-associated disorder (WAD) grades I and II that presented in the acute phase or fewer than 72 hours after collision. No acceptable studies were found regarding narcotic analgesics, psychopharmacologic therapeutics, or muscle relaxants. The literature reviewed on whiplash injuries or neck pain used salicylates,[19] NSAIDs,[37] and various other medications[36,41,62–64,69] as controls or as cotherapies and not stand-alone treatment strategies, therefore permitting only inferential conclusions to be drawn about their effectiveness.

The recommendations of the task force included the following: No medication should be prescribed for WAD grade I. Nonnarcotic analgesics and NSAIDs can be used to alleviate pain for the short term in WAD grades II and III. Their use should not be pursued for more than 3 weeks and should be weighed against possible adverse effects. Narcotic analgesics should not be prescribed for WAD grades I and II. Occasionally, they may be prescribed for pain relief in acute severe grade III but only for a limited time. Although commonly prescribed, muscle relaxants should not generally be used in the acute phase of WAD. The psychopharmacologic drugs are not recommended for use on a general basis in WAD of any duration or grade, but they may occasionally be used for symptoms such as insomnia or tension, as an adjunct to activating interventions in the acute phase (< 3 months' duration). For chronic pain in WAD (> 3 months' duration), the minor tranquilizers and antidepressants may be used.[85]

Unfortunately, the recommendations of the task force rely to a great extent on the limited scientific evidence available for whiplash at the time of the study. The only prospective randomized study[70] of drug therapy performed to date for whiplash used high-dose intravenous methylprednisolone (Medrol) for Quebec Task Force grades II and III WAD. In this trial of 40 patients, methylprednisolone, when administered within 8 hours of injury, was found to decrease the total number of sick days ($P = .01$) and sick-leave profile ($P = .003$) at 6-month follow-up compared with placebo. Disabling symptoms were also found to be less ($P = .47$) in the methylprednisolone group. This study was limited by a small number of patients. The authors do not recommend the strategy of indiscriminately prescribing steroids in light of the perceived risk over the benefits of this strategy. We believe further research is warranted in this area.

Two randomized, controlled trials describe the use of cyclobenzaprine (Flexeril) for low back and neck pain but not acute neck pain. Bercel[11] performed a study of 54 patients with osteoarthritis of the cervical or lumbosacral spine. They were treated with cyclobenzaprine or placebo for 2 weeks. A greater number of patients improved by global assessment with cyclobenzaprine as compared with placebo. Basmajian[10] compared cyclobenzaprine with diazepam (Valium) and placebo in a 2-week study for treating spasms in the neck and low back. There was a favorable response in all groups with no clinical differences. Electromyographic testing did, however, show significant improvement in muscle spasm over the Valium and placebo groups.

One possible sequela of whiplash injury is headache. These headaches often present as migraines. Retrospective data suggest that common antimigraine medications are effective in the treatment of this disorder,[50] including amitriptyline (Elavil)[90,98] and propranolol (Inderal).[98]

The extent of the literature pertaining directly to the use of medications for neck pain and whiplash injury has been presented. In light of the limited science related to medication use in neck pain or whiplash injury, it may be appropriate to apply the existing literature pertaining to low back pain as a correlate because it has been extensively studied and reviewed in this regard.[56a] In support of this contention, one can review the pathophysiology, common pain pathways, and pain-generating structures such as nerve roots, discs, zygapophyseal joints, ligaments, bones, and muscles, all of which are similar in both neck and low back pain. The remainder of this chapter applies the principles related to pharmacologic management of low back pain as a guide to management of acute neck pain after a whiplash injury. This premise, however, does need to be validated, which makes for ample research opportunities.

ACETAMINOPHEN

Acetaminophen (Tylenol) is the principle member of the group of drugs classified as paraaminophenol derivatives.[44,95] While acetaminophen's analgesic and antipyretic effects are equal to those of aspirin, its anti-inflammatory effects are weak. Its therapeutic effects appear to be secondary to an inhibition

TABLE 1. Nonsteroidal Anti-inflammatory Drugs: Dose and Cost

Drug and Family	Max Daily Dose (mg)	Usual Single Dose (mg)	Dosing	Half-Life (Hrs)	$/Month
Salicylates					
Aspirin	4000	500–1000	Q 4–6 hrs	12	1
Nonacetylated Salicylates					
Salsalate (Disalcid, others)	4000	1000	Q 8–12 hrs	16	30
Diflusinal (Dolobid)	1500	1000, 500	Q 8–12 hrs	8–12	30–45
Choline magnesium Trisalicylate	3000	1000–1500	Q 8–12 hrs	9–17	40–120
Proprionic Acids					
Ibuprofen (Motrin, others)	2400	200–400	Q 4–6 hrs	2	30–80
Flurbiprofen (Ansaid)	300	50–100	Q 6–8 hrs	5.7	50–150
Fenoprofen (Nalfon)	1200	200	Q 4–6 hrs	3	50–125
Ketoprofen (Orudis, others)	300	25–75	Q 4–8 hrs	2–4	90–180
Naproxen (Naprosyn)	1250	500, 250	Q 6–8 hrs	13	44–80
Naproxen Na (Anaprox)	1375	550, 275	Q 12 hrs	13	44–80
Indoles					
Indomethacin (Indocin)	150	25–50	Q 6–8 hrs	4.5	35–100
Sulindac (Clinoril)	400	150–200	Q 12 hrs	8	45–90
Tolmetin (Tolectin)	1800	150–600	Q 6–8 hrs	2–5	30–90
Etodolac (Lodine)	1200	200–400	Q 6–8 hrs	3–11	70–175
Fenamates					
Meclofenamate (Meclomen)	400	100	Q 6–8 hrs	2	54–162
Others					
Piroxicam (Feldene)	40	20	Q 24 hrs	50	80–160
Nalbumetone (Relafen)	2000	1000	Q 12–24 hrs	24	60–120
Ketorolac (Toradol)	40	10	Q 6 hrs	4–7	60–120
Oxaprozin (Daypro)	1800	1200	Q 24hrs	24	70–120
COX-2 Inhibitors					
Celecoxib (Celebrex)		100–200	Q 12–24 hrs		65–76
Rofecoxib (Vioxx)	25	12.5–25	Q 24 hrs	17	70

of prostaglandin biosynthesis, with a resultant increase in the pain threshold and modulation of the hypothalamic heat-regulating center. The effects of acetaminophen are noted predominantly centrally and less peripherally, where the drug serves as only a weak inhibitor of cyclooxygenase and does not inhibit the activation of neutrophils as do other NSAIDs.

In the setting of acute low back pain, acetaminophen can be effectively used as an analgesic.[14] Several studies have shown acetaminophen to be superior to placebo in the treatment of osteoarthritis pain, and because of its efficacy it has been recommended as a first-line agent in osteoarthritis treatment.[5,24,31] A 1991 study by Bradley et al[18] compared the analgesic properties of acetaminophen to ibuprofen (Motrin) in the treatment of pain associated with osteoarthritis of the knee. Over a 4-week study period, acetaminophen was found to be as efficacious as both low-dose analgesic and high-dose anti-inflammatory regimens of ibuprofen in providing pain relief and an improved functional outcome.[6] In a 1982 study, paracetamol, a compound similar to acetaminophen, was compared to diflunisal (Dolobid), an NSAID and salicylate derivative, in the treatment of chronic low back pain.[46] Thirty patients with a 6-month to several-year history of low back pain presumed secondary to facet pathology were treated in a randomized fashion for 4 weeks, and more favorable outcomes were associated with NSAID use.

The accepted oral dose of acetaminophen is 325 to 1000 mg every 4 to 6 hours, with a 24-hour use not to exceed 4000 mg. Peak plasma levels and analgesic effects are typically noted 30 to 60 minutes following ingestion. Acetaminophen is generally available without prescription and is relatively inexpensive. While erythematous or urticarial skin rashes are occasionally observed, the most serious adverse effect of acute acetaminophen overdosage is hepatotoxicity. In adults, hepatotoxicity may result from a single dose of 10 to 15 g. More chronic abuse of acetaminophen has been associated with nephrotoxicity.

Acetaminophen's analgesic effects make it an acceptable medication in the treatment of acute low back pain. It is inexpensive, and its use is typically without complications. While effective against mild to moderate pain in some acute back pain situations, it does not offer the patient other desirable effects that address inflammation, muscle spasm, or sleep disturbance. Its efficacy as an analgesic for low back disorders associated with severe pain is more questionable.

NONSTEROIDAL ANTI-INFLAMMATORY DRUGS

Aspirin is the prototypical member of the group of medications known as NSAIDs. The primary mechanism of action of NSAIDs is a reduction of cyclooxygenase activity and a resultant decrease in prostaglandin synthesis. Prostaglandins are active mediators of the inflammatory cascade that also serve to sensitize peripheral nociceptors. A reduction in their local concentration could therefore explain the combined anti-inflammatory and analgesic properties of NSAIDs.[71] In single doses, most of the NSAIDs are more effective analgesics than a single dose of acetaminophen.[1] Locally, NSAIDs are also thought to combat inflammation by inhibiting neutrophil function and interfering with the activity of enzymes such as phospholipase.[20] Most NSAIDs do not decrease the production of lipoxygenase-produced leukotrienes, which are also believed to significantly contribute to the inflammatory response.[44] A disparity between the anti-inflammatory and analgesic potencies of these agents in clinical practice has been observed, and recent data have suggested that pain relief from NSAIDs may in part be secondary to a more central antinociceptive component.[40,55,57,60] Measurable levels of anti-inflammatory agents are appreciated in the cerebrospinal fluid following short-term administration in the setting of a soft tissue injury.[39]

NSAIDs include aspirin, which inhibits cyclooxygenase irreversibly through acetylation, and several groups of organic acids, including proprionic acid derivatives, acetic acid derivatives, and enolic acids, all of which bind to and reversibly inhibit cyclooxygenase (Table 1). Elimination half-lives of these drugs range from less than 4 hours for some proprionic acid derivatives to more than 40 hours for piroxicam (Feldene).[71]

In a survey by McCormack and Brune of 26 studies investigating the role of NSAIDs in acute soft tissue injuries, 14 double-blind, placebo-controlled studies were found to demonstrate a significant difference between NSAID and

Table 2. Muscle Relaxants Used for Low Back Pain

Medication	Mechanism of Action	Dosage	Contraindications
Muscle Relaxants			
Carisoprodol (Soma)	Blockage of interneuronal activity in reticular formation and spinal cord	350 mg tid and hs	Acute intermittent porphyria
Chlorzoxazone (Parafon Forte)	Inhibition of polysynaptic reflex arcs at subcortical and spinal cord levels	250–750 mg tid–qid	
Cyclobenzaprine (Flexeril)	Inhibition of alpha and gamma motor neuron activity at brain stem	10 mg tid	Cardiac disease, hyperthyroidism, use with mono-amine oxidase (MAO) inhibitors
Methocarbamol (Robaxin)	Unknown, possible general central nervous system depression	1000–1500 mg qid	
Dantrolene (Dantrium)	Inhibits the release of calcium from the sarcoplasmic reticulum	25 mg qd	Liver disease
Lioresal (Baclofen)	Inhibits mono-and poly-synaptic reflexes at the spinal level	5–10 mg qd–tid	
Tizanidine (Zanaflex)	Alpha$_2$-adrenergic agonist in the brain stem and spinal cord	2–4 mg q6–8h	
Benzodiazepines			
Diazepam (Valium)	Depresses activity in limbic system, thalamus, hypothalamus	2–10 mg tid–qid	Acute narrow angle glaucoma

placebo for nine NSAIDs: clonixin, ketoprofen (Orudis), naproxen (Naprosyn), diclofenac (Voltaren), fenbufen, ibuprofen (Motrin), indomethacin (Indocin), piroxicam (Feldene), and azapropazone (also called apazone). In studies in which physical therapy was also administered, four NSAIDs-azapropazone, clonixin, naproxen, and ketoprofen-were demonstrated to provide unequivocal additional benefit.[61] In a similar review of investigations of NSAIDs and sports-related soft tissue injuries, Weiler concluded that benefits were typically observed among treatment groups when compared with controls. These short-term studies have found that treated athletes return to practice quicker and without any apparent significant delay in the injury healing process.[97] In 1987, Amlie et al studied the effects of 7 days of oral piroxicam treatment in 278 patients with acute low back pain.[7] Medication administration was commenced within 48 hours of symptom onset, and after 3 days of therapy patients in the treatment group revealed a significant amount of pain relief. After 7 days, the difference in pain symptoms between the treatment and control groups was no longer significant, but the treatment group demonstrated a significantly lower requirement for additional analgesics and a higher return-to-work rate.

The choice of initial anti-inflammatory agent remains largely empirical. Aspirin is generally inexpensive, and the newer NSAIDs often cost significantly more. In addition to cost considerations, patients have been observed to be more compliant with agents that require less frequent dosing.[94] Because steady states of plasma concentration are not typically observed until dosing has been continued for three to five half-lives, plateau concentrations and maximal therapeutic effects are not realized as quickly in agents with longer half-lives unless a loading dose is first prescribed.[20] By first prescribing a loading dose, which is not often done in clinical settings, and then maintaining regular dosing as indicated for each agent, adequate plasma levels will be achieved so that the antiinflammatory abilities of these medications can be realized. Prescribing NSAIDs in lower dosages and on a less regular schedule is more likely to cause only the analgesic properties of these agents to be used.[44,99] Large variations in patient response to different NSAIDs are observed even when chemically similar drugs of a common family are prescribed.[44] Over a 1- to 2-week period, the dose may be increased to the recommended maximum, and after that time, if the results remain unsatisfactory, a different agent should be tried.[20] Adverse effects generally develop within the initial weeks of treatment, although gastric complications can develop at later times. Combination therapy with more than one NSAID is to be avoided because the incidence of adverse effects is additive and there is little evidence of added benefit to the patient.[44]

Several complications are associated with NSAID use. As nonselective inhibitors of cyclooxygenase-1 (COX-1), which is responsible for thromboxane and prostaglandin synthesis and the maintenance of normal gastrointestinal mucosa, NSAIDs are commonly observed to alter gastrointestinal physiology. While dyspepsia is a common complication, erosion, ulceration, and hemorrhage may also develop—and without warning symptoms.[20,44] There is some evidence that nabumetone (Relafen), which preferentially inhibits COX-2 (mediating control of inflammation), is associated with a lower incidence of gastrointestinal adverse effects.[45] Misoprostol (Cytotec), a synthetic prostaglandin E_1 analog, has been shown to reduce the likelihood of gastroduodenal erosion during the administration of aspirin.[52]

Prostaglandins also participate in the autoregulation of renal blood flow and glomerular filtration, and numerous renal adverse effects, including acute renal failure, have been associated with NSAID use. The kidneys are most vulnerable in individuals who might enter a hypovolemic state or in whom there is preexisting renal disease.[20] While the association between NSAID use and minimal-change glomerulonephropathy has been recognized, one study suggests that nephrotic syndrome due to membranous nephropathy should also be recognized as a possible reaction to NSAID use.[74] All NSAIDs can cause central nervous system adverse effects such as drowsiness, dizziness, and confusion.[1] Blockade of platelet aggregation, inhibition of uterine contractility, interference with antihypertensive medications, and hypersensitivity reactions are also adverse effects shared by many of the commonly prescribed NSAIDs.[44]

There is some variability in adverse effects among the NSAIDs. While the nonacetylated salicylates do not prolong bleeding time and have rarely been associated with gastrointestinal complications, indomethacin has more frequently been associated with nausea, gastrointestinal bleeding, and headaches.[23] NSAIDs have less potential for abuse than opioids, and physical dependence on these medications has not been reported.[1]

***Table 3.*   Opioid Equivalents to Morphine**

Agonist Drug	Oral Dose (mg) Equianalgesic to 20–30 mg Morphine
Oxycodone (Percocet*)	20
Hydromorphone (Dilaudid)	1.5
Methadone (Dolophine)	10
Meperidine (Demerol)	75
Levorphanol (levo-Dromoran)	2

* Combination tablet contains acetaminophen.

Recent studies have investigated the effects of NSAID use on the healing process of the injured soft tissue-namely, muscle and tendon-for which NSAIDs are often prescribed. Almekinders investigated the in vitro effects of indomethacin on isolated human fibroblasts subjected to repetitive motion injury. NSAID use in this study was associated with decreased DNA synthesis during the early proliferative healing phase but with increased protein synthesis during the later remodeling phase of healing.[3] In an earlier investigation of the effects of piroxicam on the healing of rat tibialis anterior muscle subjected to strain injury, histologic observation revealed a delay in the early inflammatory reactions and regeneration within the muscle tissue of the treated group. At 11 days following injury, though, both treated and controlled groups demonstrated similar extents of regeneration and failure loads.[4] A study investigating the effects of flurbiprofen treatment on the recovery of eccentrically injured rabbit muscle revealed that treated muscles demonstrated initial histologic and contractile gains but a subsequent functional loss.[66] The effect of NSAIDs on chondrocyte function and the cartilage matrix has similarly been investigated.[23] As these apparently time-dependent effects of NSAID use on soft tissue recovery are further realized, a more scientific approach to the prescription of anti-inflammatory agents will likely arise.

A new development in NSAIDs is a class that is considered COX-2 selective. The creation of this novel group of anti-inflammatory drugs resulted from the significant morbidity and mortality caused by traditional NSAIDs.[42,101] The COX-2–selective inhibition potentiates analgesic and anti-inflammatory properties while maintaining gastric mucosa and platelet function. Siegle et al demonstrated the selective increase in COX-2 isoforms in the synovial tissue of individuals with inflammatory arthritis.[83] The COX-1–sparing properties may allow for a reduction in the leukotriene-induced asthmatic response and also allows for the concomitant use of aspirin in those with heart disease or hypercoagulable states.[81] Simon et al demonstrated no significant difference between platelet aggregation and bleeding time in patients on COX-2 selectives or placebo as compared with naproxen sodium.[84] The main potential beneficial effect of these medications is their ability to reduce the occurrence of ulcerogenic disease. Bjarnson et al demonstrated a significant reduction in endoscopically detected gastroduodenal damage of Celecoxib over naproxen sodium in a randomized, double-blind, cross-over study.[15] The potential gastrointestinal- and platelet function–sparing capabilities of these drugs make them very attractive; however, they do not appear to be superior to other NSAIDs in terms of efficacy.

MUSCLE RELAXANTS

The muscle-relaxing properties of muscle relaxants arise not from direct activity at the muscular or neuromuscular junction level but rather from an inhibition of more central polysynaptic neuronal events (Table 2). These agents have been shown in some studies to demonstrate analgesia superior to either acetaminophen or aspirin, and it remains uncertain if muscle spasm is a prerequisite to their effectiveness as analgesics. The clinical efficacy of these drugs has been the subject of significant debate, with poor selection criteria and design deficiency making results difficult to interpret.[33] Cherkin et al, in a study of 219 patients with acute low back pain, reported the best outcome in patients receiving both muscle relaxants and NSAIDs.[26] This is contrary to the Agency for Health Care Policy and Research guidelines, which reported that the combination of NSAID and muscle relaxant was not supportable by the literature.[14] In a meta-analysis, Van Tulder et al demonstrated strong evidence that muscle relaxants were more effective than placebo for acute low back pain with limited evidence for efficacy in chronic low back pain.[92] Muscle relaxants are often prescribed in the treatment of acute spinal pain in an attempt to improve the initial limitations in range of motion from muscle spasm and to interrupt the pain-spasm-pain cycle. Limiting muscle spasm and improving range of motion will prepare the patient for therapeutic exercise.[77]

In an attempt to determine the mechanism of action of carisoprodol (Soma) in the treatment of low back pain, a double-blind study was carried out comparing its effectiveness to that of a sedative control, butabarbital, and a placebo in the treatment of 48 laborers with acute lumbar pain.[47] Carisoprodol was found to be significantly more effective in providing both subjective pain relief and objective improvements in range of motion when evaluated by finger-to-floor testing. The results of this study suggest that the effects of carisoprodol are not secondary to its sedative effects alone.[47]

In 1989, Basmajian compared the effectiveness of cyclobenzaprine alone, diflunisal (Dolobid) alone, placebo, and a combination of cyclobenzaprine and diflunisal in the treatment of acute low back pain and spasm.[9] During the 10-day study period, the combined treatment group demonstrated significantly superior improvements in global ratings on day 4 but not on day 2 or 7. This study suggested some effectiveness of combined analgesic and muscle relaxant therapy when used early in the initial week of pain onset. Borenstein compared the effects of combined cyclobenzaprine and naproxen (Naprosyn) with naproxen alone and also found combination therapy to be superior in reducing tenderness, spasm, and range of motion in patients presenting with 10 days or fewer of low back pain and spasm.[16] Adverse effects, predominantly drowsiness, were noted in 12 of 20 in the combined group and in only 4 of 20 treated with naproxen alone.

Cyclobenzaprine and carisoprodol were compared in the treatment of patients with acute thoracolumbar pain and spasm rated moderate to severe and of no longer than 7 days' duration.[77] Both drugs were found to be effective, without significant differences between the treatment groups. Significant improvements were noted in physician-rated mobility and in patients' Visual Analog Scale scores on follow-up days 4 and 8. While 60% of patients experienced adverse effects in the form of drowsiness or fatigue, these differences were not significant between groups, and only 8% of patients from each group discontinued treatment. Baratta found cyclobenzaprine, 10 mg three times a day, superior to placebo in a randomized, double-blind study of 120 patients with acute low back pain presenting within 5 days of symptom onset.[8] Significant improvement was noted in range of motion, tenderness to palpation, and pain scores on follow-up days 2 to 9. Sixty percent of treatment group patients reported drowsiness or dizziness, compared with 25% of those in the placebo group. Cyclobenzaprine, as opposed to the other muscle relaxants, has been demonstrated to be effective in the treatment of more chronic disorders.[10,11,21] Cyclobenzaprine, interestingly, is chemically related to the tricyclic antidepressants, which may be at the root of this finding. Unfortunately, cyclobenzaprine has significant sedating adverse effects that limit its usefulness during the day.[8,10]

In an earlier study, diazepam (Valium) was found to offer no significant subjective or objective benefit when compared with placebo in patients treated for low back pain.[48] Carisoprodol was found to be superior to diazepam in the treatment of patients with "at least moderately severe" low back pain and spasm of no longer than 7 days' duration.[17] In this study, the overall incidence of adverse reactions was higher in the diazepam-treated group but was not of statistical significance. Methocarbamol (Robaxin) has been used since 1959 for the treatment of discomfort secondary to acute traumatic and inflammatory conditions.[30] It has been demonstrated to be superior in the treatment of painful muscle spasm.[30,88,91] However, it does have a significant potential for abuse, especially in individuals with a history of sedative or hypnotic abuse.[72]

Muscle spasm of local origin needs to be clinically differentiated from spasticity and sustained muscle contraction in the setting of central nervous system and upper motor neuron injury. Baclofen (Lioresal) and dantrolene sodium (Dantrium) are two agents whose use is indicated in the setting of spasticity of central nervous system etiology. Dantrolene sodium is of particular interest because its mechanism of action is purely at the muscular level where it serves to inhibit the release of calcium from the sarcoplasmic reticulum. Casale studied the effectiveness of dantrolene sodium, 25 mg daily, in the treatment of low back pain and found patients to demonstrate significant improvements in Visual Analog Scale scores, pain behavior, and electromyography evaluations of "antalgic reflex motor unit firing" when compared with the placebo group.[25] The findings of this study are interesting in that they demonstrate improvement secondary to a pure muscle relaxant that does not possess other outside antinociceptive properties.

Baclofen is a derivative of gamma-aminobutyric acid (GABA) and is believed to inhibit monosynaptic and polysynaptic reflexes at the spinal level. Treatment with baclofen was compared with placebo in a double-blind, randomized study of 200 patients with acute low back pain.[28] Patients with initially severe discomfort were found to benefit from baclofen, 30 to 80 mg daily, on days 4 and 10 of follow-up. Forty-nine percent of treatment patients complained of sleepiness, 38% of nausea, and 17% discontinued treatment.

Tizanidine (Zanaflex) has an interesting mechanism of action, acting as an alpha$_2$-adrenergic agonist in the brainstem and spinal cord. A dose-dependent antinociceptive effect has been demonstrated that may involve the inhibitory release of aspartic and glutamic acid, along with substance P.[27,76] Fogelholm and Murros demonstrated tizanidine to be effective in treating tension-type headaches in women.[35] Berry and Hutchinson demonstrated tizanidine to be effective for pain at rest and with movement compared with placebo in a double-blind, placebo-controlled study.[12,13] Fryda-Kaurimsky and Muller-Fassbender demonstrated tizanidine to be as effective as diazepam in treating paravertebral muscle spasm with reduced adverse effects.[38] Further research is required to validate reported antinociceptive effects of tizanidine.

Sedation is the most commonly reported adverse effect of muscle relaxant medications. These drugs should be used with caution in patients operating heavy machinery. More absolute contraindications do exist to the use of carisoprodol, cyclobenzaprine, and diazepam. Metaxalone (Skelaxin), on the other hand, also has reported efficacy in reducing muscle spasm and increasing range of motion and therapeutic response in those with acute low back pain,[34] but clinically significant sedation is uncommonly encountered with metaxalone as compared with other centrally acting muscle relaxants.[29,34] Rare idiosyncratic reactions have also been reported to carisoprodol and its metabolites such as meprobamate. Benzodiazepines have potential for abuse, and their use should be avoided. By initially prescribing muscle relaxants at bedtime, the physician might take advantage of their sedative effects and minimize daytime drowsiness. The agents reported above have been found to be effective when used either alone or in combination with an analgesic anti-inflammatory agent within 7 days of symptom onset. The prescribing physician should monitor patients receiving these medications and tailor dosages in an attempt to minimize the drowsiness and sedation often associated with their use. The use of benzodiazepines does not appear to offer any significant benefit to patients experiencing acute low back pain. Overall, the literature does support the short-term use of muscle relaxants for acute painful muscle spasm. This effect needs to be further validated in prospective, randomized clinical outcome studies.

OPIOIDS

Opioids occupy the second rung on the World Health Organization analgesic ladder in the treatment of moderate to severe cancer pain and are commonly prescribed for postoperative pain, where they have been found to successfully treat both local and more generalized pain symptoms (Table 3).[71]

Opioid drugs produce analgesia by binding to multiple types of opioid receptors, which are typically bound by endogenous opioid compounds. These receptors are generally classified as mu, kappa, and delta, but the opioid medications typically prescribed are morphine-like agonists that occupy the mu receptor. These receptors are located both peripherally, on sensory nerves and immune cells, and centrally, in the spinal cord and brainstem.[71]

In a study by Brown et al, the analgesic efficacy of diflunisal (Dolobid), 500 mg orally twice a day following a 100-mg loading dose, was compared with that of 300 mg of acetaminophen with 30 mg of codeine in the treatment of pain resulting from initial or recurrent low back strains.[22] Over this 15-day trial, the analgesic efficacy of each regimen was found to be similar, but patient acceptability and tolerance were found to be superior for diflunisal. Five of 21 patients treated with acetaminophen and codeine reported adverse effects, including drowsiness, dizziness, fatigue, and nausea, compared with 3 of 19 patients treated with diflunisal. In a study of 200 patients presenting with acute low back pain, Wiesel et al compared the analgesic efficacy of acetaminophen with both codeine and aspirin plus oxycodone.[100] While all analgesic medications considered were not shown to result in a more prompt return to work, a significantly greater pain reduction, especially within the first 3 days of treatment, was noted for individuals treated with codeine or aspirin plus oxycodone. For more opioids, peak drug effect occurs within 1.5 to 2.0 hours following oral administration, and a second opioid dose can safely be taken 2 hours after the first if adverse effects are mild at that time. Sustained-release tablets are also available and often prove beneficial in patients with more rapidly fluctuating pain.

Tramadol hydrochloride (Ultram) is a newer centrally acting analgesic that, although not chemically related to opiates, binds to mu receptors. Its mechanism of action is not completely understood but is thought to be at least in part secondary to its inhibition of the reuptake of both serotonin and norepinephrine. Tramadol has been demonstrated to provide superior analgesia to combined acetaminophen-propoxyphene in patients experiencing severe postoperative pain and to provide similar analgesia, but with greater tolerability, to morphine in patients hospitalized for cancer pain.[86,102] In a 4-week study of 390 elderly patients with chronic pain secondary to a variety of conditions, tramadol was found to provide comparable analgesia to acetaminophen with codeine without a significant difference in associated adverse effects.[75] Additional studies reveal the low abuse potential and the absence of significant respiratory depression associated with tramadol use.[49,73] Individualization of tramadol dosage is recommended for individuals over 75 years of age, those with impaired renal function, and those with significant liver disease. The goal of successful opioid prescription involves achieving a tolerable balance between analgesia and the adverse effects often associated with opioid use. Tolerance to adverse effects such as somnolence, nausea, and impaired thought processes typically occurs within days to weeks of initial opioid administration. Constipation is a more persistent adverse effect, which can be managed with stool softeners and laxatives. Accumulation of normeperidine, a metabolite of meperidine (Demerol), with repetitive dosing has been associated with the development of anxiety, tremors, myoclonus, and generalized seizures; patients with impaired renal function are at particular risk.[53] Methadone (Dolophine) demonstrates good oral potency and a plasma half-life of 24 to 36 hours. Accumulation of methadone may occur with repetitive dosing, resulting in excessive sedation on days 2 to 5.[6] Physical dependence can develop after several days of administration of opioid analgesics.[71]

Despite the stigma and fear of addiction associated with their use, when properly prescribed by a knowledgeable physician, opioid analgesics can successfully treat otherwise intractable pain. The potential role of opioids in the treatment of nonmalignant spinal pain is limited; opioids should be reserved for patients who either have failed to realize adequate analgesia from alternative medications, such as NSAIDs with or without a muscle relaxant, or have contraindications to the use of other analgesics. If opioids are prescribed, a regular, rather than an "as required" (PRN), dosing schedule should be prescribed, and their use should be limited to a short course to control pain. The prescribing physician should be aware of the possibility of dependence with more prolonged use and avoid prescribing these agents for patients with a prior history of substance abuse.

CORTICOSTEROIDS

Oral steroids are effective in the treatment of inflammatory reactions associated with allergic states, rheumatic and autoimmune diseases, and respiratory disorders. Corticosteroids interact with receptor proteins in target tissues to regulate gene expression and, ultimately, protein synthesis by the target tissue. Because these interactions and regulatory processes occur slowly, most of the effects of corticosteroids are not immediate and become apparent hours following their introduction. Recent investigations have suggested an additional and more immediate component to corticosteroid action mediated by an interaction with membrane-bound protein receptors.[44,95]

Over the past 2 decades, the biochemical contribution to sciatica and low back pain has been the focus of much attention.[68] In the late 1970s the nuclear material of the vertebral disc was found to be antigenic and capable of producing an in vitro autoimmune reaction. It was hypothesized that a chemical radiculitis might explain radicular pain in the absence of a more mechanical stressor.[58] Phospholipase A_2 (PLA_2), a potent inflammatory mediator, has been demonstrated to be released by discs following injury.[80] The anti-inflammatory and immunosuppressive effects of glucocorticoids are largely secondary to their inhibition of the immune responses of lymphocytes, macrophages, and fibroblasts. Whereas NSAIDs principally inhibit prostaglandin synthesis, corticosteroids interfere earlier in the inflammatory cascade by inhibiting PLA_2 actions and thereby curtailing both the leukotriene- and prostaglandin-mediated inflammatory response.[44]

Studies designed to investigate the use of oral steroids in the setting of acute low back pain are limited. In 1986, Haimovic and Beresford compared oral dexamethasone (Decadron) with placebo in the treatment of 33 patients with lumbosacral radicular pain.[43]

Subjects receiving dexamethasone were given a tapering dose, from 64 to 8 mg over 7 days. Early improvements (within 7 days) were not significantly different between the two groups, occurring in 7 of 21 patients in the dexamethasone group and 4 of 12 in the placebo group. In subjects initially found to have radicular-type pain on straight-leg raising, however, 8 of 19 treated with dexamethasone, compared with only 1 of 6 in the placebo group, had diminished pain on straight-leg raising repeated within 7 days. The limitations of this study include a small subject number, the use of additional analgesics that may have obscured group differences, the clinical uncertainty of a radicular process in a significant number of subjects, and the loss of several patients from follow-up after 1 year.[43]

In the setting of acute neck pain with radiculopathy, oral corticosteroids are typically prescribed in a quick tapering fashion over 1 week. Multiple adverse effects have been associated with prolonged steroid use, including suppression of the hypothalamic-pituitary-adrenal axis, immunosuppression, pseudotumor cerebri and psychoses, cataracts and increased intraocular pressure, osteoporosis, aseptic necrosis, gastric ulcers, fluid and electrolyte disturbances and hypertension, and impaired wound healing. The severity of these complications correlates with the dosage, duration of use, and potency of the steroid prescribed. While the incidence of steroid-induced myopathy does not appear to be directly related to the dosage of steroid prescribed or the duration of use, it appears to be more prevalent with the use of steroids containing a 9-alpha fluorine configuration such as triamcinolone (Aristocort). The relationship between hypertensive adverse effects and the duration of therapy is also not very clear; steroids should be prescribed with greater caution in the elderly, in individuals with known hypertension, and when compounds with greater mineralocorticoid properties are prescribed. Because hyperglycemia is a well-known complication of corticosteroid use, oral steroids should be prescribed with caution in the diabetic population.[89]

As potent anti-inflammatory agents, oral steroids represent a theoretically useful agent in the treatment of patients with radiculopathy caused by local inflammation secondary to disc injury or herniation. While many adverse effects are associated with oral steroid use, these are more frequently encountered in the setting of prolonged administration. The effectiveness of oral steroids in the acute low back pain population remains unproven; further research in this area is needed.

ANTIDEPRESSANTS

While several classes of antidepressants have been used successfully in the treatment of a variety of pain syndromes, the literature most strongly supports the analgesic efficacy of the tricyclics. Amitriptyline has been investigated as an analgesic more than the other antidepressant agents and appears to be the most popular antidepressant analgesic in the clinical setting. Migraine headaches, neuropathic pain associated with diabetic neuropathy, and postherpetic neuralgia have been found to respond favorably to antidepressant administration. These agents have also been found to alleviate the pain associated with musculoskeletal conditions such as fibromyalgia, rheumatoid arthritis, and osteoarthritis. Antidepressants have been successfully used in the treatment of cancer pain. In the cancer population, when administered concurrently with an antidepressant, opioid agents may be used at a reduced dose and with a diminished incidence of adverse effects.[54]

The analgesic abilities of antidepressants were once thought to be related to the alleviation of the depression that can often accompany persistent pain, but several antidepressants have been found to reduce pain symptoms in patients not experiencing comorbid depression.[56] These agents are now believed to have primary analgesic abilities that are most likely related to their effects on monoamines in endogenous pain pathways. The efficacy of both serotonin- and norepinephrine-selective antidepressants would suggest that effects on pathways that involve either of these transmitters might contribute to analgesia. Other suggested mechanisms of analgesia involve the antihistamine properties of some agents, increased endorphin secretion, and an increased density of cortical calcium channels.[54,71]

In a study of 44 patients admitted for low back pain, Jenkins et al compared treatment with oral imipramine (Tofranil), 25 mg three times a day, with placebo over a 4-week period.[51] After treatment, no significant difference in improvement in straight-leg raising, pain and stiffness assessments, or psychological testing was noted between the two study groups. In individuals with apparent discogenic pain, imipramine-treated patients demonstrated greater improvement in pain and stiffness, but this was not found to be statistically significant. No significant difference in adverse effects was noted between the two groups. In a study of 48 patients with chronic low back pain, treatment with imipramine was compared with placebo.[2] Seven of the patients included were determined to be clinically depressed according to standard criteria. Patients completed Beck Depression Inventory questionnaires at both the initial and final visits. Improvements in depression score, while not statistically significant, were noted in patients who benefited from imipramine treatment. Individuals treated with imipramine did demonstrate a significant improvement in both limitations of work and restrictions in normal activities. Anticholinergic adverse effects were associated with a 10% dropout rate. In a review of the literature on antidepressants in the treatment of chronic low back pain, Egbunike et al concluded that the most consistent responses were found with doxepin (Sinequan) and desipramine (Norpramin) at doses above 150 mg daily.[32] Some studies may have failed to demonstrate a response secondary to inadequate dosing. Other antidepressants were found less effective in providing analgesia. In several studies reviewed, while improvements in depression were observed, poor correlations were noted between analgesic effects and changes in the severity of depression. The relationship between pain relief and antidepressant effect remains unclear.[32]

Tricyclic antidepressants (TCAs) produce analgesia at lower dosages than are typically prescribed for the treatment of depression. The starting dose of the TCA should be low. Initial daily dosing of amitriptyline should be 10 mg in elderly patients and 25 mg in younger individuals. Every 2 to 3 days an increment in dosing equal to the initial starting dose can be made until adequate analgesia is achieved or adverse effects develop. The typical effective daily dose of amitriptyline ranges from 50 to 150 mg, although doses as low as 10 to 25 mg can be helpful in some patients. Because the TCA half-life is generally long and sedation is a common adverse effect, single nighttime dosing can be prescribed. Some patients report better pain relief and less morning drowsiness with divided daily dosing.[54,71]

Studies that have investigated the analgesic efficacy of selective serotonin reuptake inhibitors have typically involved dosages similar to those prescribed in the management of depression: 20 to 40 mg of fluoxetine (Prozac) or paroxetine (Paxil).[56,59] Further research is needed to clarify the relationship between dosage and analgesia with the serotonin-specific agents.[71]

The occurrence of serious adverse effects resulting from antidepressant administration is low. These complications would be rare at the generally lower dosages used in the treatment of pain. While cardiac adverse effects are uncommon, tricyclics are contraindicated in those individuals with heart failure or serious cardiac conduction abnormalities. Orthostatic hypotension is the most frequent cardiovascular adverse effect, and the elderly are particularly at risk. The sedating effect often observed with antidepressant use can be beneficial because patients with pain often demonstrate diminished daytime functioning from inadequate sleep. Anticholinergic adverse effects such as dry mouth, blurred vision, and urinary retention are more likely with amitriptyline use than with other TCAs. These effects are also less likely at the lower dosages used for analgesia. Nortriptyline and desipramine have been found to induce fewer anticholinergic adverse effects and are less sedating.[54,71]

While antidepressants have been demonstrated as useful adjuncts in the treatment of pain, their analgesic mechanism remains unclear. Initial dosing should be low and then slowly increased to minimize adverse effects. When taken at night, the sedating properties of these agents can be beneficial in pain patients experiencing difficulty with sleep.

GABAPENTIN

Gabapentin (Neurontin) is structurally related to the neurotransmitter GABA while not binding to GABA receptors. It is approved for use in the treatment of partial seizures in adults. It has been found to be helpful in patients with painful peripheral neuropathies.[78,82] It has also been found to be effective in the treatment of pain in patients with postherpetic neuralgia.[79]

Gabapentin has been used as an adjunctive medication in the treatment of chronic pain conditions that include a neuritic component. It has also been used to reduce radicular symptoms such as tingling and burning in patients with radicular pain who have not responded to other modes of treatment or who were hesitant to proceed with any invasive procedure. Generally, patients are started on low doses (100 mg three times daily) and gradually titrated up (usually to 300 mg three times daily but doses as high as 900 mg four times daily can be tried) until there is a therapeutic effect. A trial is aborted if there are intolerable adverse effects or if no therapeutic benefit is noted after trying the higher doses. This approach has been very effective in the authors' experience, and the medication is extremely well tolerated. Major adverse effects include sedation, dizziness, and fatigue.

MINERALS AND SUPPLEMENTS

Over the past decade the use of nontraditional treatments, including vitamins, minerals, and other supplements has rapidly increased in popularity. Unfortunately, this industry is completely unregulated, resulting in concern over safety and no assurance that what is being sold actually contains a sufficient amount of the "active" compound. In addition, the efficacy of many of these supplements is based on anecdotal evidence. Recently, however, more and more scientific research in this area has improved the scientific use of some of these agents. There is little information regarding natural supplements in the treatment of acute low back pain per se, but there is information regarding various vitamins and supplements in the treatment of pain, arthritis, fibromyalgia, and other musculoskeletal disorders. Weil suggests niacinamide beginning at 500 mg twice a day and gradually increasing to 2000 mg twice a day.[96] He also suggests ginger and *Boswellia* for generalized musculoskeletal aches and turmeric as an anti-inflammatory agent. For tissue healing, Weil recommends bromelain, which is a pineapple extract.[96] The recommended dose is 200 to 400 mg three times a day on an empty stomach. Antioxidants have also been recommended to reduce inflammatory conditions. This includes vitamin E (400–800 IU), coenzyme Q10 (30–60 mg daily), and bioflavonoids found in grape seed extract (30 mg three times daily or as a bioflavonoid complex capsule, 1000 mg twice a day).[65] Finally, white willow bark, which contains salicin, is a potent anti-inflammatory. It has similar properties to aspirin; however, it contains tannins, which protect the stomach.[65] One capsule every 3 to 4 hours is recommended as needed for pain.

For arthritic conditions, which in the spine would include facet arthropathy, lumbar spondylosis, and spinal stenosis, various supplements have been recommended. This includes the antioxidants along with glucosamine sulfate and chondroitin sulfate. These are thought to stimulate the manufacture of glycosaminoglycans, which are vital for cartilage function. In addition, glucosamine promotes the incorporation of sulfur into cartilage.[67] Studies have found glucosamine to be an effective alternative to NSAIDs.[87,93] The recommended dose for arthritis is 500 mg three times per day. Glucosamine has no significant adverse effects other than some gastrointestinal upset. It is not contraindicated in patients with a history of diabetes or allergy to sulfa.[67] For nociceptive pain conditions, a few other supplements have been recommended, including choline and B-complex (B_1, B_2, B_6) vitamins, which are thought to be important substances in the production of endorphins. D,L-phenylalanine is an amino acid that is thought to enhance the effects of natural endorphins and opioid medications. This may reduce the need for opioid medication in some patients. The recommended dose is 1 to 2 tablets every 4 hours between meals as needed for pain.[65]

The information on the scientific benefit for many minerals and supplements continues to evolve. Although relatively safe and inexpensive, these substances remain unregulated; there are concerns over purity, and possible contamination with harmful substances is a real possibility. A reputable laboratory should be used when recommending these substances. The use of most of these substances in acute low back pain is essentially unstudied and represents a fertile area for further research.

CONCLUSION

Various agents can be helpful in treating the painful phase of acute neck and low back pain after whiplash injury. Unfortunately, there is a paucity of scientific literature regarding the efficacy of these medications in acute neck pain specifically. Therefore, the literature on medications in low back pain is used as a guideline for both neck and low back pain following whiplash. A particular medication should be chosen after consideration of the (1) indications, (2) contraindications, (3) goals of treatment, such as analgesia, reduction of inflammation, and reduction of muscle spasm, and (4) the scientific and clinical evidence of their effectiveness. The goal of pharmacologic management should be to promote active treatment and functional recovery. When used purely for the treatment of pain, there is little evidence to support any significant improvement in functional outcome. Clinicians need to be cognizant of these issues and apply them to the total care of their patients.

References

1. Abramowicz M (ed): Drugs for pain. Med Lett Drugs Ther 35:1–6, 1993.
2. Alcoff J, Jones E, Rust P, Newman R: Controlled trial of imipramine for chronic low back pain. J Fam Pract 14:841–846, 1982.
3. Almekinders LC, Gilbert JA: Healing of experimental muscle strains and the effects of nonsteroidal antiinflammatory medication. Am J Sports Med 14:303–308, 1986.
4. Almekinders LC, Banes AJ, Bracey LW: An in vitro investigation into the effects of repetitive motion and nonsteroidal anti-inflammatory medications on human tendon fibroblasts. Am J Sports Med 23:119–123, 1995.
5. Amadio P Jr, Cummings DM: Evaluation of acetaminophen in the management of osteoarthritis of the knee. Curr Ther Res 34:59–66, 1983.
6. American Pain Society: Principles of Analgesic Use in the Treatment of Acute Pain and Cancer Pain, 3rd ed. Skokie, IL, American Pain Society, 1993.
7. Amlie E, Weber H, Holme I: Treatment of acute low-back pain with piroxicam: Results of a double-blind placebo-controlled trial. Spine 12:473–476, 987.
8. Baratta RR: A double blind study of cyclobenzaprine and placebo in the treatment of acute musculoskeletal conditions of the low back. Curr Ther Res 32:646–652, 1982.
9. Basmajian JV: Acute low back pain and spasm. A controlled multicenter trial of combined analgesic and antispasm agents. Spine 14:438–439, 1989.
10. Basmajian JV: Cyclobenzaprine hydrochloride effect on skeletal muscle spasm in the lumbar region and neck: two double-blind controlled clinical and laboratory studies. Arch Phys Med Rehabil 59:58–63, 1978.
11. Bercel NA: Cyclobenzaprine in the treatment of skeletal muscle spasm in osteoarthritis of the cervical and lumbar spine. Curr Ther Res Clin Exp 22:462–468, 1977.
12. Berry H, Hutchinson DR: A multicentre placebo controlled study in general practice to evaluate the efficacy and safety of tizanidine in acute low back pain. J Int Med Res 16:75–82, 1988.
13. Berry H, Hutchinson DR: Tizanidine and ibuprofen in acute low back pain: results of a double-blind multicentre study in general practice. J Int Med Res 16:83–91, 1988.
14. Bigos S, Bowyer O, Braen G, et al: Acute Low Back Problems in Adults. Clinical Practice Guideline No. 14. Rockville, MD, Agency for Health Care Policy and Research, US Department of Health and Human Services, 1994, AHCPR publication 95-0642.
15. Bjarnson I, Macpherson A, Rotman H, et al: A randomized, double blind crossover comparative endoscopy study on the gastroduodenal tolerability of a highly specific cyclooxygenase 2 inhibitor, flosulide, and naproxen. Scand J Gastroenterol 32:126–130, 1997.
16. Borenstein DG, Lacks S, Wiesel SW: Cyclobenzaprine and naproxen versus naproxen alone in the treatment of acute low back pain and muscle spasm. Clin Ther 12:125–131, 1990.
17. Boyles WF, Glassman JM, Soyka JP: Management of acute musculoskeletal conditions: thoracolumbar strain or sprain. Todays Ther Trends 1:1–16, 1983.
18. Bradley JD, Brandt KD, Katz BP, et al: Comparison of an antiinflammatory dose of ibuprofen, an analgesic dose of ibuprofen, and acetaminophen in the treatment of patients with osteoarthritis of the knee. N Engl J Med 325:87–91, 1991.
19. Brodin H: Cervical pain and mobilization. Int J Rehabil Res 7:190–191, 1984.
20. Brooks PM, Day RO: Nonsteroidal antiinflammatory drugs-differences and similarities. N Engl J Med 324:1716–1725, 1991.
21. Brown BR, Womble J: Cyclobenzaprine in intractable pain syndromes with muscle spasm. JAMA 240:1151–1152, 1978.
22. Brown FL, Bodison S, Dixon J, et al: Comparison of diflunisal and acetaminophen with codeine in the treatment of initial or recurrent low back strain. Clin Ther 9(suppl C)52–58, 1986.
23. Buckwalter JA: Current concepts review. Pharmacological treatment of soft-tissue injuries. J Bone Joint Surg Am 77:1902–1914, 1995.
24. Calin A: Pain and inflammation. Am J Med 77(suppl 3A):9–15, 1984.
25. Casale R: Acute low back pain. Symptomatic treatment with a muscle relaxant drug. Clin J Pain 4:81–88, 1988.
26. Cherkin DC, Wheal KJ, Barlow W, Deyo RA: Medication use for low back pain in primary care. Spine 23:607–614, 1998.
27. Coward DM: Tizanidine: neuropharmacology and mechanism of action. Neurology 44:6–11, 1994.
28. Dapas F, Hartman SE, Martinez L, et al: Baclofen for the treatment of acute low-back syndrome. A double-blind comparison with placebo. Spine 10:345–349, 1985.

29. Dent RW, Ervin DK: A study of metaxalone vs. placebo in acute musculoskeletal disorders: a cooperative study. Curr Ther Res 18:433–438, 1975.
30. Dent RW, Ervin DK: Relief of acute musculoskeletal symptoms with intravenous methocarbamol (Robaxin Injectable): a placebo-controlled study. Curr Ther Res Clin Exp 20:661–665, 1976.
31. Doyle DV, Lanham JG: Routine drug treatment of osteoarthritis. Clin Rheumatol Dis 10:277–291, 1984.
32. Egbunike IG, Chaffee BJ: Antidepressants in the management of chronic pain syndromes. Pharmacotherapy 10:262–270, 1990.
33. Elenbass JK: Centrally acting oral skeletal muscle relaxants. Am J Hosp Pharmacol 37:1313–1323, 1980.
34. Fathie K: A second look at a skeletal muscle relaxant: a double blind study of metaxalone. Curr Ther Res 6:677–683, 1964.
35. Fogelholm R, Murros K: Tizanidine in chronic tension-type headache: a placebo-controlled double-blind cross-over study. Headache 32:509–513, 1992.
36. Foley-Nolan D, Barry C, Coughlan, et al: Pulsed high frequency (27MHz) electromagnetic therapy for persistent neck pain. Orthopedics 13:445–451, 1990.
37. Foley-Nolan D, Moore K, Codd M, et al: Low energy high frequency pulsed electromagnetic therapy for acute whiplash injuries. Scand J Rehabil Med 24:51–59, 1992.
38. Fryda-Kaurimsky Z, Muller-Fassbender H: Tizanidine (DS 103-282) in the treatment of acute paravertebral muscle spasm: a controlled trial comparing tizanidine and diazepam. J Int Med Res 9:501–505, 1981.
39. Gaucher A, Netter P, Faure G, et al: Diffusion of oxyphenbutazone into synovial fluid, synovial tissue, joint cartilage, and cerebrospinal fluid. Eur J Clin Pharmacol 25:107–112, 1983.
40. Gebhart GF, McCormack KJ: Neuronal plasticity. Implication for pain therapy. Drugs 47(suppl 5):1–47, 1994.
41. Goldie I, Landquist A: Evaluation of the effects of different forms of physiotherapy in cervical pain. Scand J Rehabil Med 2-3:117–121, 1970.
42. Griffin MR: Epidemiology of nonsteroidal antiinflammatory drug associated injury. Am J Med 104:23–29, 1998.
43. Haimovic IC, Beresford HR: Dexamethasone is not superior to placebo for treating lumbosacral radicular pain. Neurology 36:1593–1594, 1986.
44. Hardman JG, Limbird LE (eds): Goodman and Gilman's The Pharmacological Basis of Therapeutics, 9th ed. New York, McGraw-Hill, 1996.
45. Hayllar J, Bjarnason I: NSAIDs, Cox-2 inhibitors, and the gut [commentary]. Lancet 346:521–522, 1995.
46. Hickey RFJ: Chronic low back pain: a comparison of diflunisal with paracetamol. N Z Med J 95:312–314, 1982.
47. Hindle TH: Comparison of carisoprodol, butabarbital, and placebo in the treatment of the low back syndrome. Calif Med 117:7–11, 1972.
48. Hingorani K: Diazepam in backache. A double-blind, controlled trial. Ann Phys Med 8:303–306, 1965.
49. Houmes RJ, Voets MA, Verkaaik A, et al: Efficacy and safety of tramadol versus morphine for moderate and severe postoperative pain with special regard to respiratory depression. Anesth Analg 74:510–514, 1992.
50. Jacome DE: Basilar artery migraine after uncomplicated whiplash injuries. Headache 26:515–516, 1986.
51. Jenkins DG, Ebbut AF, Evans CD: Tofranil in the treatment of low back pain. J Int Med Res 4(suppl 2):28–40, 1976.
52. Jiranek GC, Kimmey MB, Saunders DR, et al: Misoprostol reduces gastrointestinal injury from one week of aspirin: an endoscopic study. Gastroenterology 96:656–661, 1989.
53. Kaiko RF, Foley KM, Grabinski PY, et al: Central nervous system excitatory effects of meperidine in cancer patients. Ann Neurol 13:180–185, 1983.
54. King SA: Antidepressants: a valuable adjunct for musculoskeletal pain. J Musculoskel Med 12:51–57, 1995.
55. Konttinen YT, Kemppinen P, Segerberg M, et al: Peripheral and spinal neural mechanisms in arthritis with particular reference to treatment of inflammation and pain. Arthritis Rheum 37:965–982, 1994.
56. Magni G: The use of antidepressants in the treatment of chronic pain. A review of the current evidence. Drugs 42:730–748, 1991.
56a: Malanga GA, Nadler SF, Lipetz JS: Pharmacologic treatment of low back pain. PM&R: State of the Art Reviews 13(3):531–549, 1999.

57. Malmerg AB, Yaksh TL: Hyperalgesia mediated by spinal glutamate or substance P receptor blocked by spinal cyclooxygenase inhibition. Science 257:1276–1279, 1992.
58. Marshall LL, Trethewie ER, Curtain CC: Chemical radiculitis: a clinical, physiological, and immunological study. Clin Orthop 129:61–67, 1979.
59. Max MB, Lynch SA, Muir J, et al: Effects of desipramine, amitriptyline, and fluoxetine on pain in diabetic neuropathy. N Engl J Med 326:1250–1256, 1992.
60. McCormack K, Brune K: Dissociation between the antinociceptive and anti-inflammatory effects of the non-steroidal anti-inflammatory drugs. Drugs 41:533–547, 1991.
61. McCormack K, Brune K: Toward defining the analgesic role of nonsteroidal anti-inflammatory drugs in the management of acute soft tissue injuries. Clin J Sports Med 3:106–117, 1993.
62. McKinney LA: Early mobilisation and outcome in acute sprains of the neck. Br Med J 299:1006–1008, 1989.
63. McKinney LA, Dornan JO, Ryan M: The role of physiotherapy in the management of acute neck sprains following road-traffic accidents. Arch Emerg Med 6:27–33, 1989.
64. Mealy K, Brennan H, Fenelon GCC: Early mobilisation of acute whiplash injuries. Br Med J 292:656–657, 1986.
65. Mindell E: Earl Mindell's Secret Remedies. New York, Simon & Schuster, 1997.
66. Mishra DK, Friden J, Schmitz MC, Lieber RL: Anti-inflammatory medication after muscle injury. J Bone Joint Surg Am 77:1510–1519, 1995.
67. Murray MT: Encyclopedia of Nutritional Supplements. Rocklin, CA, Prima Publishing, 1996.
68. Nicholas JA, Hershman EB (eds): The Lower Extremity and Spine in Sports Medicine, Vol 2. St. Louis, Mosby, 1995.
69. Nordemar R, Thorner C: Treatment of acute cervical pain-a comparative group. Pain 10:93–101, 1981.
70. Pettersson K, Toolanen G: High dose methylprednisolone prevents extensive sick leave after whiplash injury. Spine 23:984–989, 1998.
71. Portenoy RK, Kanner RM (eds): Pain Management: Theory and Practice. Philadelphia, FA Davis, 1996.
72. Preston KL, Guarino JJ, Kirk WT, Griffiths RR: Evaluation of the abuse potential of methocarbamol. J Pharmacol Exp Ther 248:1146–1157, 1989.
73. Preston KL, Jasinski DR, Testa M: Abuse potential and pharmacological comparison of tramadol and morphine. Drug Alcohol Depend 27:7–17, 1991.
74. Radford MG, Holley KE, Grande JP, et al: Reversible membranous nephropathy associated with use of nonsteroidal anti-inflammatory drugs. JAMA 276:466–469, 1996.
75. Rauck RL, Ruoff GE, McMillen JI: Comparison of tramadol and acetaminophen with codeine for long-term pain management in elderly patients. Curr Ther Res 55:1417–1431, 1994.
76. Roberts RC, Part NJ, Pokorny R, et al: Pharmacokinetics and pharmacodynamics of tizanidine. Neurology 44:29–31, 1994.
77. Rollings HE, Glassman JM, Soyka JP: Management of acute musculoskeletal conditions-thoracolumbar strain or sprain: a double-blind evaluation comparing the efficacy and safety of carisoprodol with cyclobenzaprine hydrochloride. Curr Ther Res 34:917–927, 1983.
78. Rosner H, Rubin L, Kestenbaum A: Gabapentin adjunctive therapy in neuropathic states. Clin J Pain 12:56–58, 1996.
79. Rowbotham M, Harden N, Stacey B, et al: Gabapentin for the treatment of postherpetic neuralgia: a randomized controlled trial. JAMA 280:1837–1842, 1998.
80. Saal JS, Franson RC, Dobrow R, et al: High levels of inflammatory phospholipase A2 activity in lumbar spine disc herniations. Spine 15:674–678, 1990.
81. Schuligoi R, Amann R, Prenn C, Peskar BA: Effects of the cyclooxygenase 2 inhibitor NS-398 on thromboxane and leukotriene synthesis in rat peritoneal cells. Inflamm Res 47:227–230, 1998.
82. Siegle I, Klein T, Backman JT, et al: Expression of cyclooxygenase 1 and cyclooxygenase 2 in human synovial tissue: differential elevation of cyclooxygenase 2 in inflammatory joint diseases. Arthritis Rheum 41:122–129, 1998.
83. Simon LS, Lanza FL, Lipsky PE, et al: Preliminary study of the safety and efficacy of SC-58635, a novel cyclooxygenase 2 inhibitor: efficacy and safety in two placebo-controlled trials in osteoarthritis and rheumatoid arthritis, and studies of gastrointestinal and platelet effects. Arthritis Rheum 41:1591–1602, 1998.
84. Seidl JJ, Slawson JG: Gabapentin for painful diabetic neuropathy. J Fam Pract 48:173–174, 1999.
85. Spitzer WO, Skovron ML, Salmi LR, et al: Scientific monograph of the Quebec Task Force on Whiplash-Associated Disorders: redefining "whiplash" and its management. Spine 20(8 suppl):1S–73S, 1995.

86. Sunshine A, Olson NZ, Zighelboim I, et al: Analgesic oral efficacy of tramadol hydrochloride in postoperative pain. Clin Pharmacol Ther 51:740–746, 1992.
87. Tapadinhas MJ, Rivera JC, Bignamini AA: Oral glucosamine sulfate in the management of arthrosis: report on a multicenter open investigation in Portugal. Pharmatherapeutica 3:157–168, 1982.
88. Tisdale SA, Ervin DK: A controlled study of methocarbamol (Robaxin) in acute painful musculoskeletal conditions. Curr Ther Res 17:525–530, 1975.
89. Truhan AP, Ahmed AR: Corticosteroids: a review with emphasis on complications of prolonged systemic therapy. Ann Allerg 62:375–390, 1989.
90. Tyler GS, McNeely HE, Dick ML: Treatment of post-traumatic headache with amitriptyline. Headache 20:213–216, 1980.
91. Valtonen EJ: A double blind trial of methocarbamol versus placebo in painful muscle spasm. Curr Med Res Opin 3:382–385, 1975.
92. Van Tulder MW, Koes BW, Bouter LM: Conservative treatment of acute and chronic nonspecific low back pain: a systemic review of randomized controlled trials of the most common interventions. Spine 22:2128–2156, 1997.
93. Vaz AL: Double blind clinical evaluation of the relative efficacy of ibuprofen and glucosamine sulfate in the management of osteoarthritis of the knee in out-patients. Curr Med Res Opin 8:45–149, 1982.
94. Wasner C, Britton MC, Kraines RG, et al: Nonsteroidal antiinflammatory agents in rheumatoid arthritis and ankylosing spondylitis. JAMA 246:2168–2172, 1981.
95. Wehlig M: Novel aldosterone receptors: specificity conferring mechanism at the level of the cell membrane. Steroids 59:160–163, 1994.
96. Weil A: Spontaneous Healing. New York, Balantine Books, Random House, 1996.
97. Weiler JM: The use of nonsteroidal antiinflammatory drugs (NSAIDs) in sports soft-tissue injury. Clin Sports Med 11:625–644, 1992.
98. Weiss HD, Stern BJ, Goldberg J: Post-traumatic migraine: chronic migraine precipitated by minor head or neck trauma. Headache 31:451–456, 1991.
99. Westley GJ, Schaefer J, Sifton DW (eds): Physician's Desk Reference. 49th ed. Montvale, NJ, Medical Economics, 1995.
100. Wiesel SW, Cuckler JM, DeLuca F, et al: Acute low back pain. An objective analysis of conservative therapy. Spine 4:324–330, 1980.
101. Wilcox CM, Clark WS: Association of nonsteroidal antiinflammatory drugs with outcome in upper and lower gastrointestinal bleeding. Dig Dis Sci 42:985–989, 1997.
102. Wilder-Smith CH, Schimke J, Osterwalder B, Senn HJ: Oral tramadol, a mu-opioid monoamine reuptake-blocker, and morphine for strong cancer related pain. Ann Oncol 5:141–146, 1994.

Interventional Spine Procedures for Cervical Whiplash Management

Michael B. Furman, M.D., and Kirk M. Puttlitz, M.D.

Interventional spine procedures constitute "aggressive-conservative" treatment for whiplash. Such procedures should be employed judiciously in concert with other traditional conservative treatments such as physical therapy and oral medication.

This chapter provides a broad overview of available interventional spine procedures for whiplash, but does not explicitly teach such procedures in a how-to format. Indeed, practitioners should perform such procedures only after appropriate training. Major pain generators implicated in whiplash include the cervical zygapophyseal joint (z-joint), spinal nerve, and intervertebral disc. Consequently, procedures presented in this chapter include z-joint injection (medial branch block, third occipital nerve block, medial branch radiofrequency neurotomy, and intraarticular injection), cervical epidural steroid injection via interlaminar and transforaminal approaches, and provocative cervical discography.

PROCEDURAL CONSIDERATIONS
The patient should be thoughtfully selected for the appropriate procedure based upon available historical, physical examination, and imaging data. Informed consent should be obtained detailing risks, benefits, prognosis, and alternative treatment options. "Nothing by mouth" status is assigned if the patient is to receive intravenous conscious sedation. Blood clotting and other hematologic tests should be drawn on patients with suspected bleeding diathesis. Nonsteroidal anti-inflammatory drugs, including aspirin, as well as anticoagulants should be discontinued prior to the procedure as dictated by their half-life and pharmacologic profile. Concurrent medical conditions contraindicating invasive procedures, such as infection, fever, unstable cardiac disease, hypertension, or diabetes, should be reviewed. Sterile scrub with providone-iodine or isopropyl alcohol, as well as sterile draping, should be performed with rigorous observance of asepsis. Emergency resuscitation equipment (ie, code cart) should be available. Cardiac and pulse oximetry monitoring as well as intravenous access is recommended.

Infectious complications include local soft tissue infection, epidural abscess, meningitis, osteomyelitis, and discitis. Other complications include bleeding with hematoma formation, allergic reaction, and vasovagal syncope. Stroke and seizure may result from intravascular injection of particulate matter and local anesthetic, respectively. Spinal cord or nerve root injury, as well as pneumothorax, may result from direct needle trauma. Respiratory depression may result from oversedation or spinal anesthesia. Systemic steroid effect ("steroid flare") may result from injected corticosteroids. Scar formation and increased postprocedural pain may result from local needle-induced mechanical trauma.

Procedures should be performed under biplanar (eg, anteroposterior [AP] and lateral) fluoroscopic guidance with radiologic contrast dye enhancement to ensure delivery of injectate to the target site and to avoid vital structures (eg, spinal cord, thecal sac, vertebral artery). Furthermore, we recommend advancing the needle only in the fluoroscopic "danger view" image to avoid penetration of vital structures. Danger view is the projection that best visualizes the fluoroscopic landmarks one is trying to avoid. An example of such a danger view is when needle advancement during cervical discography is done under lateral projection, which protects against thecal sac penetration or spinal cord trauma.

ZYGAPOPHYSEAL JOINT INJECTION TECHNIQUES

Many deem the cervical z-joint as a major pain generator in whiplash. Specifically, Barnsley and colleagues determine the prevalence of cervical z-joint pain after whiplash to be 54%, with the most common symptomatic joints being C2-C3 and C5-C6.[1] Unfortunately, history and physical examination, as well as imaging studies, lack specificity in confirming cervical z-joint whiplash pain. Consequently, cervical z-joint injections, either intraarticular or medial branch blocks (MBBs), remain the gold standard in identifying a suspected z-joint as the putative pain generator.[2]

Due to the high false-positive rate (27%) seen with single z-joint injections, many advocate dual blocks, especially for MBBs, to reduce the number of placebo responders.[3,4]

Such dual blocks involve injecting two different local anesthetics with different durations of action (eg, lidocaine 1%, bupivacaine 0.5%) on two separate occasions, with the patient's reported longer-lasting relief corresponding to the longer-acting anesthetic.[5]

Specific complications of cervical facet joint injections include spinal cord, thecal sac, and vertebral artery penetration from direct needle trauma.

Zygapophyseal Joint Anatomy

Cervical z-joints exist primarily from C2-C3 to C7-T1. The more cephaladad aspect of the joint, the inferior articulating process (IAP), arises from the more cephaladad vertebral level; conversely, the more caudal aspect, the superior articulating process (SAP), originates from the more caudad vertebral level. Medial branches (MBs) of dorsal rami innervate z-joints from C3-C4 to C7-T1. Specifically, a given z-joint (eg, C4-C5) receives innervation from the MB above (eg, C4 MB) and below (eg, C5 MB). The MB (eg, C4 MB) travels posteromedially around the articular pillar's "waist" of the same numbered vertebral level (eg, C4 vertebra). The third occipital nerve (TON), implicated in whiplash pain, is the superficial MB of the C3 dorsal ramus and innervates the C2-C3 z-joint. Atlanto-occipital and atlanto-axial (C1-C2) joints receive innervation from C1 and C2 ventral rami, respectively.[6]

Cervical Medial Branch Blocks

Cervical z-joint medial branch blocks (MBBs), which block innervation to the z-joint, appear efficacious in treating whiplash-related z-joint pain. Indeed, Barnsley and Bogduk report definite or complete relief of pain with MBBs in 11 of 16 consecutive patients with motor vehicle accident–related cervical pain.[7,8] Typically, only anesthetic (ie, without corticosteroid) is injected for MBBs. Patients deriving transient relief from dual MBBs may be candidates for medial branch radiofrequency neurotomy (MBRFN), to obtain longer-lasting relief.

Cervical Medial Branch Block Technique

With the patient lying prone, a fluoroscopic AP image is obtained demonstrating the concave articular pillar "waists" where the C3-C7 MBs traverse. A spinal needle is advanced down to periosteum just medial to the articular pillar concavity. The needle is then stepped off laterally into the apex of the concavity. For the C8 MB, the needle is positioned at the cephalomedial border of the T1 spinous process. Under lateral fluoroscopic guidance, the needle tip is manipulated to lie at the center of the articular pillar, located at the intersection point of the pillar's two diagonals (Fig. 1). The notch is rotated to face medially, thereby directing injectate flow toward the MB. After negative aspirate for cerebrospinal fluid and blood, radiologic contrast dye is injected to confirm location and demonstrate nonvascular flow. Upon confirming a satisfactory contrast dye flow pattern, local anesthetic (eg, 0.5 mL bupivacaine 0.75% without epinephrine) is injected to anesthetize the MB.[2] Alternatively, lateral and supine techniques are available to approach the same anatomic structures for MBB.

Before the procedure, the patient completes a pain diary with baseline numerical pain scales (ie, pain score out of possible 10). After the procedure, the

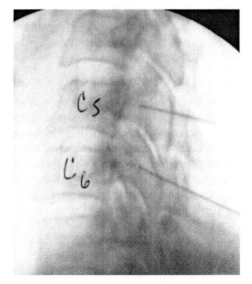

Figure 1. Lateral fluoroscopic view demonstrating correct needle placement for MBB or MBRFN at the center of the articular pillar.

patient continues the pain diary, rating the pain scale as well as percent improvement every 15 minutes for 2 hours and then every hour for 12 hours. A "successful" MBB consists of adequate analgesia, as documented in the pain diary, corresponding to the known duration of anesthetic effect (eg, bupivacaine duration of 2-4 hours). In general, 50% analgesia or greater is considered a "positive" block.

Third Occipital Nerve Block

The superficial MB of the C3 dorsal ramus innervating the C2-3 z-joint, the TON, may be associated with whiplash-related headache. Indeed, Lord and colleagues cite a prevalence of 53% for C2-C3 joint-mediated pain in whiplash-related headache.[9]

To perform MBB of the TON, a different technique is used. With the patient in the lateral position, a lateral fluoroscopic image is obtained to demonstrate the target site, a vertical line bisecting the C3 articular pillar. The needle is advanced to periosteum, and three injections are deposited along this vertical line: one cephaladad to the joint line above the subchondral plate of the C2 IAP, one directly over the joint line, and one caudad to the joint line below the subchondral plate of the C3 SAP.[2]

Cervical Medial Branch Radiofrequency Neurotomy

MBRFN appears efficacious in providing more long-term relief for those responding positively to dual MBB. Indeed, Lord and Barnsley, in their prospective, placebo-controlled, double-blinded study of percutaneous RFN for chronic motor vehicle accident–related cervical z-joint pain, demonstrate such long-lasting relief. Specifically, the median time elapsed before pain returned to at least 50% preprocedure level was 263 days in the RF group and 8 days in the control group. Of 24 patients studied, seven patients in the RF group and one patient in the control group remained pain-free at 27 weeks.[8,10] Furthermore, Wallis and colleagues, in their randomized, double-blinded, placebo-controlled trial, cite resolution of psychological distress in whiplash patients following treatment by RFN.[8,11]

Cervical Medial Branch Radiofrequency Neurotomy Technique

MBRFN coagulates MB innervation to the z- joint via RF needles that deliver high-frequency alternating current. Such alternating current induces ionic current in surrounding tissue, which, as a result of friction, generates heat. Temperatures of 70°C to 90°C are typically used to induce irreversible neurotomy. Temperature equilibrium results from maintaining such temperature for 30 to 90 seconds. Parallel, as opposed to perpendicular, needle placement ensures proper neurotomy because RF current emanates from the length of the uninsulated needle but does not project beyond the needle tip.[12] Hence, the optimal position of the cannula is parallel to the target nerve, necessitating an AP needle approach (Fig. 1). Consequently, Finch and colleagues advocate a commercially available "steerable" curved-tip needle cannula that conforms to the articular pillar contour, thereby fitting snugly in parallel against the

MB.[13] A lateral approach cannot be used for this procedure because only the AP approach places the cannula tip in the ideal position parallel to the MB.

Under fluoroscopic guidance, this curved needle cannula is steered to the chosen MB joint using the aforementioned techniques for MBB. The RF needle probe is then inserted into this cannula, and sensory/motor stimulation is performed to avoid ventral ramus or nerve root contact, manifested by radicular paresthesias or extremity myotomal contraction. The RF probe is then removed from the cannula and anesthetic (eg, lidocaine 0.5–1.0 mL) injected through the cannula to promote pain-free lesioning. The RF needle is then reinserted with heat lesioning performed as above. The cannula/probe system is repositioned along the same target to obtain three additional lesions (for a total of four) to optimize lesioning efficacy.[12]

Cervical Intraarticular Zygapophyseal Joint Injection

Intraarticular z-joint injection typically deposists both local anesthetic and corticosteroid directly into the z-joint articular space, leaving MB innervation to the z-joint intact. Unfortunately, intraarticular injection appears less efficacious in treating whiplash. For example, Barnsley and colleagues, in their randomized, double-blinded trial of local anesthetic with steroid versus local anesthetic alone, deem intraarticular steroid injection ineffective in treating whiplash-related cervical z-joint pain.[8,14] Nevertheless, some perform intraarticular injections as one of the previously mentioned dual diagnostic blocks to reduce the number of placebo responders.

Cervical Intraarticular Zygapophyseal Joint Injection Technique

Intraarticular z-joint injections may be performed using a lateral or posterior approach. For the lateral approach, the patient is placed in the side-lying position, and a lateral fluoroscopic image is obtained demonstrating the target z-joint. Unfortunately, such lateral imaging often visualizes both ipsilateral and contralateral joints. To identify the respective joints, one may rotate the image intensifier anteriorly; such rotation causes the ipsilateral joint image to appear to translate posteriorly and to a greater degree than the contralateral one, given its closer proximity to the intensifier. A needle is inserted just cephaladad to the joint line and advanced caudally into the joint. An AP fluoroscopic danger view then assists in preventing excessive medial needle advancement, with possible subsequent thecal sac penetration. After negative aspirate for cerebrospinal fluid and blood, only a small volume of radiological contrast dye (ie, 0.3–0.5 mL) is injected to avoid completely filling the joint, thereby allocating more remaining intraarticular volume to accommodate the anesthetic-corticosteroid injectate. After arthrographic, nonvascular, and nonfascial flow is demonstrated, a small volume (eg, 1 mL) of anesthetic-corticosteroid mixture is injected[2] (Fig. 2).

Alternatively, a posterior approach may be employed to avoid penetrating pleura or neurovascular structures. The patient is placed prone and an AP fluoroscopic image obtained demonstrating the target z-joint. The needle is then advanced into the joint. The lateral fluoroscopic view assists in preventing excessive anterior needle advancement into the spinal canal. Injection

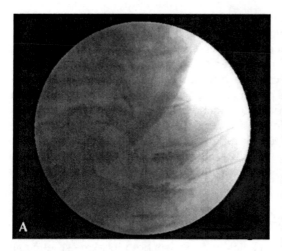

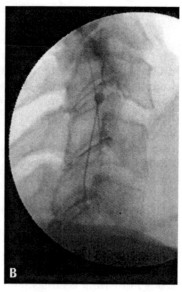

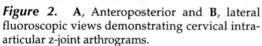

Figure 2. **A**, Anteroposterior and **B**, lateral fluoroscopic views demonstrating cervical intra-articular z-joint arthrograms.

then proceeds as above.[2] The usefulness of cervical z-joint injections has been questioned.

CERVICAL EPIDURAL STEROID INJECTION

Cervical Interlaminar Epidural Steroid Injection

Patients with cervical disc pathology typically present with radicular pain with or without neurologic compromise. Cervical disc pathology from whiplash injuries may result in compromise to the cervical nerve roots chemically or mechanically. Epidural steroid injections attempt to decrease the inflammatory response by placing steroid-anesthetic solution to the inflamed tissue. In their controlled study, Castagnera and colleagues report 79% success in a patient group that underwent cervical epidural steroid injection only for chronic cervical radicular pain, versus 80% success in a group that received steroid and morphine.[8,15]

Cervical Interlaminar Epidural Steroid Injection Technique

Cervical interlaminar steroid injection should typically be performed at the C7-T1 interlaminar space, which affords greater spinal canal diameter for epidural needle placement. The patient is placed in the prone position, and an AP fluoroscopic image is obtained demonstrating the C7-T1 interspace. Skin and soft tissues overlying the T1 lamina are locally anesthetized (eg, with 4 mL of lidocaine 1%) with a 25-gauge needle. A 22-gauge spinal needle is advanced down to the periosteum of the T1 lamina for additional local anesthetic infiltration. The 22 gauge is withdrawn, the skin nicked with an 18-gauge needle, and a 17-gauge Tuohy needle advanced down to the T1 lamina in a paramedian location. The Tuohy needle is then walked off the lamina in a medial trajectory toward the C7-T1 interlaminar space. Loss of resistance to the plunger of a 10-mL syringe filled with 3 to 5 mLof saline and the remaining volume air heralds entry into the epidural space. Biplanar imaging is used to confirm location. Needle advancement is then halted and negative aspirate for cerebrospinal fluid and blood obtained. Nonionic contrast dye is then injected demonstrating epidural, nonmyelographic, nonvascular, and nonfascial flow. A lateral fluoroscopic image confirms correct needle placement and contrast dye epidurogram. Biplanar imaging is used to confirm needle position and flow (Fig. 3). A 1- to 2-mL lidocaine 1% test dose is administered and, in the absence of apnea or upper extremity weakness, numbness, or paresthesias, an anesthetic-corticosteroid mixture (eg, 12 mg of betamethasone, 2 mL lidocaine 1%, 3 mL of normal saline) is injected.

Cervical Transforaminal Epidural Steroid Injection

Bush and Hillier report good pain relief of several months' duration in 93% of patients who underwent fluoroscopically guided transforaminal injection if they failed an initial "blind" injection.[8,16] In their retrospective analysis, Slipman and colleagues cite good to excellent outcome (with associated reduction in pain scores and medication usage) in 60% of patients with atraumatic cervical spondylotic radicular pain of 5.8 months' average duration, treated with an average of 2.2 transforaminal injections.[8,17]

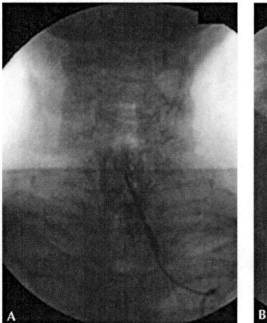
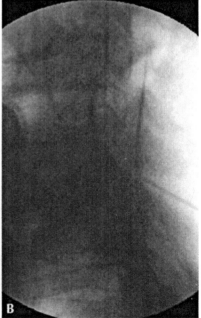

Figure 3. A, Anteroposterior and B, lateral fluoroscopic views demonstrating a typical C7–T1 epidural contrast dye pattern.

Complications include infection, epidural hematoma, thecal sac penetration, and spinal cord trauma.

Transforaminal Epidural Steroid Injection Technique

The patient is placed in a supine or lateral position, and an anterior oblique fluoroscopic image obtained demonstrating the foramen of the chosen cervical nerve to be treated. Skin and soft tissues overlying this foramen are locally anesthetized (eg, 2-3 mL of lidocaine 1%). A 25 gauge spinal needle is advanced toward the posterocaudal aspect of the foramen; indeed, the anterior aspect of the foramen is avoided, given its proximity to the vertebral artery. Under AP fluoroscopic danger view guidance, the needle is advanced medially so as not to pass beyond the "6 o'clock" (ie, midpoint) position of the lateral masses. Advancement beyond this position may result in thecal sac penetration or spinal cord trauma. Needle advancement is then halted, and negative aspirate for cerebrospinal fluid and blood is obtained. Nonionic contrast dye is then injected demonstrating flow along the nerve, nerve root sheath, and epidurally around the pedicle. Biplanar imaging is used to confirm needle position and flow (Fig. 4). A 1- to 2-mL lidocaine 1% test dose is administered and, in the

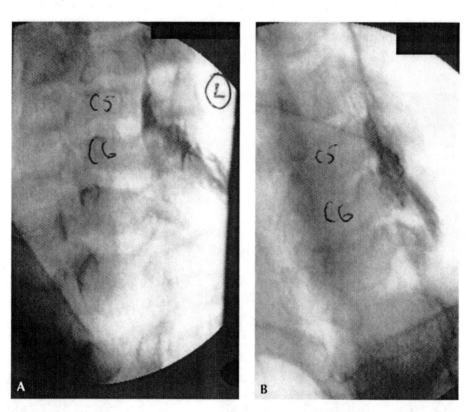

Figure 4. **A**, Anteroposterior and **B**, left anterior oblique fluoroscopic views demonstrating C6 transforaminal contrast dye pattern with flow along the nerve, nerve root sheath, and epidurally.

absence of apnea, seizures, or upper extremity weakness, numbness, or paresthesias, an anesthetic-corticosteroid mixture (eg, 12 mg of betamethasone and 1 mL of lidocaine 1%) is injected.

Furman and colleagues' study citing the incidence of vascular penetration in transforaminal cervical epidural steroid injections (19.4%) underscores the need for contrast-enhanced fluoroscopic guidance when performing this procedure. Specifically, using only "flash" (blood in the needle hub) or positive needle aspirate without contrast-enhanced fluoroscopy to predict intravascular injection was 97.0% specific but only 45.9% sensitive. Consequently, contrast-enhanced fluoroscopic guidance should minimize intravascular injection of steroid with subsequent systemic spread.[18]

Selective Nerve Blocks

When the pathological level is not clinically clear, a diagnostic block can be performed to identify the symptomatic nerve. The technique is similar to the transforaminal epidural steroid injection except that contrast and medication flow is restricted to the extraforaminal region along the exiting segmental spinal nerve or ventral ramus. Only 0.5 to 1.0 mL of anesthetic is injected. If anesthetic flows medially into the intervertebral foramen and into the epidural space, it may ascend or descend to other levels making this a nonspecific, nondiagnostic procedure. The patient is instructed to complete a pain diary.

PROVOCATIVE CERVICAL DISCOGRAPHY

Provocative discography remains the only diagnostic procedure that can confirm the suspected intervertebral disc as the putative pain generator. Consequently, discography aids presurgical fusion planning and streamlines assessment of patients mired in equivocal, inconclusive diagnostic tests.

The procedure is performed when there is predominantly axial neck pain, tenderness over the segments, magnetic resonance imaging suggesting disc desiccation and, therefore, internal disc disruption suspected. The procedure is presurgical and should be performed only to identify which, if any, cervical discs are the pain generator and circumscribe the levels.

Contraindications include midsagittal spinal canal diameter less than 12 mm and large disc herniation. Complications include discitis (0.37%),[19,20] epidural abcess,[21] spinal cord injury, nerve injury, quadriplegia,[22] stroke, and pneumothorax.

Given the relatively high frequency of multilevel symptomatic cervical discs, some advocate that discography should be performed at all accessible cervical levels.[23]

Cervical Discography Technique

The patient is placed in a supine position, and an anterior oblique fluoroscopic image is obtained demonstrating the uncinate process of the vertebral body caudal to the target intervertebral disc. Skin and soft tissues overlying this uncinate process are locally anesthetized (eg, 2-3 mL of lidocaine 1%). A 25-gauge spinal needle is stepped off medially from the uncinate process into the target disc.

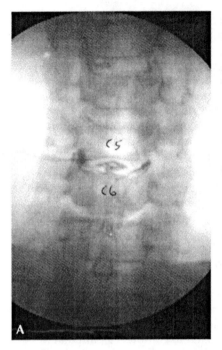

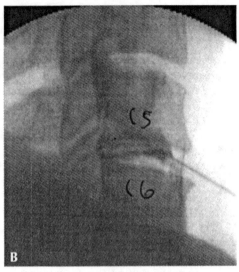

Figure 5. A, Anteroposterior and B, lateral fluoroscopic views demonstrating C5–C6 discography with posterior anular rupture and contrast extension into the epidural space.

Alternatively, a straight AP approach may be employed with the patient placed in a supine position. The esophagus and trachea are manually retracted medially and the carotid artery retracted laterally, thereby allowing a safe trajectory for needle advancement into the target disc.

The needle is then further directed into the geometric center of the disc via AP and lateral fluoroscopic guidance. A mixture of nonionic contrast dye and antibiotic (eg, cefazolin) is then injected into the disc (Fig. 5). Pain provocation, the volume injected, end point, and nucleogram are then recorded. Some discographers check each disc separately and then remove each needle. We advocate placing all needles first. Each level is subsequently checked for pain provocation. Reliability can then be assessed by repeat testing of the respective levels and performing "sham" injections. A sham injection is when the discographer feigns an injection and asks the patient for his response. Reliable responses are reproducible and supported by pain-free sham injections.

Pain provocation is graded as follows[24]:

P0   No pain response provoked.

P+/- Pain response provoked but is dissimilar, discordant, and uncharacteristic in location and quality compared to the patient's usual pain

P+   Similar pain response that mimics a fraction of patient's usual pain.

P++ Exact pain provocation concordant with the patient's usual pain.

Walsh and colleagues cite 100% specificity and a 0% false-positive rate, albeit for lumbar discography, when an abnormal nucleogram and substantial pain response defined a positive test. Criteria for substantial pain response include pain intensity of 3 out of 5 on a colored pain thermometer, two or more pain-related behaviors (ie, rubbing, grimacing, guarding/bracing/withdrawing, sighing, or verbalizing), and concordant pain.[28] Carragee describes a high rate of false positives in lumbar discography, which can be minimized by evaluating those without chronic pain and with normal psychometrics.[29]

Volume injected and end point assess anular competence. A normal cervical disc typically accepts 0.2 to 0.4 mL of injectate.[25] Abnormal discs, however, may accommodate more volume, with completely ruptured discs accepting substantial volumes (ie, even greater than 10 mL) due to injectate spilling into the epidural space. The end point feels "firm" in the normal disc, "spongy" in the disrupted disc, and "absent" in the ruptured disc.[26]

Normal nucleogram morphologies include the round "cottonball" as well as "lobular" secondary to nuclear clefts in the older, mature disc. Abnormal morphologies include "irregular," with fissures in the inner anulus, "fissured," with fissures extending to the outer anulus, and "ruptured," allowing injectate to spill into the epidural space[27] (Fig. 6).

Patients may be sent for postdiscography computed tomography scanning within 4 hours of dye injection to grade anular degeneration and disruption (Fig. 7). Specifically, Sachs and colleagues cite the contrast-enhanced CT/discography axial view (albeit for the lumbar spine) as a sensitive evaluator of

Discogram type		Stage of disc degeneration
1. Cottonball	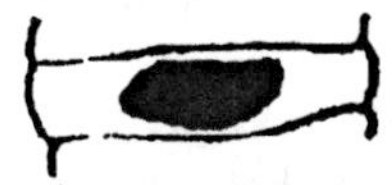	No signs of degeneration. Soft white amorphous nucleus
2. Lobular	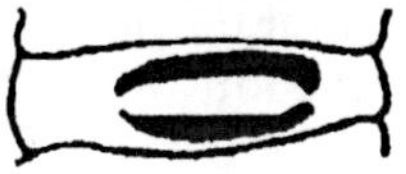	Mature disc with nucleus starting to coalesce into fibrous lumps
3. Irregular	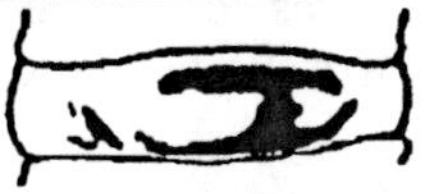	Degenerated disc with fissures and clefts in the nucleus and inner annulus
4. Fissured	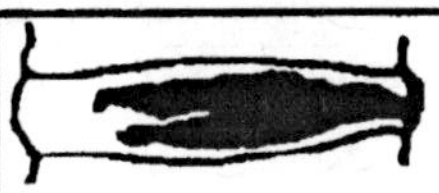	Degenerated disc with radial fissure leading to the outer edge of the annulus
5. Ruptured	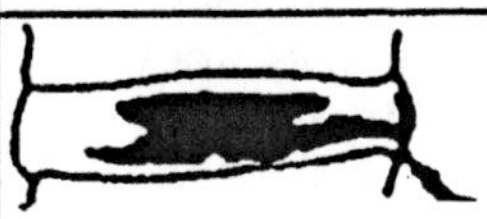	Disc has a complete radial fissure that allows injected fluid to escape. Can be in any state of degeneration.

Figure 6. Discographic contrast dye morphologies seen with fluoroscopic imaging. (From Windsor FE, Falco JE, Dreyer SJ, et al: Lumbar discography. Phys Med Rehabil Clin North Am 6:743–770, 1995, with permission; and adapted from Adams M, Dolan P, Hutton W: The stages of disc degeneration as revealed by discograms. J Bone Joint Surg Br 68:36–41, 1986, with permission.)

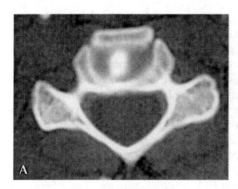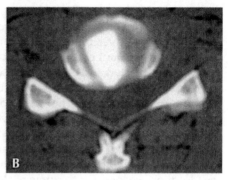

Figure 7. Postdiscography CT. **A,** A normal intranuclear injection pattern without anular spread. **B,** An abnormal discogram with contrast dye extension beyond the outer anulus (Dallas Discogram disruption—grade 3) and contrast partially filling the anular volume (Dallas Discogram degeneration—grade 2).

pathology not otherwise detected by routine AP and lateral discogram views. Although originally intended for the lumbar spine, their Dallas Discogram Description, in addition to pain and contrast volume injected, gauges morphologic degrees of anular degeneration and disruption, respectively, via contrast-enhanced axial CT.[30]

Anular degeneration is graded by the amount of contrast that fills the anulus. (Table 1).

Anular disruption is graded by degree of radial extension of contrast toward the anular margin (Table 2).

Moneta and colleagues, albeit for the lumbar spine, cite a statistically significant correlation between pain reproduction and grade 3 anular fissures.[31]

SUMMMARY

Interventional spine procedures constitute aggressive-conservative treatment for whiplash. Judicious use of these diagnostic and therapeutic procedures

Table 1. Grading of Anular Degeneration

Grade	Description
0	No change
1	Local (ie, contrast fills < 10% of the anulus)
2	Partial (ie, contrast fills < 50% of the anulus)
3	Total (ie, contrast fills > 50% of the anulus)

Table 2. Grading of Anular Disruption

Grade	Description
0	None (ie, no contrast extension)
1	Into inner anulus
2	Into outer anulus
3	Beyond outer anulus

can significantly impact on the care of appropriately selected patients. These procedures should be considered when appropriate conservative care has not resulted in functional improvement. This treatment should not be performed in isolation but instead integrated into a comprehensive program including medications and therapy.

After a thorough clinical evaluation, major pain generators to consider in patients with whiplash include the cervical z-joint, spinal nerve, and intervertebral disc. Various injection procedures can be helpful in the diagnosis and treatment of many of these disorders.

References

1. Barnsley L, Lord SM, Wallis BJ, et al: The prevalence of chronic cervical zygapophyseal joint pain after whiplash. Spine 20:20–26, 1995.
2. Dreyfuss P, Kaplan M, Dreyer SJ: Zygapophyseal joint injection techniques in the spinal axis. In Lennard T (ed): Pain Procedures in Clinical Practice. Philadelphia, Hanley & Belfus, 2000.
3. Barnsley L, Lord S, Bogduk N: Comparative local anesthetic blocks in the diagnosis of cervical zygapophyseal joint pain. Pain 55:99–106, 1993.
4. Barnsley L, Lord S, Wallis B, et al: False-positive rates of cervical zygapophyseal joint blocks. Clin J Pain 9:124–130, 1993.
5. Barnsley L, Lord SM, Wallis BJ, et al: The prevalence of chronic cervical zygapophyseal joint pain after whiplash. Spine 20:20–26, 1995.
6. Lagattuta FP, Falco JE: Assessment and treatment of cervical spine disorders. In Braddom RL (ed): Physical Medicine & Rehabilitation. Philadelphia, WB Saunders, 1996, pp 728–755.
7. Barnsley L, Bogduk N: Medial branch blocks are specific for the diagnosis of cervical zygapophyseal joint pain. Reg Anesth 18:343–350, 1993.
8. Manchikanti L, Singh V, Kloth D et al: Interventional techniques in the management of chronic pain: part 2.0. Pain Physician 4:24–96, 2001.
9. Lord S, Barnsley L, Wallis BJ, et al: Third occipital nerve headache: a prevalence study. J Neurol Neurosurg Psychiatry 57:1187–1190, 1994.
10. Lord SM, Barnsley L, Wallis BJ, et al: Percutaneous radio-frequency neurotomy for chronic cervical zygapophyseal-joint pain. N Eng J Med 335:1721–1726, 1996.
11. Wallis BJ, Lord SM, Bogduk N: Resolution of psychological distress of whiplash patients following treatment by radiofrequency neurotomy: a randomized, double-blind, placebo-controlled trial. Pain 73:15–22, 1997.
12. Dreyfuss P, Rogers CJ: Radiofrequency neurotomy of the zygapophyseal and sacroiliac joints. In Lennard T (ed): Pain Procedures in Clinical Practice. Philadelphia, Hanley & Belfus, 2000.
13. Finch PM, Racz GB, McDaniel K: A curved approach to nerve blocks and radiofrequency lesioning. Pain Digest 7:251–257, 1997.
14. Barnsley L, Lord SM, Wallis BJ, et al: Lack of effect of intra-articular corticosteroids for chronic pain in the cervical zygapophyseal joints. N Engl J Med 330:1047–1050, 1994.
15. Castagnera L, Maurette P, Pointillart V, et al: Long-term results of cervical epidural steroid injection with and without morphine in chronic cervical radicular pain. Pain 58:239–243, 1994.
16. Bush K, Hillier S: Outcome of cervical radiculopathy treated with periradicular/epidural corticosteroid injections: a prospective study with independent clinical review. Eur Spine J 5:319–325, 1996.
17. Slipman CW, Lipetz JS, Jackson HB, et al: Therapeutic selective nerve root block in the nonsurgical treatment of atraumatic cervical spondylotic radicular pain: a retrospective analysis with independent clinical review. Arch Phys Med Rehabil 81:741–746, 2000.
18. Furman MB, Giovanniello M, O'Brien E, et al: Incidence of intravascular penetration in transforaminal cervical epidural steroid injections. [abstract]. Accepted for presentation at 16th Annual Meeting of the North American Spine Society, October 31, 2001–November 3, 2001, Seattle, WA.
19. Guyer RD, Collier R, Stith WJ: Discitis after discography. Spine 13:1352–1354, 1988.
20. Grubb SA, Kelly CK: Cervical discography: clinical implications from 12 years of experience. Spine 25:1382–1389, 2000.
21. Lownie SP, Ferguson CG: Spinal subdural empyema complicating cervical discography. Spine 14:1415–1417, 1989.
22. Laun A, Lorenz R, Agnoli AL: Complications of cervical discography. J Neurosurg Sci 25:17–20, 1981.

23. Reference deleted (see ref. 20).
24. Fortin JD: Lumbar and thoracic discography with CT and MRI correlation. In Lennard T (ed): Pain Procedures in Clinical Practice. Philadelphia, Hanley & Belfus, 2000.
25. Kambin P, Abda S, Kurpicki F: Intradiskal pressure and volume recording: evaluation of normal and abnormal cervical disks. Clin Orthop 146:144–147, 1980.
26. Windsor RE, Falco JE, Dreyer SJ, et al: Lumbar discography. Phys Med Rehabil Clin North Am 6:743–770, 1995.
27. Adams M, Dolan P, Hutton W: The stages of disc degeneration as revealed by discograms. J Bone Joint Surg Br 68:36–41, 1986.
28. Walsh TR, Weinstein JN, Spratt KF, et al: Lumbar discography in normal patients. J Bone Joint Surg Am 72:1081–1088, 1990.
29. Carragee J, Tanner CM, Churana S, et al: The rates of false-positive lumbar discography in select patients without low back symptoms. Spine 25:1373–1381, 2000.
30. Sachs BL, Vanharanta H, Spivey MA, et al: Dallas Discogram Description. A new classification of CT/discography in low back disorders. Spine 12:287–293, 1987.
31. Moneta GB, Videman T, Kaivanto K, et al: Reported pain during lumbar discography as a function of annular ruptures and disc degeneration. A re-analysis of 833 discograms. Spine 17:1968–1974, 1994.

22

Complementary and Alternative Medicine in the Treatment of Whiplash-Associated Disorders

Ann C. Cotter, M.D., Pietro Memmo, M.D., and Nancy Kim, M.D.

In the last decade, complementary and alternative medicine (CAM) has received unprecedented attention by patients, physicians,[34] and researchers.[69] Approximately 42% of the population as a whole uses some sort of CAM, and 50% of physicians refer to CAM practitioners.[27] It is estimated that in 1997, patients in the United States spent more on out-of-pocket complementary medicine services and products than for physician services.[25] The group of therapies to which this heading refers are diverse and cover a wide range in terms of level of acceptance and integration into the medical mainstream. Some, such as acupuncture, are on the verge of being considered conventional and have a significant amount of research to support their efficacy. Others, such as magnet therapy, have been subject to only minimal scientific inquiry. Previously considered medically unsound, CAM was associated at best with a placebo effect and at worst with dangerous practices and unscrupulous practitioners. To improve the nation's understanding of CAM modalities, the National Center for Complementary and Alternative Medicine[69] has created a classification system for CAM modalities that is described below. Since 1983, this National Institutes of Health (NIH)-funded center has served as a clearinghouse for information on CAM and in 2001 had a budget of $70 million dedicated to funding CAM research and dissemination of CAM information to consumers.

Until recent years, whiplash as an entity remained undefined and shrouded in controversy. Expert review of existing data and consensus development among experts has done much for clarifying the definition, epidemiology, pathophysiology, and effective treatment of whiplash-associated disorder (WAD).[83] CAM is in a similar position to the position of WAD several years ago in that its place within the scope of the responsible practice of medicine is currently undergoing clarification.

Despite the fact that interest in and investigation of CAM is widespread, there are many conditions for which there are no guidelines for the use of CAM modalities. WADs fall into such a category. From 1990 to 1997, the top five reasons for seeking CAM therapies were back problems, allergies, fatigue, arthritis, and headache.[69] WADs can be associated with at least two of these five conditions.[6] Without whiplash-specific research to rely on for an overview of CAM modalities that may be effective in this area, we make inferences from the existing literature for which there is evidence supporting its use in symptoms and conditions similar to WAD. Whenever possible, reference to the Quebec Task Force Guidelines on Whiplash-Associated Disorders[83] is made (see Chapter 7).

Below is a brief description of each of the five categories within the NIH classification of CAM, with examples in each category. The modalities that are used frequently with whiplash-associated conditions are described further.

Alternative medical systems include systems of health and healing that are self-contained and exist independently of allopathic medicine. Examples include oriental medicine, ayurvedic medicine, and homeopathy

Mind-body interventions consider human beings as a continuum of body, mind, and spirit. These modalities intervene at one or more of these levels to influence the entire person. Yoga and other movement therapies, stress reduction, meditation, hypnosis and guided imagery are examples.

Biologically-based therapies include the use of biologically active natural compounds to enhance the body's ability to heal. They include herbal medicine, vitamins, and supplements as well as special diet therapies, such as macrobiotics, Ornish, fasting, and vegetarian or vegan diets.

Manipulative and body-based methods use hands-on techniques to promote circulation, balance tight tissues, and correct bony alignment to promote the body's ability to heal and maintain optimum function. They include osteopathic and chiropractic manipulation as well as massage and bodywork. Manipulation is described in Chapter 19.

Energy therapies include interventions that specifically affect the human energy field, or biofield. Magnetic therapy and biofield therapies (Therapeutic Touch, Polarity, and Reiki) are included in this category.

SELECTED MODALITIES

Acupuncture

The use of acupuncture within the Western model of illness or injury bridges Oriental medical theory and Western bioanatomic medicine. In Oriental medical theory, a vital force, or *qi*, is considered to be the foundation that powers all physiologic function. *Qi* is organized into channels or meridians that run longitudinally throughout the body, and acupuncture points are located along these meridians. A healthy person is one who is able to maintain a balanced and adequate flow of *qi* throughout the body. A second concept is that of yin and yang, the two complementary and opposite forces that constitute the energetic universe. This concept roughly corresponds to the Western concept of homeostasis. When blockage of flow in the meridians occurs, or when the balance of yin and yang is upset, acupuncture is used to effect balanced and harmonious flow of energy to positively influence health.

Western biomedical theory has neither proven nor disproven this concept of bodily energy known as *qi*, but several measurable biochemical and physiologic changes occur when acupuncture is administered. Pomeranz and Chiu[74] showed that naloxone blocked acupuncture analgesia, and Kiser[56] confirmed that relief of chronic pain symptoms correlates with increased plasma met-enkephalin. Liao[60] confirmed increased temperature in distal points after stimulation of acupuncture points. Acupuncture increases plasma adrenocorticotropic hormone levels.[62] Acupuncture points have different electrical properties than the surrounding skin, although there are no demonstrable histologic changes in the anatomic locations of acupuncture points.[44] Positron emission tomography scanning has quantified reproducible changes in cerebral metabolic functioning after acupuncture points are stimulated.[20] Thus, acupuncture may be efficacious in the treatment of whiplash by mobilizing native endorphins, improving circulation, or stimulating the release of native glucocorticoid compounds.

From a practical point of view, there is no standard protocol for acupuncture treatment of whiplash. Acupuncture is an art and a science with more than 2000 years of history, and thus there are various styles and approaches. Choice and style of treatment depends on the approach of the practitioner. One form that is readily appreciated by Western physicians is known as neuroanatomic acupuncture, in which Western anatomy and physiology is combined with Chinese medical theory.[95] Treatment of whiplash-associated symptoms would combine points chosen to stimulate anatomically relevant neural, soft tissue, and articular structures (eg, the point GB12) along with a traditional points such as the "window of the sky" point (eg, the point SI17), known to balance the flow of energy between the head and the body, and point GB34, known to benefit tendons and ligaments (Fig. 1). GB12 is chosen because it is located in the temporooccipital region posterior to the mastoid process and stimulates the suboccipital nerve and the rectus capitis muscles, often in spasm following flexion extension injury. The more traditional SI17, located posterior to the angle of the mandible and anterior to the sternocleidomastoid muscle and occipital ridge,

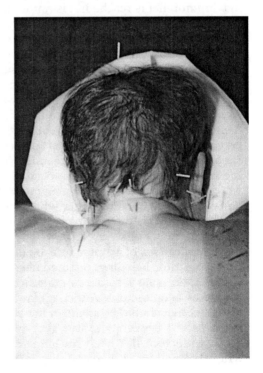

Figure 1. Treatment of whiplash-associated symptoms may include anatomically relevant points along with traditional points. (Photo courtesy of Associates in Rehabilitation, Morristown, New Jersey)

happens to stimulate the superior sympathetic ganglion,[95] something that was not known to ancient physicians but, rather, chosen empirically. GB34 is located anterior and inferior to the fibular head, and has no anatomic relationship to the cervical spine in Western terms. An acupuncturist recognizes that GB34 is located on the same meridian as the occipital points previously mentioned and that it is known to be a powerful point in treatments for musculoskeletal problems. Another form becoming popular among Western physicians is ear acupuncture, initially developed in France, which relies on stimulation of specific points on the ear to affect distal body parts. Acupuncture using meridian points may be, and often is, combined with ear acupuncture. Other forms of acupuncture are described elsewhere.[82]

After insertion, needles may be stimulated with heat, electricity, or by hand. Needles are usually left in place for 15 to 30 minutes, depending on the focus of treatment. Most studies have used a protocol of three to 16 sessions of acupuncture to demonstrate presence or lack of benefit. Patients are usually told to expect to see the beginning of pain relief after four and six sessions of acupuncture. When pain relief is experienced, the benefit is cumulative, with pain relief increasing in both degree and length of posttreatment effect with successive treatments. When a plateau of pain relief has been reached, the time between treatments is increased. In acute situations, it is not unusual to treat patients more than once per week for the first 1 or 2 weeks. In more chronic conditions, it is more usual to treat patients on a weekly basis until plateau has occurred. Afterward, treatments are spaced to a frequency of once or twice monthly until the maximum length of pain-free time between treatments is reached. After maximum relief is reached, it is not unusual for pain relief to be ongoing. In some cases, treatment may be necessary on a long-term (monthly, quarterly) basis if pain is severe and has been long-standing prior to treatment or if the patient has significant disease progression or advanced age. The American Academy of Medical Acupuncture recommends a trial of four to six sessions to evaluate efficacy. If no benefit can be documented (eg improved functional status, increased range of motion, decreased pain assessment on the Visual Analog Scale, decreased use of pain medications), it is likely that further treatment will not be of benefit. For people who are treated soon after injury, an average of 10 to 15 treatments as part of a comprehensive rehabilitation program should be sufficient. Up to 20 treatments may be necessary for persons suffering from chronic symptoms associated with whiplash injury. Regardless of chronicity, patients will better maintain their gains, require fewer sessions, and derive maximal benefit sooner when acupuncture is combined with manual and movement therapies directed at achieving an independent home maintenance program.

Complications of acupuncture are documented as low in frequency and include infection, bleeding, retained needles, perforation of an organ, and syncope.[67] There is no absolute contraindication to any medication usage during a course of acupuncture. Anticoagulants are a relative contraindication; the acupuncturist should be aware of increased bleeding risk. Delayed or blunted response may be seen with steroid or opioid medications.[44]

Acupuncture has been investigated for balance disturbance following whiplash[28] and for vertigo and dizziness of cervical origin.[43] In Fattori's study,

15 whiplash patients with balance disturbances were treated with acupuncture and compared with patients treated with medication and physical therapy.[28] Although the study showed statistically significant results in favor of acupuncture, several variables were not clarified, including the exact nature of medications taken by the control group and whether the test group received medications concurrent with acupuncture. Acupuncture was administered to a group of 15 patients with the equivalent of grade I-II injury and found to have significant effect when compared with controls.[45] More generally, acupuncture continues to be used as a remedy for headaches of multiple origins, neck stiffness, and chronic arthritic pain. Clinical trials of acupuncture and neck pain have shown positive therapeutic benefit when compared with sham acupuncture,[12] TENS,[72] standard medical treatment,[21] and physical therapy.[23] Several reviews of existing studies, however, conclude either that there is insufficient evidence to warrant recommendation to treat with acupuncture[41,57,81] or that present evidence warrants further studies.[92] These authors advocate the use of acupuncture is the manner described above.

Massage

Massage may be defined as the manipulation of soft tissue for the goal of releasing restricted tight muscular, fascial, subcutaneous, and periarticular tissues. The most common form of massage is Swedish massage, with which the common strokes known as effleurage, pétrissage, friction, and tapotement are associated. Most massage therapists in the United States practice this type of massage. In recent years, other forms of massage have become popular. Shiatsu ("finger pressure" in Japanese) and acupressure direct pressure along acupuncture points and meridians. Reflexology is confined to the feet and lower leg and uses a somatotopic map of the body on the sole of the foot to influence organs and tissues of the body. Myofascial release is directed at removing restriction in the deep fascial planes through friction techniques and was first developed as an ostepathic technique. Soft tissue massage is among the most popular of the "complementary therapies."[26] Physiologic effects of massage include increased cutaneous blood flow[39]; reduction of heart rate, blood pressure, and respiratory rate[30]; increased myofascial flexibility[15]; decreased perception of pain[33]; and decreased levels of stress hormones.[33,97]

A recent trial comparing massage, acupuncture, and self-care for persistent low back pain concluded that massage was superior in terms of cost and long-term benefit. Research on mechanisms of action and the role of massage in producing increased functional status is scant and even less available when looking at specific disorder categories, such as WAD.

A useful place for massage in the rehabilitation of WAD is for short-term use within the context of a comprehensive rehabilitation program. Massage should be directed at tissue relaxation to reduce painful spasm and myofascial restriction, with the goal of facilitating the patient's participation in active rehabilitation. A reasonable course of massage would include eight to 12 sessions as part of an active program for stretching and strengthening the cervical paraspinal and shoulder girdle musculature. Family members may be taught simple techniques to massage areas that continue to act as painful stimuli.

Movement Therapies

Movement therapies are frequently used by patients with chronic pain to reduce stress, alleviate muscular tension, and relieve pain. Five such therapies include yoga, Alexander, Feldenkrais, Trager, and Pilates techniques. Although they enjoy widespread use, these therapies have received little objective evaluation despite their potential benefits.

The movement therapies discussed here are quite distinct, yet have a number of elements in common. All use kinesthetic training as a basis for reeducating the body and mind to move without restriction and pain. Even in the well-conditioned spine, flexion/extension trauma can result in muscle spasm, guarding, and inefficient posture. Poor alignment produces chronic discomfort and decreased range of motion as well as imposing strain on structures above and below the injured area. If not interrupted early, a cycle of spasm, pain, and limited motion results. Each of the above techniques focuses on breaking patterns of poor posture and movement by teaching awareness of proper positioning and relative movement of the spine and axial skeleton. Increased awareness allows the patient to form better movement habits. Often, the floor or a table is used to help the patient experience better alignment and proprioceptive skills without the stress of gravity. As the patient lies supine, the practitioner guides him to feel what less restricted movement feels like. Later, these lessons are integrated into posture and movement. The techniques rely on combinations of conscious and unconscious learning, visualization, and breakdown of movement patterns into smaller components. Although functionally based, release of emotional patterns may occur depending on the practitioner's orientation and the needs and readiness of the client. When compared with conventional rehabilitation approaches, the methods described below take a more global approach to rehabilitation of specific conditions and seek to improve the patient's awareness of the involvement of the entire body in all movements—great or small. These therapies are suitable for patients with grade I-III complaints. Individualized therapy should be replaced by group classes when deemed safe by the supervising physician. Although individuals vary in terms of need and progress, a reasonable guideline is to prescribe up to 10 individual sessions with an emphasis on home practice. If functional status plateaus prior to 10 sessions, transition to group classes is recommended.

Yoga

Yoga is a philosophy and way of life that encompasses ethical conduct, social responsibility, nutrition, and physical health practices. It was developed in India and brought to the United States in the mid 1800s. In the West, the aspect of yoga that is most familiar is *hatha* yoga. It focuses on achieving physical, mental, and spiritual harmony via postures known as *asanas*. However, most followers concentrate on increasing strength, flexibility, and relaxation. Physical benefits from this method include the reduction of muscle tension, improvement of posture, and increase in range of motion, increase in strength and flexibility. Mental benefits from this method include the attainment of peace, well-being, body awareness, and sense of emotional balance.

Yoga is taught in a group setting that begins with stretching and centering poses. Loose and comfortable clothing are encouraged, and mats are often used. By holding a pose, physical strength, flexibility, relaxation, and energy flow (*prana*) are maximized. Emphasis is placed on attention to one's limitations and the dynamic interaction between the muscular, respiratory, and emotional balance. The instructor uses verbal direction in addition to hands-on assistance. Besides stretching and poses, relaxation techniques are taught. A variety of patients can participate because the different styles of *hatha* yoga range from vigorous to gentle exercises. Yoga can be adapted to patients with range of motion and other physical limitations and to the elderly through the use of props, such as bolsters, straps, or chairs (Fig 2).Classes are available for specific populations with disorders such as back pain, cancer, rheumatoid arthritis, and multiple sclerosis. A dedicated student of yoga practices four to six times per week, but benefits may be obtained from just one session per week.

Multiple types of yoga are available in any large and medium-sized city. They include Iyengar yoga, which focuses on precision and attention to anatomy and alignment. Specific sequences for particular ailments are used to assist in rehabilitation from a wide variety of disorders. *Kripalu* yoga focuses on compassion for self and others and may take a variety of forms, from gentle to vigorous. Integrative yoga therapy is based on *Kripalu* yoga and is designed for

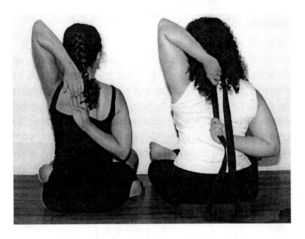

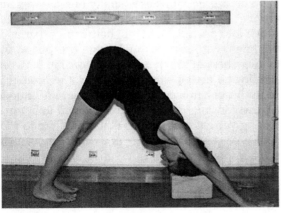

Figure 2. Yoga can be adapted to patients with ROM and other physical limitations through use of props, such as bolsters, straps, or blocks. (Photos courtesy of Madelana Ferrara, Balance and Vibration Yoga Studio, Morristown, New Jersey)

those recovering from illness. Integral yoga is an additional form of yoga that emphasizes relaxation techniques and emotional balance. *Viniyoga*, developed by TKV Desikachar, emphasizes therapeutic use of the breath with movement. It is especially adaptable to people with disabilities and, like all types of yoga, may be individualized to the particular needs of the person. *Ashtanga* yoga is a popular and vigorous set of fast-paced poses that is not advised for those recovering from musculoskeletal injuries. In the medical setting, all except the latter may be adapted to the patient recovering from cervical injury. There is no minimum training requirement for a practitioner of yoga. Clinicians should be aware of the qualifications and experience of a practitioner prior to referring a patient with cervical or any other injury.

Yoga has been used in the medical setting, specifically in patients with rheumatoid arthritis,[42] osteoarthritis,[36] chronic back pain,[77] carpal tunnel syndrome,[37] and other medical conditions.[70,80] Although there are no published studies examining the efficacy of yoga in WAD, it is clear that it is helpful in patients with chronic pain. In uncomplicated cases, yoga may be used as the primary movement modality during rehabilitation of WAD, or it may serve as a useful transition from physical therapy to independent conditioning. Specific suggestions for integrating yoga into a rehabilitation program are given below.

Alexander Technique

The Alexander technique was developed by F. M. Alexander (1869-1955), a Shakespearean actor who developed his method of self-observation and correction to help himself recover from a recurrent loss of voice that threatened his career. He discovered that his voice was inhibited by his habit of tense cervical posturing. When he was able to correct this tendency, his voice recovered. Alexander felt that habits of unnecessary and inefficient muscle tension could be broken only after they were understood and that understanding occurred with repetition of small, simple movements. He extended the technique to aid other performers as well as people with other occupation-related postural tendencies.

The foundation of this technique is to achieve a balance between the head and neck (primary control) in static and dynamic situations as well as to maintain proper breathing patterns. The patient is taught to engage the mind in choosing between beneficial versus automatic, nonbeneficial postures and to understand that there is always a choice. Sessions are usually one-on-one, but they may be done in a group format. Typically, the practitioner directs the student verbally and with light touch into postures that will help him experience the state of being in proper alignment without tension. During this phase, the patient is taught to develop an awareness of the dynamic relationship between the head, neck, and torso in static and active situations. Next, the patient is taught to sense and eliminate inhibitory muscular contractions that impede smooth movement. Lastly, the patient is taught to sense and respond to internal and external cues while performing various movements that guide him to produce smooth, coordinated actions with conscious control of an entire movement without breaking it down into component parts. In essence, this technique teaches patients to realign the spine, neck and head and to move in ways that reduce muscular tension and allow the body to move more efficiently. This increased awareness of imbalances and "habits of misuse" allows the patient to learn new ways to stand, sit, and walk by improving posture in everyday functions and reducing chronic pain.

In practice, Alexander teachers work with patients with postural difficulties, chronic and occupational back and neck pain, or for improved performance in athletics and the performing arts. This technique has been shown to be beneficial in the treatment of scoliosis,[17] for improvement in respiratory capacity,[4] Parkinson's disease,[84] stress reduction,[66,76] chronic pain,[34,85] and back pain during pregnancy.[75] Although no WAD-specific literature exists, there is enough information available on related conditions to warrant trial for those who seek an individualized, proprioceptive-based approach.

Trager Psychophysical Integration

Trager psychophysical integration was developed by Milton Trager, M.D., in the 1940s. It combines gentle hands-on tissue work, movement reeducation, and relaxation techniques. This technique emphasizes the use of the mind and body to change physical and mental patterns that interfere with ease of movement. Initially, the hands-on component is used. It involves gentle rocking, stretching, and rolling movements to aid in relaxing the tense areas of the body. Prior to working on a patient, the practitioner is trained to attain a state of calm and focus. The practitioner communicates this relaxation through the hands to the patient's body and thus "teaches" the patient in a somatic fashion the feeling of relaxation. The second aspect of the Trager method involves movement reeducation using a technique called mentastics (a combination of "mental" and "gymnastics"), which helps to facilitate light and smooth movements. It has been shown to increase the vital capacity in patients with thoracic restrictions,[93] to improve trunk mobility in cerebral palsy patients,[94] and Parkinson's disease patients.[16] There are no studies that examine the efficacy of this technique in WAD; however, Trager's work has gained popularity in the rehabilitation of chronic pain patients with musculoskeletal injuries of the head, neck, shoulder, and back.[24]

Feldenkrais Method

The Feldenkrais method was created by Moshe Feldenkrais, D.Sc., (1904-1984) who was a physicist and mechanical engineer as well as an accomplished judo practitioner. His inspiration in developing his method occurred after suffering from a chronic knee injury that interfered with his ambulation. During his recovery period, he applied his knowledge of physics, anatomy, physiology, psychology, yoga, and the Alexander technique to his observation of human movement. The result was a unique approach to movement therapy that enhanced the rehabilitation of patients with functional impairments from chronic pain. He theorized that the human mind has the ability to understand, learn, and perform new movements, unlike animals, who are more concrete and have limited choices in movement. His method guides patients in identifying and understanding their dysfunctional movement patterns and discovering alternative options to perform a single task without eliciting pain. The benefits of the Feldenkrais method include increased variety of movement patterns, increased flexibility and range of motion, improved coordination, and proper posture training. These benefits lead to the reduction of chronic pain from a wide variety of etiologies, including musculoskeletal, neurologic, and orthopedic causes.

The teaching of the Feldenkrais method can be offered in the form of *awareness through movement* (ATM) or in the form of *functional integration* (FI). Awareness through movement is often taught in groups, using verbal guidance in directing the patient in discovering alternative movements to perform functional tasks such as transferring from a wheelchair to a bed. The patients are encouraged to note the pattern of each body part during the task and encouraged to try new movements. The movements are slow and gentle, with a focus on identifying the dysfunctional movement pattern and discovering a new painless pattern. It involves multiple repetitions in order to engrave a new motor engram, encompassing the whole body in simple and complex movements. The unique aspect of this movement reeducation is that it is not a treatment but instead is considered a lesson in movement. Functional integration, the second form, is taught individually with the teacher using the hands to guide the patient through various movement sequences. Sessions are about 45 minutes.

The Feldenkrais and Alexander methods have some similarities; however, the latter can be said to concentrate somewhat more on head-to-spine relationships than the former. Feldenkrais methodology has been particularly successful in neurologic rehabilitation.[29]

Successful use of the Feldenkrais method has been reported in the rehabilitation of neurologic disorders: stroke, brain injury,[5] Parkinson's disease,[78] and spinal cord injury.[38] One study examined the efficacy of the Feldenkrais versus conventional exercises in a group of elderly patients and found no significant functional improvements in this population in contrast to the other studies. A review of the research on the Feldenkrais method in the rehabilitation setting concluded that the methodology of most of the studies was poor and that further research was needed.[49] Although there have been no published studies demonstrating the efficacy of the Feldenkrais method in patients with whiplash, it is used successfully in chronic neck and back conditions.[59] The authors recommend Feldenkrais as a reasonable choice for movement reeducation directed toward functional independence after acute issues have been addressed.

Pilates-based Methods

Joseph Pilates (1880-1967) was an athlete who studied various forms of sport as well physical and mental conditioning: yoga, Zen, modern dance, and ancient Grecian and Roman techniques. During World War I, as a prisoner of war in England, he came into contact with disabled soldiers and developed equipment to allow them to begin rehabilitation in the hospital bed as well as after they became mobile. After the war, Pilates opened a studio in New York City in the 1920s and attracted the attention of the dance community where his work has helped to train dancers ever since. In the last 15 years, his methods have come to be applied to both rehabilitation and athletic training and conditioning. The technique is characterized by an emphasis on development of a stable pelvis and trunk and on developing the ability to monitor oneself kinesthetically so that movement is as effortless as possible. A balance of eccentric and concentric muscle contractions promotes strengthening with minimal increase in bulk. The client is taught to breathe in coordination with movement to promote efficiency.

Pilates-based rehabilitation programs typically begin with exercises to enhance the awareness that the body works as a whole and that the injured area is

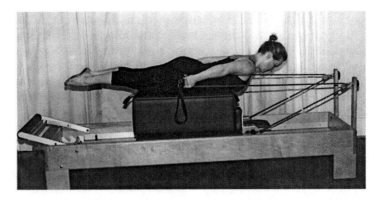

Figure 3. Dynamic scapular stabilization exercise using Pilates machine. (Photo courtesy of Atlantic Mind Body Center, Morristown, NJ)

an integral part of that whole. After the patient develops a strong pelvic and thoracic core, increased resistance and dynamic activities are added. While Pilates-based approaches are considered awareness-building techniques, they concentrate more on strengthening and form than the Feldenkrais, Alexander, and Trager methods. The equipment that Pilates designed is popular but not necessary for practice: universal reformer, the cadillac or trapeze table, and the chair. The most frequently used piece of equipment is the reformer, which consists of a flat bed on rollers with attached springs of variable resistance. Reformer exercises may be performed in a supine, prone, sitting, or standing position. Use of the reformer may be particularly useful during rehabilitation when full weightbearing or joint loading is contraindicated and for facilitation of proper form while eliminating the force of gravity. A rehabilitation program directed at the spasm, postural abnormalities, and muscle imbalance typical in chronic WAD would include Pilates-style lower abdominal strengthening and awareness exercises as well as scapular stabilization (Fig. 3). Although the beneficial use of Pilates-based rehabilitation programs has been reported for various musculoskeletal problems,[46,61,86,87] there are no published protocols for WAD specific rehabilitation. The technique is now popularized and is used by high-level athletes and performers as well as nonathletes undergoing rehabilitation. Instruction may be group or individual with or without equipment.

Pilates-based methods with specific training requirements are known as PhysicalMind The Method, and StottPilates among others. Just as in yoga, there is no minimal requirement for practitioners to use the name Pilates, and thus practitioners should be chosen with care especially when dealing with rehabilitation patients. The authors advocate introduction of a Pilates-based approach as an option for the rehabilitation of stable, chronic cervical pain (6 or more weeks) in stable rather than acutely recovering conditions.

Mind-Body Therapies

All of the mind-body uses the working principle that the mind and body are inseparable aspects of the person and that influencing one aspect has an effect on other aspects. We acknowledge that emotions, thoughts, and beliefs have an effect on health and illness, while physiological changes and illness have an effect on mood and cognitive processes. Mind-body therapies are commonly used to reduce the psychologic aspects of physical illness, including depression, anxiety, and stress. They teach the patient self directed coping strategies that increase one's perceived control over his illness in order to eliminate or at least tolerate medical symptoms, including chronic pain.

Two of the more common mind-body therapies include the relaxation response (RR) and meditation. These therapies are often taught in the context of a stress reduction group where patients learn relaxation techniques for self-control of symptoms, practice cognitive techniques to manage the psychological aspects of illness, and receive group support. These mind-body interventions can be used concurrently with conventional medical treatment. These approaches give patients tools to use in dealing with their pain, allowing them greater control and responsibility with respect to pain management.

Although there is little research specifically describing the use of these techniques with patients with whiplash, there is a growing body of evidence of their efficacy in helping patients manage chronic pain.[18] Those patients suffering from chronic, unresolved pain issues resulting from grade I-IV WAD after all indicated modalities have failed are candidates for such intervention.

Relaxation Response

The RR, a mind-body therapy designed to reduce stress, has been shown to improve the quality of life in patients with chronic pain[1,18,35] Herbert Benson pioneered the use of this technique in medical settings when he introduced the term *relaxation response* in the early 1960s. He demonstrated that inducing the RR decreased the debilitating effects of the stress or flight/fight response on the body and mind. Eliciting the RR typically decreases muscular tension and blood pressure; slows the metabolic, heart, and respiratory rates; and induces a feeling of relaxation and well-being[8]

The RR has two essential components. The first involves the repetition of a word, phrase, sound, prayer, or repetitive action such as breathing. The second involves the passive disregard or detachment from thoughts, feelings, and sensations during the practice. The RR can be induced by a variety of methods, including meditation, breathing practices, and yoga. It is typically practiced for 20 minutes a day to produce the best results. Centers throughout the United States that have adopted programs using the RR typically combine it with sessions on cognitive restructuring, or changing negative thought patterns, as well as exposure to nutritional and spiritual health. Courses that teach the RR typically span 10 sessions and are led by a trained health care professional.

Mindfulness Meditation

Mindfulness meditation, another mind-body therapy, teaches a patient to develop a sense of awareness of the present moment while becoming detached from sensations (including pain), thoughts, and feelings. This technique is rooted in the Buddhist tradition of *vispasana*, or insight meditation. Rather that fixing the mind on a single object like some other forms of meditation, students are taught to move from moment to moment with detached observation. Over a series of sessions patients are taught to observe sensations, including painful ones, without allowing the mind to become engaged with them.

The limited research into this technique focuses on patients with chronic pain. Integration of this technique into the hospital setting has been pioneered by Kabat-Zinn at the University of Massachusetts. In one study by Kabat-Zinn, 51 patients with chronic pain participated in a 10-week mindfulness meditation–based stress reduction group. Participants were asked to meditate at home on a daily basis for up to 45 minutes 6 days a week. Sixty-five percent of the subjects had more than 33% pain reduction, as measured by the Pain Rating Index. Participants also reported reduced symptoms of depression and anxiety and a greater sense of control over pain.[50] In a follow-up study of 90 subjects enrolled in another mindful meditation group, Kabat-Zinn again showed similar reductions in pain, depression, and anxiety in addition to improved feelings in body image and self-esteem and an increase in physical activity levels. A 15-month follow-up study indicated that participants maintained all improvements except present-moment pain levels, indicating that although pain may still have been present, coping and functional ability was improved.[51]

Electromagnetic Therapies

Electromagnetic therapie—magnets—operate on the premise of using energy fields, originating from either inside or outside the body, to aid in pain reduction or healing. Athletes and performers who attest to the efficacy of magnet therapy,[88,96] have made its use popular in the press. One popular use of magnets is for osteoarthitis. Magnet therapy may be divided into two types: static/time-varying magnetic fields (electromagnetic) or pulsed electromagnetic fields. Static magnetic field magnets are the most easily obtainable and less researched than electromagnetic field therapy, which requires a specialized device consisting of an electronic circuit and a power source.

Static Electromagnetic Fields

Static electromagnetic fields are generated by placement of magnetized material over an area of the body that is painful or dysfunctional. Static magnets are commercially available in the form of wraps, belts, mattresses, and jewelry. According to Vallbona,[90] both bipolar and unipolar configuration are equally effective in the control of pain, but there have been no controlled trials. There are no recorded adverse effects. Theories on the mechanisms of the biological effects of magnets include changes in the conformational state of intracellular molecules, induction of electrical currents in vascular elements, and changes in charged ions. A concise summary is offered by Vallbona.[90]

Only a small amount of evidence confirms the benefits of static electromagnetic fields in treating patients with pain. Hong found no difference between patients with chronic neck pain who wore either an active or sham magnetic necklace.[90] Colbert offered some anecdotal benefits for patients with arthritic pain,[22] and Vallbona et al showed some pain relief among postpolio patients suffering from localized pain, many of whom were likely suffering from arthritis, compared to control subjects.[89] The study reported short-term relief, and long-term follow-up was not formally recorded. Currently, the National Center for Complementary and Alternative Medicine is funding trials on magnets for a variety of conditions.[69]

With claims of extraordinary health benefits that currently go unsubstantiated by clinical trials, a healthy balance of curiosity and skepticism is recommended toward the use of magnets. It is likely that some claims will be upheld and others will be disproven. There is no evidence to date that more expensive magnets are more effective than other, less expensive types. Pending further evidence, the use of magnets for WAD is considered experimental.

TREATMENT OF WAD INTEGRATING A CAM APPROACH

In a center offering CAM modalities for rehabilitation, multiple CAM and conventional therapies may be combined for patient benefit. Like conventional modalities, CAM modalities work most efficiently with minimal delay between injury and treatment. Acute problems will require fewer sessions and less time than chronic problems.

CAM modalities are currently considered as treatments of last resort. This is unfortunate, because many of them are extremely effective in the acute phase of injury. Early use may obviate the need for more invasive, risk-prone, and expensive interventions.

In patients who have not sought treatment in the early phase of injury, or who have not received adequate relief despite timely treatment, a number of dysfunctional patterns may develop, including chronic neck stiffness, inefficient postural and movement habits to protect painful areas, involvement of the thoracic and lumbar spine, depression, and nonproductive pain behavior.

Several therapies are useful at this stage. These therapies work best when the patient is actively involved in home practice. Some practitioners consider home practice a prerequisite for work with an individual client. The goal of each of these therapies is to teach the patient to use efficient and pain-free movement patterns in daily activities and to progress to a level where individual training is no longer necessary.

The choice of CAM practitioners is important. Just as with clinicians who deliver conventional therapies, the best qualified practitioners are those who have certification in their area of expertise. In addition, practitioners should have previous experience in treating WAD and have access to, supervision by, and regular feedback with a supervising rehabilitation professional.

The algorithm illustrated in Figure 4 is a reflection of the procedure followed at the Atlantic Mind Body Center in Morristown, New Jersey. Yoga is emphasized because of the wide availability of practitioners of this modality and ease of transition from individual to group treatment. It is based on our experience with chronic and acute whiplash patients.

CONCLUSION

CAM modalities have increasingly attracted the attention of patients, health care professionals, and third-party payers. Research regarding the mechanisms of action and clinical efficacy of these modalities is in its infancy. Some have been shown to be of use in certain conditions; others continue to warrant further investigation. It is imperative that clinicians as well as those determining

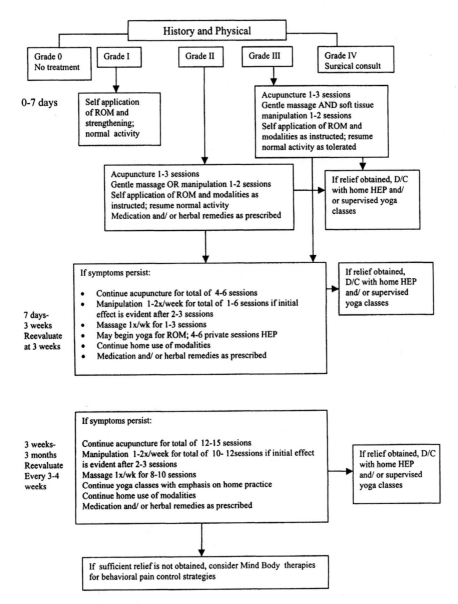

Figure 4. Algorithm for use of CAM therapies in WAD.

the expenditure of health care funds are aware of the benefits, indications, and limitations of these modalities so that they may be responsibly integrated into patient care.

References

1. Arnstein P, Caudill M, Mandle CL, et al: Self efficacy as a mediator of the relationship between pain intensity, disability and depression in chronic pain patients. Pain 80:483–491, 1999.

2. Atchison J, Stoll, S, Cotter A: Manipulation, traction and Massage in Braddom, R Physical Medicine and Rehabilitation, 2nd ed. Philadelphia, WB Saunders, 2000, pp 413–439.
3. Atchison J, Taub N, Cotter A, Tellis A: Complementary and alternative medicine treatments for low back pain. Phys Med Rehabil State of the Art Rev 13:561–586,1999
4. Austin J, Ausubul B: Enhanced respiratory muscular function in normal adults after lessons in proprioceptive musculosketal education without exercises. Chest 102:486–490, 1992.
5. Bach y Rita, Morgenstern E: New pathways in the recovery from brain injury. Somatics 3:38–47, 1981/82.
6. Barnsley L, Lord S, Bogduk N: The pathophysiology of whiplash. Spine State Art Rev 12:209–242, 1998.
7. Bassett A: Therapeutic uses of electric and magnetic fields in orthopedics. In Carpenter DO, Ayrapetyan S (eds): Biological Effect of Electric and Magnetic Fields, Vol 2. San Diego, Academic Press, 1994, pp 13–48.
8. Benson H: The relaxation response: history, physiological basis, and clinical utility. Acta Med Scand Suppl 660:231–237, 1982.
9. Berman BM, Singh BB, Lao L, et al: A randomized trial of acupuncture as an adjunctive therapy in osteoarthritis of the knee. Rheumatology 38:346–354, 1999.
10. Berman BM, Swyers JP: Establishing a research agenda for investigating alternative medical interventions for chronic pain. Prim Care 24:743–758, 1997.
11. Berman BM, Swyers JP, Ezzo J: The evidence for acupuncture as a treatment for rheumatologic conditions. Rheum Dis Clin North Am 26:103–115, 2000.
12. Birch S, Jamison RN: Controlled trial of Japanese acupuncture for chronic myofascial neck pain: assessment of specific and nonspecific effects of treatment. Clin J Pain 14:248–255, 1998.
13. Boisset M, Fitzcharles M: Alternative medicine use by rheumatology patients in a universal health care setting. J Rheumatol 21:148–152, 1994.
14. Bonneau R, Kiecolt-Glaser J, Glaser R: Stress-induced modulation of the immune response. Ann N Y Acad Sci 594:253–269, 1990.
15. Braverman D, Schulman R: Massage techniques Phys Med Rehabil Clin North Am 10:631–650, 1999.
16. Butler M: Milton Trager at the National Parkinson's Disease Foundation. Trager Network News, Mill Valley, CA, Trager Institute, 1986.
17. Caplan D: Postural Management of Scoliosis in the Adolescent and Adult Based on the Alexander Technique. American Center for the Alexander Technique, 1980.
18. Caudill M, Schnable R, Zuttermeister P, et al: Decreased clinic use by chronic pain patients: response to behavioral medicine intervention. Clin J Pain. 7:305–310, 1991.
19. Cherkin DC, Eisenberg D, Sherman KJ, et al: Randomized trial comparing traditional Chinese medical acupuncture, therapeutic massage, and self-care education for chronic low back pain. Arch Intern Med 161:1081–1088, 2001.
20. Cho ZH, Chung SC, Jones JP, et al: New findings of the correlation between acupoints and corresponding brain cortices using functional MRI. Proc Nat Acad Sci U S 95):2670–2673, 1998.
21. Coan RM, Wong G, Coan PL: The acupuncture treatment of neck pain: a randomized controlled study Am J Chin Med 9:326–332, 1981.
22. Colbert A: Magnet therapy: practical applications of magnet therapy. Presented at the 11th annual symposium of the American Academy of Medical Acupuncture, Chicago, 1999.
23. David J, Modi S, Aluko AA, et al: Chronic neck pain: a comparison of acupuncture treatment and physiotherapy. Br J Rheumatol 37:1118–1122, 1998.
24. Edwards,T: The Trager Approach [videotape]. Mill Valley, CA, Trager Institute, 1986.
25. Eisenberg DM, Davis RB, Ettner SL, et al: Trends in alternative medicine use in the United States, 1990-1997: results of a follow-up national survey. JAMA 280:1569–1575, 1998.
26. Eisenberg DM, Kessler RC, Foster C, et al: Unconventional medicine in the United States. N Engl J Med 328:246–252, 1993.
27. Ernst E, Resch KL, White AR: Complementary medicine. What physicians think of it. A meta-analysis. Arch Intern Med 155:2405–2408, 1995.
28. Fattori Br, Borsari C, Vannucci G, et al: Acupuncture treatment for balance disorders following whiplash injury. Acupunct Electrother Res 21:207–217, 1996.
29. Feldenkrais M: Body awareness as healing therapy: the Case of Nora
30. Ferrell-Tory AT, Glick OJ: The use of therapeutic massage as a nursing intervention to modify anxiety and the perception of cancer pain. Cancer Nurs 16:93–101, 1993.
31. Field T: Massage therapy effects. Am Psychol 53:1270–1281, 1998.
32. Field T, Hernandez-Reif M, Seligman S, et al: Juvenile rheumatoid arthritis: benefits from massage therapy. J Pediatr Psychology 22:607–617, 1997.

33. Field T, Peck M, Krugman S, et al: Burn injuries benefit from massage therapy. J Burn Care Rehabil 19:241–244, 1998.
34. Fisher K: Early experiences of a multidisciplinary pain management programme. Holist Med 3:47–56, 1988.
35. Friedman R, Sobel D, Myers P, et al: Behavioral medicine, clinical health psychology, and cost offset. Health Psychol 14:509–518, 1995.
36. Garfinkel MS, Schumacher HR Jr, Husain A, et al: Evaluation of a yoga based regimen for treatment of osteoarthritis of the hands. J Rheumatol 21:2341–2343, 1994.
37. Garfinkel MS, Singhal A, Katz WA, et al: Yoga-based intervention for carpal tunnel syndrome: a randomized trial. JAMA 280:1601–1603, 1998.
38. Ginsberg C: On plasticity and paraplegia Somatics 3:34–40, 1980.
39. Goats J: Massage: the scientific basis of an ancient art: part 2. Physiologic and therapeutic effects. Br J Sports Med 28:153–156, 1994.
40. Grodin A, Cantu R: Soft tissue mobilization. In Basmajian J, Nyberg R (eds): Rational Manual Therapies. Baltimore, Williams & Wilkins, 1993, pp 212–213.
41. Gross AR, Aker PD.,Goldsmith CH, Peloso P: Physical medicine modalities for mechanical neck disorders. Cochrane Database of Systematic Reviews (2):CD000961, 2000.
42. Haslock I, Monro R, Nagarathna R, et al: Measuring the effects of yoga in rheumatoid arthritis [letter]. Br J Rheumatol 33:787–788, 1994.
43. Heikkila H, Johansson M, Wenngren BI: Effects of acupuncture, cervical manipulation and NSAID therapy on dizziness and impaired head repositioning of suspected cervical origin: a pilot study. Man Ther 5:151–157, 2000.
44. Helms J: Acupuncture Energetics: A Clinical Approach for Physicians. Berkeley, Medical Acupuncture Publishers, 1995.
45. Hertz H, Meng A, Rabl V, Kern H: Treatment of whiplash injuries of the cervical spine with acupuncture. Aktuelle Traumatol 13:151–153, 1983.
46. Holmes J: The dancer's knee: ACL Injury rehabilitation using Pilates-based techniques [abstract]. Presented at the first annual meeting of the International Association for Dancemedicine and Science, San Francisco, 1991.
47. Integration of behavioral and relaxation approaches into the treatment of chronic pain and insomnia. NIH Technology Assessment Panel on Integration of Behavioral and Relaxation Approaches into the Treatment of Chronic Pain and Insomnia. Consensus Development Conference, NIH. JAMA 276):313–318, 1996.
48. Ironson G, Field T, Scafidi F, et al: Massage therapy is associated with enhancement of the immune system's cytotoxic capacity. Int J Neurosci 84: 205–217, 1996.
49. Ives J, Shelley G: The Feldenkrais method in rehabilitation: a review. Work 11: 75–90, 1988.
50. Kabat-Zinn J: An outpatient program in behavioral medicine for chronic pain patients based on the practice of mindfulness meditation: theoretical considerations and preliminary results. Gen Hosp Psychiatry 4:33–47, 1982.
51. Kabat-Zinn J, Lipworth L, Burney R: The clinical use of mindfulness meditation for the self-regulation of chronic pain. J Behav Med 8:163–191, 1985.
52. Kamenetz HL: 1History of massage. In Basmajian JV (ed): Manipulation, Traction and Massage, 3rd ed. Baltimore, Williams & Wilkins, 1985.
53. Karst M, Rollnik JD, Fink M, et al: Pressure pain threshold and needle acupuncture in chronic tension-type headache—a double-blind placebo-controlled study. Pain. 88:199–203, 2000.
54. Kemper KJ, Cassileth B, Ferris T: Holistic pediatrics: a research agenda. Pediatrics 103(4 pt 2):902–909, 1999.
55. Kiecolt-Glaser J, Glaser R: Chronic stress alters the immune response to influenza virus vaccine in older adults. Proc Nat Acad Sci U S A 93:3043–3047, 1996.
56. Kiser RS, Khatami MJ, Gatchel RJ, et al: Acupuncture relief of chronic pain syndrome correlates with increased plasma met-enkephalin concentrations. Lancet 2(8364):1394–1396, 1983.
57. Kjellman GV, Skargren EI, Oberg BE: A critical analysis of randomised clinical trials on neck pain and treatment efficacy. A review of the literature. Scand J Rehabil Med 31:139–152, 1999.
58. Krauss HH, Godfrey C, Kirk J, et al: Alternative health care: its use by individuals with physical disabilities. Arch Phys Medicine Rehabil 79:1440–1447, 1998.
59. Lake B: Acute back pain: treatment by the application of Feldenkrais principles. Aust Fam Phys 14:1175–1178, 1985.
60. Liao S, Liao M: Acupuncture and tele-electronic infra-red thermography. Acupunct Electrother Res 10:41–66, 1985.

61. Loosli A, Herold D: Knee rehabilitation for dancers using a Pilates-based technique. Kinesiol Med Dance 14(2):1–11, 1992.
62. Masala A, Satta G, Alagna S, et al: Suppression of electroacupuncture(EA)-induced beta-endorphin and ACTH release by hydrocortisone in man. Absence of effects on EA-induced anaesthesia. Acta Endocrinol 103:469–472, 1983.
63. Matsumura W: Use of acupressure techniques and concepts for nonsurgical management of TMJ disorders. J Gen Orthod 4:5–16, 1993.
64. Melzak R, Wall P: Pain mechanisms: A new theory. Science 50:971–979, 1965.
65. Nelson S: Playing with the entire self: the Feldenkrais method and musicians. Semin Neurol 9:97–104, 1989.
66. Nielsen M: The Alexander technique: a study of stress amongst professional musicians. In Stevens, C (ed): The Alexander Technique: Medical and Physiological Aspects. London, STAT Books, 1994.
67. NIH Consensus Development Conference, Statement on Acupuncture. JAMA 280:1518–1524, 1998
68. NIH: National Center for Complementary and Alternative Medicine; http://nccam.nih.gov
69. NIH/NCCAM five-year strategy, 2001–2005. 2000; http://nccam.gov/strategic
70. Ornish D, Scherwitz LW, Doody RD, et al: Effects of stress management training and dietary changes in treating ischemic heart disease JAMA 249:54–59, 1983.
71. Perry J, Jones M, Thomas L: Functional evaluation of Rolfing in cerebral palsy Develop Med Child Neurol 23:717–729, 1981.
72. Petrie JP, Langley GB: Acupuncture in the treatment of chronic cervical pain. A pilot study. Clin Exp Rheumatol 1:333–336, 1983.
73. Pomeranz B: Scientific basis of acupuncture. In Stux G, Pomeranz B (eds): Acupuncture Textbook and Atlas, 2nd ed. Berlin, Springer-Verlag, 1987, pp 1–34.
74. Pomeranz B, Chiu D: Naloxone blockade of acupuncture analgesia: endorphin implicated. Life Sci 19:1757–1762, 1976.
75. Prentice C: The pregnant patient and her partner. Occup Med State Art Rev 7:77–85, 1992.
76. Reiser S: The Alexander technique: stress reduction and optimal psychophysical functioning. Sixth International Montreux Congress on Stress [date unknown].
77. Schatz M: Back Care Basics. Berkeley, Rodmell Press, 1992.
78. Schenkman M, Tsubota J, Kluss M, et al: A management of individuals with Parkinson's disease: rationale and case studies. Phys Ther 69:944–955, 1989.
79. Shiflett S: Overview of complementary therapies in physical medicine and rehabilitation. Phys Med Rehabil Clin N Am 10:521–530, 1999.
80. Shifflett S, Schoenberger NE, Diamond B, et al: Complementary and alternative medicine. In De Lisa JA, Gans BM, et al (eds): Rehabilitation Medicine: Principals and Practice, 3rd ed. Philadelphia, Lipincott-Raven, 1998, pp 873–885.
81. Smith LA, Oldman AD, McQuay HJ, Moore RA: Teasing apart quality and validity in systematic reviews: an example from acupuncture trials in chronic neck and back pain. Pain 86:119–132, 2000.
82. Soliman N, Frank B, Nakazawa H, et al: Acupuncture reflex systems of the ear, scalp and hand. Phys Med Rehabil Clin North Am 10:547–573, 1999.
83. Spitzer WO, Skovron ML, Salmi LR, et al: Scientific monograph of the Quebec Task Force on Whiplash-Associated Disorders: redefining "whiplash" and its management. Spine 20(8 suppl):1S–73S, 1995.
84. Stallibrass C: An evaluation of the Alexander technique for the management of disability in Parkinson's disease—a preliminary study. Clin Rehabil 11:8–12, 1997.
85. Stern J: An approach to pain control. Lifeline, 1992.
86. Stolarsky L: Treating the injured dancer. PT Mag 48–54, 1993.
87. Swaim K: An alternative therapy: Pilates method. PT Magazine 55, 1993.
88. Theodosakis J, Adderly B, Fox B: Maximizing the Arthritis Cure. New York, St. Martin's Press, 1998 pp 210–212.
89. Vallbona C, Hazlewood CF, Jurida G: Response of pain to static magnetic fields in post-polio patients: a double-blind study. Arch Phys Med Rehabil 78:1200–1203, 1997.
90. Vallbona C, Richards T: Evolution of magnetic therapy from alternative to traditional medicine. Phys Med Rehabil Clin North Am 10:729–754, 1999.
91. Wharton R, Lewith G: Complementary medicine and the general practitioner. Br Med J 292:1498–1500, 1986.
92. White AR, Ernst E: A systematic review of randomized controlled trials of acupuncture for neck pain. Rheumatology (Oxford) 38:143–147, 1999.

93. Witt P, MacKinnon J: Trager psychophysical integration: a method to improve chest mobility of patients with chronic lung disease. Phys Ther 66:214–217, 1986.
94. Witt P, Parr C: Effectiveness of Trager psychophysical integration in promoting trunk mobility in a child wiyh cerebral palsy: a case report. Phys Occup Ther Pediatr 8:75–94, 1988.
95. Wong: A Manual of Neuro-Anatomical Acupuncture, Vol 1: Musculoskeletal Disorders . Toronto, Pain and Stress Clinic, 1999.
96. Zampieron E, Kamhi E: Arthritis: alternative medicine definitive guide. Tiburon, CA. AlternativeMedicine.com 1999 pp 336–339.
97. Zeitlin D, Keller SE, Shiflett SC, et al: Immunological effects of massage therapy during academic stress. Psychosom Med 62:83–84, 2000.
98. Zuck D: The Alexander technique. In Davis C: Complementary Therapies in Rehabilitation. Thorofare, NJ, Slack [date unknown].

23

Late Whiplash Syndrome: Current Psychological Theory and Practice

Roy C. Grzesiak, Ph.D., Donald S. Ciccone, Ph.D.,
and Deborah K. Elliott, B.S.

Whiplash, or acceleration-deceleration injury, occurs most commonly following motor vehicle accidents, particularly those in which the injured person's car was struck from behind. Although this is the most common mechanism of onset, virtually any situation that causes a rapid acceleration-deceleration or rotation of the head and neck can result in whiplash injury. An array of painful conditions can result from whiplash injury, including pain and tenderness in the entire upper quarter of the body, temporomandibular problems, headaches, and tinnitus. A variety of musculoskeletal problems can ensue, including myofascial pain syndrome, fibromyalgia, temporomandibular dysfunction, and headache. Additionally, many individuals with whiplash have complaints that are distinctly neuropsychological in nature. Examples include problems with attention, concentration, immediate memory, and energy level. The anatomic and pathophysiologic mechanisms of injury are described in Chapters 2 and 4.

The natural course of whiplash injury is unclear, but most individuals make a functional recovery within the first 3 months.[54] Individuals who continue to report symptoms for more than 6 months are considered to have "late whiplash injury," and their prognosis for full functional recovery is guarded.[5,69] One finds in the literature many examples of symptoms lasting for indefinite periods, in some cases for years. In a major review, Nadler and Cooke[65] found muscles, tendons, ligaments, and discs involved in the neuromusculoskeletal pains associated with whiplash. Psychological factors are often predominant in late whiplash, particularly chronic anxiety, depression, and cognitive difficulties. In many cases, these psychological features are thought to be causal because the victim's complaints are frequently out of proportion to either the nature of the objectively determined injuries or the magnitude of the accident. The above-mentioned cognitive difficulties are frequently attributed to "closed head injury" or postconcussion syndrome. On a more negative note, the continuing physical problems associated with late whiplash are frequently viewed as psychogenic, psychosomatic, or malingering. A recent article stated that psychological factors could not explain the course of recovery during the first 6 months following injury.[67] We believe that psychological factors are operative from the moment of injury and, ultimately, may prove more predictive of illness outcome than objective indications of physical pathology. After an introduction to the area of mind-body interaction and to the value of psychological and psychosocial factors in predicting chronicity, we consider the victim's psychological reaction to injury and pain. Finally, we end with an introduction to psychodiagnostic and psychotherapeutic techniques that have been found useful in dealing with trauma and chronic pain.

PAIN AND MIND-BODY ATTRIBUTION

Although the management of persistent pain has made considerable advances in the last two decades and psychological factors are now thought to be important determinants of pain-related disability and treatment seeking, there remains in clinical practice a tendency toward Cartesian dualism. Thus, many practitioners are still concerned with locating the cause of continuing pain either in the body or in the mind. This bias is frequently reflected in clinical research in which a given syndrome is characterized as either biological or psychological. Actually, psychological factors rarely, if ever, directly cause pain, though psychogenic factors can certainly amplify or maintain it indefinitely. As Dworkin[19] argued in a recent article, the presence of psychogenic pain has never been proven.

With respect to pain mechanisms, Melzack has continued to elaborate his concept of the neuromatrix. Following his work with Wall on the original gate control theory of pain,[60] Melzack has taken his early work on phantom limb phenomena and used it to develop a complex neuropsychological theory that simultaneously reflects mind and body.[57-59] According to Melzack,[59] there is a neural network within the brain that he identifies as the "body-self neuromatrix" that, although initially genetically programmed, is modifiable by sensory, cognitive, affective, and behavioral input. Perhaps the most important feature of this model is that it affords psychological processes equal weight with sensory experience. He argues that descending pathways whose function is to dampen or inhibit nociception are as important to pain expression as ascending spinocortical systems that carry nociceptive signals from the peripheral nervous system to the cortex. In a recent work, one of us (RCG) proposed an elaboration of the neuromatrix approach in which sensory experience is imbued with personal, often highly idiosyncratic meaning. Grzesiak[36] has referred to this expanded body-self matrix as the "matrix of vulnerability." He argued that some individuals are "pain-prone" or possess an unconscious propensity to suffer when faced with pain or illness in adulthood as a consequence of early adversity. Clinical pain is multidetermined and reflects the final outcome of a complex biopsychosocial process.

PSYCHOSOCIAL RISK FACTORS FOR CHRONICITY

With whiplash, as with other chronic pain problems such as low back pain, psychosocial components are important determinants of eventual outcome. Several studies of back pain patients have demonstrated that psychological factors, as opposed to the biological ones, are better predictors of chronicity.[21,73,88] There is now a similar consensus that psychological factors also play a prominent role in late whiplash syndrome.[42,52,80] Nevertheless, a number of important issues remain unresolved. In particular, a handful of studies suggest that psychological distress seen in late whiplash is a consequence of pain as opposed to a cause. As we demonstrate, multiple psychological risk factors are thought to be associated with chronic pain and disability. Some are clearly antecedent while others are consequences and still others believed to be synchronous in their clinical presentation.

There are several important categories of psychosocial risk factors for late whiplash, just as there are for other chronic pain syndromes. The first is the concept of pain-proneness. Next, we consider the possible role of psychosocial trauma and posttraumatic stress disorder and, then, litigation. In many instances, these factors coexist because of the common psychological processes they engender—namely, anxiety, depression, and somatization.

Pain-Proneness

The psychosocial risk factors for pain-proneness or "psychogenic pain" were first articulated by Engel.[24,25] Trained as an internist and psychoanalyst, Engel observed that most of his chronic pain patients (orofacial and low back) who continued to complain of pain in the absence of objective disease had similar childhood histories. Specifically, these patients reported childhood histories rife with abuse, neglect, abandonment, and substance-abusing caregivers. On the basis of these clinical (uncontrolled) observations, Engel formulated his concept of the pain-prone personality. Importantly, Engel did not propose a specific pain-prone personality but rather argued that pain-proneness was a component of many different personality types and characterologic organizations. Over the years there have been many anecdotal reports suggesting pain-prone personality as a risk factor for chronic disability following acute injury but, unfortunately, little controlled research.

Recent reports in both the clinical and research arenas suggest that pain-proneness needs more serious investigation. At present, the evidence is limited to anecdotal reports such as the two cases of chronic facial pain reported by Harness and Donlon.[40] They observed resistance to treatment until their patients admitted their injuries had been a consequence of physical abuse. Because the patients had kept this physical abuse hidden from the clinicians, they referred to this problem as "cryptotrauma" or hidden trauma. After admitting to being victims of physical abuse, each patient reportedly improved. A retrospective study by Adler et al[1] compared a group with so-called psychogenic pain with three other groups having medically explained pain or other physical problems. This study found that the psychogenic pain group was significantly different from the other three groups in that they were more likely to report (1) parents who were verbally or physically abusive of each other; (2) parents who were physically abusive of the child; (3) a history of deflecting aggression from parents to himself/herself; (4) parents who suffered from illness or pain; (5) an ill parent of the same gender as the patient suffering from pain; (6) pain of patient and parent in the same location; (7) a higher number of surgeries in adulthood; (8) disturbances in interpersonal relationships; and (9) disturbance in work life.[1] Many of these variables are consistent with Engel's earlier findings regarding the psychodynamic foundations of pain-proneness.[24,25]

The last category, disturbances in work life, deserves further exploration. In their work, Blumer and Heilbronn[8,9] described one of the characteristics of their chronic pain patients as "ergomania," which they defined as a conflicted work ethic that involves a history of excessive work performance, relentless activity, self-sacrifice, and the precocious assumption of adult responsibilities. These individuals were also found to have difficulty in interpersonal relationships, particularly around issues of trust. Similarly, Parkes[68] made similar observations in chronic pain patients and called this personality characteristic "pathological self-reliance." Another group of researchers has labeled a similar trait as "premorbid hyperactivity" or "action proneness."[92,93] Specifically attempting to provide empirical verification for Engel's risk factors, Gamsa found this ergomanic trait as well.[31,32] In a recent critical review of research on the psychosocial risk factors, Ciccone and Lenzi[18] found some support for the notion of excessive premorbid activity. From these findings, it would seem that injured individuals who are resistant to treatment efforts and therefore on the way to a chronic symptom picture may have a tendency toward perfectionism or excessive achievement. Of course, this type of individual is traditionally referred to as having "type A" personality in the cardiac literature.

Following closely the ideas promulgated to Engel, a team of researchers including spine surgeons and psychiatrists attempted to determine whether a history of childhood trauma would affect outcome of spinal surgery.[75] They operationally defined Engel's observations into the following five risk factors: (1) physical abuse by a primary caregiver; (2) sexual abuse by a primary caregiver or other adult; (3) alcohol or drug abuse in one or both primary caregivers; (4) abandonment (loss of a primary caregiver through death or abandonment of family); and (5) emotional neglect/abuse by primary caregivers. The presence or absence of these risk factors was determined by intensive psychiatric examination in 100 consecutive patients who had undergone spinal surgery. Outcome of spinal surgery was then retrospectively correlated with the presence of risk factor(s). For patients who recollected none of the risk factors, the probability of a successful outcome was 95%. On the other hand, for patients who recalled three or more of the risk factors, the success rate dropped to only 15%. This relationship was reportedly linear, with each risk factor adding incrementally to the likelihood of surgical failure.[75] Despite methodologic limitations, the study raises the possibility that early experience may influence the outcome of acute injury that occurs many years later. If replicated, the study also suggests that identical medical treatments (eg, spine operations) performed for the same medical indication may have vastly different outcomes depending on the psychological state (or pain-proneness) of the patient. As an aside, the evidence that psychological factors partially determine surgical outcomes is convincing enough that many insurance carriers, including Medicare, require a psychological clearance prior to invasive procedures such as spinally implanted stimulators or morphine pumps.

There are numerous unanswered questions about how and why some individuals are influenced by early childhood trauma while others are not. We now consider the possibility that intense anxiety associated with acute physical or psychosocial trauma may be implicated in the late whiplash syndrome.

Trauma and Posttraumatic Stress Disorder

Whiplash injuries are consequences of sudden physical trauma. The violent acceleration-deceleration or rotation of the upper torso, particularly the head and neck, causes hyperextension and hyperflexion beyond normal range of motion. These violent and unexpected directional forces injure an array of structures. In addition to the physical trauma resulting in injury, there may be psychological trauma and neurotrauma as well. One of the ingredients of psychological trauma is helplessness, the idea that one has no control over his own destiny. In an automobile accident, the situation is, by definition, out of control. The victim is powerless to influence the course of events.

Toward the end of the 19th century, there was keen interest in psychological trauma. One of the most prominent of the early trauma researchers was Pierre Janet, a neurologist who studied memory and dissociation as consequences of trauma. As van der Kolk and van der Hart[90] pointed out, Janet identified many of the emotional reactions and defensive operations, dissociation in particular, that characterize the trauma victim. Unfortunately, except for isolated pockets of research and theorizing, interest in trauma declined until the last quarter of the 20th century when the veterans of the Vietnam conflict raised an entirely new and urgent array of symptoms that required understanding and treatment. In the wake of Vietnam, posttraumatic stress took on new meaning and, despite the fact that war-related stress syndromes were familiar to professionals by names such as "shell shocked", "combat fatigue", and "war neurosis," it was not until 1980 with the publication of the third edition of the Diagnostic and Statistical Manual of the American Psychiatric Association (DSM-III)[2] that posttraumatic stress disorder (PTSD) was made an official psychiatric diagnosis.

With the publication of the fourth edition of the DSM (DSM-IV)[3] in 1994, the criteria for establishing the diagnosis of PTSD changed somewhat. The current DSM-IV diagnosis of PTSD requires the person to have been exposed to a traumatic event in which (1) the person experienced, witnessed, or was confronted with an event that involved actual or threatened death or serious injury; and (2) the person's response involved intense fear, horror, or helplessness. In the aftermath of trauma, memory for the event is often "reexperienced" in the form of intrusive recollections and recurrent dreams or nightmares. The victim is also subject to intense emotional distress or physiological reactivity when confronted with situations similar to or reminiscent of the trauma. Additionally, the person may engage in a persistent avoidance of situations associated with the trauma or experience a numbing of general responsiveness. The avoidance and numbing can include avoidance of thoughts, feelings, or conversations associated with the trauma; avoidance of activities, places, and people that recollect the trauma; gaps in memory for the traumatic event; diminished participation in activities; detachment and estrangement from others; restricted emotional range; and a foreshortened sense of future. There are persistent symptoms of increased arousal involving sleep, anger, concentration, hypervigilance, and an exaggerated startle response. If the symptoms persist for more than 1 month, the problem is labeled PTSD. It is divided into an acute (less than 3 months) and a chronic (more than 3 months) condition. There is also a delayed PTSD for symptoms that do not present until at least 6 months after the traumatic event.

In addition to PTSD, there is a diagnostic category called acute stress disorder (ASD) in which virtually all of the symptoms of PTSD are present but the time course is within the first 4 weeks of the traumatic event. From a phenomenological perspective, a major difference between PTSD and ASD is the focus on dissociative symptoms in ASD. Although dissociation is certainly a component of PTSD, it is given much more attention in the ASD criteria of DSM-IV, which notes symptoms such as "being in a daze," derealization, and depersonalization.

Both ASD and PTSD can occur following whiplash injury depending on a variety of contributing factors. The severity of the accident, the perceived threat of death, the degree of helplessness, and the severity of physical injury all play a role. However, studies that attempt to predict the occurrence of PTSD based on actual damage to the vehicle, speed at time of impact, or nature of physical injuries have not been successful. The psychological reaction to trauma is not a function of actual physical forces but is likely a function of the cognitive appraisal or perception of the event. What one thinks about the accident is based on personal meanings, rational and irrational beliefs, and perceived consequences for the individual.

Research indicates that PTSD following motor vehicle accidents occurs in approximately 25% to 33% of those who sustain physical injury.[48,55,84] What remains unclear is the percentage of individuals with PTSD who did not sustain actual physical damage in the motor vehicle accident. It is quite likely that that actual incidence of PTSD following motor vehicle accidents is unknown because, in medically oriented treatment, too little attention may be given to the person's state of mind. In psychiatric nomenclature, PTSD is considered one of the anxiety disorders. Jaspers[48] makes the point that PTSD must be identified and treated first. If the clinician does not treat the symptoms of PTSD, there is little likelihood for successful outcome and the acute whiplash has a greater probability of moving toward chronic or late whiplash syndrome.

Before moving too far afield, it is important to again consider pain-proneness. We can now elaborate on that construct by integrating what has been learned about trauma responses from the perspective of modern neuroscience. Trauma, either in childhood or in adulthood, has a neurobiological substrate that influences a wide variety of cognitive, affective, and sensory processes. Among the neurobiological consequences of trauma we find neural rewiring, "kindling," and widespread effects from brainstem to cortex, including changes in an array of neuroendocrine substances that subserve pain. How do these nervous system changes manifest themselves in clinical behavior? Examples include persistent physiological arousal/hyperarousal, including response to pain, loss of emotions as signals, loss of stimulus discrimination, and memory abnormalities.

If the above neurologic consequences of severe trauma are put in the context of pain-proneness, it is understandable how early trauma, via the matrix of vulnerability described earlier, can easily superimpose itself on adult trauma or illness. Clinically, this vulnerability is seen in chronic pain patients, including late whiplash, as an inability to cope, a tendency toward somatization, a propensity to misinterpret bodily signals, attachment issues (particularly trust), and problems in high-level cognitive processing involving attention, concentration, and immediate memory. Instead of a "mysterious leap from body to mind," clinical research is beginning to elucidate the processes by which childhood trauma influences adult-onset pain and injury. Because early trauma may occasionally be hidden, through the mechanisms of repression or dissociation, it may not be accessible to memory. However, in the wake of a new traumatic experience, it is possible that older, state-dependent memories that include anxiety and help-lessness are reactivated and thereby contribute to coping difficulty. The important point is that pain-proneness may have a neurobiological substrate and does not simply reflect psychological reactions to pain and injury.

Litigation and the Perpetuation of Whiplash

Litigation or legal pursuit of a financial damage award has been implicated as a major factor in the perpetuation of late whiplash. Prior to the mid 20th century, an accident victim could only sue for documented physical damages. Now, however, based on changes in the law, it is possible to sue for mental distress.[79] Coincidental with the acceptance of PTSD as an "official" psychiatric diagnosis, the courts now look at pain and suffering as legitimate claims that may, under certain circumstances, justify financial damages. While lawsuits have been viewed as a risk factor for chronic pain syndromes, including late whiplash, for a long time, the legitimization of PTSD and the "pain and suffering" avenue to damages has led to a psychiatric/psychological "growth industry".[79] Experts in trauma acknowledge that participation in the legal process may perpetuate trauma-related symptoms and lead to a persistence of pain-related disability.[79]

To sue for damages, with or without sustaining physical injury, requires a legal system that accommodates such lawsuits. A number of countries do not have such laws, and this has resulted in considerable controversy over the legitimacy of whiplash, particularly late whiplash, as an actual physical injury. For example, Balla[2] compared the incidence of late whiplash and chronic pain in two countries having very different legal systems regarding compensation for injury. In Australia prior to 1987, whiplash injuries were literally epidemic while in Singapore, where there is no legal recourse to compensation for damages, whiplash was virtually nonexistent. After 1987 when Australia changed the compensation system to require the claimant to bear the initial medical expenses, whiplash claims dropped significantly: 68% in the year following the change in the law. Similarly, Livingston[53] observed that despite no significant difference in the frequencies of motor vehicle accidents, whiplash claims in the United States were far ahead of those in the United Kingdom by several decades. Livingston made the point that whiplash injuries were frequently reported in the United States medical literature some three decades before the first whiplash article was published in Great Britain. As a result of studies of this nature, many concluded that whiplash injuries were more a reflection of sociocultural bias than of actual injury. Further, many blamed the legal system for prolonging lawsuits and, perhaps inadvertently, further sensitizing victims to their symptoms.

Surprisingly, few authors have taken the position that the chronic whiplash victim in litigation is maintaining his symptoms merely for compensation or malingering his symptoms for secondary gain. In a thoughtful commentary, Ferrari and Russell[26] reviewed these findings and suggested that the chronic pain seen in late whiplash is predominantly a function of psychological factors. They suggest that the length of litigation allows for symptom expectations and fear to lead to enhanced somatization and symptom amplification. Commenting on their paper, Radanov,[71] a psychiatrist, notes that psychological reactions cannot be viewed as isolated from the initial neck injury and that prognosis for recovery from whiplash injury is significantly related to the initial severity of injury. Furthermore, Radanov notes that two recent studies[61,76] have indicated that the negative impact of compensation on symptom persistence has been overestimated. A particularly intriguing paper by Schrader et al[76] compared the evolution of late whiplash syndrome in a cohort study of injury victims and uninjured age- and sex-matched controls. They looked at neck pain, headache, subjective cognitive dysfunction, psychological disorders, and low back pain and found no significant differences between the groups. However, those patients with chronic complaints frequently had similar preexisting symptoms but now attributed their causation to the trauma. These papers suggest the importance of early detection and intervention for both physical injury and psychological reaction. In particular, the value of multidisciplinary assessment and timely intervention is suggested as a means to forestall chronic complications.

On the basis of the above studies, we do not believe we can state with any degree of certainty that litigation is always associated with exaggerated symptom reporting or abnormal illness behavior in the form of nonorganic (pain-related) disability. However, it is probable that litigation may be implicated in such behavior for certain vulnerable individuals. We suggest that timely psychological assessment and intervention can make a difference. With respect to litigation, it does appear that those countries that have made lawsuits impossible or placed limitations on damages enjoy a lower (reported) rate of late whiplash.

PSYCHOLOGICAL REACTIONS TO PAIN AND INJURY

In this section, we return to some of the basic psychological factors that enhance or maintain pain. Specifically, we review the mechanisms involved in anxiety, depression, and somatization as they impact on symptom presentation. Current evidence seems to suggest that acute injury and pain are more likely associated with anxiety, whereas chronic pain and disability are more typically associated with depression. Also, individuals who have been injured and continue to experience pain and discomfort for long periods but who continue most or all of their premorbid activities are psychologically different from individuals who become physically inactive, give up their jobs, abdicate marital and parental responsibilities, withdraw from social and interpersonal activities, and pursue compensation through the legal system.

Anxiety

Although anxiety has been less systematically researched in clinical pain, there is a substantial literature on the subject. Anxiety is the immediate reaction to any real or imagined threat to one's bodily or psychological integrity. In effect, anxiety usually serves an adaptive function by mobilizing resources for "flight or fight." In our opinion, the potentially damaging consequences of anxiety that can occur in the immediate aftermath of injury are often overlooked.

Anxiety is an autonomic nervous system response and, as such, it shares many of the same pathways as nociception or pain transmission. Anxiety is the initial emotional or affective component of pain.[81] It has also been shown to heighten pain sensation, and a significant amount of the variance in pain ratings can be accounted for by anxiety.[13,28,44] Chronic pain patients have been found to be more anxious than the general population.[4] Although anxiety is often thought to be reflexive, it is more accurately thought of as a learned response. The concept of "fear avoidance" refers to the learned avoidance of activities expected to increase pain that leads to diminished activity, physical deconditioning, and reduced confidence or self-efficacy. This is turn tends to perpetuate further inactivity and avoidance. In a study of acute low back pain patients that attempted to predict chronicity, fear avoidance alone predicted chronic status at 12 months 66% of the time.[50]

The cognitive style called catastrophizing has been studied extensively in pain populations. We have previously referred to such thinking as "awfulizing"[14] and defined it as an exaggerated appraisal of threat. Recent studies have demonstrated that catastrophic thinking is common in depressed pain patients. We believe that such thinking may ultimately lead to depression, fear avoidance, and coping failure. In a study investigating cognitive beliefs, catastrophizing, and coping style in temporomandibular disorders, the results indicated that, although all three are important in terms of disability, pain beliefs and catastrophizing appeared more predictive than coping style. In particular, the authors noted that changing one's belief that pain is disabling is critical.[87] In one of the first attempts at a prospective investigation of chronic pain, Dworkin and associates[21] found anxiety to be a significant predictor of subsequent postherpetic neuralgia in a sample of patients with shingles.

As a number of investigators have pointed out, most psychosocial research on chronic pain is performed in tertiary pain centers or other specialized health care clinics. As such, participants come from a skewed population with an increased prevalence of psychiatric illness and a predisposition to seeking treatment. Therefore, these studies are not likely to enhance our understanding of the transition from acute to chronic pain. As this section on anxiety has demonstrated, more attention needs to be paid to psychological events that occur in the immediate aftermath of injury, that is, to psychological factors occurring during the acute phase. Anxiety, often an adaptive response to acute trauma, may have deleterious consequences when sustained at high levels by vulnerable individuals. To prevent chronicity, the role of the psychologist should ideally encompass interventions at the acute stage of injury.

Depression

The role of depression in chronic pain has been the subject of extensive study. Clinical depression can be a cause, consequence, or concomitant of chronic pain. In the early years of multidisciplinary pain management, the successful treatment of many pain problems with tricyclic antidepressants led some to believe that chronic pain was a variant of depression. Only later did pain management professionals realize that antidepressants, prescribed in subtherapeutic doses, improved and stabilized sleep patterns and, in some cases, provided a mild analgesic benefit as well. Living with persistent pain that is unresponsive to conventional medical treatment can lead to a profound sense of hopelessness and helplessness that, in turn, may precipitate an episode of clinical depression.

In patients with chronic pain, Hendler[43] considers depression to be a "normal illness behavior." However normative it may be, depression often assumes clinical proportions in patients with chronic pain and may significantly interfere with daily functioning. In two studies summarized by Krishnan, France, and Davidson,[51] the prevalence of major depression was highest in an inpatient pain management program (43%). The rate of major depression among outpatients was found to be 21%. Interestingly, in both samples, the percentage of patients without a depressive diagnosis was the same (21%). Assessment of depression in medically ill patients, including those with chronic pain, may be confounded by reliance on vegetative symptoms that may be the result of illness-related factors or medication. Neurovegetative signs and symptoms—sleep, appetite, weight stability, and libido—may thus be unreliable indicators of clinical depression. In our experience, the assessment of sleep pattern is especially difficult with pain patients because sleep onset, early awakening, and hypersomnia are all affected by pain and comfort level. Disturbed sleep is common in pain patients and, as noted by Moldofsky and associates,[63] the lack of necessary non-rapid-eye-movement sleep contributes to generalized musculoskeletal pain in both fibromyalgia patients and normal controls. In any event, assessment of the cognitive/affective components of depression is critical to appropriate management of the chronic pain patient. A depression diagnosis may signal the need for antidepressant medication and for concomitant psychotherapy aimed at addressing the precipitating factors such as pain and loss of physical function.

Coping failure is typically the result of one or more erroneous beliefs or a lack of effective coping skills. Among the former we would include the concept of catastrophizing.[14,15] The presence of depression in late whiplash is best addressed within the context of a multidisciplinary pain team that includes a mental health professional. Failing that, frequent psychiatric or psychological consultation should be considered a minimum standard of care.

From a behavioral perspective, chronic pain behavior may be viewed as a consequence of maladaptive response-reward contingencies in the patient's social and occupational environments. The chronic pain patient may no longer be rewarded for adaptive or positive behaviors (such as work) but instead receive increased attention and support that are contingent on continued pain and suffering. These maladaptive reward patterns are most effectively addressed within the context of an intensive outpatient or inpatient pain rehabilitation program.

Somatization

Somatization may be defined as a psychological tendency to interpret benign physiologic sensations as symptoms of medical illness or injury. Katon et al,[48a] among others,[22] have shown that medically unexplained symptoms are associated with an increased risk of disability and with an increased prevalence of psychiatric disorders. We are using the term *somatization* to describe a psychological process or tendency as opposed to a formal psychiatric disorder (also called somatization disorder). Simon[78] has suggested four approaches to understanding somatization. Somatization can represent a nonspecific amplification of distress so that aversive psychological states may lead to heightened awareness of bodily sensations and to increased symptom reporting. Somatization can also be viewed as a psychological defense in that pain or bodily symptoms may serve to circumvent psychological conflict. Another approach to somatization involves a tendency to seek medical reassurance for stress-related or otherwise benign physical sensations and symptoms. This process of social reinforcement may lead to an excessive reliance on the health care system. Finally, Simon suggested that somatization may be a consequence of health care utilization in that medical providers may focus exclusively on physical symptoms at the expense of obvious psychological distress. In other words, somatization may be iatrogenic. Dworkin and associates[22] have suggested that somatization may be a risk factor for chronic pain (including whiplash). Specifically, they state: "The most important reason for considering the relationship between pain complaint and somatization relates to the possibility that when chronic pain complaints increase in number, nonspecific factors in the person may require more attention than the physical condition. Thus, the presence of numerous physical complaints, including pain, may be telling us more about the emotional and mental state of the person than the physical status."[22] Anxiety, depression, and somatization are integral components of pain and suffering, and all three are common in patients with late whiplash syndrome.

THE PSYCHOLOGICAL EVALUATION: AN OVERVIEW

For the clinician working with the late whiplash patient, the same questions need to be asked that would be asked of any chronic pain patient or trauma victim. It is important for the clinician to be aware of early signs and symptoms that augur poorly for successful rehabilitation. Elsewhere, we have spelled out in some detail many of the components of psychological evaluation.[15,17,20,36,37,39] Because most patients with intractable pain have met with numerous treatment failures, many are mistrustful of physicians and mental health providers and believe their physical complaints may not be taken seriously. It may be helpful to reassure these patients that the mental health clinician does not believe that pain is "all in the mind." The clinician could also note that most patients with painful injuries such as whiplash inevitably suffer from some degree of depression or anxiety.

The psychological evaluation is composed of any or all of the following components: clinical interview, psychological testing, and psychophysiologic assessment. Some clinicians use interview findings only, while others combine interview findings with test results. A much smaller number add psychophysiologic assessment to the initial clinical evaluation. Psychophysiologic assessment can be very useful if the patient is presenting with a musculoskeletal pain syndrome, such as whiplash or cervical headache.

The Clinical Interview

Ciccone and Grzesiak[17] have offered a set of evaluative questions the clinician can use to screen for psychological problems in chronic pain patients. These evaluative questions can be broken down into three domains: (1) inappropriate illness behavior, (2) emotional disorder, and (3) premorbid risk factors.

Regarding inappropriate or abnormal illness behavior, the questions asked involve the following: Has the pain persisted beyond expected healing time? Has a medical or biological cause of pain been clearly identified? Is the patient's disability out of proportion to the physical pathology? Are the patient's complaints diffuse (nonspecific) or localized? Does the patient receive financial or social reward contingent on pain and suffering? Who performs the routine household chores? Is there evidence of excessive alcohol use or compulsive (addictive) drug use?

The presence of emotional disorder is assessed by asking questions such as the following: Does the patient report prolonged periods (2 weeks or longer) of depression or anxiety? Does he express feelings of hopelessness or helplessness? Is the patient anhedonic, guilt-ridden, or anergic? Does the patient catastrophize pain and pain-related disability? Does the patient express active or passive suicidal ideation?

The existence of premorbid risk factors is still controversial, but a few questions may provide useful information: Does the patient report a history of compulsive work behavior (type A) before the onset of pain? Does the patient report being the victim of sexual or physical violence during childhood? Does the patient report being the victim of violence during adulthood? Is there a history of premorbid psychiatric illness? Is there a history of previous pain complaints or a history of unexplained medical illness (eg, irritable bowel syndrome, chronic fatigue)?

Psychological Testing

Unfortunately, few psychological assessment instruments have been developed expressly for use with pain patients. In recent years there has been both refinement of old instruments and new tests that do address issues of pain and trauma. These psychometric instruments add a more formal and, some would say, more objective dimension to clinical assessment. Because space is limited, some but not all of the psychological tests in use with pain and trauma patients are presented.

The Pain Visual Analog Scale (VAS) is the most popular pain assessment technique in use today. The VAS is not actually a psychometric "instrument" although its psychometric properties have been well researched. The VAS is usually a 10-cm line anchored at one end as "no pain" and at the other end by "unbearable pain" or "pain as bad as can be." The patient, with the assistance of the examiner if necessary, marks a spot on the line that indicates his subjective pain rating, and this is converted into a 0-to-10 or a 0-to-100 numerical score. Although variations of the VAS have been tried, Huskisson[46] has argued that leaving the scale rather pure with only its anchor terms allows the scale to have greater sensitivity and psychometric purity. The VAS can serve as a useful measure of pain as well as a repeated measure of therapeutic change. The VAS can be used to separately assess the sensory dimension of pain (related to intensity) and the affective dimension (related to level of unpleasantness or suffering). Certain patients may be greatly distressed about a problem that involves relatively little pain while, on the other hand, others may not be distressed about a problem even though it involves high levels of pain. In addition, it is often useful to elicit numerical ratings for pain at the present time, for the usual or typical level of pain over the past week, for the lowest level of pain over the past week and, finally, for the highest level of pain over the past week.

The McGill Pain Questionnaire was constructed by Melzack[56] in the 1970s as an approach to assessing the pain patient based on his model of pain experience; it incorporated both sensory and affective/motivational components. The McGill Pain Questionnaire is a semistructured interview that includes an array of verbal descriptors that classify the experience of pain into sensory, affective, and cognitive components. Analysis of the verbal descriptors provides three scores reflecting a pain rating index, number of words chosen, and present pain intensity. One can assess the relative relationship of the sensory, affective, and cognitive components of pain to determine how the individual is perceiving his pain experience.

The Psychosocial Pain Inventory (PPI)[41] was designed specifically for the assessment of pain patients. As its name suggests, the PPI was designed to determine the impact of pain on the\tpsychosocial aspects of a patient's functioning and, as such, it serves a complementary role to some of the other psychometric instruments described here. The PPI provides information on pain experience, psychosocial factors, pain-related treatments, secondary gain, interpersonal factors, and premorbid job satisfaction.

The Multidimensional Pain Inventory (MPI)[49] was initially called the West Haven–Yale Multidimensional Pain Inventory. The MPI was designed to supplement behavioral and psychophysiologic information. The MPI provides three categories of information: pain intensity and pain-related interference, social responses to pain behavior by significant others, and ability to perform household chores and other functional activities. The MPI is widely used in clinical practice and research.

The Pain Patient Profile (P-3)[85] was developed to assess anxiety, depression, and somatization in pain patients. In addition to assessing these processes in a normal population, the P-3 provides normative responses on the anxiety, depression, and somatization scales based on a clinical sample of chronic pain patients. This scale thus provides information enabling the clinician to compare his pain patient with results drawn from clinical as well as nonclinical samples.

The Minnesota Multiphasic Personality Inventory (MMPI, MMPI-2) is one of the older personality tests still in use. It has been updated and includes a subscale for PTSD. The MMPI was not developed for use with pain patients but, based on extensive research, it has shown some utility in the psychometric evaluation of pain patients. The MMPI and MMPI-2 have validity scales as well as clinical scales and an array of highly specific experimental scales for use with various clinical populations. There is extensive research on the MMPI in pain that may be useful to the clinician. However, because of space limitations, we only cite the studies of Bradley and associates,[11,70] who completed the first multivariate analysis of MMPI data on pain patients. This study demonstrated a lack of homogeneity among pain patients and emphasized the observations of Sternbach[82] that pain patients are not unique but bring to the clinical situation their premorbid personality styles and character traits.

Because we have emphasized the interactive effects of pain and trauma, we now offer two psychometric instruments designed specifically to assess the impact of trauma. Our choice of the scales is based on personal experience and does not reflect a judgment about the relative merits of other instruments.

Impact of Event Scale-Revised (IES-R)[94] is a revised version of the oldest and most widely used measure of trauma responses, the IES.[45] This scale is self-report and short, providing scaled scores for the major components of trauma: intrusion, avoidance, and hyperarousal. Both the IES and IES-R have been used extensively in research studies, and the IES-R is in clinical use as well.

The Trauma Symptom Inventory[12] is a 100-item rating scale that provides a number of scales related to trauma response as well as self-references. The Trauma Symptom Inventory also has three validity scales. The 10 clinical scales are as follows: anxious arousal, depression, anger/irritability, intrusive experiences, defensive avoidance, dissociation, sexual concerns, dysfunctional sexual behavior, impaired self-reference, and tension-reduction behavior.

Psychophysiologic Assessment

The third area of psychological assessment is that of psychophysiologic evaluation. More commonly referred to as biofeedback, physiologic assessment of the pain patient may prove useful in localizing the patient's sympathetic response to pain or in understanding the mechanical reasons for chronic myofascial pain (eg, postural defect, bracing, muscle guarding). The latter form of feedback, called surface electromyography (EMG), may be especially useful in patients with whiplash, tension and migraine headache, orofacial pain of myofascial origin, and other problems involving overuse or misuse of superficial muscle. Of all the parameters that can be assessed in psychophysiologic profiling, only two are discussed here: the electrodermal response and surface EMG.

Electrodermal assessment of sympathetic activity is based on a measure of skin conduction. These responses are significantly correlated with self-reported measures of anxiety and therefore are useful in the management of pain-related distress such as anxiety. We have already emphasized how important we think anxiety management is in the early care of whiplash patients. Anxiety is one of the critical parameters that may set the stage for a chronic adaptation.

EMG responses reflecting the strength of muscle contraction are measured by surface electrodes. EMG assessment and feedback can play an important role in the multidisciplinary management of whiplash but, as Middaugh and Kee[62] have emphasized, static assessment of muscle tension is often inaccurate and may be misleading. They argue for an approach based on "dynamic assessment" of the affected muscle, that is, assessment of muscle activity before, during, and after the performance of functional work-related tasks. The dynamic psychophysiologic assessment of muscle activity may offer a promising technique for understanding the mechanical basis of late whiplash syndrome. An overview of this subject is beyond the scope of the present chapter, and the reader is referred to summaries of these techniques by Middaugh and Kee[62] or Ciccone and Grzesiak.[16]

We briefly return to biofeedback in the section on psychological treatment. To summarize, clinical psychologists may elicit verbal reports of pain, behavior, and mood during a clinical interview, diagnose mental illness based on current case definitions, administer and interpret standardized tests, and perform psychophysiologic assessment as part of their initial evaluation. These sources of data provide important clinical information that may be useful in the interdisciplinary management of patients with acute and late whiplash syndrome.

PSYCHOLOGICAL TREATMENT: AN OVERVIEW

The professional roles of the psychologist include both assessment and treatment. A variety of treatment approaches have been applied to patients with pain, trauma, and whiplash. The treatment modalities described in this section are summarized in capsule form because of space limitations. For pragmatic purposes, the treatments are divided into two broad categories: psychotherapy and the self-regulatory approaches.

Psychotherapy

Under the rubric of psychotherapy, we present introductory material on behavioral management, cognitive-behavioral therapy (CBT), and integrative psychodynamic psychotherapy.

Behavioral Management

These approaches to the patient with chronic pain were originally introduced by Fordyce.[29] The primary tenet of the behavioral approach lies in Fordyce's observation that pain behavior is an "operant", that is, behavior under the control of its consequences. Thus, chronic avoidance behavior becomes chronic because it is reinforced (socially or financially) while efforts to maintain premorbid function may be ignored or even punished. When this happens, the probability of engaging in avoidance behavior is increased (or strengthened) while that of approach behavior is decreased (or weakened). The behavioral treatment of pain calls for a reversal of these maladaptive response-reward contingencies in the patient's environment. Fordyce offers a detailed program for managing self-defeating pain behavior such as avoidance or excessive inactivity.[29] Many of the principles of behavioral pain treatment have been incorporated into the practice of multidisciplinary pain clinics. For example, the suggestion that patients should not discuss their pain at length with a (solicitous) spouse because this elicits increased attention which, in turn, increases the probability of future symptom reporting is essentially an operant concept that has been incorporated in most interdisciplinary pain clinics.

Cognitive-Behavioral Psychotherapy

CBT has become the most prevalent therapeutic approach used to treat pain and maladaptive illness behavior. A specific version of CBT, designed for patients with chronic pain, was developed by Turk, Meichenbaum, and Genest.[86] Rather than attempt to provide specific techniques, we describe the basic philosophy underlying CBT. The central assumption is that one's cognitive interpretation (or perception) of painful injury will largely determine one's emotional and behavioral response. As Turk and associates[86] reported, "affect and behavior are largely determined by the way in which the individual construes the world." They note that patients often maintain inner dialogues, have automatic thoughts, make self-statements, and hold private conceptualizations that add to their symptomatic distress. Similarly, Ciccone and Grzesiak[14,15] have suggested that irrational beliefs and dysfunctional cognitive styles (faulty thinking) lead to much of the emotional distress and behavioral difficulty found in chronic patients. Consequently, changing how one thinks about pain can lead to improvement in emotions, behavior, and psychophysiologic functioning. Another useful comprehensive cognitive approach has been put forth by Eimers,[23] who used the acronym "PADDS" to describe his approach to pain and illness behavior: Pacing, Anxiety management, Distraction, Disputation of negative thoughts, and Stopping negative thoughts and images through a cognitive technique called thought stopping.

The major focus of all the cognitive techniques is on improving coping and enabling people to develop a sense of control over what is happening to them. When faced with pain and injury, individuals often perceive themselves as helpless to alter their life circumstances. This faulty belief may serve to increase depression and further magnify the problem. Cognitive restructuring or disputing techniques attempt to identify faulty thinking habits, teach the patient alternative coping statements, and facilitate more active coping through the use of frequent behavioral homework assignments. The approach does not emphasize insight into faulty or maladaptive thinking but instead is aimed at achieving concrete changes in behavior and reduced patient suffering. These changes occur when patients accept responsibility for their maladaptive responses to pain rather than shifting responsibility to their health care provider. By promoting self-responsibility, focusing on current emotional disturbance, increasing activity level, and fostering cognitive restructuring of faulty beliefs about pain, CBT has become an integral component of the multidisciplinary approach to chronic pain management.

Integrative Psychodynamic Psychotherapy

This approach[20,39] to pain and illness-related problems is an attempt to integrate CBT techniques with a psychodynamic understanding of how idiosyncratic beliefs or assumptions about pain and suffering may be confounding their recovery and adaptation.

Guidelines for Psychotherapeutic Intervention

Regardless of therapeutic modality, psychotherapy for patients with chronic pain and disability should endeavor to identify specific behavioral objectives (eg, returning to work, reducing depression) that are mutually agreed upon by therapist and patient. The framework of therapy is thus circumscribed rather than open-ended, and often the preferred approach is time-limited. Unless patients are demonstrating tangible progress toward achieving stated objectives, such as increasing activity level, there may be little justification for continuing psychological intervention. At times it may be necessary to make psychotherapy contingent on behavioral progress or else run the risk of implicitly encouraging (or enabling) patients who may be committed to a disability lifestyle. The risk of such iatrogenic therapy may be higher when treatment is provided in isolation rather than as a component of a comprehensive rehabilitation program.

In addition to psychotherapy as discussed above, self-regulatory techniques (see below) may be appropriate, though rarely as stand-alone modalities for patients with chronic whiplash. The psychological needs of the recently injured or chronic pain patient may vary considerably. Consequently, the psychological interventions that are appropriate vary as well. Some recently injured individuals may profit from brief psychotherapy while others with a premorbid vulnerability to pain (ie, pain-prone) may benefit from more intensive psychotherapeutic intervention. Such intervention is not usually indicated for patients with acute injury but may be applicable to those with premorbid psychopathology or personality disorder.

Self-Regulatory Approaches: Relaxation, Biofeedback, and Hypnosis

A number of psychological interventions fall under the broad heading of self-regulatory techniques. We present three of these techniques. Generally, relaxation approaches and biofeedback are commonly used to treat behavioral and psychophysiologic symptoms of chronic pain and are far less often applied to patients with acute injury. An exception would be an acutely injured patient with persistent symptoms of anxiety or excessive avoidance behavior. While often including a relaxation component, hypnotic techniques may include other self-regulatory instructions.

Relaxation training is probably the most common psychological intervention used to treat patients with neck or cervical injury. Relaxation techniques are so common in psychological practice that they are referred to as the "aspirin of behavioral medicine."

The central objective of most relaxation training is to elicit an active "relaxation response," that is, to actively inhibit sympathetic responding or, alternatively, promote parasympathetic responding. This usually entails the use of self-instructional phrases that are repeated over and over, such as "I feel more and more at peace" or "I can feel the tension leaving my lower back." Relaxation training may prove more acceptable to patients who are not appropriate for psychotherapy or who demonstrate resistance to psychological intervention. As with most of the psychological techniques used in pain management, however, relaxation training is not usually recommended as a stand-alone technique but rather as a component of a more comprehensive multidisciplinary treatment program.

Muscle relaxation training has its origins in the work of Jacobson[47] although few practitioners actually use the training scheme devised by him because it is extremely time-consuming and ill-suited to the typical, short-term interventions required in pain and trauma management settings. The technique requires patients to alternately tense and then relax specific muscles until all voluntary muscle groups have been treated. Most psychologists who conduct relaxation training use one of the abbreviated formats such as that suggested by Bernstein and Borkovec,[7] who divided the body's musculature into 16 major groups. Grzesiak[34] has provided a short version in which a meditation/imagery component is added. Relaxation induction protocols are readily available in the literature. Relaxation approaches have been found to be useful adjunctive treatments in the management of cervical headache, migraine, back pain, and in most syndromes that involve a chronic myofascial component.[38]

Biofeedback approaches were covered briefly in the section on psychophysiologic assessment. The premise of biofeedback is that electronic amplification of unconscious physiologic activity, such as heart rate or muscle tension, provides patients with conscious awareness of abnormal bodily events they could not previously feel or perceive. After achieving awareness of these "abnormal" responses, such as chronic elevation of muscle tension in the upper trapezius, individuals can acquire voluntary control over them. This control is achieved with aid of near real-time feedback in the form of visual or auditory cues indicating whether the target response is increasing, decreasing, or holding steady.

In a brief review of biofeedback in pain management, Grzesiak[35] pointed out that biofeedback can be viewed as involving either of two strategies. The first entails the use of biofeedback as a form of general relaxation training. Patients are taught how to monitor and reduce various sympathetic responses that may be associated with anxiety or arousal (eg, skin conductance responding, heart rate, respiration rate). In addition to reducing sympathetic nervous system activity, the biofeedback paradigm teaches the patient that he can control his physiologic responding. This may contribute to a sense of self-efficacy and thereby facilitate the process of cognitive restructuring.

The second approach to biofeedback is to target specific areas of physiologic dysfunction believed to play a causal role in generating pain. For example, sustained muscle tension in the upper trapezius and cervical paraspinal muscles is widely believed to result in chronic neck and head pain. Earlier, we noted the importance of using dynamic psychophysiologic assessment to identify abnormal muscle activity during the performance of work-related tasks. There is an extensive literature on biofeedback suggesting that surface EMG may be of tangible benefit to patients with late whiplash syndrome. However, these benefits may be restricted to those who actually demonstrate abnormal muscle function on dynamic EMG assessment.

In any event, the relationship between muscle tension and muscle pain is far from clear. As Nouwen and Bush[66] have demonstrated, many of the principles that underlie EMG biofeedback are equivocal at best. Their findings do, however, confirm the importance of a dynamic approach to biofeedback assessment as discussed earlier. Biofeedback should probably not be used alone, but rather included within a comprehensive pain treatment program.

Hypnosis remains a controversial modality despite an abundance of clinical and anecdotal evidence that it may be useful in the management of chronic pain. Wolskee[95] suggested that there are four domains of hypnotic suggestion. The first involves direct suggestion of analgesia. The second set of suggestions involves approaches to filtering or modifying the pain sensation. The third group of suggestions refers to those that facilitate a dissociative response by which painful sensation is moved away from the body. Finally, the fourth domain of suggestions refers to displacing pain sensations from one part of the body to the other. Hypnotic techniques are often combined with other forms of psychological treatment. Just as with the psychodynamic psychotherapies, hypnotherapy and hypnoanalysis can be used to ascertain and process the personal meanings and other idiosyncratic aspects of the patient's pain experience.

SUMMARY

We have argued that late whiplash syndrome is not a purely medical problem and that effective clinical management requires an interdisciplinary team approach. Because acute whiplash injury is largely self-limiting, considerable doubt has been cast on the medical "validity" of chronic whiplash. Still, most specialists do not believe that these patients are consciously malingering or feigning symptoms for financial or social gain. On the other hand, many believe that an array of psychological reactions to neck injury, including prolonged litigation, overly solicitous spouses, and aggressive health care providers, can sensitize patients to benign physical sensations and unwittingly promote anxiety, depression, and unnecessary illness behavior. Anxiety, in particular, appears to be underappreciated in the recently injured person undergoing treatment for traumatic-onset soft tissue strain or sprain. We have endeavored to demonstrate some of the psychological vulnerabilities to pain and suffering, such as pain-proneness and posttraumatic responses. Both anxiety and depression can lead to somatization and generalized somatic preoccupation that forestall improvement in pain and suffering. Like many chronic pain problems, we have argued that late whiplash syndrome is as much a psychological problem as a biological one. Appropriate focus on psychological factors in the treatment of acute whiplash is critical to the prevention of most late whiplash syndromes. We have also summarized the various psychological evaluation and treatment approaches currently used with chronic pain patients. Throughout this review, we have stressed the need for early psychological intervention and the importance of using a multidisciplinary approach to manage pain and suffering.

References

1. Adler RH, Zlot S, Horny C, Minder C: Engel's "psychogenic pain and the pain-prone patient." A retrospective controlled clinical study. Psychosom Med 51:87–101, 1989.
2. American Psychiatric Association: Diagnostic and Statistical Manual of Mental Disorders, 3rd ed, rev. Washington, DC, American Psychiatric Association, 1987.
3. American Psychiatric Association: Diagnostic and Statistical Manual of Mental Disorders, 4th ed. Washington, DC, American Psychiatric Association, 1994.
4. Asmundson GJ, Norton GR, Allerdings MD: Fear and avoidance in dysfunctional chronic back pain patients. Pain 69:231–236, 1997.
5. Balla JI: The late whiplash syndrome: a study of an illness in Australia and Singapore. Cult Med Psychiatry 6:191–210, 1982.
6. Bellissimo A, Tunks E: Chronic Pain: The Psychotherapeutic Spectrum. New York, Praeger, 1984.
7. Bernstein DA, Borkovec TD: Progressive Relaxation Training. Champaign, IL, Research Press, 1973.
8. Blumer D, Heilbronn M: Chronic pain as a variant of depressive disease: the pain-prone disorder. J Nerv Ment Dis 170:381–405, 1982.
9. Blumer D, Heilbronn M: Dysthymic pain disorder: the treatment of chronic pain as a variant of depression. In Tollison CD (ed): Handbook of Chronic Pain Management. Baltimore, Williams & Wilkins, 1989, pp 197–209.
10. Boissevain MD, McCain GA: Toward an integrated understanding of fibromyalgia syndrome: psychological and phenomenological aspects. Pain 45:239–248, 1991.
11. Bradley LA, Prokop CK, Margolis R, Gentry WD: Multivariate analysis of the MMPI profiles of low back pain patients. J Behav Med 1:253–272, 1978.
12. Briere J: Trauma Symptom Inventory Professional Manual. Odessa, FL, Psychological Assessment Resources, 1995.
13. Brown FF, Robinson ME, Riley JL, Gremillion HA: Pain severity, negative affect, and micostressors as predictors of life interference in TMD patients. Cranio 14:63–70, 1996.

14. Ciccone DS, Grzesiak RC: Cognitive dimensions of chronic pain. Soc Sci Med 19:1339–1345, 1984.
15. Ciccone DS, Grzesiak RC: Cognitive therapy: an overview of theory and practice. In Lynch NT, Vasudevan SV (eds): Persistent Pain: Psychosocial Assessment and Intervention. Boston, Kluwer, 1988, pp 133–161.
16. Ciccone DS, Grzesiak RC: Chronic musculoskeletal pain: a cognitive approach to psychophysiologic assessment and intervention. In Eisenberg MG, Grzesiak RC (eds): Advances in Clinical Rehabilitation, Vol 3. New York, Springer, 1990, pp 197–215.
17. Ciccone DS, Grzesiak RC: Psychological dysfunction in chronic cervical pain: an introduction to clinical assessment. In Tollison CD, Satterthwaite JR (eds): Painful Cervical Trauma: Diagnosis and Rehabilitative Treatment of Neuromusculoskeletal Injuries. Baltimore, Williams & Wilkins, 1992, pp 79–92.
18. Ciccone DS, Lenzi V: Psychosocial vulnerability to chronic dysfunctional pain: a critical review. In Grzesiak RC, Ciccone DS (eds): Psychological Vulnerability to Chronic Pain. New York, Springer, 1994, pp 153–178.
19. Dworkin RH: What do we really know about the psychological origins of chronic pain? Am Pain Soc Bull 1(5):7–11, 1991.
20. Dworkin RH, Grzesiak RC: Chronic pain: on the integration of psyche and soma. In Stricker G, Gold GR (eds): Comprehensive Handbook of Psychotherapy Integration. New York, Plenum, 1993, pp 365–384.
21. Dworkin RH, Hartstein G, Rosner HL, et al: A high-risk method for studying psychosocial antecedents of chronic pain: the prospective investigation of herpes zoster. J Abnorm Psychol 101:200–205, 1992.
22. Dworkin SF, Wilson L, Massoth DL: Somatizing as a risk factor for chronic pain. In Grzesiak RC, Ciccone DS (eds): Psychological Vulnerability to Chronic Pain. New York, Springer, 1994, pp 28–54.
23. Eimers BN: Psychotherapy for chronic pain: a cognitive approach. In Freeman A, Simon KM, Beutler LA, et al (eds): Comprehensive Handbook of Cognitive Therapy. New York, Plenum, 1989, pp 440–465.
24. Engel GL: Primary atypical facial neuralgia: an hysterical conversion symptom. Psychosom Med 13:375–396, 1951.
25. Engel GL: "Psychogenic" pain and the pain-prone patient. Am J Med 26:899–918, 1959.
26. Ferrari R, Russell AS: The whiplash syndrome—common sense revisited [editorial]. J Rheumatol 24:618–623, 1997.
27. Fishbain DA, Cutler R, Rosomoff HL, Rosomoff RS: Chronic pain-associated depression: antecedent or consequence of chronic pain? A review. Clin J Pain 13:116–137, 1997.
28. Fishbain DA, Goldberg M, Meagher BR, Steele R: Male and female chronic pain patients categorized by DSM-III psychiatric diagnostic criteria. Pain 26:181–197, 1986.
29. Fordyce WE: Behavioral Methods for Chronic Pain and Illness. St. Louis, Mosby, 1976.
30. Freud S: Fragment of an analysis of a case of hysteria. In Jones E (ed): Sigmund Freud: Collected Papers, Vol 3. New York, Basic Books, 1955 (orig. pub. 1905), pp 13–145.
31. Gamsa A: Is emotional disturbance a precipitator or a consequence of chronic pain? Pain 42:183–195, 1990.
32. Gamsa A, Vikis-Freibergs V: Psychological events are both risk factors in, and consequences of, chronic pain. Pain 44:271–277, 1991.
33. Goldstein JA: Betrayal by the Brain: The Neurologic Basis of Chronic Fatigue Syndrome, Fibromyalgia Syndrome, and Related Neural Network Disorders. New York, Haworth, 1996.
34. Grzesiak RC: Relaxation techniques in treatment of chronic pain. Arch Phys Med Rehabil 58:270–272, 1977.
35. Grzesiak RC: Biofeedback in the treatment of chronic pain. Curr Concepts Pain 2:3–8, 1984.
36. Grzesiak RC: The matrix of vulnerability. In Grzesiak RC, Ciccone DS (eds): Psychological Vulnerability to Chronic Pain. New York, Springer, 1994, pp 1–27.
37. Grzesiak RC: Psychological considerations in myofascial pain, fibromyalgia, and related musculoskeletal pain. In Rachlin ES (ed): Myofascial Pain and Fibromyalgia: Trigger Point Management. St. Louis, Mosby, 1994, pp 61–90.
38. Grzesiak RC, Ciccone DS: Relaxation, biofeedback and hypnosis in the management of pain. In Lynch NT, Vasudevan SV (eds): Persistent Pain: Psychosocial Assessment and Intervention. Boston, Kluwer, 1988, pp 163–188.
39. Grzesiak RC, Ury GM, Dworkin RH: Psychodynamic psychotherapy with chronic pain patients. In Gatchel RJ, Turk DC (eds): Psychological Approaches to Pain Management: A Practitioner's Handbook. New York, Guilford, 1996, pp 148–178.

40. Harness DM, Donlon WC: Cryptotrauma: the hidden wound. Clin J Pain 4:257–260, 1988.
41. Heaton RK, Lehman RAW, Getto CJ: Psychosocial Pain Inventory. Odessa, FL, Psychological Assessment Resources, 1980.
42. Heikkila H, Heikkila E, Eisemann M: Predictive factors for the outcome of a multidisciplinary pain rehabilitation programme on sick leave and life satisfaction in patients with whiplash trauma and other myofascial pain: a follow-up study. Clin Rehabil 12:487–496, 1998.
43. Hendler N: Diagnosis and Nonsurgical Management of Chronic Pain. New York, Raven, 1981.
44. Holzberg AD, Robinson ME, Geisser ME, Gremillion HA: The effects of depression and chronic pain on psychosocial and physical functioning. Clin J Pain 12:118–125, 1996.
45. Horowitz MJ, Wilner N, Alvarez D: Impact of Event Scale: A study of subjective stress. Psychosom Med 41: 209–218, 1979.
46. Huskisson EC: Measurement of pain. Lancet 2(7889):1127–1131, 1974.
47. Jacobson E: Modern Treatment of Tense Patients. Springfield, IL, Charles C Thomas, 1964.
48. Jaspers JP: Whiplash and post-traumatic stress disorder. Disabil Rehabil 20:397–404, 1998.
48a. Katon W, Lin E, Von Korff M, et al: Somatization: A spectrum of severity. Am J Psychiatry 148:34–40, 1991.
49. Kerns RD, Turk DC, Rudy TE: The West Haven-Yale Multidimensional Pain Inventory. Pain 23:345–356, 1985.
50. Klenerman L, Slade PD, Stanley IM, et al: The prediction of chronicity in patients with an acute attack of low back pain in a general practice. Spine 20:478–484, 1995.
51. Krishnan KRR, France RD, Davidson J: Depression as a psychopathological disorder in chronic pain. In France RD, Krishnan KRR (eds): Chronic Pain. Washington, DC, American Psychiatric Press, 1988, pp 142–193.
52. Lee J, Giles K, Drummond PD: Psychological disturbances and an exaggerated response to pain in patients with whiplash injury. J Psychosom Res 37:105–110, 1993.
53. Livingston M: Whiplash injury: misconceptions and remedies [letter]. Aust Fam Physician 21:1642–1644, 1992.
54. Maimaris C, Barnes MR, Allen MJ: Whiplash injuries of the neck: a retrospective study. Injury 19:393–396, 1988.
55. Mayou R, Bryant B, Duthrie R: Psychiatric consequences of road traffic accidents. BMJ 307:647–651, 1993.
56. Melzack R: The McGill Pain Questionnaire: major properties and scoring methods. Pain 1:277–299, 1975.
57. Melzack R: Central pain syndromes and theories of pain. In Casey KL (ed): Pain and the Central Nervous System: The Central Pain Syndromes. New York, Raven, 1991, pp 59–64.
58. Melzack R: Phantom limbs. Sci Am 266:120–126, 1992.
59. Melzack R: From the gate to the neuromatrix. Pain Suppl 6:S121–S126, 1999.
60. Melzack R, Wall PD: Pain mechanisms: a new theory. Science 150:971–979, 1965.
61. Meldelson G: "Compensation neurosis" revisited: outcome studies of the effects of litigation. J Psychosom Res 39:695–706, 1995.
62. Middaugh SJ, Kee WG: Advances in electromyographic monitoring and biofeedback in the treatment of chronic cervical and low back pain. In Eisenberg MG, Grzesiak RC (eds): Advances in Clinical Rehabilitation, Vol 1. New York, Springer, 1987, pp 137–172.
63. Moldofsky H, Scarisbrick P, England R, et al: Musculoskeletal symptoms and nonREM sleep disturbance in patients with "fibrositis" syndrome and healthy subjects. Psychosom Med 37:341–351, 1975.
64. Moldofsky H, Wong MTH, Lue FA: Litigation, sleep, symptoms and disabilities in postaccident pain (fibromyalgia). J Rheumatol 20:1935–1940, 1993.
65. Nadler S, Cooke P: Myofascial pain in whiplash injuries: diagnosis and treatment. Spine State Art Rev 12(2): 357–376, 1998.
66. Nouwen A, Bush C: The relationship between paraspinal EMG and chronic low back pain. Pain 20:109–123, 1984.
67. Olsnes BT: Neurobehavioral findings in whiplash patients with long-standing symptoms. Acta Neurol Scand 80:584–588, 1989.
68. Parkes CM: Factors determining the persistence of phantom limb pain in the amputee. J Psychosom Res 17:97–108, 1973.
69. Pearce JMS: Whiplash injury: a reappraisal. J Neurol Neurosurg Psychiatry 52:1329–1331, 1989.
70. Prokop CK, Bradley LA, Margolis R, Gentry WD: Multivariate analysis of the MMPI profiles in multiple pain patients. J Pers Assess 44:246–252, 1980.
71. Radanov BP: Common whiplash - research findings revisited [editorial]. J Rheumatol 24: 623–625, 1997.

72. Radanov BP, DiStefano G, Schnidrig A, Ballinari P: Role of psychosocial stress in recovery from common whiplash. Lancet 338:712–715, 1991.
73. Rudy TE, Turk DC, Zaki HS, Curtin HD: An empirical taxometric alternative to traditional classification of temporomandibular disorders. Pain 36:311–320, 1989.
74. Sarno JE: The Mindbody Prescription. New York, Warner Books, 1998.
75. Schofferman J, Anderson D, Hines R, Smith G, White A: Childhood psychological trauma correlates with unsuccessful lumbar spine surgery. Spine 17(suppl): S138–S144, 1992.
76. Schrader H, Obelieniene D, Bovim G, et al: Natural evolution of the late whiplash syndrome outside of the medicolegal context. Lancet 347:1207–1211, 1996.
77. Schwartzman LC, Teasell RW, Shapiro AP, McDermid AJ: The effect of litigation status on adjustment to whiplash injury. Spine 21:53–58, 1996.
78. Simon GE: Somatization and psychiatric disorders. In Kirmayer LJ, Bobbins JM (eds): Current Concepts in Somatization: Research and Clinical Perspectives, 31st ed. Washington DC, American Psychiatric Press, 1991, pp 37–62.
79. Simon RI (ed): Posttraumatic Stress Disorders in Litigation. Washington, DC, American Psychiatric Press, 1995.
80. Soderlund A, Olerud C, Lindberg P: Acute whiplash-associated disorders (WAD): the effects of early mobilization and prognostic factors in long-term symptomatology. Clin Rehabil 14:457–467, 2000.
81. Sternbach RA: Pain: A Psychophysiological Analysis. New York, Academic Press, 1968.
82. Sternbach RA: Pain Patients: Traits and Treatment. New York, Academic Press, 1974.
83. Sternbach RA: Clinical aspects of pain. In Sternbach RA (ed): The Psychology of Pain, 2nd ed. New York, Raven, 1986, pp 223–239.
84. Teasell RW, McCain GA: Clinical spectrum and management of whiplash injuries. In Tollison CD, Satterthwaite JR (eds): Painful Cervical Trauma: Diagnosis and Rehabilitative Treatment of Neuromusculoskeletal Injuries. Baltimore, Williams & Wilkins, 1992, pp 292–318.
85. Tollison CD, Langley JC: Pain Patient Profile Manual. Minneapolis, National Computer Systems, 1992.
86. Turk DC, Meichenbaum D, Genest M: Pain and Behavioral Medicine: A Cognitive-Behavioral Perspective. New York, Guilford, 1983.
87. Turk DC, Rudy TE: Toward an empirically derived taxonomy of chronic pain patients: integration of psychological assessment data. J Consult Clin Psychol 56:233–238, 1988.
88. Turner JA, Dworkin SF, Manel L, et al: The roles of beliefs, catastrophizing, and coping in the functioning of patients with temporomandibular disorders. Pain 92:41–51, 2001.
89. van der Kolk BA: The body keeps the score: memory and the evolving psychobiology of PTSD. Harvard Rev Psychiatry 1:253-265, 1994.
90. van der Kolk BA, van der Hart O: Pierre Janet and the breakdown of adaptation in psychological trauma. Am J Psychiatry 146:1530–1540, 1989.
91. van der Kolk BA, van der Hart O: The intrusive past: the flexibility of memory and the engraving of trauma. Am Imago 48:425–454, 1991.
92. VanHoudenove B: Prevalence and psychodynamic interpretation of premorbid hyperactivity in patients with chronic pain. Psychother Psychosom 45:195–200, 1986.
93. VanHoudenove B, Stans L, Verstraeten D: Is there a link between "pain-proneness" and "act-proneness?" Pain 29:113–117, 1987.
94. Weiss DS, Marmar CR: The Impact of Event Scale-Revised. In Wilson J, Keane TM (eds): Assessing Psychological Trauma and PTSD. New York, Guilford, 1996, pp 399–411.
95. Wolskee PJ: Psychological therapy for chronic pain. In Wu W (ed): Pain Management: Assessment and Treatment of Chronic and Acute Syndromes. New York, Human Sciences Press, 1987, pp 201–215.

24

Surgical Indications Following Whiplash Injury

Robert F. Heary, M.D., and Christopher M. Bono, M.D.

Whiplash is a common mechanism of injury in patients involved in motor vehicle accidents. Although not a diagnosis itself, the term "whiplash" has become synonymous with the clinical sequelae of an acute hyperflexion or hyperextension injury of the cervical spine. Injuries can vary from mild sprains to unstable ligamentous disruptions,[28] with an estimated incidence of 1 million cases per year.[23] Traditionally, fractures and dislocations are not considered whiplash injuries. By convention, cervical whiplash injuries display minimal to no acute plain radiographic findings.[19] It has been described less frequently in the lumbar spine.[11,12] Management of whiplash sequelae is challenging. Nonoperative measures are the mainstay of treatment, including rest, nonsteroidal anti-inflammatory medications, short-term bracing, physical therapy, and rehabilitation. In some cases, minimally invasive procedures such as spinal injections can be helpful.

In rare instances of prolonged symptoms, operative intervention can be contemplated. Effective operative treatment relies on a thorough understanding of the rationale, indications, limitations, preoperative assessment, and available surgical options. Goals of surgery can be neuroablative, decompressive, or stabilizing and can focus on the anterior or posterior elements of the spine. It is the authors' intention to increase the readers' understanding of these and other issues relevant to the operative management of whiplash injury.

RATIONALE

Treatment is focused on the amelioration of symptoms. In rare cases, high-energy mechanisms can produce spinal cord injury. Most commonly, symptoms are pain, headache, spasm, and dysfunction but may also consist of dizziness, paresthesias, or cognitive impairment.[9] Pain is the most frequent complaint following whiplash.[9] Pain can be from muscle, ligament, or skeletal damage. The practitioner's first challenge is to determine the origin of symptoms, which is often elusive. If this can be determined with reasonable confidence, surgery is directed toward the responsible anatomic structure(s). Injury can be detected at the level of the intervertebral disc, the anterior ligamentous complex, the facet joints, the neuroforamina, or the posterior ligamentous complex (PLC).

Anterior Structures

Anatomy and Injury Mechanism

The anterior longitudinal ligament (ALL) spans the ventral surface of the cervical vertebral bodies. It serves to limit extension as a "check-rein" and can be injured with severe, abrupt hyperextension. These are most common with acceleratory mechanisms such as rear-end collisions. The anulus fibrosus of the intervertebral disc supplements the ALL against these forces and can be similarly injured. Reports of intervertebral disc avulsion have been reported.[8,14] In addition, the outer anulus resists rotational forces and can be damaged with sudden torque, but this is not a common mechanism of whiplash.

The nucleus pulposus is the gel-like core of the intervertebral disc. Contained by the fixed boundaries of the multilayered anulus fibrosus, it becomes pressurized under compressive loads along the anterior spine. Abrupt hyperflexion can lead to pressures that exceed the capacity of the anulus to contain the nucleus. Microscopic tears in this layered-wall structure of the anulus can occur, but they are exceedingly difficult to detect acutely; magnetic resonance (MR) images can be negative in the first few weeks.[26] In some cases, intradiscal degeneration can be detected as a so-called "black disc" on T2-weighted MR images, which may present weeks to the months after the accident.

Pain Generation

It is commonly held that a posttraumatic degenerative disc can act as a pain source. Anatomically, the disc receives nociceptive branches from the dorsal root ganglion.[5] Indirect clinical evidence exists in the discography literature. Discograms are performed to help determine symptomatic levels of degenerative disease. A positive discogram, with a correlative MR imaging (MRI) scan indicating degeneration at the same level, is a reasonably good indicator of favorable clinical results after fusion.[20,30] Motimaya et al[20] reported 79% good or excellent results in 14 patients who had cervical interbody fusion based on a positive discogram. Likewise, Siebenrock and associates[30] documented 73% good to excellent results in 27 fusions. Interestingly, results were better in patients who reported no pain before the whiplash injury. From these data, it can be inferred that the cervical disc was a significant pain generator that responded well to treatment.

Instability

An unstable spine can result from acute traumatic disruption of one or more of the stabilizing ligamentous structures. In the anterior spine, injury to the ALL or anterior disc can lead to instability. After whiplash injury, cervical instability usually presents late. In actuality, cervical instability after whiplash is likely a result of a combination of ligamentous damage and incompetence of the posterior facet complex. This is best detected on dynamic lateral flexion-extension radiographs. These should always be performed in an awake patient under volitional control. Unfortunately, pain and muscle spasms in the neck occur acutely after a whiplash injury. As a result, adequate dynamic flexion-extension radiographs may not be obtained until these symptoms improve over the course of weeks to even months.

Posterior Structures

Anatomy and Injury Mechanism

The integrity of the zygapophyseal (facet) joints helps to stabilize the posterior aspect of the cervical spine. With hyperflexion mechanisms, the facet joint capsule is stretched and may tear.[35] The bones of the facet joints are more frequently injured with hyperextension forces.[36] Hyperextension briefly impacts the apposed articular surfaces. Articular cartilage damage can predispose to posttraumatic arthritis, which is often reported after whiplash injuries.[16,17] Sensory innervation from branches of the dorsal root ganglion to the facet joints can transmit arthritic pain.

The PLC consists of interspinous and supraspinous structures that are tensioned with flexion of the neck. Hyperflexion with high-energy front-end motor vehicle collisions can disrupt the PLC. The posterior longitudinal ligament (PLL) is the weakest of the spinal ligaments and contributes little to stability of the cervical spine. The PLL may be damaged by retropulsed fragments of herniated disc material from anterior compressive loads.

Pain Generation

The facet joint, like the intervertebral disc, receives pain sensory innervation from the dorsal root ganglion. This is the proposed nociceptive pathway of posttraumatic facet arthritis after whiplash injury. This is evidenced by the effectiveness of anesthetic blocks injected into the zygapophyseal joints. Numerous randomized controlled studies have demonstrated significant pain relief with facet injections in some patients after whiplash.[2,3,15] Although not every patient will have facet-generated pain, this information lends strong support to the facet joint as a pain generator following whiplash injury.

Instability

The facet joint contributes to rotational stability of the spine, while the PLC is a major restraint to distractive forces along the posterior elements. Disruption or attenuation of one or both of these structures can yield to clinical instability. With whiplash injury, these may appear late as mild subluxations on flexion-extension views of the cervical spine.

DIAGNOSIS

Clinical Assessment

The patient's recollection of the inciting event and whether rear-end or front-end collision occurred is important in clinical assessment. Rear-end collision results in sudden forward acceleration of the car. The inertia of the patient's head to maintain its position acts to hyperextend the neck. As discussed above, this places distractive anterior forces and posterior compressive forces that may result in particular injury patterns. The presence or absence of a headrest can influence the amount of hyperextension. In contrast, a front-end collision results in abrupt deceleration, causing the neck to hyperflex and, thus, compression anteriorly and distraction posteriorly. A history of preinjury pain is helpful because it can indicate preexisting cervical spondylosis. Preinjury spondylosis can negatively influence the surgical results after interbody fusion for postwhiplash disc degeneration.[30]

In the acute setting, the patient must be carefully examined, including a systematic neurologic evaluation. Subtle signs, such as ankle clonus or a positive Babinski response, can indicate spinal cord trauma without focal neurologic deficits. Radicular symptoms or signs can suggest foraminal encroachment. In most cases, cervical range of motion should not be tested at the time of injury. A hard cervical collar should remain in place until the initial pain and spasm subside. Spasm can mask occult instability or subluxation of the vertebral column, which is more safely assessed 1 to 2 weeks after the injury. Palpation of the spine can reveal tenderness at the injured level.

Surgical assessment usually occurs months after the accident when pain is no longer ameliorated by other measures. With chronic whiplash injury, the patient may be able to localize the approximate anatomic region (ie, upper cervical, lower cervical) or provocative motions (ie, flexion versus extension). In most cases, however, symptoms are more generalized along the entire neck. Attempts to discern midline tenderness from paraspinal tenderness can help differentiate vertebral versus paraspinal pathology.

A complete physical examination is mandatory. In both the acute and chronic situation, the practitioner must keep a differential diagnosis in mind. Pain from underlying infection and tumor can first manifest after a low-energy whiplash-type mechanism. Careful inspection of radiographs or advanced imaging studies is useful in ruling these processes out. Nonspinal etiologies of pain must also be considered, such as tracheal or esophageal tears, mediastinitis, thyroid lesions, or brachial plexopathies.[27,31]

Imaging

Plain Radiography

Plain films of the cervical spine are initially obtained. Anteroposterior and lateral views are the minimum. Emergency patients sustaining acute trauma should have every cervical level visualized clearly. Often, the lateral radiograph is inadequate for the more cranial and caudal segments. A "swimmer's view" offers better visualization of the cervicothoracic junction. Open-mouth views give excellent visualization of the odontoid process and lateral masses of C1 and C2.

In general, plain radiographs after whiplash are usually normal. In some cases, a loss of normal cervical lordosis can be appreciated. It is thought that loss of lordosis is secondary to muscular spasm after trauma. However, this may reflect normal variation in spinal posture. Matsumoto and associates[18] prospectively compared the radiographs of 488 whiplash-injured patients with 495 asymptomatic control subjects and found no difference in the incidence of nonlordotic curves between the two groups.

Lateral flexion-extension views of the cervical spine can help detect dynamic instability not otherwise detectable on static films. Without other evidence of fracture, instability is attributed to ligamentous attenuation or frank disruption. Of 451 patients imaged with static and flexion-extension views, Brady et al[7] detected 11 cases of subluxation on dynamic imaging that were not detected on static films alone. Overall, patients with normal static roentgenograms were less likely to demonstrate instability on the dynamic films. Criteria for clinically significant cervical instability are 3.5 mm of translation or 11 degrees of angulation change between the flexion and extension views.

Advanced Imaging

Although computed tomography (CT) and MRI are of great benefit in cases of higher-energy cervical trauma, their utility in the acute evaluation of whiplash injury has not been demonstrated. Without evidence of fracture on plain radiographs, there is little role for CT in evaluating whiplash injury.[33] Likewise, MRI is of low value in the early management of whiplash.[6,25] Because of the high sensitivity of MR, a large number of false-positive MR results are obtained immediately following the accident. Findings include muscle contusions, disc herniations, spondylosis, and disc changes.[6,25] Unfortunately, investigators have found that MR findings have little to no correlation with clinical findings. Most authors would agree that MRI is best reserved for the chronic setting in patients with long-standing symptoms after whiplash injury.[24,25]

MRI is the modality of choice for preoperative evaluation of posttraumatic degeneration from whiplash. Its advantage over CT is superior visualization of soft tissues, including muscle, nerve, ligament, and disc. The disc, normally exhibiting a bright central signal on T2-weighted images, can be dark. This can indicate disc degeneration. Compression of the neural elements, either central or radicular, can be noted in the spinal canal or the neural foramina, respectively. The PLC and ALL can also be visualized and inspected for laxity, redundancy, or incompetence. Ligamentum flavum hypertrophy and facet joint overgrowth, usually present prior to the whiplash injury, can encroach the spinal canal posteriorly. In addition, the integrity of the articular cartilage of the zygapophyseal joint as well as eburnation, osteophytes, and joint space collapse can all be detected with high-resolution MR images.

SURGICAL OPTIONS

The indications for surgery after whiplash injury are limited. Procedures can be categorized as decompressive, stabilizing, or neuroablative. In the acute setting, clear documentation of a progressive neurologic deficit warrants urgent decompression. Likewise, radiographic evidence of instability may warrant early operative stabilization. This is most concerning with ligamentous injuries in the upper cervical spine, particularly the atlantoaxial junction. Chronically, sustained discogenic or facetogenic pain can warrant discectomy or fusion in a select group of patients. However, the indications for these procedures continue to evolve. Similarly, clinical manifestation of root compression may be alleviated with foraminal decompression with or without arthrodesis. In some patients with primarily arthritic facet pain, percutaneous neurotomy can be effective.[16] Operative management must be considered carefully because surgical complications can occur.[22]

Radiofrequency Neurotomy

The facet joint has been implicated as a major source of chronic pain after whiplash.[15] With radiographic and MR evidence of posttraumatic articular degeneration, the diagnosis of facet arthritis can be strengthened with pain relief after selective injections of the facet joint.[2,3] Although injections can sometimes give long-lasting relief, minimally invasive neuroablative procedures have been developed for resistant cases.

Radiofrequency neurotomy involves percutaneous insertion of an electrode that is directed toward the facet joint. The heat at the electrode can obliterate the nociceptive sensory innervation from the dorsal rami. This acts as a longer-lasting facet joint injection. Recent results with this technique for whiplash have been promising.[16,17]

In a double-blind randomized study, Lord et al[17] used this method in chronic whiplash patients. Twelve patients who underwent the procedure had at least 50% pain relief for a median of 263 days, while a control group reported only 8 days of relief. Interestingly, some patients in the neurotomy group complained of numbness in the region of the procedure. This is most likely secondary to denervation of some of the dorsal rami branches to the posterior skin of the neck. No other neurologic complications were reported.

This procedure is indicated for patients with intractable facet joint pain after whiplash with documented short-term relief with selective injections.[16,17] In the authors' opinion, the diagnosis of facet joint pain should be supported with radiographic or other imaging evidence of degeneration in the region. Disc pathology can be a contraindication for neurotomy; however, if the facet joint injection offers significant relief, the disc may not be a substantial pain generator. The advantages of radiofrequency neurotomy are that it is minimally invasive with few, if any, significant complications and does not require cervical collar immobilization. Also, it does not preclude other surgical procedures such as posterior or anterior fusion if pain progresses. Disadvantages are that it is not permanent because of the regenerative properties of the sensory peripheral nerves to the facet joint.

Anterior Discectomy Without Fusion

Discectomy without fusion is rarely performed in the cervical spine. However, it has been reported as a treatment for chronic discogenic or radicular pain after whiplash injury. The rationale for this technique is that the disc is the pain source; thereby, with its removal, the pain should be relieved. Also, bulging regions of disc can impinge on nerve roots, which can cause dermatomal symptoms.

Algers et al[1] reported on 20 patients surgically treated with anterior discectomy and/or discectomy with fusion for chronic pain after whiplash injury. Only two cases of discectomy without fusion were reported. The indications were a herniated disc documented by myelography or MRI. Surgical outcome was fair in one case and poor in the other. Only one of the patients reported relief of the radicular symptoms, while the other continued to have daily complaints. Although the numbers are small, these results are not encouraging. Importantly, the authors reported no use of preoperative discography or selective injections to deduce or confirm the symptomatic levels of disease.

In the authors' opinion, discectomy alone has no role in the treatment of whiplash injury. Even if radicular symptoms are the only finding, a discectomy should be followed by anterior interbody fusion (see below). In reported series of discectomy without fusion for other degenerative processes, continued complaints of neck pain are common.[4,13,34] Without fusion, instability at the operative level can potentiate osteophyte formation, which can lead to further nerve root compression and radicular pathology. Additionally, collapse of the disc space will usually occur following an anterior discectomy without fusion, which can cause symptomatic narrowing of the neural foramina and late radiculopathy. Fortunately, up to 72% of levels with discectomy alone can autofuse.[21]

Anterior Discectomy and Interbody Fusion

The rationale for anterior discectomy for whiplash injury sequelae relies on the idea that the disc is a major pain generator. In addition, the disc or its counterparts (PLL) can contribute to anterior compression on the spinal elements. Sometimes, a frank herniated disc can compress a single nerve root. In most situations after whiplash, the disc exhibits evidence of decreased elasticity and resiliency against compressive anterior loads. The dorsal rami branches that enter the posterior aspect of the disc are thought to be the transmitters of discogenic pain.

Anterior discectomy and fusion (ACDF) is the most commonly reported fusion procedure for whiplash injury.[1,10,12,22,29,32] Although a number of techniques of anterior fusion exist, an in-depth description of each is beyond the scope of this chapter. Regardless of the method employed, vital structures must be protected during the procedure. Of note, the carotid sheath is retracted laterally for protection. Also at risk is the recurrent laryngeal nerve, which may be at greater risk with right-sided approaches than left-sided ones.[22] The sympathetic plexus lies on the belly of the longissimus colli and is in danger with overzealous lateral dissection on the muscle.

After careful dissection and stable retraction, the ALL is visualized. The correct disc space is identified using a cross-table lateral radiograph intraoperatively. With the correct site confirmed, the ALL is incised along the superior and inferior borders of the neighboring vertebrae. The disc is then removed piecemeal until the PLL can be visualized. Adequate visualization and lighting is essential to the safe performance of an ACDF procedure. While loupe magnification with a headlight is used by some surgeons, the authors prefer to use the operating microscope. Using microsurgical techniques, the posterior anulus fibrosus of the intervertebral disc and the PLL are resected. This allows for a safe exposure of the ventral dura and absolute confirmation that an adequate decompression has been accomplished.

After the discectomy has been completed, a block of structural bone graft is inserted into the empty disc space. Iliac crest autograft or allograft from a variety of sources has been used successfully. Fixation with an anterior cervical plate can sometimes be used. If stable fixation can be achieved, this practice can minimize the length of postoperative collar immobilization. However, good results and fusion rates can be expected after both instrumented and noninstrumented fusions.

Several authors have reported on the results of ACDF for whiplash injury. Surgical outcomes have varied. Algers et al[1] documented 4-year follow-up of

18 patients who underwent uninstrumented ACDF for painful sequelae after whiplash injury. Patients had a combination of isolated discogenic neck pain with or without radicular symptoms. Symptoms persisted between 1 and 25 years before surgery was contemplated. Preoperative discography was used in only two cases. The authors reported two good, eight fair, and eight poor results.

To determine the frequency that fusion is performed in whiplash-injured patients, Hamer et al[10] retrospectively reviewed all cases of ACDF over a 3-year period. Thirty (14%) of the 215 patients had a history of whiplash. The whiplash patients had surgery at a significantly younger age (P<.001). Fusion was commonly performed at the C5-C6 level, with frequent surgical findings being chronic disc herniation and osteophytes. To compare, they polled 800 control

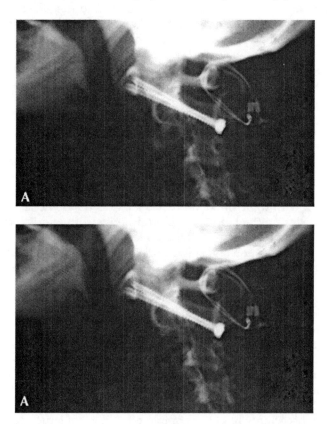

Figure 1. Whiplash injury in a 48-year-old man following a rear-end motor vehicle accident resulted in an injury to the transverse atlantal ligament and a C1-C2 subluxation. **A,** Plain film (lateral view). Stabilization and fusion accomplished with C1-C2 transarticular screws (Magerl technique) and a posterior Gallie-type fusion using a sublaminar cable beneath the C1 posterior arch and wrapping around the spinous process of C2; autologous structural iliac crest graft is interposed between the posterior bony elements of the atlas and the axis. **B,** Plain film (anteroposterior view). Well-positioned screws placed via a posterior approach to appose the lateral masses of C1 and C2.

subjects, noting that 40 patients (5%) reported a history of cervical trauma. The authors concluded that whiplash-injured patients undergo ACDF at a higher rate than the general population. They inferred that structural damage that occurs at the time of injury is responsible for this disparity.

Hohl[12] reviewed the long-term prognosis of 146 patients who sustained a whiplash injury after an automobile accident. Although most responded to nonoperative measures, three patients eventually had a surgical procedure. An anterior fusion was performed in each, with or without posterior decompression for radicular complaints. Two had good pain relief, while one reported no improvement. Likewise, Squires[32] reviewed the records of 40 cases of whiplash-injured patients. Two eventually underwent an ACDF. One had complete alleviation of symptoms, and the other remained symptomatic.

The use of cervical discography as a preoperative tool may improve surgical results from ACDF by better patient selection. Motimaya and associates[20] documented 79% good to excellent results in necks fused by ACDF for discogenic pain after whiplash injury. Similarly, Siebenrock and Aebi[30] reported 73% overall good to excellent results. Interestingly, outcomes were better in patients who reported no preinjury neck pain. Contraintuitively, single-level fusions had worse outcomes than two-level procedures. These values are substantially higher than previously reported for ACDF after whiplash.

It is the authors' feeling that ACDF should be reserved for a select group of patients with pain secondary to whiplash injury. The best results have been documented in conjunction with discography that localizes the painful disc level. With supportive discographic, MRI, and radiographic findings and failure of prolonged nonoperative and minimally invasive measures including injections, ACDF may be contemplated. The authors usually wait at least 1 year before first discussing surgical options with the patient. In addition, the authors are reluctant to progress toward surgery if litigation or workers' compensation issues are pending. Absolute indications for ACDF are a progressive neurologic deficit, either central or radicular, with MR-documented pathology. Although no series of cases of cervical instability after whiplash injury exist, spines with more than 3.5 mm of translation or 11 degrees of angulation difference between flexion and extension views, with associated symptoms, can also be an indication for an ACDF.

A successful ACDF requires demonstration of no motion between the posterior bony elements on dynamic flexion-extension radiographs as well as bridging trabeculae of bone spanning the discectomy defect. In most cases, the involved facet joints will also demonstrate fusion when a solid anterior fusion has occurred. This demonstration of a solid fusion on dynamic imaging is usually evident 3 to 12 months postoperatively depending on whether autograft or allograft bone was used in the procedure. Typically, autograft bone fuses more quickly; however, the use of autograft is associated with persistence of pain from the donor harvest site in some cases.

Posterior Decompression and Fusion

An extensive review of the literature reveals no reports of isolated posterior fusion procedures in the treatment of whiplash injury. Some isolated reports of posterior laminectomy for decompression have been accompanied by ACDF.[12] This brings up an interesting topic of discussion. There is a large body of evidence to support facet injury after whiplash. Facet injection and neurotomy studies have documented good pain relief. It is likely that some of the patients who have undergone ACDF have had concomitant facet pain. It is the authors' belief that fusion of the anterior spine diminishes or eliminates motion in the involved posterior spine region as well. Therefore, an ACDF could address facet arthritis in addition to discogenic pain. An important question is whether isolated facet pain without disc pathology, documented by MRI and discography, could be successfully treated with an isolated posterior fusion of the zygapophyseal joint. This option remains to be explored in a clinical study.

Atlantoaxial Instability

The atlanto-dens articulation is stabilized by a number of important ligaments. These can be injured with no radiographic or CT evidence of fracture. Disruption of one or more of these ligamentous structures can result in clinical instability. Atlantoaxial instability can be detected by flexion-extension films, which should be delayed for at least 1 week after the motor vehicle injury to allow spasm to subside. The normal atlanto-dens interval is 2 to 3 mm in

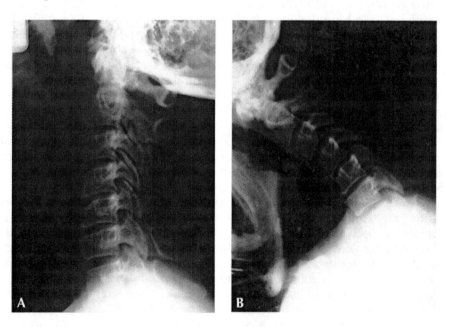

Figure 2. Whiplash injury in a 45-year-old woman following a front-end collision resulted in significant axial neck pain and persistent headaches. Plain film radiographs (lateral views) *obtained 3 years after the motor vehicle accident*—**A,** On extension, a slight loss of cervical lordosis is seen. Film is otherwise normal. **B,** On flexion, focal instability is demonstrated at the C4-C5 level, with a 2-mm anterolisthesis and widening of the posterior elements (indicative of posterior ligamentous instability.) *(Continued on next page.)*

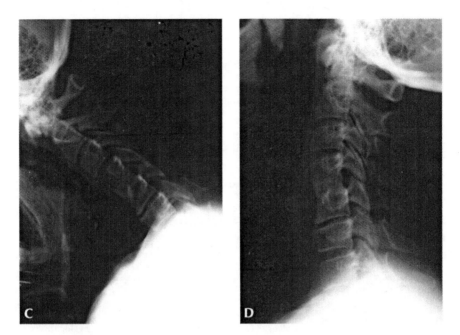

Figure 2 *(Continued).*   Plain-film radiographs *obtained 6 months after an anterior cervical discectomy and fusion with autologous iliac crest bone graft—C,* On extension, solid fusion is demonstrated. **D,** On flexion, the posterior elements are well aligned. There is no motion between the posterior elements of C4 and C5, which indicates the presence of a solid fusion. The patient's neck pain and headaches had completely resolved.

adults. Following cervical trauma, intervals greater than 5 mm may be considered unstable. In this situation, a posterior C1-C2 fusion may be indicated to prevent spinal cord compression, chronic neck pain, or persistent suboccipital region headaches. A number of techniques are available. The surgical goal is a stable and solid fusion of the two vertebrae to prevent translation and, thus, diminution of the space available for the spinal cord.

SUMMARY
Whiplash injury can result in chronic discogenic and facet pain. Although nonsurgical measures are helpful in most cases, some patients continue to be symptomatic. With positive responses to injections, prolonged facet pain can be treated with percutaneous neurotomy. Open anterior surgery should not be contemplated for at least 1 year after injury. Surgical indications must be stringent. With a history and physical findings that support the diagnosis, an MRI study indicating disc degeneration, and lack of an acceptable response to a prolonged course of conservative therapy, the option of an ACDF can be addressed. The patient, family, and surgeon must have frank discussions about the less-than-optimal reported surgical outcomes and potential complications.[22] In some patients, ACDF can yield long-standing pain relief from discogenic and facet-related pain after whiplash injury to the cervical spine.

References

1. Algers G, Pettersson K, Hildingsson C, et al: Surgery for chronic symptoms after whiplash injury. Follow-up of 20 cases. Acta Orthop Scand 64:654–656, 1993.
2. Barnsley L, Lord S, Bogduk N: Comparative local anaesthetic blocks in the diagnosis of cervical zygapophsial joint pain. Pain 55:99–106, 1993.
3. Barnsley L, Lord S, Wallis B, et al: The prevalence of chronic cervical zygapophysial joint pain after whiplash. Spine 20:20–25, 1995.
4. Benini A, Krayenbuhl H, Bruderl R: Anterior cervical discectomy without fusion: microsurgical technique. Acta Neurochir (Wien) 61:105–110, 1982.
5. Bogduk N, Windsor M, Omgos A: The innervation of the cervical intervertebral discs. Spine 13:2–8, 1988.
6. Borchgrevink G, Smevik O, Nordby A, et al: MR imaging and radiography of patients with cervical hyperextension-flexion injuries after car accidents. Acta Radiol 36:425–428, 1995.
7. Brady W, Moghtader J, Cutcher D, et al: ED use of flexion-extension cervical spine radiography in the evaluation of blunt trauma. Am J Emerg Med 17:504–508, 1999.
8. Davis S, Teresi L, Bradley W, et al: Cervical spine hyperextension injuries: MR findings. Radiology 180:245–251, 1991.
9. Evans R: Some observations on whiplash injuries. Neurol Clin 10:975–997, 1992.
10. Hamer AJ, Gargan MF, Bannister GC, et al: Whiplash injury and surgically treated cervical disc disease [see comments]. Injury 24:549–550, 1993.
11. Hildingsson C, Toolanen G: Outcome after soft-tissue injury of the cervical spine. Acta Orthop Scand 61:357–359, 1990.
12. Hohl M: Soft tissue injuries of the neck in automobile accidents: factors influencing prognosis. J Bone Joint Surg Am 56:1675–1682, 1974.
13. Hukuda S, Mochizuki T, Ogata M, et al: Operations for cervical spondylotic myelopathy: a comparison of the results of anterior and posterior procedures. J Bone Joint Surg Br 67:609–615, 1985.
14. LaRocca H, Butler J, Whitecloud T: Cervical acceleration injuries: diagnosis, treatment, and long-term outcome. In Frymoyer J (ed): The Adult Spine. Philadelphia, Lippincott-Raven, 1997, pp 1235–1243.
15. Lord S, Barnsley L, Wallis B, et al: Chronic cervical zygapophysial joint pain after whiplash. Spine 21:1737–1745, 1996.
16. Lord SM, Barnsley L, Bogduk N: Percutaneous radiofrequency neurotomy in the treatment of cervical zygapophysial joint pain: a caution. Neurosurgery 36:732–739, 1995.
17. Lord SM, Barnsley L, Wallis BJ, et al: Percutaneous radio-frequency neurotomy for chronic cervical zygapophyseal-joint pain [see comments]. N Engl J Med 335:1721–1726, 1996.
18. Matsumoto M, Fujimura Y, Suzuki N, et al: Cervical curvature in acute whiplash injuries: prospective comparative study with asymptomatic subjects. Injury 29:775–778, 1998.
19. McDowell G, Cammisa F, Eismont F: Hyperextension injuries of the cervical spine. In Levine A, et al (ed): Spine Trauma. Philadelphia, WB Saunders, 1998, pp 380–384.
20. Motimaya A, Arici M, George D, et al: Diagnostic value of cervical discography in the management of cervical discogenic pain. Conn Med 64:395–398, 2000.
21. Murphy M, Gado M: Anterior cervical discectomy without interbody bone graft. J Neurosurg 37:71–74, 1972.
22. Muzumdar DP, Deopujari CE, Bhojraj SY: Bilateral vocal cord paralysis after anterior cervical discoidectomy and fusion in a case of whiplash cervical spine injury: a case report. Surg Neurol 53:586–588, 2000.
23. O'Neill B, Haddon W, Kelly A, et al: Automobile head restraints-frequency of neck injury claims in relation to the presence of head restraints. Am J Public Health 62:403, 1972.
24. Pettersson K, Hildingsson C, Toolanen G, et al: Disc pathology after whiplash injury. A prospective magnetic resonance imaging and clinical investigation. Spine 22:283–287, 1997.
25. Pettersson K, Hildingsson C, Toolanen G, et al: MRI and neurology in acute whiplash trauma. No correlation in prospective examination of 39 cases. Acta Orthop Scand 65:525–528, 1994.
26. Ronnen H, deKorte P, Brink P, et al: Acute whiplash injury: is there a role for MR imaging?—a prospective study of 100 patients. Radiology 201:93–96, 1996.
27. Rotstein O, Rhame F, Molina E, et al: Mediastinitis after whiplash injury. Can J Surg 29:54–56, 1986.
28. Schweighofer F, Ranner G, Schleifer P, et al: [Hyperextension injury of the lower cervical spine and diagnosis of dorsal unstable motion segments]. Langenbecks Arch Chir 380:162–165, 1995.
29. Senter BS: Cervical discogenic syndrome: a cause of chronic head and neck pain. J Miss State Med Assoc 36:231–234, 1995.

30. Siebenrock K, Aebi M: Cervical discography in discogenic pain syndrome and its predictive value for cervical fusion. Arch Orthop Trauma Surg 113:199–203, 1994.
31. Splener C, Benfield J: Esophageal disruption from blunt and penetrating external trauma. Arch Surg 111:663–667, 1976.
32. Squires B, Gargan M, Bannister G: Soft-tissue injuries of the cervical spine. J Bone Joint Surg Br 78:955–957, 1996.
33. Van Goethem JW, Biltjes IG, van den Hauwe L, et al: Whiplash injuries: is there a role for imaging? Eur J Radiol 22:30–37, 1996.
34. Wilson D, Campbell D: Anterior cervical discectomy without bone graft: report of 71 cases. J Neurosurg 47:551–555, 1977.
35. Winkelstein B, Nightingale R, Richardson W, et al: The cervical facet capsule and its role in whiplash injury: a biomechanical investigation. Spine 25:1238–1246, 2000.
36. Yoganandan N, Pintar F, Klienberger M: Cervical spine vertebral and facet joint kinematics under whiplash. J Biomech Eng 120:305–307, 1998.

25

The Legal System and Soft Tissue Injuries

Richard Rubenstein, J.D.

The volumes devoted to the civil trial of automobile accident cases would fill an entire room.[*1] However, a trial is a failure, in a sense. It results from an inability to persuade either the plaintiff or the defendant of a reasonable solution to a thorny problem: the seriousness of an injury. The limited ability of the medical arts to prove or measure the existence or degree of objective injury and subjective reaction creates this thorny problem of evaluation. Complicating matters, the tort system often demands that medicine be practiced in a way that emphasizes the forensic over the curative.

The paradox of the system is that it both facilitates very thorough diagnostic and curative care and creates a motivation for gainsaying the success of the care. The tort system, with consideration of insurance coverage and proof of damages, exerts both subtle and overt pressure on the victims of soft tissue injuries, their treating physicians, and their counsel. Conversely, the twin, opposing concerns of treat–cost containment and the defense of proofs of damage can obstruct and occlude a clear, accurate picture of the effects of injuries.

This chapter provides the reader with an understanding of the effects of litigation on victims of soft tissue injuries as well as a modest ethical philosophy and framework for representing the victim of a soft tissue injury up to trial. The actual conduct of a trial is beyond the scope of this volume.

THE ATTORNEY'S RESPONSIBILITY

The philosophy of an attorney charged with representing an injured person is circumscribed by the rules of professional conduct of the state in which the practice is conducted. The rules are largely uniform from state to state. While there are subtle differences, the New York Canon is instructive to this inquiry[2]:

EC 7-1 The duty of a lawyer, both to the client and to the legal system, is to represent the client zealously within the bounds of the law, which includes Disciplinary Rules and enforceable professional regulations.

The mission of the Association of Trial Lawyers of America is as follows[3]:
- To uphold the honor and dignity of the legal profession and the highest standards of ethical conduct and integrity.

---

* While an exhaustive bibliography is beyond the scope of this chapter, a suggested reading is Wecht and Preiser.[1]

- Promote the public good through concerted efforts to secure safe products, a safe workplace, a clean environment, and quality health care.
- Inspire excellence in advocacy through training and education.
- Champion the cause of those who deserve redress for injury to person or property.

While the ATLA is a purely voluntary organization closely identified with the plaintiff's bar, its mission is an eloquent description of the ideal agenda of the claimant's counsel.

One dilemma of the modern personal injury litigator is the collision of the ethical obligation for zeal and the trial lawyer's mission to assist his client in avoiding unnecessary consequences of the original mishap. Is there an inherent conflict between the demands of legal proof and the accomplishment of a successful medical result for the client? It may well be that the rise of the no-fault system created this dilemma or at least exacerbated it.

INSURANCE, THE TORT SYSTEM, AND TREATMENT

The Tort System

State automobile liability insurance laws currently fall into four general types: (1) those based solely on the traditional, fault-based tort liability system; (2) those that require an insurance company to pay first-party (policy-holder) benefits, regardless of who was at fault in the accident, but retain the right to sue as in traditional states; (3) those that provide no-fault first-party benefits but restrict the right to sue except under enumerated conditions; and (4) those that provide a contractual choice between the traditional liability system and a no-fault system.

The system of valuing soft tissue claims upon "special damages" preexisted the no-fault systems that have dominated state tort laws for three decades. At the time of this writing, 24 states have full or modified no-fault systems. No state has enacted a no-fault system since 1976. Arizona voters rejected a no-fault ballot measure in 1990 by 85.1% to 14%. A "pure" no-fault ballot measure was placed before California voters in March 1996; it was rejected by 65% of voters despite a $19 million campaign in its favor. In Hawaii, a pure no-fault measure sponsored by State Farm Insurance was approved by the legislature but vetoed by the governor. Indeed, the emphasis in no-fault states has shifted to *repealing* no-fault. Since 1988, there have been serious efforts to repeal no-fault laws in at least six states; three were successful. Nevada, Georgia, and Connecticut repealed their no-fault laws.

Prior to no-fault, the "tortfeasor," or negligent driver, bore the responsibility for paying the medical bills of the injured plaintiff if found liable for the accident that occasioned the injury. In the absence of collateral sources of coverage, the accrual of these medical bills could be economically devastating to the accident victim. It was widely believed by proponents of no-fault that the number of liability claims would decline if medical bills were not an issue. A number of social and scientific factors impacted to bring about an opposite result, not the least of which was the growth of sophisticated diagnostic methods that tended to provide further proof of soft tissue injuries.

New Jersey, a state with traditionally high automobile insurance premiums, is an instructive example in charting the effect of the tort system on medical handling of soft tissue cases. New Jersey has been a no-fault state since 1973, the second state in the nation to adopt the policy.[4] In 1973, the legal requirement to exercise the right to sue another party was contingent upon the accrual of $200 in medical bills for curative treatment. In 1984, the legislature increased the amount to $1500, with an annual increase that continued for several years. The net effect of this 1984 amendment was to direct claimants to physicians who would enable them to accrue bills and thus receive financial redress for their injuries. Bills continued to escalate upward until the monetary requirement for suit was superseded by a "verbal" requirement that required the establishment of objective evidence of permanent injury. As a result, the use of multiple sophisticated diagnostic tests (which might not be strictly medically indicated) became necessary for forensic and legal purposes. Costs continued to escalate.

The conventional wisdom regarding valuation of soft tissue injuries is that the frequency and regularity of medical or chiropractic treatment, demonstrated through treatment or billing records, bear a direct consequence in the appraisal of the case. Thus, plaintiffs' attorneys disapproved of treatment by physicians who did not administer or prescribe physical therapy or advanced diagnostic methods, fearing that the proofs necessary to document claims would not be available to them regardless of the damage to the client. Insurance companies fueled the fire by valuing claims on the basis of medical bills, or "special damages."

The insurance industry practice with respect to soft tissue injuries was to multiply the medical bills by a factor of three, where there was no economic (wage) loss. Thus, the attorney would receive one-third of the settlement, the plaintiff one-third, and the medical bills would be paid with the final third. In different regions, and with different insurance carriers, the multiplier could be higher or lower.

With the advent of no-fault insurance, wherein the injured party's own insurance policy paid the bills for medical treatment, the logical basis for the multiplier system ceased to exist, but the practice did not. Lacking a reliable means for evaluating the probable jury verdicts, and wishing to stabilize costs, insurance carriers continued their prior evaluation methods for soft tissue injuries. The cycle continued.

Current Trends

For many years, the "soft tissue" automobile accident case was the bread and butter of the general practice attorney. No special expertise was required, at least as many general practitioners believed. Diagnostic tests such as computed tomography and magnetic resonance imaging were not yet in wide use. Cases were handled as a volume business, with settlements representing the aforementioned, nearly arbitrary multiple of medical bills. The client was not so much *represented* as *processed* by the attorney.

Ironically, the system of arbitrary multiples has given way to an even more insidious method of claims handling: so-called "artificial intelligence." A number of software developers have produced applications that value claims based upon an algorithm with many variables, including:

- Emergency department visit
- Ordering of x-rays
- Lapse between emergency department visit and first visit with the physician
- Administration of prescription medication
- Time lost from work
- Number of physical therapy visits
- Number of epidural or trigger point injections.

The applications vary widely in their ability to assess the individualized claim. It can be argued that the intent is not to fairly assess damages but to create a self-fulfilling prophesy of a sort: The computer values the case according to incomplete or invalid criteria, but the computer's valuation becomes objective truth because it becomes part of the database, and we accept it as reliable regardless of its validity. Like all "learning programs," the bias of the person entering the data becomes the determiner of the result. This process of reification of values may prove to be reliable but of questionable validity.

Ultimately, the cycle will recur: Trial and error will teach attorneys and claimants what steps to take to document treatment or injuries to maximize claim value. Because there is little likelihood that the *best* medical practices will also be the ones that maximize claim value, medical judgment will once again be subjugated to the tort system.

Claim Building versus Cost Containment: Danger from Two Directions

The clash between claimants and insurance companies continued into the late 1990s with the adoption of peer [paper] reviews, independent medical examinations, and care paths.

Peer Reviews and Medical Necessity

The concept of medical peer review is not a new one. The American College of Surgeons created the first accreditation program, including peer review, in 1918, with respect to hospital care. This evolved into the Joint Commission on Accreditation of Health Care Organizations. Over time, the insurance community has employed the concept of peer review for both risk management (validation of care) and cost containment (denial of unnecessary care).

A number of criticisms have been leveled at peer review systems in recent years. First, in the context of a first-party benefits insurance system, peer review implicates a hired-gun concepts, where physicians paid by interests adverse to claims payment decide on the necessity of care. Second, peer review is inherently conservative: It adopts and protects the conventional wisdom at the expense of advancements in medicine. Third, the lack of a physician-patient relationship between the claimant and reviewer, and the legal immunities of reviewers, conferred by legislation, prevent true accountability for the reviewer.[5]

On the other hand, unfettered access to unlimited modalities is an economic disaster for insurance carriers, particularly given the litigation-based incentive to seek or render treatment.

The trend toward peer review, either embodied in first-party insurance policies or legislation, will no doubt continue. In the current system of litigation, however, the peer review, conducted on paper, will never have the credibility before an adjudicator of a living, breathing, treating physician who has actually examined and treated the patient. Unlike the moderately successful peer reviewing in academia, particularly hard sciences, the exposure of medical practices to the court system necessarily limits the efficacy of cold, paper reviews as a limitation on treatment.

In practical terms, insurance carriers employ peer reviews for the purpose of excluding charges that are not medically necessary. The concept of medical necessity, like the concept of "maximum benefit of medical treatment," is not part of a traditional medical school curriculum. They have their roots in cost containment and litigation systems, not the Hippocratic oath. Here again, we see physicians being asked to take on the mantle of another art or discipline to lend legitimacy to the agenda of insurance claims and subsequent litigation. The alliance is an uneasy one.

Legislatures in several states have created fee schedules for medical and chiropractic charges to limit costs and prevent the practice of unbundling.[6] Outright exclusions for certain diagnostic practices have been imposed by policy language.[7]

Independent Medical Examinations: Causal Relationship and Further Treatment

First-party insurers generally have a contractual right to conduct examinations of claimants to determine the need for further treatment or to exclude covered losses as the legal or proximate causes for claimed injuries.[8] Some insurance carriers simply draw from a list of physicians, choosing based upon specialty and region. Other companies wish to insulate themselves from allegations of overreaching. They employ third-party vendors who choose examining physicians and often format their reports. Arguably, physicians who are chosen and paid by insurance carriers are not "independent" in any meaningful sense of the word. On the other hand, there is no other readily apparent means of clinical oversight for treating physicians.

The use of the independent medical examination has polarized the medicolegal community more than ever before. Fundamental disagreements have never been more apparent concerning bedrock issues: How long should a person be treated? What modalities or combination of modalities should be employed? Should a physician treat a soft tissue injury on the basis of subjective complaints, where objective findings are mild or inconsistent? Can there be permanent impairment or disability from a soft tissue injury? Issues of a causal relationship between accident and injury have required the employment of biomechanical engineers at great cost.

The clash is typically between the treating physician, who maintains a physician-patient relationship, and the examining physician, who does not. Physicians who perform large numbers of independent medical examinations tend to orient themselves toward a brief regimen of physical therapy, anti-inflammatory drugs, reassurance, and release. Their orientation is not without some, arguable medical basis.[9] One source of conflict between treating physicians and independent medical evaluators is over definition. First-party benefits such as health insurance and no-fault personal injury protection depend only on a causal link founded in reasonable probability between an accident and aggravation or acceleration of a condition as well as "creation" of the condition. Often, an examining expert will apply a higher, more stringent standard to causality, causing a denial of benefits. Denials based upon preexisting conditions seldom prevail, because the burden would ordinarily be on the provider to prove a negative (the *lack* of trauma) or that the preexisting condition would inexorably lead to the present condition without the intervening trauma—and in the same time frame.

Care Paths and Cost Control

The costs of medical treatment have been borne by no-fault insurers subject to several controls. In the early no-fault era, there were few deductibles or copayments on no-fault policies. Premiums began to rise rather quickly and, after several years, most states instituted modest deductibles and copayments as a method of reducing premiums and deterring insureds from seeking marginally necessary care.

Administration of a no-fault system is a primary cost. In fact, one study conducted by AIS Risk Consultants showed that approximately 45% of collected no-fault premiums are allocated to overhead expenses for carriers, not claim payments.[10]

In the face of the diminishing coverage and rising administrative costs, the trend has been to adopt a system akin to health maintenance organizations, which, ironically, have been subject to the same problems in recent years, without a solution in sight.

One health maintenance organization-like aspect of the reform trend is the adoption of care paths. A flowchart of clinical and diagnostic choices is created and applied through regulations and policy language to neck and back injuries. There is a diagram of treatment patterns and projected norms for utilization of both diagnostic and curative methods.

While there can be deviation from the flowchart to meet the needs of individual patients, justification (to the insurance company) of significant reasons for deviation must be supplied. Preexisting conditions and comorbidities would ostensibly be considered.[11] Other cost-containment devices include precertification requirements for diagnostic and surgical procedures, decision-point referrals for insurance oversight of continuing treatment, and networked providers for durable medical equipment.

Medical Necessity and Clinical Support

The underpinning of most first-party medical benefits in automobile accident policies is the need for medical necessity for treatment or diagnostics. Insurance policies and state insurance regulations have been rewritten to limit overtesting. Precertification plans provide that a treating physician must supply clinical findings before ordering sophisticated or expensive diagnostic tests. The insurance provider will then consult care paths and guidelines to determine the necessity for the test. Exclusions are generally written into the regulations so that emergent necessity allows for testing.

The New Jersey regulations are, depending on the point of view of the reader, either a model of objectivity or a vague straightjacket for diagnostic investigation. The concept of clinical support is defined by regulation. Under N.J.R. 11:3-4.2, clinically supported treatments or diagnostic tests must pass a threshold. The provider must have:

1. Personally examined the patient to ensure that the proper medical indications exist to justify ordering the treatment or test;
2. Physically examined the patient including making an assessment of any current and/or historical subjective complaints, observations, objective findings, neurologic indications, and physical tests;
3. Considered any and all previously performed tests that relate to the injury and the results and which are relevant to the proposed treatment or test; and
4. Recorded and documented these observations, positive and negative findings, and conclusions on the patient's medical records.

The concept of medical necessity is itself defined by the regulations in New Jersey. It means that "the medical treatment or diagnostic test is consistent with the clinically supported symptoms, diagnosis or indications of the injured person, and:

1. The treatment is the most appropriate level of service that is in accordance with the standards of good practice and standard professional treatment protocols [ratified by the State];
2. The treatment of the injury is not primarily for the convenience of the injured person or provider;
3. Does not include unnecessary testing or treatment [N.J.R. 11.3-4.3]."

A critical look at the definition above yields little of substance unfortunately. The first paragraph incorporates the much-criticized "care path" system into the definition of medical necessity. Because a single committee that included actuaries and nonmedical personnel created the care paths, it is quite open to attack from physicians. Additionally, it leaves no room to recognize changes in custom or protocol that may evolve more quickly than government agencies revise their regulations.

The second paragraph of the definition is inexplicable. It appears to be a precious and opaque manner in which to define treatment for the purpose of "building up" litigation expenses by way of treatment as unnecessary.

The third paragraph is a circular tautology. Essentially, the adopting agency defines medical necessity as the employment of modalities that are not unnecessary. No additional information is provided the reader beyond the obvious redundancy contained within the "definition."

A cynical reader might conclude that the drafters lacked the fortitude or mandate to dictate the practice of medicine to physicians. A cynical writer might point out that neither of these shortcomings will necessarily work to the prejudice of either physicians or patients. The fact, however, remains that none of the no-fault states have adopted a definition of medical necessity that overcomes the problems of vagueness or circularity and, thus, the decision as to medical necessity will rely upon the decisions of courts and the testimony of physicians and patients, as before.

PERMANENT INJURY: A LEGAL QUESTION
WITH A MEDICAL ANSWER

Schools of Thought

Proof of permanent injury is either a threshold question for a patient's financial recovery, or the most important part of the summation, in the end. In a number of states, notably Michigan, New Jersey, New York, and Florida, legislatures have established a set of standards for proof to be applied in automobile accident cases, requiring medical evidence of a permanent injury for a meaningful financial recovery. Each state asks a different question of the physician, and each state asks the physician the question as if medical school training imbued the practitioners with some special power to divine the nature and extent of a permanent injury.

A search of medical school curricula discloses no mandatory course designed to determine or define injuries or conditions as permanent in any meaningful legal sense. Physicians are not schooled in the forensic prognostication of soft tissue injuries in a classroom or clinical setting, because curative medicine rather than forensic medicine is the emphasis in medical school. Yet orthopedists, neurologists, neurosurgeons, physiatrists, and general practitioners are called upon every day for their expert medical advice to define and quantify "permanent injuries." In theory, the determination of permanency is partially philosophical and partially semantic.

Several philosophical schools have evolved with respect to the permanent injury prognosis. The most partisan experts define soft tissue injuries as nonpermanent by *nature*. That is, they rely upon a physiologic principle that sprains and strains of muscles and ligaments, even superimposed upon tissues with some level of preexisting morbidity, cannot give rise to permanent injury. The muscles heal, they observe, and most complaints are subjective. While these practitioners commonly *treat* patients on the basis of subjective complaints, they are ironically unwilling to credit those complaints with probity when it comes to prognosis.

A second school, on the other extreme, is that by definition a sprain results in the tearing or rending of soft tissues and the resulting healing process creates scar tissue that lacks the elasticity and vigor of the original tissues. Armed with this conclusory physiologic syllogism, every sprain becomes a permanent injury in some measure.

In the center is a school that refuses to attribute permanency on the basis of theoretical anatomic proofs and prefers to rely upon clinical and radiologic tests. The problem therein is that they usually lack a baseline for comparison. For instance, a vigorous and athletic patient might have a painless range of motion at the extremes of normal. A traumatic accident might reduce the clinical findings to barely normal. Employing the talisman of a "normal range of motion," the examining physician would relate no basis for a finding of permanent injury. Although impairment has been suffered from which no further improvement is likely, the examination would read *normal*, except for subjective complaints discounted by the examiner as without correlation.

Framing the Question: Threshold

Attorneys, insurance companies, and physicians are concerned about the question of permanent injury for two significant and distinct reasons. First, several states require a threshold showing of permanent injury to reach a jury on issues of pain and suffering or permanent disabilities.[12] The New Jersey law, now modeled after the Florida statute, is instructive, mandating that no person covered by the threshold law can recover noneconomic (non–wage loss) damages . . .

> as a result of bodily injury, arising out of the ownership, operation, maintenance or use of such automobile in this State, unless that person has sustained a bodily injury which results in death; dismemberment; significant disfigurement or significant scarring; displaced fractures; loss of a fetus; or a permanent injury within a reasonable degree of medical probability, other than scarring or disfigurement. An injury shall be considered permanent when the body part or organ, or both, has not healed to function normally and will not heal to function normally with further medical treatment. NJSA 39:6a-8(a).

The Michigan law is distinctly different:

> 500.3135. (1) A person remains subject to tort liability for noneconomic loss caused by his or her ownership, maintenance, or use of a motor vehicle only if the injured person has suffered death, serious impairment of body function, or permanent serious disfigurement.

> 7) As used in this section, "serious impairment of body function" means an objectively manifested impairment of an important body function that affects the person's general ability to lead his or her normal life.

New York employs a multipronged test to the right to recover noneconomic damages, with only one prong requiring analysis of the permanency of injuries:

> (d) "Serious injury" means a personal injury which results in death; dismemberment; significant disfigurement; a fracture; loss of a fetus; permanent loss of use of a body organ, member, function or system; permanent consequential limitation of use of a body organ or member; significant limitation of use of a body function or system; or a medically determined injury or impairment of a non-permanent nature which prevents the injured person from performing substantially all of the material acts which constitute such person's usual and customary daily activities for not less than ninety days during the one hundred eighty days immediately following the occurrence of the injury or impairment.[13]

Note that the New York standard emphasizes permanent loss of "use" or "consequential limitation," which implicates more than simply objective testing but, rather, *context* necessitating consideration of patient lifestyle.

The discussion of case law that has evolved, and will evolve, from these three statutes, would fill volumes. In the context of the discussion herein, it is notable that the New Jersey law did not adopt a purely objective standard for permanent injury, did not adopt the necessity for proof of loss of a "general ability to lead his or her normal life," and did not define the need for an "important" bodily function. Each of these states asks the permanency question differently.

Framing the Question: Summation

The report of the treating physician, addressing the threshold question of permanent injury, is the key to the courthouse door in states that require proof of permanent injury to reach a jury on the question of general damages. However, the opinion of the physician then becomes important for a second reason after the trial begins: Pain and suffering and permanent injury are neither presumed nor subject to bare speculation.

After the testifying physician offers testimony as to the permanency of a condition, an attorney may employ this evidence in summation to form a rational basis for a calculation of damages. This technique, often known as the "time-unit" rule, will allow argument to a jury based upon a multiplier. The jury is asked to evaluate the permanent injury as a per diem value. A mortality chart is then introduced, and the jury may multiply the per diem value by the days, weeks, or months of a plaintiff's life expectancy. It is therefore critical that degree of permanent disability be explained to the jury so that the per diem half of the equation is given meaningful foundation and context. Even without the application of multipliers, the extent and nature of permanent loss of function can be the linchpin of an argument for hedonic damages or future wage loss.

Physicians: Adversaries or Allies?

The Medicolegal Report

Many practitioners assume that there is some form book for medical reports upon which treating physicians draw for their own narratives. Quite often, this is far from the case. Every physician should receive a comprehensive request for a narrative report from the attorney, enclosing a police report, interrogatory answers if they exist, and the records of any emergency department or consulting physician.

The systems in states that maintain tort limitation laws require much more specific language than others.[14] Physicians in those states must affirm that injuries are permanent to some degree, depending on the statute. New Jersey and Florida have similar requirements for those upon whom the threshold is imposed: An injury to a bodily system must not be likely to heal to its prior state of function, even with further medical treatment.[15] Even given that somewhat vague requirement, attorneys must be vigilant to ask the question directly of physicians, lest they receive a report without such a conclusion. Attorneys should forward charts describing any preexisting conditions to treating physicians for both forensic and therapeutic benefit to their clients.

It is therefore essential that there be dialogue between physician and counsel. Although physicians who treat automobile accident patients have some familiarity with the legal systems, it cannot be assumed that their familiarity is either current or correct. Physicians quite commonly employ boilerplate language in reports that ignore the underlying facts of the accident, the preaccident lifestyle or job of the patient, and the changes in lifestyle that an accident can create.

It is therefore suggested that attorneys draft requests for narrative reports, which address specific needs relevant to the theory of the case:

- Discuss the nature of the impact.
- Discuss the correlation between emergency department complaints and current complaints.
- Discuss medical history to exclude allegations of symptomatic preexisting morbidity.
- Discuss compliance with course of treatment and effect of treatment.
- Discuss, in factual detail, the preaccident lifestyle of the patient, along with both personal and physiologic postaccident changes. Weight, hobbies, work habits, social habits, and family life all constitute verifiable and objective correlations with diagnosis and prognosis.

It is submitted that most physicians will welcome specific guidance from counsel and patients so that reports will be complete and accurate, preventing time-consuming revisions. The request for the report should thus predate the discharge of the patient so that the physician will have the opportunity to gather information relevant to his determinations from the patient directly at discharge, as opposed to from counsel.

SUMMARY

The soft tissue, or "whiplash," injury will always be controversial when placed in the adversarial context of insurance. Seemingly endless debates over necessity of treatment and objectivity of evidence will no doubt outlive the current debaters by generations. The conventional wisdom about how professionals look at these injuries will continue to be formed by economic concerns about cure or palliation.

The challenge for attorneys is to maximize their clients' recoveries without subjugating their care to the Scylla and Charybdis of insurance cost versus overutilization, which can transform the client into a chronic pain patient. It is submitted that ethical representation can be pursued by developing those proofs that are relevant to the client's condition, as opposed to endless referrals for that positive but nontherapeutic test result.

References & Notes

1. Wecht CH, Preiser SE, Preiser ML: Handling Soft Tissue Injury Cases. Charlottesville, Virginia: The Michie Company, 1993.
2. New York State Bar Association: The Lawyers' Code of Professional Responsibility. Adopted by the NYSBA, as amended, June 30, 1999.
3. ATLA Desk Reference Supplement, 1999–2000.
4. N.J.S.A. 39:6A-1, et seq.
5. Scheutzow SO: State medical peer review: High cost but no benefit—Is it time for a change? Am J Law Med 25(1):7–60, 1999.
   Also: Pennsylvania Code/69.51.
   Also: Erhard GD: The Peer Review Masquerade: Disguising Healthcare Rationing Under the Pennsylvania Auto Review Law. 57 U. Pitt. L. Rev. 959, Summer 1996.
6. Several states, New Jersey and New York included, have actually imposed regionalized rates that differ within the state.
7. New Jersey, for instance, excludes surface EMG testing, spinal diagnostic ultrasound, reflexology, iridology, brain-mapping, mandibular tracking and simulation, and surrogate arm mentoring in the standard auto policy.
8. See, for example, Rutgers Casualty Insurance Company Standard No Fault Automobile Insurance Policy, which is an Insurance Services Organization standard policy: Cherry Hill, New Jersey, 2001.
9. Laborde JM: Biomechanics of minor automobile accidents: Treatment implications for associated chronic spine symptoms. J South Orthop Assoc 9*3):187–192, 2000.

26

The Future of Whiplash-Associated Injuries

Gerard A. Malanga, M.D., and Scott F. Nadler, D.O.

What is the future of whiplash-associated injuries? Ideally, the future would have a head and neck support system along with other car design and material technology that would entirely eliminate spine and other injuries that now occur after motor vehicle accidents. The current deficiencies in this area (and a possible solution) have been reviewed in Chapter 6. Much of the motivation to aggressively find newer head and neck restraint systems is related to economics. Who should pay for the cost of the development and production of these new systems? Should it be the automobile industry, the health insurance industry, the federal government, or the consumer? This same issue of cost is problematic in many other areas of health care as well. Ultimately, it seems that everyone who is impacted by this problem should share the cost to treat these injuries. Overall, through better preventive care we can reduce health care costs, decrease lost wages from disability, and allow society as a whole to enjoy better health when these injuries are avoided.

Short of preventing whiplash-associated injuries, what else can we expect in the future? When an injury occurs, the clinician should be able to quickly and efficiently evaluate and diagnose injuries and initiate an active treatment program that enhances recovery and minimizes disability. This would begin with a detailed history and physical examination. Those with obvious neurologic, orthopedic, or other abnormalities would be quickly referred to an appropriate specialist. At present, these injuries are usually appropriately addressed and are not the main factors driving up cost and disability. Patients with more subtle injuries and pathology ("soft tissue injuries") represent the major area in which current evaluation and treatment paradigms have been unsatisfactory. This book reviews the pathophysiology, prognosis, and current available literature regarding treatment of these various whiplash-associated disorders (WADs).

Although the literature is not complete and definitive, it does contain information to guide the thoughtful practitioner. Appropriate diagnostic evaluation and treatment of patients with WADs has been nicely documented in the literature to provide an evidenced-based approach to care. It is clear that not all patients with spine or jaw pain benefit from magnetic resonance imaging; the indiscriminate use of this test for these conditions has weakened its clinical utility. Likewise, it is also clear that electrodiagnostic studies should not be performed in every individual complaining of extremity pain and most likely not at all in individuals with pure axial pain. Use should be based on both subjective and objective findings in a circumstance in which it will modify the treatment program.

In regard to treatment strategies, the benefits and limitations of physical therapy, chiropractic treatment, injection procedures, and surgery have been established in the scientific literature and nicely outlined in this text. Any treatment strategy used in the care of WAD patients should be used to ultimately address function. Treatment strategies focusing on the amelioration of pain alone may validate a "sick role" and lead to a poor functional outcome. The appropriate management of the WAD patient should provide for a rapid progression to active treatment stressing normalization of activity and deemphasizing passive treatment focusing on pain reduction. While this treatment approach has already been validated, it remains to be fully embraced by health care providers. Scientific literature has established that recommending rest, collars, and prolonged passive treatment promotes a view of the patient as disabled, leading to increased long-term disability. This represents the poorest outcome in WADs.

Using this evidenced-based approach in the evaluation and treatment of patients with WADs will likely result in a decrease in the number of patients who suffer from long-term disability following these injuries. The current and prevalent treatment of these patients with chronic symptoms also remains flawed. Bogduk and colleagues have reviewed the literature in this area and have noted the prevalence of cervical zygapophyseal pain in many patients in this group and have described a meticulous method for the evaluation and treatment of this difficult problem. Patients with chronic pain who are not appropriate candidates for this treatment should be treated in a multidisciplinary manner that includes appropriate pharmacologic intervention, functional rehabilitation, and behavioral techniques to improve the patient's ability to self-manage his or her symptoms. It is clear that prolonged passive therapy, modalities, and multiple injections will not be helpful and only reinforce disability behavior and a self-perception of being disabled.

The development of new technologies and techniques in the treatment of acute and chronic WADs must be carefully assessed. History has taught us that the newest treatments are not necessarily the best or most useful treatments. Many of these treatments initially report fantastic results only to be proven essentially useless when subjected to rigorous scientific evaluation. When scientifically validated, however, this information must be quickly disseminated to clinicians in practice. In the future, this will occur with relative ease through the Internet. This will ensure that patients with a particular disorder are afforded the most up-to-date treatment throughout the world. As clinicians are informed of what is appropriate for their patients, useless treatment will be abandoned so that available resources can be allocated to treatments that have been demonstrated to be both efficient and effective.

Newer treatments will likely be less invasive and less destructive. Treatment will be geared toward enhancing tissue healing through the use of gene therapy along with strategies that help activate normal biological healing. Through science we will be able to treat conditions before they become chronic, and before central sensitization of the brain occurs, to ultimately decrease long-term disability.

This future view of WADs could be achieved, in part, today. There is literature regarding the appropriate use of imaging and other diagnostic studies. The knowledge of what is and is not currently effective is available and should guide treatment. There are ongoing developments in head and neck restraints, materials, and automotive design. Ultimately, the future of WADs will require the coordinated efforts of the automotive, insurance, government, and medical industries along with the support of the general public. If selfish interest is abandoned, future prospects for WAD will greatly improve, to everyone's benefit.

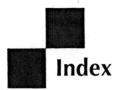

Index

Page references in *italic* denote figures; page references with a "t" denote tables.

10. Andres K before the New Jersey Joint Committee on Auto Insurance Reform, 1/22/98: www.njleg.state.nj.us/pubhear/012298dt.htm.
11. See, for example, 30 N.J.R. 4413.
12. Among the examples are New York, New Jersey, Florida, Pennsylvania, and Michigan.
13. NY Consolidated Laws/5103(d).
14. Examples are New York, New Jersey, Florida, Pennsylvania, and Michigan, among others.
15. N.J.S.A. 39:6A01, et seq.
    Also: Florida Statutes Annotated/627.737.

CPSIA information can be obtained at www.ICGtesting.com
Printed in the USA
LVOW10*0904211113

362177LV00002B/13/P